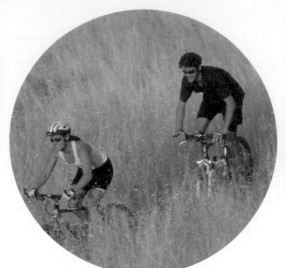

Principles and Labs For Fitness and Wellness

SIXTH EDITION

Werner W.K. Hoeger
Boise State University

Sharon A. Hoeger
Fitness & Wellness, Inc.

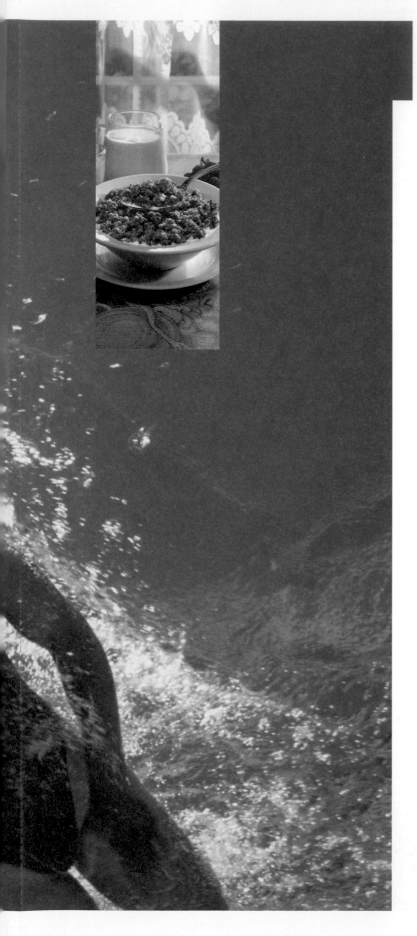

WADSWORTH
™
THOMSON LEARNING

Australia • Canada
Mexico • Singapore
Spain • United Kingdom
United States

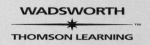

WADSWORTH

THOMSON LEARNING

Publisher: Peter Marshall
Associate Editor: April Lemons
Assistant Editor: John Boyd
Editorial Assistant: Andrea Kesterke
Marketing Manager: Joanne Terhaar
Marketing Assistant: Megan Hansen
Advertising Project Manager: Brian Chaffee
Project Manager: Sandra Craig
Print/Media Buyer: Karen Hunt

Permissions Editor: Stephanie Keough-Hedges
Production and Composition: Ash Street Typecrafters
Text and Cover Designer: Norman Baugher
Photo Researcher: Myrna Engler
Copy Editor: Carol Lombardi
Cover Images: **Large photo:** © 2001 Stone/David Madison; fruit inset: © Lois Ellen Frank/CORBIS; skinfold text inset: © Fitness & Wellness, Inc.
Printer: Transcontinental Printing

Printed in Canada
1 2 3 4 5 6 7 05 04 03 02 01

For permission to use material from this text, contact us by
Web: http://www.thomsonrights.com
Fax: 1-800-730-2215
Phone: 1-800-730-2214

Library of Congress Cataloging-in-Publication Data

Hoeger, Werner W. K.
    Principles and labs for fitness and wellness / Werner W. K. Hoeger, Sharon A. Hoeger. — 6th ed.
        p.   cm.
    Includes bibliographical references and index.
    ISBN 0-534-58950-2
    1. Physical fitness. 2. Health. I. Hoeger, Sharon A.
        II. Title.

RA781 .H59 2001
613.7—dc21

Wadsworth/Thomson Learning
10 Davis Drive
Belmont, CA 94002-3098
USA

For more information about our products, contact us:
Thompson Learning Academic Resource Center
1-800-423-0563
http://www.wadsworth.com

International Headquarters
Thomson Learning
International Division
290 Harbor Drive, 2nd Floor
Stamford, CT 06902-7477
USA

UK/Europe/Middle East/South Africa
Thomson Learning
Berkshire House
168-173 High Holborn
London WC1V 7AA
United Kingdom

Asia
Thomson Learning
60 Albert Street, #15-01
Albert Complex
Singapore 189969

Canada
Nelson Thomson Learning
1120 Birchmount Road
Toronto, Ontario M1K 5G4
Canada

2001016241

Contents in Brief

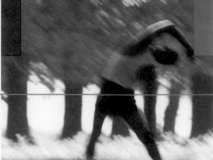

Table of Contents

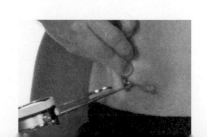

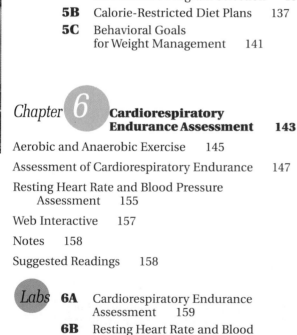
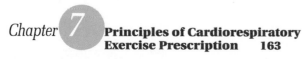

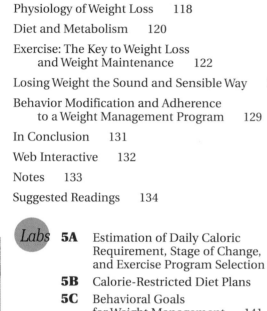

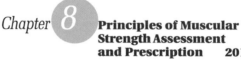

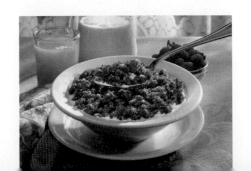

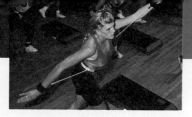

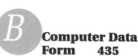
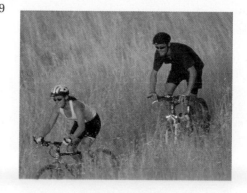

THE CURRENT North American way of life does not provide the human body with sufficient physical activity to maintain adequate health and improve quality of life. Many present lifestyle patterns are such a serious threat to our health that they actually increase the deterioration rate of the human body and often lead to premature illness and death.

People who lead an active and healthy lifestyle live longer and enjoy a better quality of life. Thus, healthy lifestyle programs have become a trend that is now very much a part of the American way of life. Many people, however, do not reap the benefits because they are either led astray by a multi-billion-dollar "quick fix" fad industry or they simply do not know how to develop their own program. The information in this book has been written to provide readers with the necessary tools and guidelines for a lifetime exercise program and a healthy lifestyle.

Principles and Labs for Fitness and Wellness contains 16 chapters and 33 labs that serve as a guide to implement a complete lifetime fitness and wellness program. The book points out the need to go beyond the basic components of fitness to achieve total well-being. Physical fitness, including all health- and skill-related components, is thoroughly discussed. In addition, extensive, up-to-date information is provided on behavior modification, nutrition, weight management, stress management, cardiovascular disease and cancer risk reduction, exercise and aging, prevention of sexually transmitted diseases, and substance abuse control (including tobacco, alcohol, and other psychoactive drugs).

As you work through the various chapters and labs in the book, you will be able to develop and regularly update your own lifetime program to improve fitness components and personal wellness. The emphasis throughout the book is on teaching you how to take control of your own personal health and lifestyle habits so that you can make a continuing, deliberate effort to stay healthy and achieve the highest potential for well-being.

New and Enhanced Features of the Sixth Edition

All chapters in this edition of *Principles and Labs for Fitness and Wellness* have been revised and updated to include new information reported in literature and at professional health, physical education, and sports medicine meetings. The most significant changes include the following:

■ In Chapter 1 the discussion on the six dimensions of wellness has been expanded, including the information on spirituality. The latter information, along with the section on accident prevention and personal safety, has been moved to this chapter from Chapter 16. The concept of "healthy life expectancy," as opposed to just life expectancy, with year 2000 statistics, is introduced in this chapter. A discussion of Healthy People 2010 has also been included. An update on health care costs throughout the world and the lack of preventive approaches is also discussed in Chapter 1. A newly developed wellness questionnaire that includes questions on all dimensions of wellness was incorporated as Lab 1A.

■ In Chapter 2 corrections were made to the sixth stage of the Transtheoretical Model of behavioral change. Instead of the termination stage it is now referred to as the termination/adoption stage. *Termination* is used for undesirable behaviors that are permanently eliminated, while the term *adoption* is used for positive behaviors that have been successfully embraced.

■ In addition to extensive updates to the topic of Chapter 3, nutrition, information has been added on the Dietary Reference Intakes (DRIs), the 2000 Dietary Guidelines for Americans, creatine supplementation, vegetarian diets, ethnic diets, antioxidant nutrients, dietary benefits of nuts and soy, and FDA-approved health claims that link foods and disease.

- Statistical updates on mortality rates based on Body Mass Index (BMI) and the ever-growing obesity epidemic are discussed in Chapters 4 and 5. A new section, "The Diet Craze," that discusses myths and detrimental effects of popular diets on the market today is included in Chapter 5. The glycemic index, effects of high-intensity versus low-intensity exercise in weight loss, and additional tips for behavior modification have all been added to this chapter.

- The list of suggestions to help motivate individuals to start and adhere to exercise has been expanded in Chapter 7. New questions were added to the Specific Exercise Considerations section, including the 2000 American College of Sports Medicine (ACSM) exercise guidelines for diabetics. The section on Exercise and Aging was also updated and moved from Chapter 16 to this chapter.

- The concepts of positive and negative resistance (concentric and eccentric muscle contractions), and guidelines for strength-training exercises were added to Chapter 8. Other additions include differences in strength training between free weights and machines, new free-weight strength-training exercises, and graphic illustration of muscles exercised with each exercise.

- The benefits of flexibility training have been revised in Chapter 9, and the section on the prevention and treatment of low-back pain has been enhanced.

- Information on the effects of hostile behaviors on health has been added to Chapter 11, the stress management chapter. This information is complemented by a questionnaire in Lab 11B.

- Revisions were made to Chapter 12, on cardiovascular disease prevention, to incorporate advances in this area, including information on strokes, diabetes, treatment of high blood lipids, the metabolic syndrome (Syndrome X), homocysteine, effects of soy foods on cardiovascular risk, benefits of strength training on heart health and hypertension, new blood pressure classification guidelines, and the healthy lifestyle approach to the treatment of high blood pressure. The chapter also includes statistical updates from the American Heart Association and new graphs on the incidence of cardiovascular diseases and high blood pressure in the United States.

- All cancer statistics were updated in Chapter 13. The general guidelines for cancer prevention were revised along with risk factors, prevention, and warning signals for each specific cancer site in this chapter. The previously used cancer questionnaire by the Preventive Medicine Institute/Strang Clinic has been replaced by a questionnaire produced by the Texas Division of the American Cancer Society, a more practical tool for cancer prevention.

- The contents on substance abuse previously found in Chapter 15 were combined with the information on freedom from tobacco to form Chapter 14. This chapter is now entitled "Addictive Behavior and Wellness." Information on heroin and methamphetamine was also added to the chapter.

- Chapter 15, completely updated, is now fully devoted to the topic of sexually transmitted diseases and their prevention.

- Chapter 16 now includes two new sections on life expectancy and physiological age and on complementary and alternative medicine. A thorough 46-question lab that can be used to predict life expectancy and physiological age, based on lifestyle factors discussed throughout the book, is introduced in Lab 16A. This lab provides a good summary of many of the fitness and wellness concepts learned by students throughout the course.

- Many of the labs have been rearranged and edited to make the experiences more practical, meaningful, and educational. Additional questions have been added to foster critical thinking on the part of students and help them analyze and summarize the principles learned in each chapter and the respective labs.

- New photography, new graphs, and data for various ethnic groups are included throughout the book.

Ancillaries

- **Instructor's Manual with Test Bank.** The Instructor's Manual with Test Bank helps instructors plan and coordinate their lectures by offering detailed outlines of each chapter with specific transparency and PowerPoint references. A Lab list accompanies Instructor's Activities for each chapter. These activities offer instructors ideas for incorporating the material into classroom activities and discussions. A set of Key Point Transparencies is provided. A full test bank containing approximately 50

questions per chapter is also provided.

- **Transparencies.** Approximately 80 color transparency acetates of graphs, tables, and illustrations from the text can be used to enhance lectures. The transparencies will also be available on the Web and on a CD-ROM. Also provided is a set of Key Point Transparencies—text-only transparencies that list important terms from each chapter.

- **Profile Plus 2002.** This interactive CD-ROM includes study guides, quizzes, lecture outlines, and digital video clips. The CD allows students to generate personalized fitness and wellness programs, conduct self-assessments, analyze their diets, and keep an exercise log.

- **Diet Analysis Plus 5.0 CD-ROM.** This interactive nutrition learning tool allows students to create personal profiles and determine the nutritional value of their diet. The program calculates nutrition intakes, goal percentages, and actual percentages of nutrients, vitamins, and minerals, customized according to the student's profile. The information is displayed in colorful, easy-to-read graphs, charts, and spreadsheets.

- **ExamView ®—Computerized Testing.** Create, deliver, and customize tests and study guides (both print and online) in minutes with this easy-to-use assessment and tutorial system. ExamView offers both a Quick Test Wizard and an Online Test Wizard that guide you step-by-step through the process of creating tests, while its unique "WYSIWYG" capability allows you to see the test you are creating on the screen exactly as it will print or display online.

- **Presentation CD-ROM for Introduction to Fitness and Wellness.** More than 100 Power Point® slides, featuring art from the text and additional sources, are available to adopters.

- **CNN Today: Fitness and Wellness Video.** Launch your lectures with riveting footage from CNN, the world's leading 24-hour global news television network. The CNN Today: Fitness and Wellness Video allows you to integrate the news gathering and programming power of CNN into the classroom to show students the relevance of course topics to their everyday lives. Organized by topics introduced in the text, the clips are presented in short 2–5 minute segments, and a new video is available each year.

- **Wadsworth Video Library for Fitness, Wellness, and Personal Health.** A comprehensive library of videos is available to adopters of this textbook. Topics include weight control and fitness, AIDS, sexual communication, peer pressure, compulsive and addictive behaviors and the relationship between alcohol and violence. Contact your local Wadsworth/ Thomson Learning representative for a detailed list of video options.

- **Personal Daily Log.** This log contains an exercise pyramid, ethnic foods pyramid, time management strategies and goal setting worksheets, cardiorespiratory exercise record forms, strength training forms, and much more.

- **Wellness Worksheets.** Forty detachable self-assessments and a complete wellness inventory are included.

- **Trigger Video Series.** Exclusive to Wadsworth/ Thomson Learning! This video is designed to promote classroom discussion on a variety of important topics related to physical fitness and stress. Each 60-minute video contains five 8–10 minute clips, followed by questions for answer or discussion and material appropriate to the chapters in Hoeger and Hoeger's text.

- **InfoTrac® College Edition.** This extensive online library gives professors and students access to the latest news and research articles online—updated daily and spanning four years! Conveniently accessible from students' own computers or the campus library, InfoTrac College Edition opens the door to the full text of articles from hundreds of scholarly and popular journals and publications.

- **The Wadsworth Health & Wellness Resource Center Web Site:**

  http://health.wadsworth.com

  When you adopt *Principles and Labs for Fitness and Wellness*, you and your students will have access to a rich array of teaching and learning resources you won't find anywhere else. This outstanding site features both student and instructor resources for this text, including self-quizzes, Web links, suggested online readings, and discussion forums for students—as well as downloadable supplementary resources, PowerPoint® presentations, and more for instructors.

- **Thomson Learning WebTutor™.** Available on WebCT or Blackboard! This content-rich, Web-based teaching and learning tool is rich with study and mastery tools, communication tools, and course content. WebTutor is filled with

pre-loaded content and is ready to use as soon as you and your students log on. At the same time, you can customize the content in any way you choose, from uploading images and other resources, to adding Web links, to creating your own practice materials.

Acknowledgments

This book is dedicated to Joanne Saliger. Her friendship and unconditional support and sacrifice have made our books the finest available during the past fifteen years. Joanne, we are forever indebted to you for all you have done in our behalf.

We wish to extend special gratitude to Amber Lee Fawson for her valuable editorial comments and assistance with the revisions of Chapters 14 and 15. Thanks are also expressed to Brent Fawson, Dr. Elaine Long, Chuck Scheer, Dr. James Hesson, Dr. Ross Vaughn, Dr. Norman Kaluhiokalani, and Brandi Hagemann for their personal contributions and continued support of our scholarly endeavors.

Finally, we would like to thank the reviewers for their valuable comments and contributions to the Sixth Edition:

Andrea Abercrombie, Clemson University
Helaine Cigal, CUNY John Jay College of Criminal Justice
Dale Devoe, Colorado State University
John Hammett, Jacksonville State University
Paul Krack, University of Southern Indiana
Lance Lamport, St. Petersburg Junior College
Julie Lombardi, Millersville University
Sharon Milligan, University of Findlay
Alison Nye, Cape Fear Community College
Linda Rosskopf, Georgia State University
Tammy Sabourin, Valencia Community College
Al Thompson, Kalamazoo Valley Community College
Glenda Warren, Cumberland College
Roy Wohl, Washburn University
Cheryl Yoder, Umpqua Community College

Photo Credits

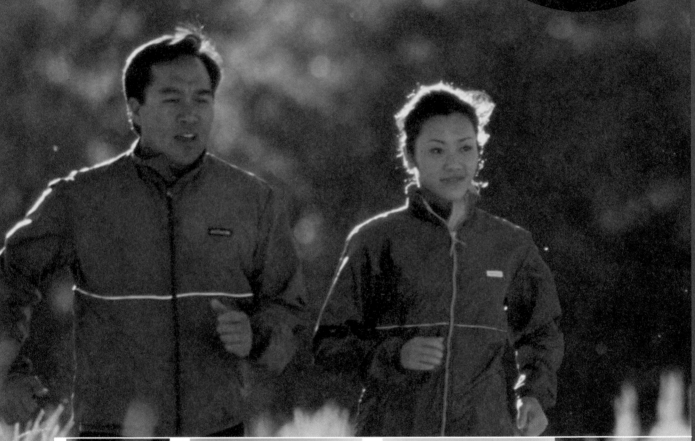

Chapter 1

Physical Fitness and Wellness

Objectives

- Define wellness and list its dimensions.

- Define physical fitness and list health-related and skill-related fitness components.

- State the differences between physical fitness and wellness.

- Distinguish between health fitness standards and physical fitness standards.

- Identify the major health problems in the United States.

- Understand the benefits and the significance of participating in a lifetime fitness and wellness program.

- Identify lifestyle factors that improve health and longevity.

- Identify risk factors that may interfere with safe participation in exercise.

1

Widespread interest in **health** and preventive medicine over the last three decades has led to a tremendous increase in the number of people participating in fitness and wellness programs. From an initial fitness fad in the early 1970s, physical activity and wellness programs became a trend that now is very much a part of the North American way of life. The growing number of participants is attributed primarily to scientific evidence linking regular physical activity and positive lifestyle habits to better health, longevity, quality of life, and total well-being.

Research findings in the last few years have shown that physical inactivity and a negative lifestyle seriously threaten health and hasten the deterioration rate of the human body. Physically active people live longer than their inactive counterparts, even if activity begins later in life. Current U.S. estimates indicate that more than 250,000 deaths yearly are attributed to lack of regular physical activity.[1] Most industrialized nations throughout the world show similar trends.

The human organism needs movement and activity to grow, develop, and maintain health. Advances in modern technology, however, have almost completely eliminated the necessity for physical exertion in daily life. The automated society in which we live no longer provides us with enough activity to ensure adequate health.

At the beginning of the 20th century, **life expectancy** for a child born in the United States was only 47 years. The most common health problems in the Western world were infectious diseases, such as tuberculosis, diphtheria, influenza, kidney disease, polio, and other diseases of infancy. Progress in the medical field largely eliminated these diseases. Then, as more North American people started to enjoy the "good life" (sedentary living, alcohol, fatty foods, excessive sweets, tobacco, drugs), we saw a parallel increase in the incidence of chronic diseases such as hypertension, coronary heart disease, atherosclerosis, strokes, diabetes, cancer, emphysema, and cirrhosis of the liver (see Figure 1.1).

As the incidence of **chronic diseases** climbed, we recognized that prevention is the best medicine. Consequently, a fitness and wellness movement developed gradually at the end of the 20th century. People began to realize that good health is mostly self-controlled and that the leading causes of premature death and illness in North America could be prevented by adhering to positive lifestyle habits. Whereas we all desire to live a

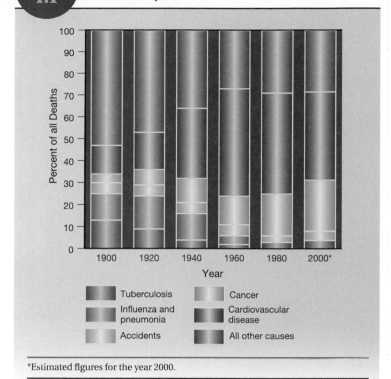

> ## Figure 1.1
> **Causes of deaths in the United States for selected years.**
>
> Legend:
> - Tuberculosis
> - Influenza and pneumonia
> - Accidents
> - Cancer
> - Cardiovascular disease
> - All other causes
>
> *Estimated figures for the year 2000.
>
> **Source:** National Center for Health Statistics, Division of Vital Statistics.

Daily lifestyle habits have a lot more to do with what makes a person sick and when he dies than all of the influence of medicine.

long life, wellness programs focus on enhancing the overall *quality* of life—for as long as we live.

Presently, the average life expectancy in the United States is 76 years (73 for men and 80 for women). In a break with tradition, however, for the first time in the year 2000, the World Health Organization (WHO) calculated **healthy life expectancy** (HLE) estimates for 191 nations. (This figure is obtained by subtracting the years of ill health from total life expectancy.) The United States ranked 24th in this report with a HLE of 70 years; Japan was first with a HLE of 74.5 years (see Figure 1.2). The U.S. ranking was a major surprise, given its status as a developed country with one of the best medical care systems in the world. The rating indicates that Americans die earlier and spend more time disabled than people in most other advanced countries. The WHO report points to several factors that may account for this unexpected finding:

1. The extremely poor health of some groups, such as Native Americans, rural African Americans, and the inner-city poor. Their health status is more characteristic of poor developing nations rather than a rich industrialized country.
2. The HIV epidemic, which causes more U.S. deaths and disability than in other developed nations.

Figure 1.2 Life expectancy (top values) and healthy life expectancy (bottom values) for selected countries.

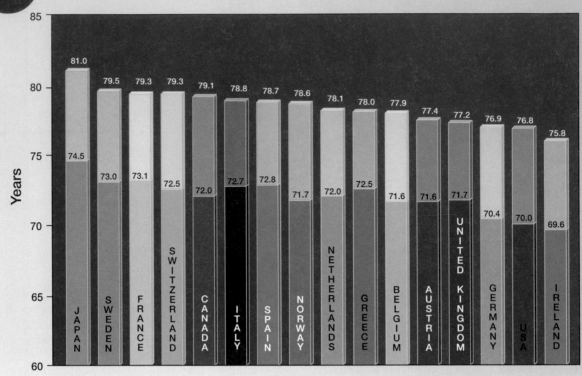

Source: World Health Organization, http://www.who.int/inf-pr-2000/en/pr2000-life.html. Retrieved June 4, 2000.

3. The high incidence of tobacco use.
4. The high incidence of coronary heart disease.
5. Fairly high levels of violence, notably homicides, compared with other developed countries.

Physical Activity Versus Exercise

Physical inactivity and a sedentary lifestyle seriously threaten our health and hasten the deterioration rate of the human body.

Based on the abundance of scientific research on physical activity and exercise over the last three decades, a clear distinction has been established between physical activity and exercise. **Physical activity** is bodily movement produced by skeletal muscles. It requires energy expenditure and produces progressive health benefits.[2] Typical examples of physical activity include walking to and from work, taking the stairs instead of elevators and escalators, gardening, doing household chores, dancing, and washing the car by hand. Physical inactivity, on the other hand, implies a level of activity that is lower than that required to maintain good health.

Exercise is a type of physical activity that requires "planned, structured, and repetitive bodily movement to improve or maintain one or more

Health A state of complete well-being, and not just the absence of disease or infirmity.

Life expectancy Number of years a person is expected to live based on the person's birth year.

Chronic diseases Illnesses that develop and last a long time.

Healthy Life Expectancy (HLE) Number of years a person is expected to live in good health. This number is obtained by subtracting ill-health years from the overall life expectancy.

Physical activity Bodily movement produced by skeletal muscles; requires expenditure of energy and produces progressive health benefits.

Exercise A type of physical activity that requires planned, structured, and repetitive bodily movement with the intent of improving or maintaining one or more components of physical fitness.

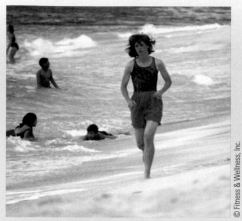
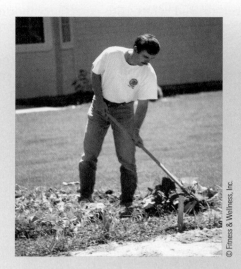
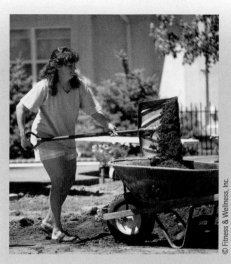

Exercise and an active lifestyle increases health, quality of life, and longevity.

components of physical fitness."[3] Examples of exercise are walking, running, cycling, aerobics, swimming, and strength training.

Surgeon General's Report on Physical Activity and Health

In 1996, the U.S. Surgeon General released a landmark report on the influence of regular physical activity on health.[4] The significance of this historic document cannot be underestimated. Until 1996, the Surgeon General had released only two other such reports—one on smoking and health in 1964, and a second one on nutrition and health in 1988. The 1996 document on physical activity and health summarized more than 1,000 scientific studies from the fields of epidemiology, exercise physiology, medicine, and the behavioral sciences.

According to the 1996 report, poor health because of the lack of physical activity is a serious public health problem that we must meet head-on at once. More than 60 percent of adults do not achieve the recommended amount of physical activity (see Table 1.1), and 25 percent are not physically active at all. Further, almost half of all people between 12 and 21 years of age are not vigorously active on a regular basis. The report also stated that physical inactivity is more prevalent in

1. Women than men
2. African Americans and Hispanic Americans than whites
3. Older than younger adults
4. Less affluent than more affluent people
5. More educated than less educated adults

Furthermore, the number of people who are not physically active is more than twice the number of people who suffer from hypertension, have high cholesterol, or smoke cigarettes. This report became a nationwide call to action.

The report states that regular **moderate physical activity** can prevent premature death, unnecessary illness, and disability. It could provide substantial benefits in health and well-being for the vast majority of people who are not physically active. Among these benefits are significantly reduced risks for developing or dying from heart disease, diabetes,

Table 1.1 Percent of Total U.S. Adult Population that Regularly Participates in Physical Activity

	Moderate Intensity*	High Intensity**
Overall	20%	14%
By Gender		
Men	21	13
Women	19	16
By Ethnicity		
White	21	15
African American	15	9
Hispanic American	20	12

* A minimum of 5 days per week for at least 30 minutes per session.

** A minimum of 3 days per week for a minimum of 20 minutes.

Source: U.S. Department of Health and Human Services, *Physical Activity and Health: A Report of the Surgeon General* (Atlanta: Centers for Disease Control and Prevention, National Center for Chronic Disease Prevention and Health Promotion, 1996).

colon cancer, and high blood pressure. Regular physical activity also is important for the health of muscles, bones, and joints, and it seems to reduce symptoms of depression and anxiety, improve mood, and enhance the ability to perform daily tasks throughout life. Individuals who are already moderately active can achieve greater health benefits by increasing the amount of physical activity. It also can help control health-care costs and help to maintain a high quality of life into old age.

The report defined moderate physical activity as using 150 calories of energy per day, or 1,000 calories per week. It recommended that people strive to achieve at least 30 minutes of physical activity per day most days of the week. Examples of moderate physical activity (generally more strenuous than the typical examples previously listed) are walking, cycling, playing basketball or volleyball, swimming, water aerobics, dancing fast, pushing a stroller, raking leaves, shoveling snow, washing or waxing a car, washing windows or floors, and even gardening.

A Healthy Lifestyle

Most people recognize that participating in fitness programs improves their quality of life. In recent years, however, we came to realize that improving physical fitness alone was not always sufficient to lower the risk for disease and ensure better health. For example, individuals who run 3 miles (about 5 km) a day, lift weights regularly, participate in stretching exercises, and watch their body weight might be easily classified as having good or excellent fitness. Offsetting these good habits, however, might be **risk factors**, including high blood pressure, smoking, constant stress, drinking excessive alcohol, and eating too many fatty foods. These factors place people at risk for cardiovascular disease and other chronic diseases of which they may not be aware.

One of the best examples that good fitness does not always provide a guarantee of a healthy and productive life was the tragic death in 1984 of Jim Fixx, author of the best-selling book *The Complete Book of Running*. More than one million copies of this book were sold. At the time of his death by heart attack, Fixx was 52 years old. He had been running between 60 and 80 miles a week and believed that his high level of fitness would prevent dying from heart disease.

At age 36, Jim Fixx smoked two packs of cigarettes per day, weighed about 215 pounds, did not participate in regular physical activity, and had a family history of heart disease. His father, having had a first heart attack at age 35, later died at age 43. Perhaps in an effort to lessen his risk for heart disease, Fixx began to raise his level of fitness. He started to jog, lost 50 pounds, and quit smoking. On

several occasions, though, Fixx declined to have an exercise electrocardiogram (ECG) test, which likely would have revealed his cardiovascular problem. His unfortunate death illustrates that an exercise program by itself will not make high-risk people immune to heart disease, though it may delay the onset of a serious or fatal problem.

Wellness

Even though most people are aware of their unhealthy behaviors (smoking, inactivity, high-fat diets, excessive stress), they seem satisfied with life as long as they are free from symptoms of disease or illness. They do not contemplate change until they suffer a major health problem. Present lifestyle habits, however, dictate the health and well-being of tomorrow.

Good health is no longer viewed as simply the absence of illness. The notion of good health has evolved notably in the last few years and continues to change, as scientists learn more about lifestyle factors that bring on illness and affect wellness. Furthermore, once the idea took hold that fitness by itself would not always decrease the risk for disease and ensure better health, the wellness concept developed in the 1980s.

The term **wellness** covers several components that are conducive to health. Wellness living requires implementing positive programs to change behavior to improve health and quality of life, prolong life, and achieve total well-being.

Wellness has seven dimensions: physical, emotional, mental, social, environmental, occupational, and spiritual (see Figure 1.3). These dimensions are interrelated: One frequently affects the others. For example, a person who is emotionally down often has no desire to exercise, study, socialize with friends, attend church, and may be more susceptible to illness and disease.

The seven dimensions of wellness show how the concept clearly goes beyond the absence of disease. Wellness incorporates factors such as adequate fitness, proper nutrition, stress management, disease prevention, spirituality, not smoking or abusing drugs, personal safety, regular physical examinations, health education, and environmental support (see Figure 1.4).

Moderate physical activity Activity that uses 150 calories of energy per day, or 1,000 calories per week.

Risk factors Characteristics that predict the development of certain diseases.

Wellness The constant and deliberate effort to stay healthy and achieve the highest potential for well-being. It encompasses seven dimensions—physical, emotional, mental, social, environmental, occupational, and spiritual—and integrates them all into a quality life.

Figure 1.3

Dimensions of wellness.

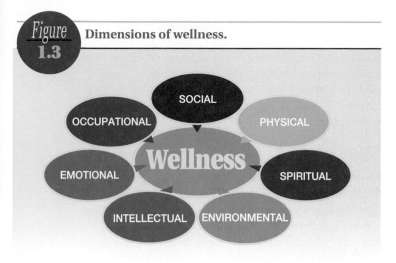

The Seven Dimensions of Wellness*

Physical

Physical wellness is the dimension most commonly associated with being healthy. Physically well individuals are physically active, exercise regularly, eat a well-balanced diet, maintain recommended body weight, get sufficient sleep, practice safe sex, minimize exposure to environmental contaminants, avoid harmful drugs (including tobacco and excessive alcohol), and seek medical care and exams as needed. Physically well people also exhibit good cardiorespiratory endurance, adequate muscular strength and flexibility, proper body composition, and the ability to carry out ordinary and unusual demands of daily life safely and effectively.

Emotional

Emotional wellness involves the ability to understand your own feelings, accept your limitations, and achieve emotional stability. Furthermore, it implies the ability to express emotions appropriately, adjust

For a wellness way of life, not only must individuals be physically fit and manifest no signs of disease, but they must also be free of risk factors for disease (such as hypertension, hyperlipidemia, cigarette smoking, negative stress, faulty nutrition, careless sex). The relationship between adequate fitness and wellness is illustrated in the continuum in Figure 1.5. Even though an individual tested in a fitness center may demonstrate adequate or even excellent fitness, indulgence in unhealthy lifestyle behaviors will still increase the risk for chronic diseases and diminish the person's well-being.

* Adapted from W.W.K. Hoeger, L. W. Turner, and B. Q. Hafen. *Wellness: Guidelines for a Healthy Lifestyle.* Belmont, CA: Wadsworth/Thomson Learning, 2002.

Figure 1.4

Selected wellness components.

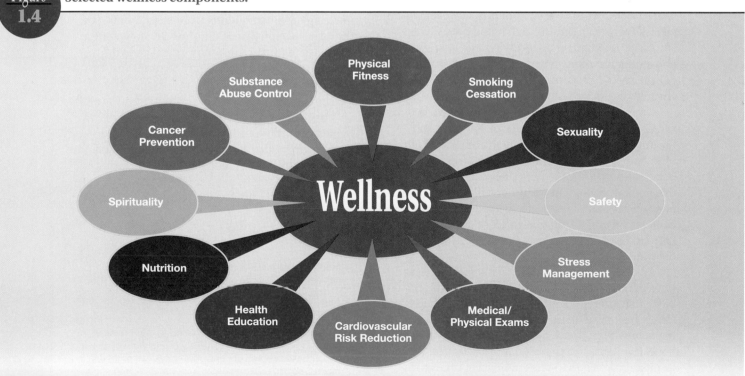

Figure 1.5 Wellness continuum.

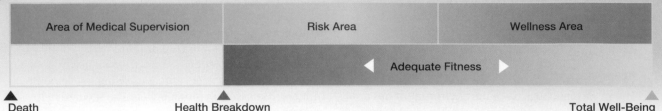

Area of Medical Supervision	Risk Area	Wellness Area

◄ Adequate Fitness ►

▲ Death   ▲ Health Breakdown   ▲ Total Well-Being

to change, cope with stress in a healthy way, and enjoy life despite its occasional disappointments and frustrations.

Emotional wellness brings with it a certain stability, an ability to look both success and failure squarely in the face and to keep moving along a predetermined course. When success is evident, the emotionally well person radiates the expected joy and confidence. When failure seems evident, the emotionally well person responds by making the best of circumstances and moving beyond the failure. Wellness enables you to move ahead with optimism and energy instead of spending time and talent worrying about failure. You learn from it, identify ways to avoid it in the future, and then go on with the business at hand.

Mental

Mental wellness, also referred to as intellectual wellness, implies that you can apply the things you have learned, create opportunities to learn more, and engage your mind in lively interaction with the world around you. When you are mentally well, you are not intimidated by facts and figures with which you are unfamiliar, but you embrace the chance to learn something new. Your confidence and enthusiasm enables you to approach any learning situation with eagerness that leads to success.

Mental wellness brings with it vision and promise. More than anything else, mentally well people are open-minded and accepting of others. Instead of being threatened by people different from themselves, they show respect and curiosity without feeling they have to conform. They are faithful to their own ideas and philosophies and allow others the same privilege. Their self-confidence guarantees that they can take their place among others in the world without having to give up part of themselves and without requiring others to do the same.

Emotional wellness also involves happiness— an emotional anchor that gives meaning and joy to life. Happiness is a long-term state of mind that permeates the various facets of life and influences our outlook. Although there is no simple recipe for

creating happiness, researchers agree that happy people are usually part of a family; they are partners, parents, or children; they love others, and they feel loved themselves. Healthy, happy people enjoy friends, work hard at something fulfilling, get plenty of exercise, and enjoy play and leisure time. They know how to laugh, and they laugh often. They give of themselves freely to others and seem to have found deep meaning in life.

An attitude of true happiness signals freedom from the tension and depression that many people endure. Emotionally well people are obviously subject to the same kinds of depression and unhappiness that occasionally plague us all, but the difference lies in their ability to bounce back. Well people take minor setbacks in stride and have the ability to enjoy life despite it all. They don't waste energy or time recounting the situation, wondering how they could have changed it, or dwelling on the past.

Social

Social wellness, with its accompanying positive self-image, endows you with the ease and confidence to be outgoing, friendly, and affectionate toward others. Social wellness involves not only a concern for oneself, but also an interest in humanity and the environment as a whole.

One of the hallmarks of social wellness is the ability to relate to others and to reach out to other people, both within one's family and outside it. Similar to emotional wellness, it involves being

Physical wellness Good physical fitness and confidence in one's personal ability to take care of health problems.

Emotional wellness The ability to understand your own feelings, accept your limitations, and achieve emotional stability.

Mental wellness A state in which your mind is engaged in lively interaction with the world around you.

Social wellness The ability to relate well to others, both within and outside the family unit.

comfortable with your emotions and thus helps you understand and accept the emotions of others. Your own balance and sense of self allows you to extend respect and tolerance to others. Healthy people are honest and loyal. This dimension of wellness leads to the ability to maintain close relationships with other people.

Environmental

The man-made toxicity of the environment has a direct effect on personal wellness. To enjoy health, we require clean air, pure water, quality food, adequate shelter, satisfactory work conditions, personal safety, and healthy relationships. Health is negatively affected when we live in a polluted, toxic, unkind, and unsafe environment. To enjoy **environmental wellness**, it is our personal responsibility not only to educate and protect ourselves against environmental hazards, but also to protect the environment so that we, our children, and future generations can enjoy a safe and clean environment.

Occupational

Occupational wellness is not tied to high salary, prestigious position, or extravagant working conditions. Any job can bring occupational wellness if it provides rewards that are important to the individual. Salary might be the most important factor to one person, whereas another might place a much greater value on creativity. A person who is occupationally well has his or her own "ideal" job, which allows them to thrive.

People with occupational wellness face demands on the job, but they also have some say over demands that are placed on them. Any job has routine demands, but occupational wellness means that routine demands are mixed with new, unpredictable challenges that keep a job exciting. Occupationally well people are able to maximize their skills, and they have the opportunity to broaden existing skills or gain new ones. Their occupation offers opportunity for advancement and recognition for achievement. Occupational wellness encourages collaboration and interaction among co-workers, which fosters a sense of teamwork and support.

Spiritual

Spiritual wellness provides a unifying power that integrates all dimensions of wellness. Basic characteristics of spiritual people include a sense of meaning and direction in life and a relationship to a higher being. Pursuing these may lead to personal freedom, prayer, faith, love, closeness to others, peace, joy, fulfillment, and altruism.

Several studies have reported positive relationships among spiritual well-being, emotional well-being, and satisfaction with life. People who attend church and regularly participate in religious organizations enjoy better health, have a lower incidence of chronic diseases, handle stress more effectively, and seem to live longer.

Although the ways that religious affiliation enhances wellness are difficult to determine, possible reasons include the promotion of healthy lifestyle behaviors, social support, assistance in times of crisis and need, and counseling to overcome one's weaknesses. Spiritual beliefs also seem to help people overcome crises and aid them in developing better coping techniques to deal with future trauma.

Altruism, a key attribute of spiritual people, seems to enhance health and longevity. Studies indicate that people who perform regular volunteer work live longer. Doing good for others is good for oneself, especially for the immune system. Research has found that health benefits of altruism to be so powerful that simply watching films of altruistic endeavors enhances the formation of an immune system chemical that helps fight disease.

Wellness requires a balance among all of its seven dimensions. The relationship between spirituality and wellness, therefore, is meaningful in our quest for a better quality of life. As with other parameters listed above, optimum wellness requires development of the spiritual dimension to its fullest potential.

Wellness, Fitness, and Longevity

During the 1960s and 1970s, we began to realize the importance of good fitness and improved lifestyle in the fight against chronic diseases, particularly those of the cardiovascular system. Because of more participation in wellness programs, cardiovascular mortality rates dropped: The decline began in about 1963, and between 1960 and 2000 the incidence of cardiovascular disease dropped by 26 percent. This decrease is credited to higher levels of wellness and better health care in the United States. More than half of the decline is specifically attributed to improved diet and reduction in smoking.

Furthermore, several studies have shown an inverse relationship between physical activity and premature cardiovascular mortality rates. In a study conducted among 16,936 Harvard alumni linking physical activity habits and mortality rates, as the amount of weekly physical activity increased, the risk of cardiovascular deaths decreased.[5] The largest decrease in cardiovascular deaths was observed among alumni who used more than 2,000 calories per week through physical activity. Figure 1.6 graphically illustrates the study results.

Another major study, conducted by Dr. Steve Blair and associates, upheld the findings of the

Figure 1.6

Death rates by physical activity index.

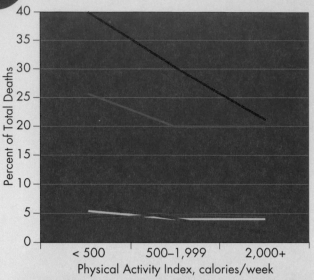

Note: The graph represents cause-specific death rates per 10,000 man-years of observation among 16,936 Harvard alumni, 1962–1978, by physical activity index; adjusted for differences in age, cigarette smoking, and hypertension.

Source: R. S. Paffenbarger, R. T. Hyde, A. L. Wing, and C. H. Steinmetz, "A Natural History of Athleticism and Cardiovascular Health," *Journal of the American Medical Association* 252 (1984): 491–495. Used by permission.

Harvard alumni study.[6] Based on data from 13,344 people followed over an average of 8 years, the results confirmed that the level of physical activity is related to mortality from all causes. The study revealed a graded and consistent inverse relationship between physical activity levels and mortality, regardless of age and other risk factors. As illustrated in Figure 1.7, the higher the level of physical activity, the longer the lifespan. The death rate during the 8-year study from all causes for the least-fit (group 1) men was 3.4 times higher than that of the most-fit men. For the least-fit women, the death rate was 4.6 times higher than that of most fit women.

This study also reported a greatly reduced rate of premature death, even at moderate fitness levels that most adults can achieve easily. Greater protection is attained by combining higher fitness levels with reduction in other risk factors such as hypertension, serum cholesterol, cigarette smoking, and excessive body fat.

A 5-year research study into fitness and mortality found a substantial (44 percent) reduction in mortality risk when people abandoned a **sedentary** lifestyle and become moderately fit.[7] The lowest death

rate was found in people who were fit at the start of the study and remained fit; and the highest death rate was found in men who were unfit at the beginning of the study and remained unfit (see Figure 1.8).

Subsequent research published in 1995 substantiated previous findings and indicated that primarily **vigorous activity** is associated with greater longevity.[8] Vigorous activity was defined as any activity that requires a MET level equal to or greater than 6 METs (21 ml/kg/min—see Health Fitness Standards on page 12) or briefly, an activity that provides a substantial challenge to the cardiorespiratory system. One MET is the energy expenditure at rest, or approximately 3.5 ml/kg/min. Six or more METs represents exercising at an oxygen uptake (VO_2) equal to or greater than 6 times the resting energy requirement (briefly, any activity that provides a "substantial challenge" to the participant). Examples of vigorous activities in this study include brisk walking, jogging, swimming laps, squash, racquetball, tennis, and shoveling snow. Also, vigorous exercise was found to be as important as maintaining recommended weight and not smoking. (See also the detailed discussion of MET and oxygen uptake in Chapter 7.)

In another major research study, a healthy lifestyle was shown to contribute to some of the lowest mortality rates ever reported in the literature.[9] The investigators in this study looked at three general health habits among the participants: regular physical activity, sufficient sleep, and lifetime abstinence from smoking. Additionally, study participants abstained from alcohol, caffeine, drugs, and all forms of tobacco.

Compared with the general white population, this group of over 10,000 people had much lower cancer, cardiovascular, and overall death rates. Men in the study had one-third the death rate from cancer, one-seventh the death rate from cardiovascular disease, and one-fifth the rate of overall

Environmental wellness The capability to live in a clean and safe environment that is not detrimental to health.

Occupational wellness The ability to perform one's job skillfully and effectively under conditions that provide personal and team satisfaction and adequately reward each individual.

Spiritual wellness The sense that life is meaningful, that life has purpose, and that some power brings all humanity together; the ethics, values, and morals that guide us and give meaning and direction to life.

Altruism True concern for the welfare of others.

Sedentary A person who is relatively inactive and whose lifestyle is characterized by a lot of sitting.

Vigorous activity Any activity that requires a MET level equal to or greater than 6 METs (21 ml/kg/min); 1 MET = energy expenditure at rest, 3.5 ml/kg/min.

Figure
1.7

Death rates by physical fitness groups.

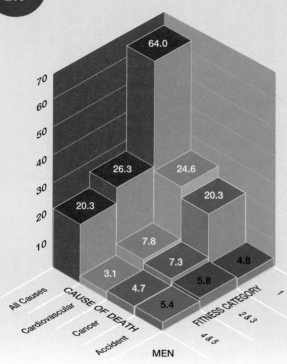
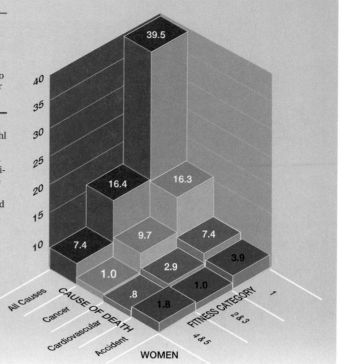

Numbers on top of the bars are all-cause death rates per 10,000 person-years of follow-up for each cell; 1 person-year indicates one person who was followed up one year later.

Source: Based on data from S. N. Blair, H. W. Kohl III, R. S. Paffenbarger, Jr., D. G. Clark, K. H. Cooper, and L. W. Gibbons, "Physical Fitness and All-Cause Mortality: A Prospective Study of Healthy Men and Women," *Journal of the American Medical Association* 262 (1989): 2395–2401.

Fitness Category
Least fit group = 1
Most fit group = 5

MEN

WOMEN

Figure
1.8

Five-year follow-up in mortality rates associated with maintenance and improvements in fitness.

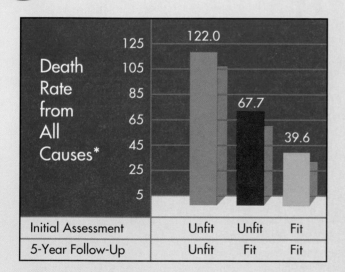

| | Initial Assessment | Unfit | Unfit | Fit |
| 5-Year Follow-Up | Unfit | Fit | Fit |

Death Rate from All Causes*

122.0
67.7
39.6

* Death rate per 10,000 man-years observation. Based on data from "Changes in Physical Fitness and All-Cause Mortality: A Prospective Study of Healthy Men," *Journal of the American Medical Association* 273 (1995): 1193–1198.

Source: S. N. Blair, H. W. Kohl III, C. E. Barlow, R. S. Paffenbarger, Jr., L. W. Gibbons, and C. A. Macera, "Changes in Physical Fitness and All-Cause Mortality: A Prospective Study of Healthy and Unhealthy Men," *Journal of the American Medical Association* 273 (1995): 1193–1198.

mortality. Women had about half the rate of cancer and overall mortality and one-third the death rate from cardiovascular disease. Life expectancies for 25-year-olds who adhered to the three health habits were 85 and 86 years, respectively, compared with 74 and 80 for the average U.S. white man and woman. The additional 6 to 11 "golden years" are precious—and more enjoyable—for those who maintain a lifetime wellness program.

The results of these studies clearly indicate that fitness improves wellness, quality of life, and longevity. Vigorous exercise is preferable to the extent of one's capabilities because it is most clearly associated with longer life.

If you don't make time to be physically active, sooner or later you will need to make time to treat illness.

Physical Fitness

As the fitness concept grew during the 1970s, it became clear that a battery of tests was necessary to assess physical fitness, because several specific components contribute to an individual's overall level of fitness.

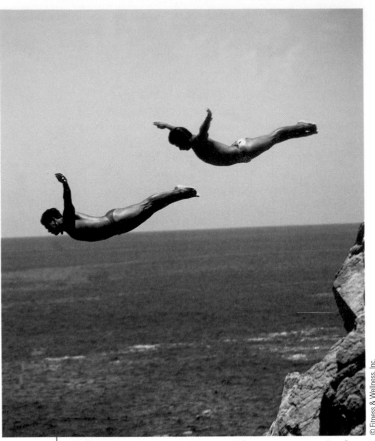

Physical fitness can be classified into health-related and motor skill-related fitness. The four **health-related fitness** components are cardio-respiratory (aerobic) endurance, muscular strength and endurance, muscular flexibility, and body composition (Figure 1.9). **Skill-related fitness** components consist of agility, balance, coordination, power, reaction time, and speed (Figure 1.10). The latter are aimed primarily at succeeding in athletics and may not be as crucial to better health. In terms of preventive medicine, the main emphasis of fitness programs should be on the health-related components. Nevertheless, total fitness is achieved by taking part in specific programs to improve both health-related and skill-related components.

Good health- and skill-related fitness are required to participate in highly skilled activities.

© Fitness & Wellness, Inc.

Physical fitness The ability to meet the ordinary as well as the unusual demands of daily life safely and effectively without being overly fatigued and still have energy left for leisure and recreational activities.

Health-related fitness Fitness programs that are prescribed to improve the overall health of the individual.

Skill-related fitness Fitness programs that are used to improve athletic ability.

Figure 1.9 Health-related components of physical fitness.

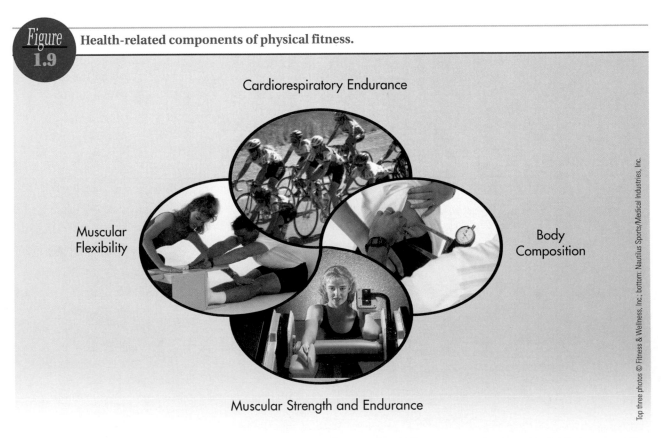

Cardiorespiratory Endurance

Muscular Flexibility

Body Composition

Muscular Strength and Endurance

Top three photos © Fitness & Wellness, Inc.; bottom: Nautilus Sports/Medical Industries, Inc.

Figure
1.10

Motor skill-related components of physical fitness.

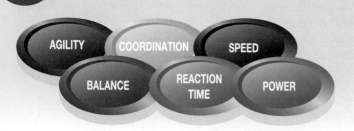

Fitness Standards: Health Versus Physical Fitness

The discussion of health-related fitness assessment in Chapters 4, 6, 7, 8, and 9 describe several tests to assess fitness. A meaningful debate regarding age- and gender-related fitness standards for the general population has resulted in the two standards: a health fitness standard (also referred to as criterion-referenced) and a physical fitness standard.

Health Fitness Standards

The **health fitness standards** proposed here are based on data linking minimum fitness values to disease prevention and health. Attaining the health fitness standard requires only moderate physical activity. For example, a 2-mile walk in less than 30 minutes, 5 to 6 times per week, seems to be sufficient to achieve the health-fitness standard for cardiorespiratory endurance.

As illustrated in Figure 1.11, significant *health* benefits can be reaped with such a program,

although *fitness* (expressed in terms of oxygen uptake, VO_{2max}—see discussion on cardiorespiratory endurance below) improvements are not as notable. These improvements are quite striking, and only slightly greater benefits are obtained with a more intense exercise program. These benefits include reduction in blood lipids, lower blood pressure, weight loss, stress release, decreased risk for diabetes, and lower risk for disease and premature mortality.

More specifically, improvements in the **metabolic profile** (better insulin sensitivity and glucose tolerance and improved cholesterol levels) can be notable despite little or no improvement in aerobic capacity or weight loss. **Metabolic fitness** can be attained through an active lifestyle and moderate physical activity.

Another assessment of health related fitness uses **cardiorespiratory endurance,** measured in terms of the maximal amount of oxygen the body is able to utilize per minute of physical activity (maximal oxygen uptake, or VO_{2max})—essentially, a measure of how efficiently your heart, lungs, and muscles can operate during maximal exertion (see Chapter 6). VO_{2max} is commonly expressed in milliliters (ml) of oxygen (volume of oxygen) per kilogram (kg) of body weight per minute (ml/kg/min). Individual values can range from about 10 ml/kg/min in cardiac patients to over 80 ml/kg/min in world-class runners, cyclists, and cross-country skiers.

Research data from the study presented in Figure 1.7 reported that achieving VO_{2max} values of 35 and 32.5 ml/kg/min for men and women, respectively, may be sufficient to lower the risk for all-cause mortality significantly. Although greater improvements in fitness yield a slightly lower risk for premature death, the largest drop is seen between the least fit (group 1) and the moderately fit (groups 2

Figure
1.11

Health and fitness benefits based on the type of lifestyle and physical activity program.

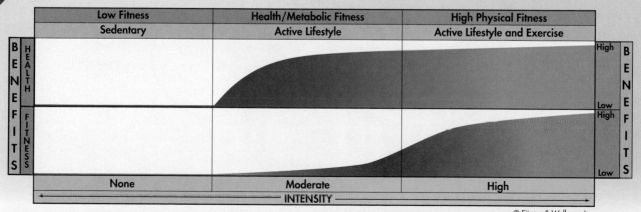

© Fitness & Wellness, Inc.

and 3). Therefore, the 35 and 32.5 ml/kg/min values could be selected as the health fitness standards.

Physical Fitness Standards

Physical fitness standards are set higher than the health fitness standards and require a more vigorous exercise program. Physically fit people of all ages have the freedom to enjoy most of life's daily and recreational activities to their fullest potential. Current health fitness standards may not be enough to achieve these objectives.

Sound physical fitness gives the individual a degree of independence throughout life that many people in the United States no longer enjoy. Most older people should be able to carry out activities similar to those they conducted in their youth, though not with the same intensity. These standards do not require being a championship athlete, but activities such as changing a tire, chopping wood, climbing several flights of stairs, playing basketball, mountain biking, playing soccer with grandchildren, walking several miles around a lake, and hiking through a national park do require more than the current "average fitness" level in the United States.

If the main objective of one's fitness program is to lower the risk of disease, attaining the health fitness standards may be enough to ensure better health. If, however, the individual wants to participate in moderate to vigorous fitness activities, achieving a high physical fitness standard is recommended. This book gives both health fitness and physical fitness standards for each fitness test. Your own personal objectives will determine the fitness program you use.

Leading Health Problems in the United States

The leading causes of death in the United States today are largely lifestyle-related (see Figure 1.12). Nearly 64 percent of all deaths in the United States are caused by cardiovascular disease and cancer.[10] Nearly 80 percent of these deaths could be prevented through a healthy lifestyle program. The third and fourth leading causes of death are chronic and obstructive pulmonary disease (COPD) and accidents.

The most prevalent degenerative diseases in the United States are those of the cardiovascular system. More than 40 percent of all deaths in this country are attributed to diseases of the heart and blood vessels. According to the American Heart Association, 58.8 million people in the United States were afflicted with diseases of the cardiovascular system in 1999, including 50 million with hypertension (high blood pressure) and 12 million with coronary heart disease

(many of these people have more than one type of cardiovascular disease). About 1.1 million people have heart attacks each year, and more than 350,000 of them die as a result. The estimated cost of heart and blood vessel disease in 2000 exceeded $326 billion.[11] A complete cardiovascular disease prevention program is outlined in Chapter 12.

The second leading cause of death in the United States is cancer. Unlike cardiovascular disease, the mortality rate for cancer has increased steadily over the last few decades (see Figure 1.1). In 1996, the cancer rate declined slightly for the first time. Even though cancer is not the number-one killer, it is the number-one health fear of the American people.

About 23 percent of all deaths in the United States are attributable to cancer. More than 550,000 people died from this disease in 2000, and an estimated 1,220,100 new cases were reported the same year.[12] The major contributor to the increase in the incidence of cancer during the last five decades is lung cancer. Without lung cancer, cancer mortality rates would have decreased by 14 percent between 1950 and 1990.

The American Cancer Society maintains that the most influential factor in fighting cancer today is prevention through health education programs. Evidence indicates that as much as 80 percent of all human cancer can be prevented through positive lifestyle behaviors. A comprehensive cancer prevention program is presented in Chapter 13.

The third cause of death, chronic and obstructive pulmonary disease, (COPD) is related mostly to tobacco use (see Chapter 14).

Accidents are the fourth leading cause of death. Even though not all accidents are preventable, many are. Fatal accidents are often related to abusing drugs and not wearing seat belts.

Health fitness standards The lowest fitness requirements for maintaining good health, decreasing the risk for chronic diseases, and lowering the incidence of muscular-skeletal injuries.

Metabolic profile A measurement to assess risk for diabetes and cardiovascular disease through plasma insulin, glucose, lipid, and lipoprotein levels.

Metabolic fitness Denotes improvements in the metabolic profile through a moderate-intensity exercise program in spite of little or no improvement in physical fitness standards.

Cardiorespiratory endurance The ability of the lungs, heart, and blood vessels to deliver adequate amounts of oxygen to the cells to meet the demands of prolonged physical activity.

Physical fitness standards A fitness level that allows a person to sustain moderate to vigorous physical activity without undue fatigue and the ability to closely maintain this level throughout life.

Figure
1.12
Leading causes of death in the United States in 1998.

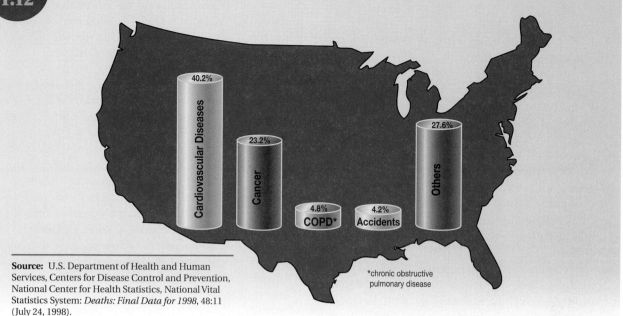

Source: U.S. Department of Health and Human Services, Centers for Disease Control and Prevention, National Center for Health Statistics, National Vital Statistics System: *Deaths: Final Data for 1998*, 48:11 (July 24, 1998).

*chronic obstructive pulmonary disease

Most people do not perceive accidents as a health problem. Even so, accidents affect the total well-being of millions of Americans each year. Accident prevention and personal safety are part of a health enhancement program aimed at achieving a better quality of life. Proper nutrition, exercise, stress management, and abstinence from cigarette smoking are of little help if the person is involved in a disabling or fatal accident as a result of distraction, a single reckless decision, or not wearing safety seat belts properly.

Accidents do not just happen. We cause accidents and we are victims of accidents. Although some factors in life, such as earthquakes, tornadoes, and airplane crashes, are completely beyond our control, more often than not, personal safety and accident prevention are a matter of common sense. Most accidents stem from poor judgment and confused mental states. Accidents frequently happen when people are upset, are not paying attention to the task at hand, or are abusing alcohol or other drugs.

Alcohol abuse is the number-one cause of all accidents, and alcohol intoxication is the leading cause of fatal automobile accidents. Other commonly abused drugs alter feelings and perceptions, generate mental confusion, and impair judgment and coordination, greatly enhancing the risk for accidental morbidity and mortality (see Chapter 14).

The underlying causes of death in the United States (see Figure 1.13) indicate that 8 of the 9 causes are related to lifestyle and lack of common sense. The "big three"—tobacco use, poor diet and

inactivity, and alcohol abuse—are responsible for some 800,000 deaths each year.

Lifestyle as a Health Problem

As the incidence of chronic diseases rose, it became obvious that prevention was—and remains —the best medicine. Estimates indicate that more than half of disease is lifestyle-related, a fifth is attributed to the environment, and a tenth is influenced by the health care the individual receives. Only 16 percent is related to genetic factors (see Figure 1.14).[13] Thus, the individual controls as much as 84 percent of disease and quality of life. Further, according to estimates, 83 percent of deaths before age 65 are preventable. In essence, most people in the United States are threatened by the very lives they lead today.

Ideally, healthy lifestyle habits should be taught and reinforced in early youth. Unfortunately, many young people are in such poor physical condition that they will add to national health concerns in years to come. Surveys conducted during the past decade have raised public concern regarding the fitness level of American youth. As compared to the 1960s and 1970s, cardiorespiratory endurance and upper body strength have decreased and body fat has increased. These findings suggest that current physical education programs are not promoting lifetime fitness and wellness adequately.

Because of the unhealthy lifestyles that many young adults lead, their bodies may be middle-aged or older! Healthy choices made today influence health for decades. Many physical education

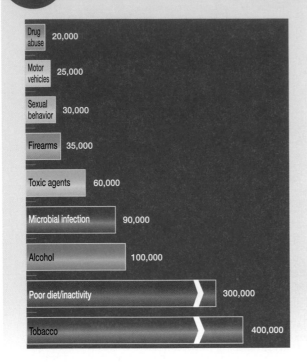

Figure 1.13 Underlying causes of death in the United States.

Drug abuse	20,000
Motor vehicles	25,000
Sexual behavior	30,000
Firearms	35,000
Toxic agents	60,000
Microbial infection	90,000
Alcohol	100,000
Poor diet/inactivity	300,000
Tobacco	400,000

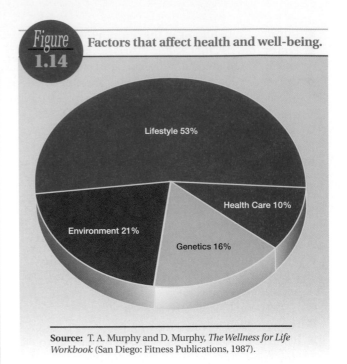

Figure 1.14 Factors that affect health and well-being.

Lifestyle 53%
Health Care 10%
Environment 21%
Genetics 16%

Source: T. A. Murphy and D. Murphy, *The Wellness for Life Workbook* (San Diego: Fitness Publications, 1987).

> *Over 50 percent of the people who die in this country each year die because of what they do.*
>
> —David Satcher, U.S. Surgeon General

programs do not emphasize the skills necessary for youth to maintain a high level of fitness and health throughout life. The intent of this book is to provide those skills and help to prepare you for a lifetime of physical fitness and wellness. A healthy lifestyle is self-controlled, and people can learn how to be responsible for their own health and fitness.

Benefits of a Comprehensive Wellness Program

A most inspiring story illustrating what fitness can do for a person's health and well-being is that of George Snell from Sandy, Utah. At age 45, Snell weighed approximately 400 pounds, his blood pressure was 220/180, he was blind because of undiagnosed diabetes, and his blood glucose level was 487.

Snell had determined to do something about his physical and medical condition, so he started a walking/jogging program. After about 8 months of conditioning, Snell had lost almost 200 pounds, his

eyesight had returned, his glucose level was down to 67, and he was taken off medication. Two months later, less than 10 months after beginning his personal exercise program, he completed his first marathon, a running course of 26.2 miles!

Health Benefits

Most people exercise because it improves their personal appearance and makes them feel good about themselves. Although many benefits accrue from participating in a regular fitness and wellness program and active people generally live longer, the greatest benefit of all is that physically fit individuals enjoy a better quality of life. These people live life to its fullest, with fewer health problems than inactive individuals (who may also indulge in other negative lifestyle behaviors). Although compiling an all-inclusive list of the benefits reaped from participating in a fitness and wellness program is difficult, the following list summarizes many of them:

- Improves and strengthens the cardiorespiratory system.
- Maintains better muscle tone, muscular strength, and endurance.
- Improves muscular flexibility.
- Enhances athletic performance.
- Helps maintain recommended body weight.
- Helps preserve lean body tissue.
- Increases resting metabolic rate.
- Improves the body's ability to use fat during physical activity.
- Improves posture and physical appearance.

- Improves functioning of the immune system.
- Lowers the risk for chronic diseases and illness (such as cardiovascular diseases and cancer).
- Decreases the mortality rate from chronic diseases.
- Thins the blood so it doesn't clot as readily (thereby decreasing the risk for coronary heart disease and strokes).
- Helps the body manage cholesterol levels more effectively.
- Prevents or delays the development of high blood pressure and lowers blood pressure in people with hypertension.
- Helps prevent and control diabetes.
- Helps achieve peak bone mass in young adults and maintain bone mass later in life, thereby decreasing the risk for osteoporosis.
- Helps people sleep better.
- Helps prevent chronic back pain.
- Relieves tension and helps in coping with life stresses.
- Raises levels of energy and job productivity.
- Extends longevity and slows down the aging process.
- Promotes psychological well-being; better morale, self-image, and self-esteem.
- Reduces feelings of depression and anxiety.
- Motivates a person toward positive lifestyle changes (improving nutrition, quitting smoking, controlling alcohol and drug use).
- Speeds recovery time following physical exertion.
- Speeds recovery following injury or disease.
- Regulates and improves overall body functions.
- Improves physical stamina and counteracts chronic fatigue.
- Helps to maintain independent living, especially in older adults.
- Enhances quality of life: People feel better and live a healthier and happier life.

Economic Benefits

Sedentary living can have a strong impression on a nation's economy. As the need for physical exertion in Western countries decreased steadily during the last century, health-care expenditures increased dramatically. Health-care costs in the United States rose from $12 billion in 1950 to $1.2 trillion in 2000 (Figure 1.15). At the present rate of escalation, health-care expenditures will reach $1.6 trillion by the year 2002. In 1995, health care costs represented about 14 percent of the gross national product (GNP). They are projected to reach about 18 percent by the year 2002 and 37 percent by 2030.

In terms of yearly health care costs per person, as illustrated in Figure 1.16, the United States spends more per person ($3,724) than any other industrialized

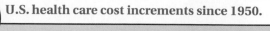

U.S. health care cost increments since 1950.

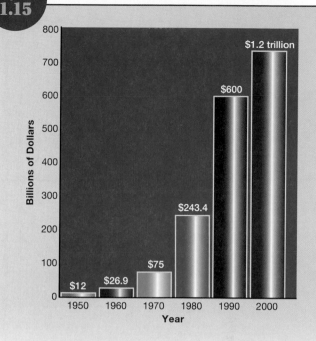

Figure 1.15

Source: "Daten Der Woche," Welt am Sonntag 25 (1991): 35. World Health Organization, *The World Health Report 2000—Health Systems: Improving Performance*, (2000): Annex Table 8.

nation, yet, overall, the health care system ranks only 37th in the world. One of the reasons for the low overall ranking is the overemphasis on state-of-the art cures instead of prevention programs. The United States is the best place in the world to treat someone once they are sick, but the system does a poor job at keeping people healthy in the first place. The United States also fails to provide good health care for all: Forty-four million residents do not have health insurance.

Unhealthy behaviors are contributing to the staggering U.S. health care costs. Risk factors for disease carry a heavy price tag (see Figure 1.17). According to estimates, 1 percent of the people account for 30 percent of these costs.[14] Half of the people use up about 97 percent of health-care dollars. Furthermore, the average health-care cost per person in the United States is almost twice as high as for most other industrialized nations.[15]

Strong scientific evidence now links participation in fitness and wellness programs not only to better health but also to lower medical costs and higher job productivity. Most of this research is being conducted and reported by organizations that already have implemented fitness or wellness programs.

As a result of the recent staggering rise in medical costs, many organizations are beginning to

Figure
1.16

Estimated 1997 and 1989 health-care costs per person for selected countries (bottom value represents the 1989 cost).

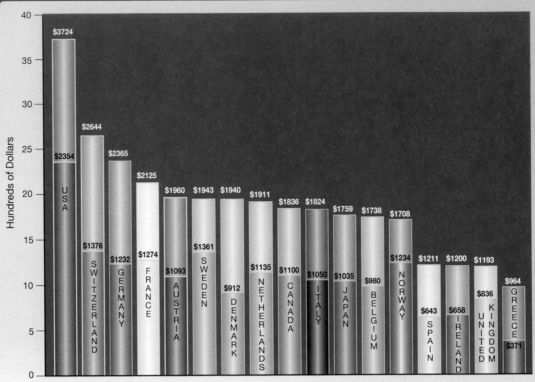

Sources: "Daten Der Woche", *Welt am Sonntag* 25 (1991): 35. World Health Organization, *The World Health Report 2000—Health Systems: Improving Performance* (2000): Annex Table 8.

Figure
1.17

Average annual health care costs for leading risk factors.

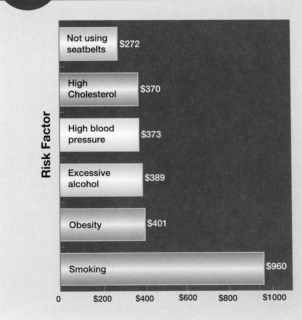

Source: *Journal of Occupational Medicine*, November 1991.

realize that keeping employees healthy costs less than treating them once they are sick. A survey by the American Institute for Preventive Medicine found that large corporations are reaping health-cost savings by implementing health promotion programs.[16] A sample return on investment per dollar spent is provided in Figure 1.18. Containing the costs of health care through fitness and wellness programs has become a major issue for many organizations around the United States.

Another reason some organizations are offering wellness programs to their employees—overlooked by many because it does not seem to affect the bottom line directly—is simply concern by top management for employees' physical well-being. Whether the program lowers medical costs is not the main issue. The main reason to top management is that wellness programs help individuals feel better about themselves and improves their quality of life.

In addition to the financial and physical benefits, some corporations are offering health promotion programs as an incentive to attract, hire, and retain employees. Many executives believe that an on-site health promotion program is the best fringe benefit they can offer at their company. Young executives are looking for organizations such as

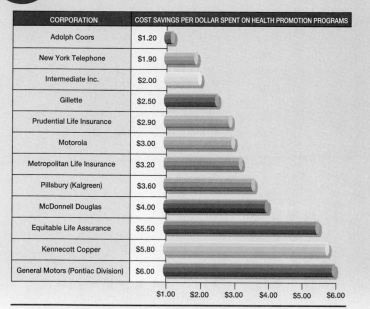

Figure 1.18 Health care cost savings by selected corporations per dollar spent on health promotion programs.

CORPORATION	COST SAVINGS PER DOLLAR SPENT ON HEALTH PROMOTION PROGRAMS
Adolph Coors	$1.20
New York Telephone	$1.90
Intermediate Inc.	$2.00
Gillette	$2.50
Prudential Life Insurance	$2.90
Motorola	$3.00
Metropolitan Life Insurance	$3.20
Pillsbury (Kalgreen)	$3.60
McDonnell Douglas	$4.00
Equitable Life Assurance	$5.50
Kennecott Copper	$5.80
General Motors (Pontiac Division)	$6.00

Source: 1991 Survey by the American Institute for Preventive Medicine, Southfield, Michigan.

these, not only for the added health benefits but also because the corporate officers are showing an attitude of concern and care.

The Wellness Challenge of the 21st Century

Because a better and healthier life is something every person should strive for, our biggest challenge, as we begin the new century, is to teach people how to take control of their personal health habits and adhere to a positive lifestyle. Considering the wealth of information available on the benefits of fitness and wellness programs, improving the quality and possible length of our lives is a matter of personal choice.

Research indicates that accomplishing the following changes will significantly improve health and extend life:

1. Participate in a lifetime physical activity program. Exercise regularly at least 3 times per week and try to accumulate a minimum of 30 minutes of physical activity each day of your life. The exercise program should consist of 20 to 30 minutes of aerobic exercise, along with some strengthening and stretching exercises.

2. Do not smoke cigarettes. Cigarette smoking is the largest preventable cause of illness and premature death in the United States. If we include all related deaths, smoking is responsible for more than 400,000 unnecessary deaths each year.

3. Eat right. Eat a good breakfast and two additional well-balanced meals every day. Unless snacks consist of healthy foods, refrain from snacking between meals. Avoid eating too many calories and foods with a lot of sugar, fat, and salt. Increase your daily consumption of fruits, vegetables, and whole-grain products.

4. Maintain recommended body weight through adequate nutrition and exercise. This is important in preventing chronic diseases and in developing a higher level of fitness.

5. Get enough rest. Sleep 7 to 8 hours each night.

6. Lower your stress levels. Reduce your vulnerability to stress and practice stress management techniques as needed.

7. Be wary of alcohol. Drink alcohol moderately or not at all. Alcohol abuse leads to mental, emotional, physical, and social problems.

8. Surround yourself with healthy friendships. Unhealthy friendships contribute to destructive behaviors and low self-esteem. Associating with people who strive to maintain good fitness and health reinforces a positive outlook in life and encourages positive behaviors. Constructive social interactions enhance well-being.

9. Be informed about the environment. Seek clean air, clean water, and a clean environment. Be aware of pollutants and occupational hazards: asbestos fibers, nickel dust, chromate, uranium dust, and so on. Take precautions when using pesticides and insecticides.

10. Take personal safety measures. Although not all accidents are preventable, many are. Taking simple precautionary measures, such as using seat belts and keeping electrical appliances away from water, lessens the risk for avoidable accidents.

Thanks to current scientific data and the fitness and wellness movement of the past three decades, most Americans now see a need to participate in programs that improve and maintain health. The typical American, however, is not a good role model when cardiorespiratory fitness is concerned. Almost 60 percent of U.S. adults engage in little or no leisure-time physical activity. In fact, 25 percent of the adult population is not active at all.

Aerobic activities are the most popular form of exercise, so an even lower percentage of the population probably engages in and derives benefits from strength and flexibility programs. In addition, an estimated half or more of the adult population in

the United States has a weight problem, and a third of all adults are considered obese.

Even though people in the United States believe a positive lifestyle has a great impact on health and longevity, most do not reap the benefits because they don't know how to implement a safe and effective fitness and wellness program. Others are exercising incorrectly and, therefore, are not reaping the full benefits of their program.

National Health Objectives for the Year 2010

Every 10 years, the U.S. Department of Health and Human Services releases a list of objectives for preventing disease and promoting health. Since its initiation in 1980, this 10-year plan has helped instill a new sense of purpose and focus for public health and preventive medicine. These national health objectives are intended to be realistic goals to improve the health of all Americans. Two unique goals of the new 2010 objectives emphasize increased quality and years of healthy life and seek to eliminate health disparities among all groups of people (see Figure 1.19). The objectives address three important points:[17]

> *The nation's top health goals as we begin the new millennium are: exercise, increased consumption of fruits and vegetables, smoking cessation, and the practice of safe sex.*
> —David Satcher, U.S. Surgeon General

1. Personal responsibility for health behavior. Individuals need to become ever more health-conscious. Responsible and informed behaviors are the key to good health.
2. Health benefits for all people and all communities. Lower socioeconomic conditions and poor health often are interrelated. Extending the benefits of good health to all people is crucial to the health of the nation.
3. Health promotion and disease prevention. A shift from treatment to preventive techniques will drastically cut health-care costs and help all Americans achieve a better quality of life.

Development of these health objectives usually involves more than 10,000 people representing 300 national organizations, including the Institute of Medicine of the National Academy of Sciences, all state health departments, and the federal Office of Disease Prevention and Health Promotion. A summary of key 2010 objectives is provided in Figure 1.20.

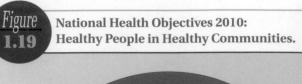

Figure 1.19 National Health Objectives 2010: Healthy People in Healthy Communities.

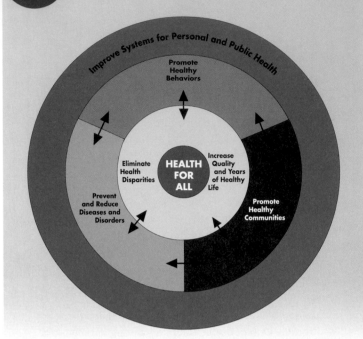

Living the fitness and wellness principles provided in this book not only will enhance the quality of your life but also will allow you to be an active participant in achieving the Healthy People 2010 Objectives.

Wellness Education

Most people go to college to learn how to make a living, but a fitness and wellness course will teach you how to live—how to truly live life to its fullest potential. Some people seem to think that success is measured by how much money they make. Making a good living will not help you unless you live a wellness lifestyle that will allow you to enjoy what you have.

Although everyone would like to enjoy good health and wellness, most people don't know how to reach this objective. Lifestyle is the most important factor affecting personal well-being. Granted, some people live long because of genetic factors, but quality of life during middle age and the "golden years" is more often related to wise choices initiated during youth and continued throughout life.

In a few short years, lack of wellness leads to a loss of vitality and gusto for life, as well as

> *Your wellness lifestyle today will determine the health and quality of your life tomorrow.*

Figure 1.20 Selected Health Objectives for the Year 2010.

SELECTED HEALTH OBJECTIVES
FOR THE YEAR 2010

1. Increase quality and years of healthy life.
2. Eliminate health disparities.
3. Improve the health, fitness, and quality of life of all Americans through the adoption and maintenance of regular, daily physical activity.
4. Promote health and reduce chronic disease risk, disease progression, debilitation, and premature death associated with dietary factors and nutritional status among all people in the United States.
5. Reduce disease, disability, and death related to tobacco use and exposure to secondhand smoke.
6. Increase the quality, availability, and effectiveness of educational and community-based programs designed to prevent disease and improve the health and quality of life of the American people.
7. Promote health for all people through a healthy environment.
8. Reduce the incidence and severity of injuries from unintentional causes, as well as violence and abuse.
9. Promote worker health and safety through prevention.
10. Improve access to comprehensive, high quality health care.
11. Ensure that every pregnancy in the United States is intended.
12. Improve maternal and pregnancy outcomes and reduce rates of disability in infants.
13. Improve the quality of health-related decisions through effective communication.
14. Decrease the incidence of functional limitations due to arthritis, osteoporosis, and chronic back conditions.
15. Decrease cancer incidence, morbidity, and mortality.
16. Promote health and prevent secondary conditions among persons with disabilities.
17. Enhance the cardiovascular health and quality of life of all Americans through prevention and control of risk factors, and promotion of healthy lifestyle behaviors.
18. Prevent HIV transmission and associated morbidity and mortality.
19. Improve the mental health of all Americans.
20. Raise the public's awareness of the signs and symptoms of lung disease.
21. Increase awareness of healthy sexual relationships and prevent all forms of sexually transmitted diseases.
22. Reduce the incidence of substance abuse by all people, especially children.

premature **morbidity** and mortality. The Wellness Lifestyle Questionnaire given in Lab 1A will provide an initial rating of your current efforts to stay healthy and well. The components of a wellness lifestyle are discussed in subsequent chapters of this book.

Because fitness and wellness needs vary significantly from one individual to another, all exercise and wellness prescriptions must be personalized to obtain best results. The information in the following chapters and their respective laboratory experiences set forth the necessary guidelines that will allow you to develop a personal lifetime program to improve fitness and promote preventive health care and personal wellness.

The laboratory experiences have been prepared on tear-out sheets so they can be turned in to class instructors. As you study this book and complete the respective worksheets, you will learn to do the following:

- Implement motivational and behavior modification techniques to help you adhere to a lifetime fitness and wellness program.
- Determine whether medical clearance is needed for your safe participation in exercise.
- Conduct nutritional analyses and follow the recommendations for adequate nutrition.
- Write sound diet and weight-control programs.
- Assess the health-related components of fitness (cardiorespiratory endurance, muscular strength

and endurance, muscular flexibility, and body composition).
- Write exercise prescriptions for cardiorespiratory endurance, muscular strength and endurance, and muscular flexibility.
- Assess the skill-related components of fitness (agility, balance, coordination, power, reaction time, and speed).
- Determine your levels of tension and stress, lessen your vulnerability to stress, and implement a stress management program if necessary.
- Determine your potential risk for cardiovascular disease and implement a risk-reduction program.
- Follow a cancer risk reduction program.
- Implement a smoking cessation program, if applicable.
- Avoid chemical dependency and know where to find assistance if needed.
- Learn the health consequences of sexually transmitted diseases, including HIV/AIDS, and guidelines for preventing STDs.
- Discover the relationship between fitness and aging.
- Write objectives to improve your fitness and wellness and learn how to chart a wellness program for the future.
- Differentiate myths and facts of exercise and health-related concepts.

Exercise Safety

Even though testing and participation in exercise are relatively safe for most apparently healthy individuals under age 45, the reaction of the cardiovascular system to higher levels of physical activity cannot be totally predicted.[18] Consequently, a small but real risk exists for exercise-induced abnormalities in people with a history of cardiovascular problems and those who are at higher risk for disease. These include abnormal blood pressure, irregular heart rhythm, fainting, and, in rare instances, a heart attack or cardiac arrest.

Before you start to engage in an exercise program or participate in any exercise testing, you should fill out the questionnaire in Lab 1B. If your answer to any of the questions is yes, you should see a physician before participating in a fitness program. Exercise testing and participation is not wise under some of the conditions listed in Lab 1B and may require a stress electrocardiogram (ECG) test. If you have any questions regarding your current health status, consult your doctor before initiating, continuing, or increasing your level of physical activity.

An exercise tolerance test (stress test) with 12-lead electrocardiographic monitoring may be required of some individuals prior to initiating an exercise program.

Morbidity A condition related to or caused by illness or disease.

Web Interactive

- Healthy People 2010. Healthy People is a national health promotion and disease prevention initiative that lists a series of national goals for improving health of all Americans by the year 2010.

  http://www.health.gov/healthypeople

- National Wellness Institute. The premier site for college and university wellness programs and assessment tools.

  http://www.nationalwellness.org

- Exercise Encyclopedia. This site features aerobic exercises, strength training and bodybuilding information as well as a comprehensive exercise library.

  http://www.fitnesslink.com/exercise

- Surgeon General Statement regarding Physical Fitness. A series of interesting fact sheets prepared by the U.S. Surgeon General reporting on national findings regarding physical activity facts and benefits, and suggestions for communities. Information concerning the following demographic groups are listed: Adolescents and Young Adults, Adults, Older Adults, Persons with Disabilities, and women

  http://www.cdc.gov/nccdphp/sgr/fact.htm

- CDC's National Physical Activity Initiative. The Centers for Disease Control and Prevention provides scientific and technical leadership and assistance and promotes physical activity through the National Physical Activity Initiative reflecting the CDC's continuing commitment to reduce the major risk factors for chronic disease in the United States.

  http://www.cdc.gov/nccdphp/sgr/npai.htm

Interactive Sites:

- Thriveonline Personal Health Assessments. This comprehensive site features many interactive assessments in a variety of health topics: medical (lifestyle assessment, pregnancy calculator, asthma trigger zapper, pollen map), fitness (calorie and activity calculator, fitness planner, park and trail guide, and target heart rate calculator), sexuality (contraceptive chooser, ovulation calculator, and STD map), nutrition (recipe finder, vitamin guide), serenity (assess your stress, sleep test, poetry in motion), and weight (BMI calculator).

  http://thriveonline.oxygen.com

- Lifescan Health Risk Appraisal. This site was created by Bill Hettler, M.D. of the National Wellness Institute and features a series of questions to help you identify what specific lifestyle factors can impair your health and longevity.

  http://wellness.uwsp.edu/Health_Service/Services/lifescan/lifescan.shtml

- Your Personalized Health Portrait. Take this confidential health questionnaire to determine your personal lifestyle score, featuring a list of health habits to change, in order of importance. You will also receive a list of screening tests and immunizations to ask your doctor about.

  http://www.thriveonline.com/cgi-bin/hmi/healthportrait.cgi

- Select Your Health Quiz: Test your general health and medical knowledge; select the "Conventional", "Advanced", and/or "Extreme" Health Quiz.

  http://www.mededge.com/quizbb.htm

Notes

1. U.S. Centers for Disease Control and Prevention and American College of Sports Medicine, "Summary Statement: Workshop on Physical Activity and Public Health," *Sports Medicine Bulletin* 28, no. 4 (1993): 7.

2. National Institutes of Health, *Consensus Development Conference Statement: Physical Activity and Cardio-vascular Health* (Washington, DC: NIH, December 18–20, 1995).

3. See note 2.

4. U.S. Department of Health and Human Services, *Physical Activity and Health: A Report of the Surgeon General* (Atlanta: Centers for Disease Control and Prevention, National Center for Chronic Disease Prevention and Health Promotion, 1996).

5. R. S. Paffenbarger, Jr., R. T. Hyde, A. L. Wing, and C. H. Steinmetz, "A Natural History of Athleticism and Cardiovascular Health," *Journal of the American Medical Association* 252 (1984): 491–495.

6. S. N. Blair, H. W. Kohl III, R. S. Paffenbarger, Jr., D. G. Clark, K. H. Cooper, and L. W. Gibbons, "Physical Fitness and All-Cause Mortality: A Prospective Study of Healthy Men and Women," *Journal of the American Medical Association* 262 (1989): 2395–2401.

7. S. N. Blair, H. W. Kohl III, C. E. Barlow, R. S. Paffenbarger, Jr., L. W. Gibbons, and C. A. Macera, "Changes in Physical Fitness and All-Cause Mortality: A Prospective Study of Healthy and Unhealthy Men," *Journal of the American Medical Association* 273 (1995): 1193–1198.

8. I. Lee, C. Hsieh, and R. S. Paffenbarger, Jr., "Exercise Intensity and Longevity in Men: The Harvard Alumni Health Study," *Journal of the American Medical Association* 273 (1995): 1179–1184.

9. J. E. Enstrom, "Health Practices and Cancer Mortality Among Active California Mormons," *Journal of the National Cancer Institute* 81 (1989): 1807–1814.

10. U.S. Department of Health and Human Services, Centers for Disease Control and Prevention, National Center for Health Statistics, National Vital Statistics System: *Deaths, Final Data for 1998* 48, no. 11 (July 24, 2000).

11. *2000 Heart and Stroke Statistical Update* (Dallas: American Heart Association, 2000).

12. American Cancer Society, *2000 Cancer Facts and Figures* (New York: ACS, 2000).

13. T. A. Murphy and D. Murphy, *The Wellness for Life Workbook* (San Diego: Fitness Publications, 1987).

14. "Wellness Facts," *University of California at Berkeley Wellness Letter* (Palm Coast, FL: The Editors, April 1995).

15. "Daten Der Woche," *Welt am Sonntag* 25, no. 35 (1991).

16. Robert C. Chadbourne, "Fit for Hire," *Fitness Management* 12, no. 2 (1996): 28–30.

17. U. S. Department of Health and Human Services. *Healthy People 2010.* (Washington DC: U.S. Government Printing Office, November 2000).

18. American College of Sports Medicine, *Guidelines for Exercise Testing and Prescription* (Baltimore: Williams & Wilkins, 2000).

Suggested Readings

American College of Sports Medicine. "Position Stand: The Recommended Quantity and Quality of Exercise for Developing and Maintaining Cardiorespiratory and Muscular Fitness, and Flexibility in Healthy Adults." *Medicine and Science in Sports and Exercise* 30 (1998): 975–991.

Blair, S. N. "C.H. McCloy Research Lecture: Physical Activity, Physical Fitness, and Health." *Research Quarterly for Exercise and Sport* 64 (1993): 365–376.

Blair, S. N., et al. "Influences of Cardiorespiratory Fitness and Other Precursors on Cardiovascular Disease and All-cause Mortality in Men and Women." *Journal of the American Medical Association* 276 (1996): 205–210.

Booth, F. W., and B. S. Tseng. "America Needs to Exercise for Health." *Medicine and Science in Sports and Exercise* 27 (1995): 462–465.

Hoeger, W. W. K., L. W. Turner, and B. Q. Hafen. *Wellness: Guidelines for a Healthy Lifestyle* (Belmont, CA: Wadsworth/Thomson Learning, 2002).

Nieman, D. C. *The Exercise-Health Connection.* (Champaign, IL: Human Kinetics, 1998).

Pate, R., et al. "Physical Activity and Public Health." *Journal of the American Medical Association* 273 (1995): 402–407.

U.S. Department of Health and Human Services, *Physical Activity and Health: A Report of the Surgeon General.* (Atlanta: Centers for Disease Control and Prevention, National Center for Chronic Disease Prevention and Health Promotion, 1996).

U. S. Department of Health and Human Services, Public Health Service, *Healthy People 2010: Conference Edition.* (http://www.health.gov/healthypeople/Document/tableofcontents.htm).

Lab 1A

WELLNESS LIFESTYLE QUESTIONNAIRE

Name: _____ Date: _____ Grade: _____

Instructor: _____ Course: _____ Section: _____

Necessary Lab Equipment
None.

Objective
To analyze current lifestyle habits and help determine changes necessary for future health and wellness.

Instructions
Check the appropriate answer to each question and obtain a final score according to the guidelines provided at the end of the questionnaire.

	Always	Nearly always	Often	Seldom	Never
1. I participate in vigorous aerobic activity for 20 minutes on three or more days per week, and I accumulate at least 30 minutes of moderate intensity physical activity on a minimum of three additional days per week.	5	4	3	2	1
2. I participate in strength training exercises, using a minimum of eight different exercises, two or more days per week.	5	4	3	2	1
3. I perform flexibility exercises a minimum of three days per week.	5	4	3	2	1
4. I maintain recommended body weight (includes avoidance of excessive body fat, excessive thinness, or frequent fluctuations in body weight).	5	4	3	2	1
5. Every day, I eat three regular meals that include a wide variety of foods.	5	4	3	2	1
6. I limit the amount of fat and saturated fat in my diet on most days of the week.	5	4	3	2	1
7. I eat a minimum of five servings of fruits and vegetables and six servings from grain products on a daily basis.	5	4	3	2	1
8. I regularly avoid snacks, especially those that are high in calories and fat and low in nutrients and fiber.	5	4	3	2	1
9. I do not smoke cigarettes or use tobacco in any other form.	5	4	3	2	1
10. I do not drink alcoholic beverages. If I drink, I do so in moderation (one daily drink for women and two for men), and I do not combine alcohol with other drugs.	5	4	3	2	1
11. I do not use addictive drugs or needles used by others.	5	4	3	2	1
12. I use prescription drugs and over-the-counter drugs sparingly, only when needed, and I follow all directions for their proper use.	5	4	3	2	1
13. I readily recognize when I am under excessive tension and stress (distress).	5	4	3	2	1
14. I am able to perform effective stress management techniques.	5	4	3	2	1
15. I have close friends and relatives that I can discuss personal problems with and approach for help when needed, and with whom I can express my feelings freely.	5	4	3	2	1
16. I spend most of my daily leisure time in wholesome recreational activities.	5	4	3	2	1
17. I sleep 7 to 8 hours each night.	5	4	3	2	1
18. I floss my teeth every day and brush them at least twice daily.	5	4	3	2	1
19. I avoid overexposure to the sun, and I use sunscreen and appropriate clothing when I am out in the sun for extended periods of time.	5	4	3	2	1
20. I avoid using products that have not been shown by science to be safe and effective (this includes anabolic steroids and unproven nutrient or weight loss supplements).	5	4	3	2	1
21. I know the warning signs for heart attack, stroke, and cancer.	5	4	3	2	1

	Always	Nearly always	Often	Seldom	Never
22. I practice monthly breast/testicle self-exams, get recommended screening tests (blood lipids, blood pressure, Pap tests), and seek a medical evaluation when I am not well or disease symptoms arise.	5	4	3	2	1
23. I have a dental checkup at least once a year, and I get regular medical exams according to age recommendations.	5	4	3	2	1
24. I am not sexually active / I always practice safe sex.	5	4	3	2	1
25. I can effectively deal with disappointments and temporary feelings of sadness, loneliness, and depression. If I am unable to deal with these feelings, I seek professional help.	5	4	3	2	1
26. I can work out emotional problems without turning to alcohol or other drugs.	5	4	3	2	1
27. I associate with people who have a positive attitude about life.	5	4	3	2	1
28. I respond to temporary setbacks by making the best of the circumstances and by moving ahead with optimism and energy. I do not spend time and talent worrying about failures.	5	4	3	2	1
29. I wear a seatbelt whenever I am in a car, I ask others in my vehicle to do the same, and I make sure that children are in an infant seat or wear a shoulder harness.	5	4	3	2	1
30. I do not drive under the influence of alcohol or other drugs, and I make an effort to keep others from doing the same.	5	4	3	2	1
31. I avoid being alone in public places, especially after dark; I seek escorts when I visit or exercise in unfamiliar places.	5	4	3	2	1
32. I seek to make my living quarters accident-free, and I keep doors and windows locked, especially when home alone.	5	4	3	2	1
33. I try to minimize environmental pollutants, and I support community efforts to minimize pollution.	5	4	3	2	1
34. I keep my living quarters clean and organized.	5	4	3	2	1
35. I study and/or work in a clean environment (including avoidance of second-hand smoke).	5	4	3	2	1
36. I participate in recycling programs for paper, cardboard, glass, plastic, and aluminum.	5	4	3	2	1

How to Score

Enter the score you have circled for each question in the spaces provided below. Next, total the score for each specific wellness lifestyle category and obtain a rating for each category according to the criteria provided below.

	Health-Related Fitness	Nutrition	Avoiding Chemical Dependency	Stress Management	Personal Hygiene/ Health	Disease Prevention	Emotional Well-being	Personal Safety	Environmental Health & Protection
	1.	5.	9.	13.	17.	21.	25.	29.	33.
	2.	6.	10.	14.	18.	22.	26.	30.	34.
	3.	7.	11.	15.	19.	23.	27.	31.	35.
	4.	8.	12.	16.	20.	24.	28.	32.	36.
Total:									
Rating:									

Category Rating

Excellent (E) = ≥17 Your answers show that you are aware of the importance of this category to your health and wellness. You are putting your knowledge to work for you by practicing good habits. As long as you continue to do so, this category should not pose a health risk. You are also setting a good example for family and friends to follow. Because you got a very high test score on this part of the test, you may want to consider other categories where your score indicates room for improvement.

Good (G) = 13–16 Your health practices in this area are good, but there is room for improvement. Look again at the items you answered with a 4 or below and identify changes that you can make to improve your lifestyle. Even small changes can often help you achieve better health.

Needs Improvement (NI) ≤12 Your health risks are showing. You may be taking serious and unnecessary risks with your health. Perhaps you are not aware of the risks and what to do about them. Most likely you need additional information and help in deciding how to successfully make the changes you desire. You can easily get the information that you need to improve, if you wish. The next step is up to you.

Please note that no final overall rating is provided for the entire questionnaire, because it may not be indicative of overall wellness. For example, an excellent rating in most categories will not offset the immediate health risks and life-threatening consequences of using addictive drugs and not wearing a seatbelt.

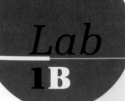

Name: _____ Date: _____ Grade: _____

Instructor: _____ Course: _____ Section: _____

Necessary Lab Equipment
None.

Objective
To determine the safety of exercise participation.

Introduction
Although exercise testing and exercise participation are relatively safe for most apparently healthy individuals under the age of 45, the reaction of the cardiovascular system to increased levels of physical activity cannot always be totally predicted. Consequently, there is a small but real risk of certain changes occurring during exercise testing and participation. Some of these changes may be abnormal blood pressure, irregular heart rhythm, fainting, and in rare instances a heart attack or cardiac arrest. Therefore, you must provide honest answers to this questionnaire. Exercise may be contraindicated under some of the conditions listed below; others may simply require special consideration. **If any of the conditions apply, consult your physician before you participate in an exercise program.** Also, promptly report to your instructor any exercise-related abnormalities that you may experience during the course of the semester.

A. Have you ever had or do you now have any of the following conditions?

   1. A myocardial infarction.

   2. Coronary artery disease.

   3. Congestive heart failure.

   4. Elevated blood lipids (cholesterol and triglycerides).

   5. Chest pain at rest or during exertion.

   6. Shortness of breath.

   7. An abnormal resting or stress electrocardiogram.

   8. Uneven, irregular, or skipped heartbeats (including a racing or fluttering heart).

   9. A blood embolism.

  10. Thrombophlebitis.

  11. Rheumatic heart fever.

  12. Elevated blood pressure.

  13. A stroke.

  14. Diabetes.

  15. A family history of coronary heart disease, syncope, or sudden death before age 60.

  16. Any other heart problem that makes exercise unsafe.

B. Do you have any of the following conditions?

   1. Arthritis, rheumatism, or gout.

   2. Chronic low-back pain.

   3. Any other joint, bone, or muscle problems.

   4. Any respiratory problems.

   5. Obesity (more than 30 percent overweight).

   6. Anorexia.

   7. Bulimia.

   8. Mononucleosis.

   9. Any physical disability that could interfere with safe participation in exercise.

C. Do any of the following conditions apply?

   1. Do you smoke cigarettes?

   2. Are you taking any prescription drug?

   3. Are you 45 years or older?

D. Do you have any other concern regarding your ability to safely participate in an exercise program? If so, explain:

_____

_____

Student's Signature: _____ Date: _____

Personal Challenge

In your own words, indicate what the Wellness Lifestyle Questionnaire in Lab 1A tells you about your current state of wellness. Also, identify categories where you can personally make changes in the next few months and indicate what may help you accomplish your goals.

Lab 1A suggests that _____

_____

_____

_____

_____

I can make these changes in the next few months: _____

_____

_____

_____

_____

The following could help me accomplish my goals: _____

_____

_____

_____

_____

Do you feel that it is safe for you to proceed with an exercise program? Explain any concerns or limitations that you may have regarding your safe participation in a comprehensive exercise program that will target cardiorespiratory, muscular strength, and flexibility.

I believe it is / is not safe for me to exercise. I have the following concerns or limitations: _____

_____

_____

_____

_____

Behavior Modification

Objectives

- Learn the effects of environment on human behavior.

- Understand obstacles that hinder the ability to change behavior.

- Understand the concepts of motivation and locus of control.

- Identify the stages of change.

- Become familiar with the processes of change.

- Learn techniques that will facilitate the process of change.

- Learn the role of goal setting in the process of change.

- Be able to write specific objectives for behavioral change.

Research studies during the last three decades have convincingly documented the benefits of physical activity and healthy lifestyles. Although the scientific evidence continues to mount each day and the data are impressive, most people are still unable to implement or adhere to a healthy lifestyle program.

The information in this book will be of little value to you if you are unable to abandon negative habits and adopt new, healthy behaviors. Before looking at physical fitness and wellness guidelines, you will need to take a critical look at your behaviors and lifestyle—and most likely make some permanent changes to promote overall health and wellness.

The science of behavioral therapy has established that most of the behaviors we adopt in life are a product of our environment—the forces of social influences and the thought processes we go through. This environment includes family, friends, peers, homes, schools, workplaces, television, radio, and movies, as well as our communities, country, and culture in general.

Unfortunately, when it comes to fitness and wellness, we live in a "toxic environment." From a young age, parents, relatives, and friends drive us nearly any place we need to go. We also watch them drive short distances to run errands. We see them take escalators and elevators and ride moving sidewalks at malls and airports. We notice that they use remote controls, pagers, and cellular phones. We observe as they stop at fast-food restaurants and pick up super-sized, calorie-dense, high-fat meals. They watch television and surf the Net for hours at a time. Some smoke, some drink heavily, and some have hard-drug addictions. Others engage in risky behaviors by not wearing seat belts, drinking and driving, and having unprotected sex.

Elevators and escalators are often of the finest workmanship and located in convenient places. Many of our best and finest shopping centers and convention centers don't provide accessible stairwells, so people are all but forced to ride escalators. If they want to walk up the escalator, they can't because the people in front of them obstruct the way. Entrances to buildings provide electric sensors and automatic door openers. Without a second thought, people walk through automatic doors instead of taking the time to push a door open.

Walking, jogging, and bicycle trails are too sparse in our cities, further discouraging physical

> *We have very few inferior people in the world. We have lots of inferior environments. Try to enrich your environments.*
> —*Frank Lloyd Wright*

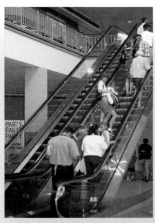
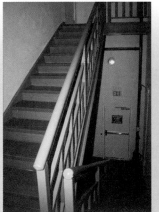
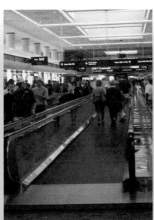

Our environment is not conducive to a healthy, physically active lifestyle.

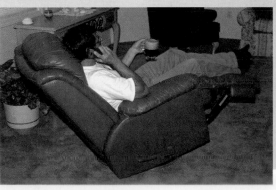
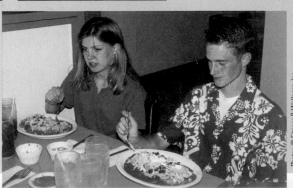

Photos © Fitness & Wellness Inc.

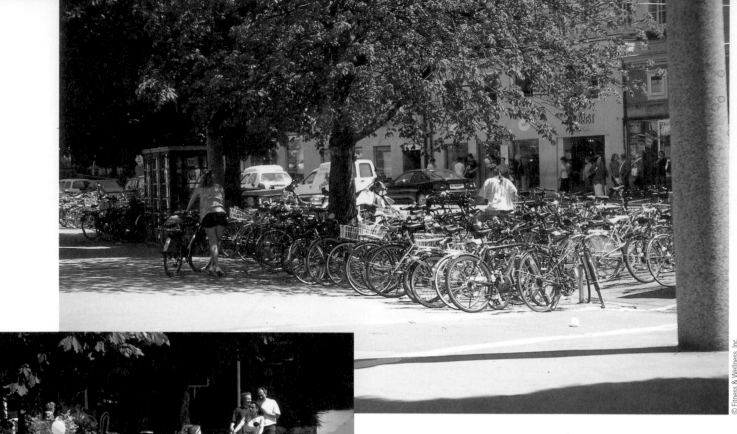

© Fitness & Wellness, Inc.

Salzburg, Austria: Bicycles are the preferred mode of transportation in this large European city.

activity. Places for safe exercise are a concern in many metropolitan areas. Many people remain indoors during leisure hours for fear for their personal safety and well-being.

In recent years the food portion sizes have substantially increased at restaurants. Patrons consume huge amounts of food, almost as if it were the last meal they will ever have. They drink entire pitchers of soda pop or beer instead of the traditional 8-ounce cup size. Most restaurants are colorful, well-lit, and nicely decorated to enhance comfort and appetite and increase the length of stay to entice more eating.

All of the these examples influence our thought process and hinder our ability to be physically active and adopt healthy behaviors. From childhood through young adulthood, we observe, we learn, we emulate, and gradually, without realizing it, we incorporate many of these unhealthy behaviors into our personal lifestyle.

Let's look at weight gain. Most people do not start life with a weight problem. By age 20, a man may weigh 160 pounds. A few years later, the weight starts to climb and may reach 170 pounds. He now adapts and accepts 170 pounds as his weight. The person may "go on a diet" but not make the necessary lifestyle changes. Gradually the weight continues to climb to 180, 190, 200 pounds. Although he may not like it and would like to weigh less, once again he adapts and accepts 200 pounds as his stable weight.

The time comes, usually around middle age, when most people want to make changes in their lives but find this difficult to accomplish, illustrating the adage that "old habits die hard." Acquiring positive behaviors that will lead to better health and well-being is a long-lasting process and requires continual effort. Understanding why most people are unsuccessful at changing their behaviors and are unable to live a healthy lifestyle may increase your readiness and motivation for change. The next sections will examine barriers to change, what motivates people to change, the various stages of change, the process of change, techniques for change, and actions required to make permanent changes in behavior.

Barriers to Change

In spite of best intentions, people make unhealthy choices daily. The most common reasons are

1. Procrastination. People seem to think that tomorrow, next week, or after the holiday is the best time to start change.

   Tip to initiate change. Ask yourself: Why wait until tomorrow when you can start changing today? Lack of motivation is a key factor in procrastination (motivation is discussed later in this chapter).

2. Preconditioned cultural beliefs. If we accept the principle that we are a product of our environment, our cultural beliefs and our physical surroundings pose significant barriers to change. In the culture of Salzburg, Austria, people of both genders and all ages use bicycles as a primary mode of transportation. In the United States, few people other than children ride bicycles.

   Tip to initiate change. In the pre-Columbian era, people thought the world was flat. Few dared to sail long distances for fear that they would fall off the edge. If your health and fitness are at stake, preconditioned cultural beliefs shouldn't keep you from making changes. Finding people who are willing to "sail" with you will help overcome this barrier.

3. Gratification. People prefer instant gratification to long-term gratification. Therefore, they will overeat (instant pleasure) instead of using self-restraint to eat moderately to prevent weight gain (long-term satisfaction). We love tanning (instant gratification) without paying much attention to skin cancer (long-term consequence).

   Tip to initiate change. Think ahead and ask yourself the following questions: How did you feel the last time you engaged in this behavior? How did it affect you? Did you really feel good about yourself or about the results? In retrospect, was it worth it?

4. Risk complacency. Consequences of unhealthy behaviors often don't manifest themselves until years later. People will tell themselves, "If I get heart disease, I'll deal with it then. For now, let me eat, drink, and be merry."

   Tip to initiate change. Ask yourself these questions: How long do you want to live? How do you want to live the rest of your life and what type of health do you want to have? What do you want to be able to do when you are 60, 70, or 80 years old?

5. Complexity. People think the world is too complicated, with too much to think about. If you are living the typical lifestyle, you may feel overwhelmed by everything that seems to be required to lead a healthy lifestyle, for example:

   - Getting exercise
   - Eating low-fat/high-fiber meals and cutting total calories
   - Controlling use of substances
   - Managing stress
   - Wearing seat belts
   - Practicing safe sex
   - Getting medical physicals, including blood tests, Pap smears, and so on
   - Taking nutrient supplements if indicated
   - Fostering spirituality

   Tip to initiate change. Take it one step at a time. Work only on one or two behaviors at a time so the task at hand won't feel insurmountable.

6. Indifference and helplessness. Our thought process often takes over, and we may believe that the way we live won't really affect our health, that we have no control over our health, or that our destiny is all in the genes (also see discussion of locus of control, later in this chapter).

   Tip to initiate change. As much as 84 percent of the leading causes of death in the United States are preventable. Realize that only you can take control over your personal health and lifestyle habits and affect the quality of your life.

7. Rationalization. Even though people are not practicing healthy behaviors, they often tell themselves that they get sufficient exercise, that their diet is fine, that they have good solid relationships, or that they really don't smoke/drink/get high enough to affect their health.

   Tip to initiate change. Rationalizing in this manner will not right the wrong. You need to face up to the fact that you have a problem and commit to change. Your health and your life are at stake.

8. Illusions of invincibility. At times people believe that unhealthy behaviors will not harm them. Young adults often have the attitude that, "I can smoke now, and in a few years I'll quit before it causes any damage." When it comes to cigarettes, nicotine is one of the most addictive drugs known to us. Quitting smoking is not an easy task (see Chapter 14). Health problems may arise before you quit, and the risk of lung cancer lingers for years after you quit. Drinking and driving is another example. The feeling of "I'm in control" or "I can handle it" while under the influence is a deadly proposition.

   Others perceive low risk when engaging in negative behaviors with people they like (for example, sex with someone you've recently met

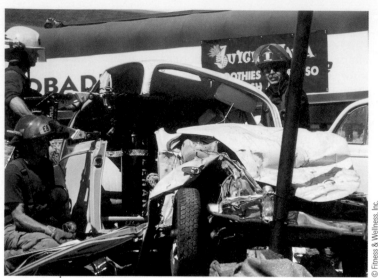

© Fitness & Wellness, Inc.

Feelings of invincibility are a strong barrier to change that can bring about life-threatening consequences.

and feel attracted to), but perceive themselves at risk just by being in the same classroom with an HIV-infected person.

Tip to initiate change. No one is immune to sickness, disease, and tragedy. The younger you are when you implement a healthy lifestyle, the better your odds for a long and healthy life.

When health and appearance begin to deteriorate—usually around middle age—people seek out health care professionals in search of the "magic pill" to reverse and cure the many ills accumulated during years of abuse and overindulgence. The sooner we implement a healthy lifestyle program, the greater will be the health benefits and quality of life that lie ahead.

Motivation and Locus of Control

Motivation is often the explanation given for why some people succeed and others do not. Although motivation comes from within, external factors trigger the inner desire to accomplish a given task. These external factors, then, control behavior.

When studying motivation, understanding **locus of control** is helpful. People who believe they have control over events in their lives are said to have an internal locus of control. People with an external locus of control believe that what happens to them is a result of chance or the environment and is unrelated to their behavior. People with an internal locus of control generally are healthier and have an easier time initiating and adhering to a wellness program than those who perceive that they have no

control and think of themselves as powerless and vulnerable. The latter people also are at greater risk for illness. When illness does strike, restoring a sense of control is vital to regain health.

Few people have either a completely external or a completely internal locus of control. They fall somewhere along a continuum. The more external one's locus of control, the greater the challenge to change and adhere to exercise and other healthy lifestyle behaviors. Fortunately, developing a more internal locus of control can be accomplished. Understanding that most events in life are not determined genetically or environmentally helps people pursue goals and gain control over their lives. Three impediments, however, can keep people from taking action: lack of competence, confidence, and motivation.[1]

1. Problems of competence. Lacking the skills to get a given task done leads to less competence. If your friends play basketball regularly but you don't know how to play, you might not be inclined to participate. The solution to this problem of competence is to master the skills you need to participate. Most people are not born with all-inclusive natural abilities, including playing sports.

   Another alternative is to select an activity in which you are skilled. It may not be basketball, but it well could be aerobics. Don't be afraid to try new activities, though. Similarly, if your body weight is a problem, you could learn to cook low-fat meals. Try different recipes until you find foods that you like.

2. Problems of confidence. Problems with confidence arise when you have the skill but don't believe you can get it done. Fear and feelings of inadequacy often interfere with ability to perform the task. You shouldn't talk yourself out of something until you have given it a fair try. If the skills are there, the sky is the limit. Initially, try to visualize yourself doing the task and getting it done. Repeat this several times, then actually try it. You will surprise yourself.

   Sometimes lack of confidence arises when the task seems insurmountable. In these situations, dividing a goal into smaller, more realistic objectives helps to accomplish the task. You may know how to swim, but to swim a continuous mile may take several weeks to accomplish. Set up your training program so you swim a little farther each day until you are able to swim the entire mile. If you don't meet your objective on

Motivation The desire and will to do something.

Locus of control A concept examining the extent to which a person believes he or she can influence the external environment.

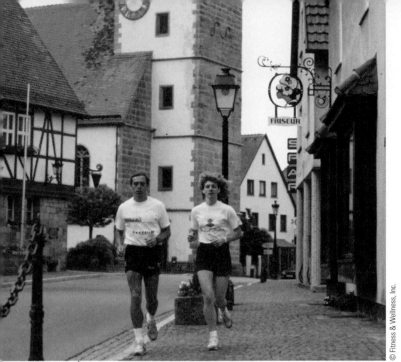

The higher quality of life experienced by people who are physically fit is hard to explain to someone who has never achieved good fitness.

a given day, try it again, reevaluate, cut back a little, and, most important, don't give up.

3. Problems of motivation. In problems of motivation, both the competence and the confidence are there, but individuals are unwilling to change because the reasons to change are not important to them. For example, people begin contemplating a smoking cessation program only when the reasons for quitting outweigh the reasons for smoking. When considering quality of life, the primary causes of unwillingness to change are lack of knowledge and lack of goals. Knowledge often determines goals, and goals determine motivation. How badly you want something dictates how hard you'll work at it. Many people are unaware of the magnitude of the benefits of a wellness program. When it comes to a healthy lifestyle, however, you may not get a second chance. A stroke, a heart attack, or cancer can have irreparable or fatal consequences. Greater understanding of what leads to disease may be all that is needed to initiate change.

Also, feeling physically fit is difficult to explain unless you have experienced it yourself. Feelings of fitness, self-esteem, confidence, health, and quality of life cannot be conveyed to someone who is constrained by sedentary living. In a way, wellness is like reaching the top of a mountain. The quietness, the clean air, the lush vegetation, the flowing water in the river, the wildlife, and the majestic valley below are difficult to explain to someone who has spent a lifetime within city limits.

Changing Behavior

Psychotherapy has been used successfully to help change behavior. The great majority of people, however, do not seek professional help. They usually attempt change by themselves with limited or no knowledge of the process itself.

The simplest model of change is the two-stage model of unhealthy behavior and healthy behavior. This model states that either you do it or you don't. Most people who use this model attempt self-change but end up asking themselves why they just can't do it (exercise) or not do it (smoke). The intention to change may be good, but to do so, knowledge about how to achieve change is needed.

The Transtheoretical Model

For most people, changing chronic/unhealthy behaviors to stable/healthy behaviors is a challenging process. Change usually does not happen all at once. It is a gradual process that involves several stages. To aid with the process of self-change, psychologists James Prochaska, John Norcross, and Carlo DiClemente developed the Transtheoretical Model of Stages of Change.[2]

The Transtheoretical Model incorporates six stages that are important in understanding the process of willful change. These stages describe underlying processes that people go through to change most problem behaviors and adopt healthy behaviors. Most frequently, the model is used to change health-related behaviors such as physical inactivity, smoking, poor nutrition, weight problems, stress, and alcohol abuse.

The six stages of change in the Transtheoretical Model are precontemplation, contemplation, preparation, action, maintenance, and termination/adoption (see Figure 2.1). After years of study, researchers found that applying specific behavioral-change processes during each stage of the model increases the success rate for change. Understanding each stage of this model will help you determine where you are in relation to your personal healthy-lifestyle behaviors. It will also help you identify processes to make successful changes.

Precontemplation

People in the **precontemplation stage** are not considering or do not want to change a given behavior. They typically deny having a problem and have no intent to change in the immediate future. These people are usually unaware or underaware of the problem. Other people around them, including family, friends, health care practitioners, and

Figure 2.1

Stages of change model.

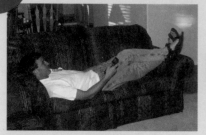
Precontemplation

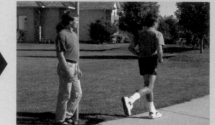
Contemplation

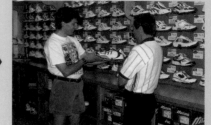
Preparation

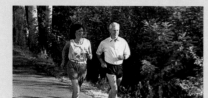
Termination/Adoption

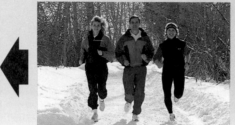
Maintenance

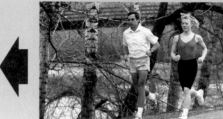
Action

Photos © Fitness & Wellness, Inc.

co-workers, however, identify the problem clearly. Precontemplators do not care about the problem behavior and may even avoid information and materials that address the issue. They tend to avoid free screenings and workshops that might help identify and change the problem, even if they receive financial compensation for attendance. These people frequently have an active resistance to change and seem resigned to accept the unhealthy behavior as their "fate."

> *People don't contemplate change until they begin to feel uncomfortable with their lifestyle habits.*

Precontemplators are the most difficult people to reach for behavioral change. They often think that change isn't even a possibility. Educating them about the problem behavior is critical to help them start contemplating the process of change. Knowledge is power. The challenge is to find ways to help them realize that they are ultimately responsible for the consequences of their behavior. Typically, they initiate change only when others pressure them.

Contemplation

In the **contemplation stage**, people acknowledge that they have a problem and begin to seriously think about overcoming it. Although they are not quite ready for change, they are weighing the pros and cons of changing. Even though people may remain in this stage for years, in their minds they are planning to take some action within the next 6 months. Education and peer support are valuable during this stage.

Preparation

In the **preparation stage**, people are seriously considering and planning to change a behavior within the next month. They are taking initial steps for change and may even try the new behavior for a short while, such as stopping smoking for a day or exercising a few times during the month. During this stage, people define a general goal for

> *Self-defeating behaviors can be defeated.*
> —David J. Lieberman

Precontemplation stage Stage of change in which people are unwilling to change behavior.

Contemplation stage Stage of change in which people are considering changing behavior in the next 6 months.

Preparation stage Stage of change in which people are getting ready to make a change within the next month.

behavioral change (to quit smoking by the last day of the month) and write specific objectives to accomplish this goal (see goal setting discussion later in this chapter). Continued peer and environmental support are helpful during the preparation phase.

Action

This stage requires the greatest commitment of time and energy on the part of the individual. Here people are actively doing things to change or modify the problem behavior or to adopt a new health behavior. The **action stage** requires that the person follow the specific guidelines set forth for that behavior. For example, a person has actually stopped smoking completely, is exercising aerobically 3 times per week according to exercise prescription guidelines, or is maintaining a diet that derives less than 30 percent of its calories from fat. Relapse is common during this stage, and the individual may regress to previous stages. Once people maintain the action stage for 6 consecutive months, they move into the maintenance stage.

Maintenance

During the **maintenance stage**, the person continues to maintain the behavioral change for up to 5 years. The maintenance phase requires continued adherence to the specific guidelines that govern the behavior (such as complete smoking cessation, exercising aerobically 3 times per week, practicing proper stress management techniques). At this time the person works to reinforce the gains made through the various stages of change and strives to prevent lapses and relapse.

Termination/Adoption

Once a behavior has been maintained for more than 5 years, a person is said to be in the **termination** or **adoption** phase and exits from the cycle of change without fear of **relapse**. In the case of negative behaviors that are terminated, the stage of change is referred to as termination. If a positive behavior has been successfully "adopted" for over 5 years, this stage is designated as the adoption stage. Some researchers have also labeled this stage the "transformed" stage of change because the word literally means "to have changed."[3]

Many experts believe that, once an individual enters the termination/adoption stage, former addictions, problems, or lack of compliance with healthy behaviors no longer present an obstacle in the quest for wellness. The change has now become a part of one's lifestyle. This phase is the ultimate goal for all people searching for a healthier lifestyle.

For addictive behaviors like alcoholism and hard drugs, many health care practitioners believe that the individual never enters the termination stage.

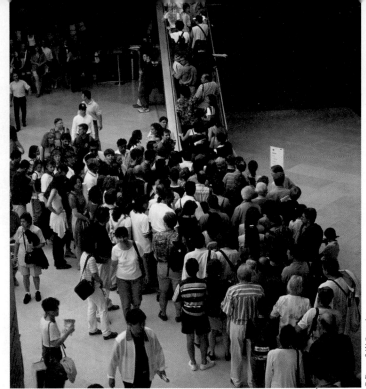

© Fitness & Wellness, Inc.

Advances in modern technology have almost completely eliminated the necessity for physical exertion in daily life.

Chemical dependency is so strong that most former alcoholics and hard-drug users must make a lifetime effort to prevent relapse. Similarly, some behavioral scientists suggest that the adoption stage may not be applicable to health behaviors like exercise and weight control, because the likelihood for relapse is always high.[4]

Use the form in Lab 2A to determine where you stand in respect to behaviors you want to change or new ones you wish to adopt. As you use this form, you will realize that you might be at different stages for different behaviors. For instance, you may be in the preparation stage for aerobic exercise and smoking, in the action stage for strength training, but only in the contemplation stage for a healthy diet. Realizing where you are at with respect to different behaviors will help you design a better action plan for a healthy lifestyle.

Relapse

After getting out of the precontemplation stage, relapse may occur at any level of the model. Even individuals in the maintenance and termination stages may regress to any of the first three stages of the model (see Figure 2.2). Relapse, however, does not mean failure. Failure comes to those who give up and don't use prior experiences as a building block for future success. The chances of moving back up to a higher stage of the model are far better for someone who has previously made it into one of those stages.

Figure
2.2
Model of progression and relapse.

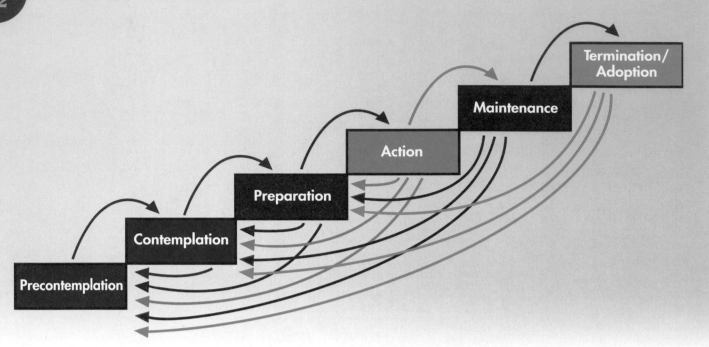

The Process of Change

Using the same plan for every individual who wishes to change a behavior will not work. With exercise, we provide different prescriptions to people of varying fitness levels (see Chapter 7). The same prescription would not provide optimal results for a person who has been inactive for 20 years, compared with one who walks regularly 3 times each week. This principle also holds true for people who are attempting to change behaviors.

Timing is important in the process of willful change. People respond more effectively to selected **processes of change** according to the stage of change they have reached at any given time.[5] Thus, applying specific processes at each stage of change enhances the likelihood of changing behavior permanently. The following description of 14 of the most common processes of change will help you develop a personal plan for change. The respective stages of change where each process works best are summarized in Table 2.1.

Consciousness-Raising

The first step in a **behavior modification** program is consciousness-raising. This process involves obtaining information about the problem so you can make a better decision about the problem behavior. For example, the problem could be physical inactivity. Learning about the benefits of exercise or the difference in benefits between physical activity and exercise (see Chapter 1) can help you decide the type of fitness program (health or physical) that you want to pursue. It is also possible that you don't even know that a certain behavior is a problem, such as unawareness of fat content in many fast food items. This is part of the precontemplation stage.

Action stage Stage of change in which people are actively changing a negative behavior or adopting a new, healthy behavior.

Maintenance stage Stage of change in which people maintain behavioral change for up to 5 years.

Termination/adoption stage Stage of change in which people have eliminated an undesirable behavior or maintained a positive behavior for over 5 years.

Relapse To slip or fall back into unhealthy behavior(s) or failure to maintain healthy behaviors.

Process of change Actions that help you achieve change in behavior.

Behavior modification The process to permanently change negative behaviors in favor of positive behaviors that will lead to better health and well-being.

Table 2.1

Applicable Processes of Change During Each Stage of Change

Precontemplation	Contemplation	Preparation	Action	Maintenance	Termination/Adoption
Consciousness-raising	Consciousness-raising	Consciousness-raising			
Social liberation	Social liberation	Social liberation	Social liberation		
	Self-analysis	Self-analysis			
	Emotional arousal	Emotional arousal			
	Positive outlook	Positive outlook	Positive outlook		
		Commitment	Commitment	Commitment	Commitment
		Behavior analysis			
		Goal setting	Goal setting	Goal setting	
		Self-reevaluation	Self-reevaluation	Self-reevaluation	
			Countering	Countering	
			Monitoring	Monitoring	Monitoring
			Environment control	Environment control	Environment control
			Helping relationships	Helping relationships	Helping relationships
			Rewards	Rewards	Rewards

Source: Adapted from J. O. Prochaska, J. C. Norcross, and C. C. DiClemente, *Changing for Good,* (New York: William Morrow, 1994); and W. W. K. Hoeger and S. A. Hoeger, *Fitness & Wellness* (Englewood, CO: Morton Publishing, 1999).

Social Liberation

Social liberation stresses external alternatives that make you aware of problem behaviors and contemplate change. Examples of social liberation include pedestrian-only traffic areas, nonsmoking areas, health-oriented cafeterias and restaurants, advocacy groups, civic organizations, policy interventions, and self-help groups. Social liberation often provides opportunities to get involved, stir up emotions, and enhance self-esteem—helping you gain confidence in your ability to change.

Self-Analysis

The second step in modifying behavior is a decisive desire to do so, called self-analysis. If you have no interest in changing a behavior, you won't do it. You will remain a precontemplator or a contemplator. A person who has no intention of quitting smoking will not quit, regardless of what anyone may say or how strong the evidence in favor of quitting. In your self-analysis, you may want to prepare a list of reasons for continuing or discontinuing the behavior. When the reasons for changing outweigh the reasons for not changing, you are ready for either the contemplation stage or the preparation stage.

Emotional Arousal

In emotional arousal, a person experiences and expresses feelings about the problem and its solutions. Also referred to as "dramatic release," this process often involves deep emotional experiences. Watching a loved one die from lung cancer caused by cigarette smoking may be all that is needed to make a person quit smoking. Other examples of emotional arousal are dramatizations of the consequences of drug use and abuse and a film about a person undergoing open-heart surgery.

Positive Outlook

Having a positive outlook means taking an optimistic approach from the beginning and believing in yourself. Following the guidelines in this chapter will help you design a plan so you can work toward change and remain enthused about your progress. Also, you may become motivated by looking at the outcome—how much healthier you will be, how much better you will look, or how far you will be able to jog.

Commitment

Upon making a decision to change, you now accept the responsibility to change and believe in your

ability to do so—you've begun the preparation stage. During this process, you may draw up a specific plan of action. Write down your goals and, preferably, share them with others. In essence you are signing a behavioral contract for change. You will be more likely to adhere to your program if others know you are committed to change.

Behavior Analysis

Now determine the frequency, circumstances, and consequences of the behavior to be altered or implemented. If the desired outcome is to consume less fat, you must first find out what foods in your diet are high in fat, when you eat them, and when you don't eat them—all part of the preparation stage. Knowing when you don't eat them points to circumstances under which you exert control of your diet and will help as you set goals.

Goal Setting

Goals motivate change in behavior. The stronger the goal or desire, the more motivated you'll be either to change unwanted behaviors or to implement new, healthy behaviors. The discussion on goal setting (page 38) will help you write goals and prepare an action plan to achieve those goals. This will aid with behavior modification.

Self-Reevaluation

During this process, individuals analyze their feelings about a problem behavior. The pros and cons or advantages and disadvantages of a certain behavior can be reevaluated at this time. For example, you may decide that strength training will help you tone up and boost your metabolism, but implementing this change will require you to stop watching an hour of TV 3 times per week. If you presently have a weight problem and you are unable to lift certain objects around the house, you may feel good about weight loss and enhanced physical capacity as a result of a strength-training program. You may also visualize what it would be like if you were successful at changing.

Countering

The process whereby you substitute healthy behaviors for a problem behavior is known as countering. This process is critical in changing behaviors as part of the action and maintenance stages. You need to replace unhealthy behaviors with new, healthy ones. You can use exercise to combat sedentary living, smoking, stress, or overeating. You

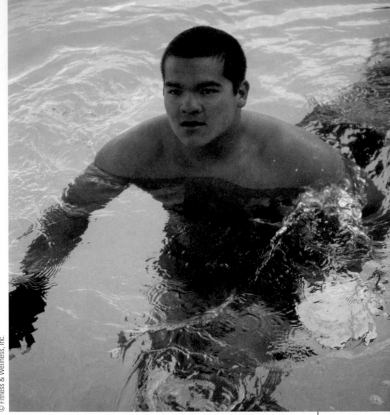

© Fitness & Wellness, Inc.

Countering: Replacing healthy behaviors for problem behaviors facilitates change.

may also use exercise, diet, yardwork, volunteer work, or reading to prevent overeating and achieve recommended body weight.

Monitoring

During the action and maintenance stages, continuous behavior monitoring increases awareness of the desired outcome. Sometimes this process in itself is sufficient to cause change. For example, keeping track of daily food intake reveals sources of fat in the diet. This can help you cut down gradually or completely eliminate high-fat foods. If the goal is to increase daily intake of fruit and vegetables, keeping track of the number of servings consumed each day raises awareness and may help increase intake.

Environment Control

In environment control, the person restructures the physical surroundings to avoid problem behaviors and decrease temptations. If you don't buy alcohol, you can't drink any. If you shop on a full stomach, you can reduce impulse-buying of junk food.

Similarly, you can create an environment where exceptions become the norm and then the norm can flourish. Instead of bringing home cookies for snacks, bring fruit. Place notes to yourself on the

refrigerator and pantry to avoid unnecessary snacking. Place baby carrots or sugarless gum where you used to place cigarettes. Post notes around the house to remind you of your exercise time. Leave exercise shoes and clothing by the entry way so they are visible as you walk into your home. Put an electric timer on the TV so it will shut off automatically at 7:00 PM. All of these tactics will be helpful throughout the action, maintenance, and termination/adoption stages.

Helping Relationships

Surrounding yourself with people who will work toward a common goal with you or those who care about and will encourage you along the way will be helpful during the action, maintenance, and termination/adoption stages. Attempting to quit smoking, for instance, is easier when a person is around others who are trying as well. The person could also get help from friends who have quit already.

Peer support is a strong incentive for behavioral change. During this process, the individual should avoid people who will not be supportive. Friends who have no desire to quit smoking may tempt one to smoke and encourage relapse into unwanted behaviors. People who have achieved the same goal already may not be supportive either. For instance, someone may say, "I can do six consecutive miles." The response should be, "I'm proud that I can jog three consecutive miles."

Rewards

People tend to repeat behaviors that are rewarded and disregard those that are not rewarded or are punished. Rewarding oneself or being rewarded by others is a powerful tool during the process of change in all stages. If you have successfully cut down your fat intake during the week, reward yourself by going to a show or buying a new pair of shoes. Do not reinforce yourself with destructive behaviors such as eating a high-fat dinner. If you fail to change a desired behavior (or to implement a new one), you may want to put off buying those new shoes you had planned for that week. When a positive behavior becomes habitual, give yourself an even better reward. Treat yourself to a weekend away from home, or buy a new bicycle.

Techniques of Change

Not to be confused with the processes of change, within each process you can apply any number of **techniques of change** that help you through that particular process (see Table 2.2). For example, following dinner, people with a weight problem often can't resist continuous snacking during the rest of the evening until it is time to retire for the night. Using the process of countering, you can use various techniques to avoid unnecessary snacking. Examples include: going for a walk, flossing and brushing your teeth right after dinner, going for a drive, playing the piano, going to a show, or going to bed earlier.

As you develop your behavior modification plan, you need to identify specific techniques that may work for you within each process of change. A list of techniques for each process is provided in Table 2.2. This is only a sample list; dozens of other techniques may be used as well. For example, Behavior Modification and Adherence to a Weight Management Program is found on page 129, Getting Started and Adhering to a Lifetime Exercise Program is presented on page 184, stress management techniques are provided in Chapter 11, and tips to help stop smoking on pages 378–379. Some of the techniques can also be used with more than one process, such as visualization in emotional arousal and self-reevaluation.

Goal Setting

To initiate change, goals are essential. **Goals** motivate behavioral change and provide a plan of action. Goals are most effective when they are

1. Well planned. Only a well-conceived action plan will help you attain your goal. The items below (as well as others discussed in following chapters) will help you design your plan of action. You also should write specific objectives to help you reach each goal.

   The specific **objectives** are the steps required to reach a goal. For example, a goal might be to achieve recommended body weight. Several specific objectives could be to (a) lose an average of 1 pound (or 1 fat percentage point) per week (b) monitor body weight before breakfast every morning (c) assess body composition every 2 weeks (d) limit fat intake to less than 25 percent of total calories (e) eliminate all pastries from the diet during this time, and (f) exercise in the proper target zone for 45 minutes, 5 times per week.
2. Personalized. Goals that you set for yourself are more motivational than goals that someone else sets for you.
3. Written. An unwritten goal is simply a wish. A written goal, in essence, becomes a contract with yourself. Show this goal to a friend or an instructor and have him or her witness the contract you made with yourself by signing alongside your signature.
4. Realistic. Goals should be within reach. If you currently weigh 190 pounds and your target

Table 2.2

Sample Techniques for Use With Processes of Change

Process	Techniques
Consciousness-Raising	Become aware that there is a problem, read educational materials about the problem behavior or about people who have overcome this same problem, find out about the benefits of changing the behavior, watch an instructional program on television, visit a therapist, talk and listen to others, ask questions, take a class.
Social Liberation	Seek out advocacy groups (Overeaters Anonymous, Alcoholics Anonymous), join a health club, buy a bike, join a neighborhood walking group, work in nonsmoking areas.
Self-Analysis	Question yourself on the problem behavior, express your feelings about it, become aware that there is a problem, analyze your values, list advantages and disadvantages of continuing (smoking) or not implementing a behavior (exercise), take a fitness test, do a nutrient analysis.
Emotional Arousal	Practice mental imagery of yourself going through the process of change, visualize yourself overcoming the problem behavior, do some role-playing in overcoming the behavior or practicing a new one, watch dramatizations (a movie) of the consequences or benefits of your actions, visit an auto salvage yard or a drug rehabilitation center.
Positive Outlook	Believe in yourself, know that you are capable, know that you are special, draw from previous personal successes.
Commitment	Just do it, set New Year's resolutions, sign a behavioral contract, set start and completion dates, tell others about your goals, work on your action plan.
Behavior Analysis	Prepare logs of circumstances that trigger or prevent a given behavior and look for patterns that prompt the behavior or cause you to relapse.
Goal Setting	Write goals, objectives, and design a specific action plan.
Self-Reevaluation	Determine accomplishments and evaluate progress, rewrite goals and objectives, list pros and cons, weigh sacrifices (can't eat out with others) versus benefits (weight loss), visualize continued change, think before you act, learn from mistakes, and prepare new action plans accordingly.
Countering	Seek out alternatives: Stay busy, walk (don't drive), read a book (instead of snacking), attend alcohol-free socials, carry your own groceries, mow your yard, dance (don't eat), go to a movie (instead of smoking), practice stress management.
Monitoring	Use exercise logs (days exercised, sets and resistance used in strength training), keep journals, conduct nutrient analyses, count grams of fat, number of consecutive days without smoking, days and type of relaxation technique(s) used.
Environment Control	Rearrange your home (no TVs, ashtrays, large-sized cups), get rid of unhealthy items (cigarettes, junk food, alcohol), then avoid unhealthy places (bars, happy hour), avoid relationships that encourage problem behaviors, use reminders to control problem behaviors (post notes indicating "don't snack after dinner" or "lift weights at 8:00 P.M."). Frequent healthy environments (a clean park, a health club, restaurants with low-fat/low-calorie/nutrient-dense menus, friends with goals similar to yours).
Helping Relationships	Associate with people who have and want to overcome the same problem, form or join self-help groups, join community programs specifically designed to deal with your problem (eating disorders, substance abuse control, smoking cessation).
Rewards	Go to a movie, buy a new outfit or shoes, buy a new bike, go on a weekend get-away, reassess your fitness level, use positive self-talk ("good job," "that felt good," "I did it," "I knew I'd make it," "I'm good at this").

weight (at 22 percent body fat) is 140 pounds, setting a goal to lose 50 pounds in 2 months would be unsound, if not impossible. This program would not allow implementation of adequate behavior modification techniques or ensure weight maintenance at the target weight. Unattainable goals lead to discouragement and loss of interest.

Techniques of change Methods or procedures used to aid with each process of change.

Goal The ultimate aim toward which effort is directed.

Objectives Steps required to reach a goal.

At times problems arise even with realistic goals. Try to anticipate potential difficulties as much as possible and plan for ways to deal with them. If your goal is to jog for 30 minutes on 6 consecutive days, what are the alternatives if the weather turns bad? Possible solutions are to jog in the rain, find an indoor track, jog at a different time of day when the weather improves, or participate in a different aerobic activity such as stationary cycling, swimming, or step aerobics.

5. Short-term and long-term. If the long-term goal is to attain recommended body weight and you are 50 pounds overweight, you might set a short-term goal of losing 10 pounds and write specific objectives to accomplish this goal. Then the task will not seem as overwhelming and will be easier.

6. Measurable. Whenever possible, goals and objectives should be measurable. For example, "to lose weight" is not measurable. If the goal is to achieve recommended body weight, this implies lowering your body weight (fat) to the recommended percent body fat standard given in Table 4.9 (page 104). For a 19-year-old female, the high fitness recommended fat percent would be in the range of 17 to 27 percent.

To be more descriptive, the goal could be reworded to read "Reduce body weight to 22 percent body fat." Also note that all of the sample specific objectives a through f given in Item 1 are measurable. For instance, you can figure out easily whether you are losing a pound or a percentage point per week; you can conduct a nutrient analysis to assess your average fat intake; or you can monitor your weekly exercise sessions to make sure you are meeting this specific objective.

7. Time-specific. A goal always should have a specific date set for completion. To simply state, "I will decrease body fat to 22 percent" is not time-specific. The chosen date should be realistic but not too distant in the future. With a deadline, a task is much easier to work toward.

8. Monitored. Monitoring your progress as you move toward a goal reinforces behavior. Keeping an exercise log or doing a body composition assessment periodically enables you to determine your progress at any given time.

9. Evaluated. Periodic reevaluations are vital for success. You may find that a goal is unreachable. If so, reassess the goal. On the other hand, if a goal is too easy, you may lose interest and stop working toward it. Once you achieve a goal, set a new one to improve upon or maintain what you have achieved. Goals keep you motivated.

Recognize that you will face obstacles, and you will not always meet your goals. Use your setbacks and learn from them. Rewrite your goal and create a plan that will help you get around self-defeating behaviors in the future.

Now that you have read this chapter, use Figure 2.3 and Lab 2A to identify two problem behaviors

---

Figure 2.3 **Stage of change identification and behavior modification outline.**

Please indicate which response most accurately describes your current [_____] behavior (in the blank space identify the behavior: smoking, physical activity, stress, nutrition, weight control). Next, select the statement below (select only one) that best represents your current behavior pattern. To select the most appropriate statement, fill in the blank for one of the first three statements if your current behavior is a problem behavior. (For example, you may say, "I currently smoke and I do *not* intend to change in the foreseeable future," or "I currently *do not exercise* but I am contemplating changing in the next 6 months.") If you have already started to make changes, fill in the blank in one of the last three statements. (In this case, you may say: "I currently *eat a low-fat diet* but I have only done so within the last 6 months," or "I currently *practice adequate stress management techniques* and I have done so for over 6 months.") As you can see, you may use this form to identify your stage of change for any type of health-related behavior.

1. I currently [_____], and I do not intend to change in the foreseeable future.

2. I currently [_____], but I am contemplating changing in the next 6 months.

3. I currently [_____] regularly, but I intend to change in the next month.

4. I currently [_____], but I have done so only within the last 6 months.

5. I currently [_____], and I have done so for more than 6 months.

6. I currently [_____], and I have done so for more than 5 years.

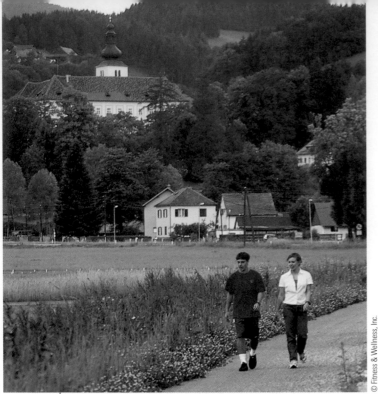

Rewarding oneself when a goal is achieved, such as a weekend getaway, is a powerful tool during the process of change.

in your life. In this worksheet you will be asked to determine your stage of change for each behavior according to six standard statements. Based on your selection, determine the stage of change classification according to the ratings provided in Table 2.3. Identification of stages of change for other fitness and wellness behaviors are also provided in subsequent worksheets in this book.

Table 2.3 Stage of Change Classification

Selected Statement (see Figure 2.3)	Classification
1	Precontemplation
2	Contemplation
3	Preparation
4	Action
5	Maintenance
6	Termination/Adoption

Web Interactive

- The Transtheoretical Model. This excellent site features self-assessment tools to help you personally determine what stage of change you are in based on the transtheoretical model for the following behaviors: Smoking, exercise, eating and diet, alcohol and drug behaviors, and condoms and HIV prevention.

  http://www2.msstate.edu/~bhunt/Stages_of_Change_Theory/transtheoretical.html

- Cancer Prevention Research Center. This site describes the ten processes of changes, activities and experiences that individuals engage in when they attempt to modify problem behaviors. The ten processes of change include consciousness raising, counter-conditioning, dramatic relief, environmental reevaluation, helping relationships, reinforcement management, self-liberation, self-reevaluation, social liberation, and stimulus control.

  http://www.uri.edu/research/cprc/TTM/ProcessesOfChange.htm

- Behavior Change Theories. A very comprehensive site by the Department of Health Promotion at Cal Poly Pomona University describes all of the various theories of behavioral change, including Learning Theories, Transtheoretical Model, Health Belief Model, Relapse Prevention Model, Reasoned Action and Planned Behavior, Social Learning/Social Cognitive Theory, and Social Support.

  http://www.csupomona.edu/~jvgrizzell/best_practices/bctheory.html

- How to Fit Exercise into Your Daily Routine. This site sponsored by the Centers for Disease Control and Prevention describes how you can incorporate simple exercises into your daily schedule, while at home, work, or spending time away with the family. Make time to exercise.

  http://www.cdc.gov/nccdphp/dnpa/phys_act.htm

Interactive Sites:

- Personalized Fitness Planner. This visually-appealing site has five interactive assessments, each of which allows you to set your personal fitness goals. The assessments include flexibility and balance, strength, cardiovascular, body composition, and total fitness. The site also features a glossary and an index of exercises.

  http://thriveonline.oxygen.com/fitness/planner

- Create Your Personal Contract to Healthy Behavior Change. This site allows you to put your goals to become a healthier you into writing. Print out your personal contract and have a friend sign it for validation! You can do it.

  http://www.thriveonline.com/seasonal/new_year/resolutions/contract.html

Notes

1. G. S. Howard, D. W. Nance, and P. Myers, *Adaptive Counseling and Therapy* (San Francisco: Jossey-Bass, 1987).

2. J. O. Prochaska, J. C. Norcross, and C. C. DiClemente, *Changing for Good* (New York: William Morrow, 1994).

3. B. J. Cardinal, "Extended Stage Model of Physical Activity Behavior," *Journal of Human Movement Studies* 37 (1999): 37–54.

4. See note 3.

5. See note 2.

Also in B. H. Marcus et al., "Evaluation of Motivationally Tailored vs. Standard Self-help Physical Activity Interventions at the Workplace," *American Journal of Health Promotion* 12 (1998): 246–253.

Suggested Readings

Bouchard, C., et al. *Exercise, Fitness, and Health: A Consensus of Current Knowledge.* Champaign, IL: Human Kinetics, 1990.

Bouchard, C., et al. *Physical Activity, Fitness, and Health.* Champaign, IL: Human Kinetics, 1994.

Cardinal, B. J. and S. S. Levy. "Are Sedentary Behaviors Terminable?" *Journal of Human Movement Studies* 38 (2000): 137–150.

Dishman, R. *Exercise Adherence.* Champaign, IL: Human Kinetics, 1988.

Dishman, R. "Increasing and Maintaining Exercise and Physical Activity." *Behavioral Therapy* 22 (1991): 345–378.

Guttman, M. "The New Science of Risky Behavior." *USA Weekend* (March 6–8, 1998): 4–5.

Marcus, B. and L. Simkin. "The Stages of Exercise Behavior." *Journal of Sports Medicine and Physical Fitness* 33 (1993): 83–88.

Marcus, B., et al. "The Stages and Processes of Exercise Adoption and Maintenance in a Worksite Sample." *Health Psychology* 11 (1992): 386–395.

Prochaska, J. O., and B. H. Marcus. "The Transtheoretical Model: Applications to Exercise." In *Advances in Exercise Adherence,* edited by R. K. Dishman, 161–180. Champaign, IL: Human Kinetics, 1994.

Prochaska, J. O., J. C. Norcross, and C. C. DiClemente. *Changing for Good.* New York: William Morrow, 1994.

Prochaska, J. O., and W. F. Velcier. "The Transtheoretical Model of Health Behavior Change." *American Journal of Health Promotion* 12 (1997): 38–48.

Samuelson, M. "Stages of Change: From Theory to Practice." *The Art of Health Promotion* 2 (1998): 1–7.

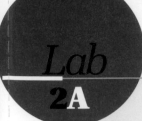

Lab 2A

BEHAVIOR MODIFICATION:
STAGES, PROCESSES, AND TECHNIQUES FOR CHANGE

Name: _____   Date: _____   Grade: _____

Instructor: _____   Course: _____   Section: _____

Necessary Lab Equipment
None required.

Lab Preparation
Chapter 2 must be read prior to this lab.

Objective
To help you identify the stage of change for two problem behaviors and the processes and techniques for change.

I. Stages of Change Instructions

Please indicate which response most accurately describes your current _____ behavior (in the blank space identify the behavior: smoking, physical activity, stress, nutrition, weight control). Next, select the statement below (select only one) that best represents your current behavior pattern. To select the most appropriate statement, fill in the blank for one of the first three statements if your current behavior is a problem behavior. For example, you may say:

> "I currently <u>smoke</u>, and I do not intend to change in the foreseeable future" or

> "I currently <u>do not exercise</u>, but I am contemplating changing in the next 6 months."

If you have already started to make changes, fill in the blank in one of the last three statements. In this case you may say:

> "I currently <u>eat a low-fat diet</u>, but I have only done so within the last 6 months" or

> "I currently <u>practice adequate stress management techniques</u>, and I have done so for over 6 months."

You may use this form to identify your stage of change for any health-related behavior. After identifying two problem behaviors, look up your stage of change for each one using Table 2.3 (on page 41).

Behavior #1. Fill in only one blank.

☐   1. I currently _____, and do not intend to change in the foreseeable future.

☐   2. I currently _____, but I am contemplating changing in the next 6 months.

☐   3. I currently _____ regularly, but I intend to change in the next month.

☐   4. I currently _____, but I have only done so within the last 6 months.

☐   5. I currently _____, and I have done so for over 6 months.

☐   6. I currently _____, and I have done so for over 5 years.

Stage of change: _____ (see Table 2.3 on page 41).

Behavior #2. Fill in only one blank.

☐ 1. I currently _____ , and do not intend to change in the foreseeable future.

☐ 2. I currently _____ , but I am contemplating changing in the next 6 months.

☐ 3. I currently _____ regularly, but I intend to change in the next month.

☐ 4. I currently _____ , but I have only done so within the last 6 months.

☐ 5. I currently _____ , and I have done so for over 6 months.

☐ 6. I currently _____ , and I have done so for over 5 years.

Stage of change: _____ (see Table 2.3 on page 41).

II. Processes of Change

According to your stage of change for the two behaviors identified above, list the processes of change that apply to each behavior (see Table 2.1 on page 36).

Behavior #1: _____

Behavior #2: _____

III. Techniques for Change

List a minimum of three techniques that you will use with each process of change (see Table 2.2 on page 39).

Behavior #1: 1. _____

2. _____

3. _____

Behavior #2: 1. _____

2. _____

3. _____

Today's date: _____ Completion Date: _____ Signature: _____

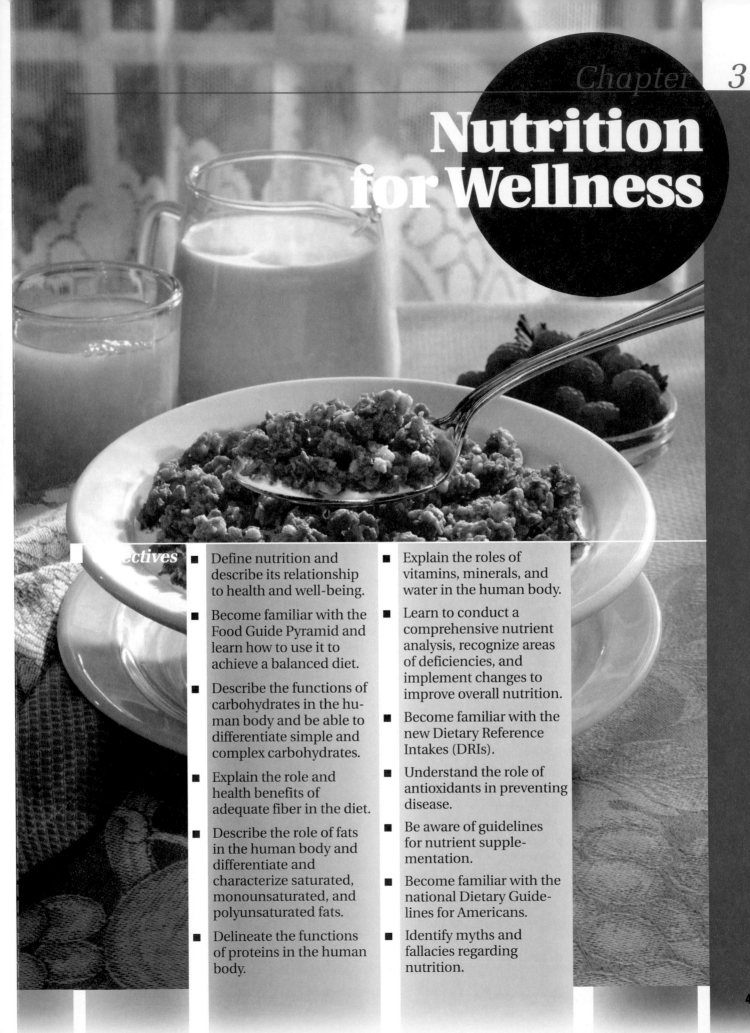

Chapter 3

Nutrition for Wellness

Objectives

- Define nutrition and describe its relationship to health and well-being.

- Become familiar with the Food Guide Pyramid and learn how to use it to achieve a balanced diet.

- Describe the functions of carbohydrates in the human body and be able to differentiate simple and complex carbohydrates.

- Explain the role and health benefits of adequate fiber in the diet.

- Describe the role of fats in the human body and differentiate and characterize saturated, monounsaturated, and polyunsaturated fats.

- Delineate the functions of proteins in the human body.

- Explain the roles of vitamins, minerals, and water in the human body.

- Learn to conduct a comprehensive nutrient analysis, recognize areas of deficiencies, and implement changes to improve overall nutrition.

- Become familiar with the new Dietary Reference Intakes (DRIs).

- Understand the role of antioxidants in preventing disease.

- Be aware of guidelines for nutrient supplementation.

- Become familiar with the national Dietary Guidelines for Americans.

- Identify myths and fallacies regarding nutrition.

Scientific evidence has long linked good **nutrition** to overall health and well-being. Proper nutrition means that a person's diet supplies all the essential nutrients needed to carry out normal tissue growth, repair, and maintenance. These nutrients should be obtained from a wide variety of sources. Figure 3.1 shows the Food Guide Pyramid with the recommended number of servings from each food group for proper nutrition. The diet also should provide enough **substrates** to produce the energy necessary for work, physical activity, and relaxation.

Too much or too little of any nutrient can precipitate serious health problems. The typical U.S. diet is too high in calories, sugar, fat, saturated fat, and sodium, and not high enough in fiber—factors that undermine good health. Food availability is not the problem. The problem is overconsumption.

According to the 1988 report on nutrition and health issued by the U.S. Surgeon General—the first ever of its kind—diseases of dietary excess and imbalance are among the leading causes of death in the United States.[1] Similar trends are observed in developed countries throughout the world. In the report, based on more than 2,000 scientific studies, the Surgeon General said that dietary changes can bring better health to all Americans. Other surveys reveal that, on a given day, nearly half of the people in the United States eat no fruit and almost a fourth eat no vegetables.

Diet and nutrition often play a crucial role in the development and progression of chronic diseases. A diet high in saturated fat and cholesterol increases the risk for atherosclerosis and coronary heart disease. In sodium-sensitive individuals, high salt intake has been linked to high blood pressure. Some researchers believe that 30 to 50 percent of all cancers are diet-related. Obesity, diabetes, and osteoporosis also have been associated with faulty nutrition.

To lower the risk for chronic disease, an effective wellness program must incorporate the dietary recommendations for Americans, as follows:

- Let the Food Pyramid guide your food choices.
- Eat a variety of foods daily, especially grains, fruits, and vegetables. Many of these foods are high in nutrients, starch, and fiber.
- Avoid too much fat, saturated fat, and cholesterol.
- Avoid too much sugar and sodium.
- Maintain adequate calcium intake.
- Keep food safe to eat—which means that the food poses little risk of food-borne illness.
- Maintain recommended body weight.
- Drink alcoholic beverages in moderation, if at all.

These guidelines will be discussed throughout this chapter and in later chapters of this book.

Nutrients

The essential **nutrients** the human body requires are carbohydrates, fat, protein, vitamins, minerals, and water. The first three are called "fuel nutrients" because they are the only substances the body uses to supply the energy (commonly measured in calories) needed for work and normal body functions. The three others—vitamins, minerals, and water—are regulatory nutrients. They have no caloric value, but still are necessary for a person to function normally and maintain good health. Many nutritionists add a seventh nutrient to this list: fiber. This nutrient has received a great deal of attention recently. Recommended amounts appear to provide protection against several diseases, including cardiovascular disease and some cancers.

Carbohydrates, fats, proteins, and water are termed "macronutrients" because we need them in proportionately large amounts daily. Vitamins and minerals are required in only small amounts—grams, milligrams, and micrograms instead of, say, ounces—and nutritionists therefore refer to them as "micronutrients."

Depending on the amount of nutrients and calories they contain, foods can be classified by their **nutrient density**. Foods that contain few or a moderate number of calories but are packed with nutrients are said to have high nutrient density. Foods that have a lot of calories but few nutrients are of low nutrient density and are commonly called "junk food."

A **calorie** is the unit of measure indicating the energy value of food to the person who consumes it. It is also used to express the amount of energy a person expends in physical activity. Technically, a kilocalorie (kcal), or large calorie, is the amount of heat necessary to raise the temperature of 1 kilogram of water 1 degree Centigrade. For simplicity, people call it a calorie rather than a kcal. For example, if the caloric value of a food is 100 calories (kcal), the energy in this food would raise the temperature of 100 kilograms of water 1 degree Centigrade. Similarly, walking 1 mile would burn about 100 calories.

Nutrition Science that studies the relationship of foods to optimal health and performance.

Substrate Substance acted upon by an enzyme (examples: carbohydrates and fats).

Nutrients Substances found in food that provide energy, regulate metabolism, and help with growth and repair of body tissues.

Nutrient density A measure of the amount of nutrients and calories in various foods.

Calorie The amount of heat necessary to raise the temperature of 1 gram of water 1 degree Centigrade; used to measure the energy value of food and cost (energy expenditure) of physical activity.

Figure 3.1 Food Guide Pyramid.

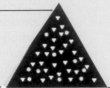

Fats, Oils, and Sweets
USE SPARINGLY

KEY
● Fat and oils (naturally occurring and added)
▼ Sugars (added)

These symbols show fats, oils, and added sugars in foods.

Milk, Yogurt, and Cheese Group
2–3 SERVINGS

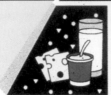
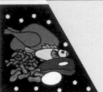

Meat, Poultry, Fish, Dry Beans, Eggs, and Nuts Group
2–3 SERVINGS

Vegetable Group
3–5 SERVINGS

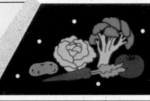
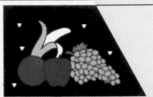

Fruit Group
2–4 SERVINGS

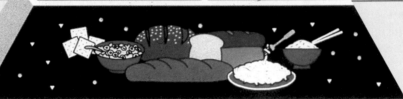

Bread, Cereal, Rice, and Pasta Group
6–11 SERVINGS

What counts as one serving?

Breads, Cereals, Rice, and Pasta
1 slice of bread
1/2 cup of cooked rice or pasta
1/2 cup of cooked cereal
1 ounce of ready-to-eat cereal

Vegetables
1/2 cup of chopped raw or cooked vegetables
1 cup of leafy raw vegetables

Fruits
1 piece of fruit or melon wedge
3/4 cup of juice
1/2 cup of canned fruit
1/4 cup of dried fruit

Milk, Yogurt, and Cheese
1 cup of milk or yogurt
1½ to 2 ounces of cheese

Meat, Poultry, Fish, Dry Beans, Eggs, and Nuts
2½ to 3 ounces of cooked lean meat, poultry, or fish
Count 1/2 cup of cooked beans, or 1 egg, or 2 tablespoons of peanut butter as 1 ounce of lean meat (about 1/3 serving)

Fats, Oils, and Sweets
LIMIT CALORIES FROM THIS GROUP especially if you need to lose weight

The amount you eat may be more than one serving. For example, a dinner portion of spaghetti would count as two or three servings of pasta.

How many servings do you need each day?

	Women and some older adults	Children, teen girls, active women, most men	Teen boys and active men
Calorie level*	about 1,600	about 2,200	about 2,800
Bread group	6	9	11
Vegetable group	3	4	5
Fruit group	2	3	4
Milk group	2–3**	2–3**	2–3**
Meat group	2, for a total of 5 ounces	2, for a total of 6 ounces	3, for a total of 7 ounces

* These are the calorie levels if you choose low-fat, lean foods from the 5 major food groups and use foods from the fats, oils, and sweets group sparingly.

** Women who are pregnant or breastfeeding, teenagers, and young adults to age 24 need 3 servings.

A Closer Look at Fat and Added Sugars

The small tip of the pyramid shows fats, oils, and sweets. These are foods such as salad dressings, cream, butter, margarine, sugars, soft drinks, candies, and sweet desserts. Alcoholic beverages are also part of this group. These foods provide calories but few vitamins and minerals. Most people should go easy on foods from this group.

Some fat or sugar symbols are shown in the other food groups. That's to remind you that some foods in these groups can also be high in fat and added sugars, such as cheese or ice cream from the milk group, or french fries from the vegetable group. When choosing foods for a healthful diet, consider the fat and added sugars in your choices from all the food groups, not just fats, oils, and sweets from the pyramid tip.

Carbohydrates

Carbohydrates constitute the major source of calories the body uses to provide energy for work, maintain cells, and generate heat. They also help regulate fat and metabolize protein. Each gram of carbohydrates provides the human body with 4 calories. The major sources of carbohydrates are breads, cereals, fruits, vegetables, and milk and other dairy products. Carbohydrates are classified into simple carbohydrates and complex carbohydrates (Figure 3.2).

Simple Carbohydrates

Often called "sugars," **simple carbohydrates** have little nutritive value. Examples are candy, soda, and cakes. Simple carbohydrates are divided into monosaccharides and disaccharides. These carbohydrates—whose names end with –"-ose"—often take the place of more nutritive foods in the diet.

Monosaccharides The simplest sugars are **monosaccharides**. The three most common monosaccharides are glucose, fructose, and galactose:

1. Glucose is a natural sugar found in food; it also is produced in the body from other simple and complex carbohydrates. It is used as a source of energy, or it may be stored in the muscles and liver in the form of glycogen (a long chain of glucose molecules hooked together). Excess glucose in the blood is converted to fat and stored in **adipose tissue**.
2. Fructose, or fruit sugar, occurs naturally in fruits and honey and is converted to glucose in the body.
3. Galactose is produced from milk sugar in the mammary glands of lactating animals and is converted to glucose in the body.

Disaccharides The three major **disaccharides** are

1. Sucrose or table sugar (glucose + fructose).
2. Lactose (glucose + galactose).
3. Maltose (glucose + glucose).

These disaccharides are broken down in the body and the resulting simple sugars are used as indicated above.

Complex Carbohydrates

Complex carbohydrates are also called "polysaccharides." Anywhere from about ten to thousands of monosaccharide molecules can unite to form a single polysaccharide. Examples of complex carbohydrates are starches, dextrins, and glycogen.

1. Starch is the storage form of glucose in plants, needed to promote their earliest growth. Starch is commonly found in grains, seeds, corn, nuts, roots, potatoes, and legumes. In a healthful diet, grains, the richest source of starch, should supply most of the energy. Once eaten, starch is converted to glucose for the body's own energy use.
2. Dextrins are formed from the breakdown of large starch molecules exposed to dry heat, such as in baking bread or producing cold cereals. These complex carbohydrates of plant origin provide many valuable nutrients and can be an excellent source of fiber.
3. Glycogen is the animal polysaccharide synthesized from glucose and is found only in tiny amounts in meats—in essence, we manufacture it; we don't consume it. **Glycogen** constitutes the body's reservoir of glucose. Thousands of glucose molecules are linked to be stored as glycogen in liver and muscle. When a surge of energy is needed, enzymes in the muscle and the liver break down glycogen and thus make glucose readily available for energy transformation. (This process is discussed under "Nutrition for Athletes," page 73.)

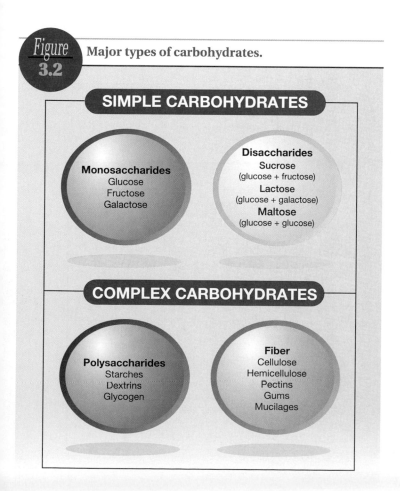

Figure 3.2 Major types of carbohydrates.

SIMPLE CARBOHYDRATES

Monosaccharides
Glucose
Fructose
Galactose

Disaccharides
Sucrose
(glucose + fructose)
Lactose
(glucose + galactose)
Maltose
(glucose + glucose)

COMPLEX CARBOHYDRATES

Polysaccharides
Starches
Dextrins
Glycogen

Fiber
Cellulose
Hemicellulose
Pectins
Gums
Mucilages

Fiber

Fiber is a form of complex carbohydrate. A high-fiber diet gives a person a feeling of fullness without added calories. **Dietary fiber** is present mainly in plant leaves, skins, roots, and seeds. Processing and refining foods removes almost all of the natural fiber. In our diet, the main sources of fiber are whole-grain cereals and breads, fruits, vegetables, and legumes. Fiber is important in the diet because it decreases the risk for cardiovascular disease and cancer. Increased fiber intake also may lower the risk of coronary heart disease, because saturated fats often take the place of fiber in the diet, increasing the absorption and formation of cholesterol. Other health disorders that have been tied to low intake of fiber are constipation, diverticulitis, hemorrhoids, gallbladder disease, and obesity.

The recommended amount of fiber intake is about 25 to 30 grams per day. Most people in the United States eat only 10 to 12 grams of fiber per day, putting them at increased risk for disease. A person can increase fiber intake by eating more fruits, vegetables, legumes, grains, and cereals. A 6-year follow-up study provided further evidence linking increased fiber intake (to 30 grams per day) to a significant reduction in heart attacks, cancer of the colon, breast cancer, diabetes, and diverticulitis.[2] Table 3.1 provides the fiber content of selected foods.

Fibers typically are classified according to their solubility in water. Soluble fiber dissolves in water and forms a gel-like substance that encloses food particles. This property allows soluble fiber to bind and excrete fats from the body. This type of fiber has been shown to lower blood cholesterol and blood sugar levels. Soluble fibers are found primarily in oats, fruits, barley, and legumes.

Insoluble fiber is not easily dissolved in water, and the body cannot digest it. This type of fiber is important because it binds water, causing a softer

Table 3.1	**Dietary Fiber Content of Selected Foods**	
Food (gm)	**Serving Size**	**Dietary Fiber**
Almonds, shelled	¼ cup	3.9
Apple	1 medium	3.7
Banana	1 small	1.2
Beans (red, kidney)	½ cup	8.2
Blackberries	½ cup	4.9
Beets, red, canned (cooked)	½ cup	1.4
Brazil nuts	1 oz	2.5
Broccoli (cooked)	½ cup	3.3
Brown rice (cooked)	½ cup	1.7
Carrots (cooked)	½ cup	3.3
Cauliflower (cooked)	½ cup	5.0
Cereal		
All Bran	1 oz	8.5
Cheerios	1 oz	1.1
Cornflakes	1 oz	0.5
Fruit and Fibre	1 oz	4.0
Fruit Wheats	1 oz	2.0
Just Right	1 oz	2.0
Wheaties	1 oz	2.0
Corn (cooked)	½ cup	2.2
Eggplant (cooked)	½ cup	3.0
Lettuce (chopped)	½ cup	0.5
Orange	1 medium	4.3
Parsnips (cooked)	½ cup	2.1
Pear	1 medium	4.5
Peas (cooked)	½ cup	4.4
Popcorn (plain)	1 cup	1.2
Potato (baked)	1 medium	4.9
Strawberries	½ cup	1.6
Summer squash (cooked)	½ cup	1.6
Watermelon	1 cup	0.1

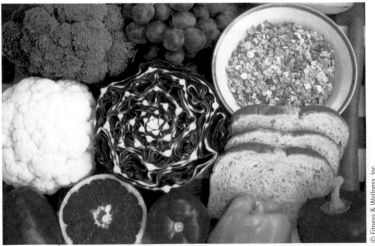

High-fiber foods are essential in a healthy diet.

© Fitness & Wellness, Inc.

Carbohydrates A classification of dietary nutrient containing carbon, hydrogen, and oxygen; the major source of energy for the human body.

Simple carbohydrates Formed by simple or double sugar units with little nutritive value; divided into monosaccharides and disaccharides.

Monosaccharides The simplest carbohydrates (sugars) formed by five- or six-carbon skeletons. The three most common monosaccharides are glucose, fructose, and galactose.

Adipose tissue Fat cells in the body.

Disaccharides Simple carbohydrates formed by two monosaccharide units linked together, one of which is glucose. The major disaccharides are sucrose, lactose, and maltose.

Complex carbohydrates Carbohydrates formed by three or more simple sugar molecules linked together; also referred to as "polysaccharides."

Glycogen Form in which glucose is stored in the body.

Dietary fiber A complex carbohydrate in plant foods that is not digested but is essential to the digestion process.

and bulkier stool that increases **peristalsis**—involuntary muscle contractions of intestinal walls that force the stool through the intestines and enable quicker excretion of food residues. Speeding up passage of food residues through the intestines seems to lower the risk for colon cancer, mainly because it reduces the amount of time that cancer-causing agents are in contact with the intestinal wall. Insoluble fiber also is thought to bind with carcinogens (cancer-producing substances), and more water in the stool may dilute the cancer-causing agents, lessening their potency. Sources of insoluble fiber include wheat, cereals, vegetables, and skins of fruits.

The most common types of fiber are

1. Cellulose, water-soluble fiber found in plant cell walls.
2. Hemicellulose, water-soluble fiber found in cereal fibers.
3. Pectins, water-insoluble fiber found in vegetables and fruits.
4. Gums and mucilages, water-insoluble fiber is also found in small amounts in foods of plant origin.

Surprisingly, too much fiber can be detrimental to health. It can produce loss of calcium, phosphorus, and iron, not to mention gastrointestinal discomfort. If you increase the fiber in your diet, do so gradually over several weeks to avoid gastrointestinal disturbances. While increasing fiber intake, be sure to drink more water to avoid constipation and even dehydration.

Fats

The human body uses **fats** as a source of energy. Fat is the most concentrated energy source. Each gram of fat supplies 9 calories to the body (in contrast to 4 for carbohydrates). Fats are a part of the cell structure. They are used as stored energy and as an insulator to preserve body heat. They absorb shock, supply essential fatty acids, and carry the fat-soluble vitamins A, D, E, and K. Fats can be classified into three main groups: simple, compound, and derived (Figure 3.3). The most familiar sources of fat are whole milk and other dairy products, and meats and alternatives such as eggs and nuts.

Simple Fats

A simple fat consists of a glyceride molecule linked to one, two, or three units of fatty acids. According to the number of fatty acids attached, simple fats are divided into monoglycerides (one fatty acid), diglycerides (two fatty acids), and triglycerides (three fatty acids). More than 90 percent of the weight of fat in foods and more than 95 percent of the stored fat in the human body are in the form of triglycerides.

The length of the carbon atom chain and the amount of hydrogen saturation (that is, the number

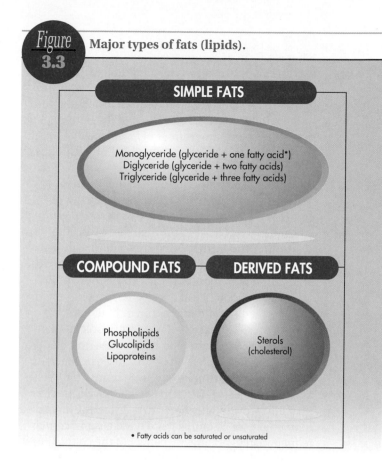

Figure 3.3 Major types of fats (lipids).

SIMPLE FATS

Monoglyceride (glyceride + one fatty acid*)
Diglyceride (glyceride + two fatty acids)
Triglyceride (glyceride + three fatty acids)

COMPOUND FATS

Phospholipids
Glucolipids
Lipoproteins

DERIVED FATS

Sterols
(cholesterol)

* Fatty acids can be saturated or unsaturated

of hydrogen molecules attached to the carbon chain) in fatty acids vary. Based on the extent of saturation, fatty acids are said to be saturated or unsaturated. Unsaturated fatty acids are classified further into monounsaturated and polyunsaturated. Saturated fatty acids are mainly of animal origin; unsaturated fats are found mostly in plant products.

Saturated Fats

In saturated fatty acids, the carbon atoms are fully saturated with hydrogen atoms; only single bonds link the carbon atoms on the chain (see Figure 3.4). These saturated fatty acids often are called saturated fats. Foods high in saturated fatty acids are meats, meat fat, lard, whole milk, cream, butter, cheese, ice cream, hydrogenated oils (a process that makes oils saturated), coconut oil, and palm oils. Saturated fats typically do not melt at room temperature. Coconut and palm oils are exceptions. In general, saturated fats raise the blood cholesterol level.

Unsaturated Fats

In unsaturated fatty acids (unsaturated fats), double bonds form between the unsaturated carbons. In monounsaturated fatty acids (MUFA), only one double bond is found along the chain. Examples of monounsaturated fatty acids are olive, canola, rapeseed, peanut, and sesame oils. Polyunsaturated

Figure 3.4

Chemical structure of saturated and unsaturated fats.

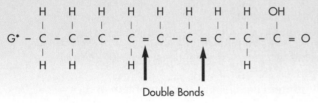

Saturated Fatty Acid

Monounsaturated Fatty Acid

Double Bond

Polyunsaturated Fatty Acid

Double Bonds

*Glyceride component

fatty acids (PUFA) contain two or more double bonds between unsaturated carbon atoms along the chain. Corn, cottonseed, safflower, walnut, sunflower, and soybean oils are high in polyunsaturated fatty acids. Unsaturated fats usually are liquid at room temperature. Shorter fatty acid chains also tend to be liquid at room temperature.

Polyunsaturated and monounsaturated fats tend to lower blood cholesterol. When unsaturated fats replace saturated fats in the diet, the former tend to stimulate the liver to clear cholesterol from the blood.

Earlier studies had suggested that polyunsaturated fats also seemed to cause reduction of "good" (HDL) cholesterol and a high HDL-cholesterol level is desirable because it helps to decrease the risk of diseases of the cardiovascular system. Additional research, however, does not support the lowering effect on HDL-cholesterol.[3] At typical levels found in the diet, both polyunsaturated and monounsaturated fats now seem to have similar effects on blood cholesterol.

Other Fatty Acids

Hydrogen often is added to monounsaturated and polyunsaturated fats to increase shelf life and to solidify them so they are more spreadable. During this process of partial hydrogenation, the position of hydrogen atoms may be changed along the carbon chain, transforming the fat into a **transfatty acid**.

Margarine and spreads, crackers, cookies, and french fries often contain transfatty acids. Health-conscious people minimize the intake of these types of fats, because studies suggest that diets high in transfatty acids elevate LDL cholesterol and lower HDL cholesterol to the same extent as saturated fats.[4] Paying attention to food labels is important, because the words "partially hydrogenated" and "transfatty acids" indicate that the product carries a health risk just as high as that of saturated fat.

One type of polyunsaturated fatty acids that gained attention in recent years is **omega-3 fatty acids**, which seem to decrease cancer risk and lower triglycerides (which are a risk factor for coronary heart disease). Fish—especially fresh or frozen mackerel, herring, tuna, salmon, and lake trout—and flaxseed contain omega-3 fatty acids. Canned fish is not recommended for this purpose, because the canning process destroys most of the omega-3 oil. These fatty acids also are found, but to a lesser extent, in canola oil, walnuts, soybeans, and wheat germ.

Some data suggest that eating one or two servings of fish weekly lessens the risk for coronary heart disease. People who have diabetes or a history of hemorrhaging or strokes, who are on aspirin or blood-thinning therapy, and who are presurgical patients should not consume fish oil except under a physician's instruction.

Compound Fats

Compound fats are a combination of simple fats and other chemicals. Examples are

1. Phospholipids—similar to triglycerides, except that choline (or another compound) and phosphoric acid take the place of one of the fatty acid units.
2. Glucolipids—a combination of carbohydrates, fatty acids, and nitrogen.
3. Lipoproteins—water-soluble aggregates of protein and triglycerides, phospholipids, or cholesterol.

Lipoproteins (a combination of lipids and proteins) are especially important because they

Peristalsis Involuntary muscle contractions of intestinal walls that facilitate excretion of wastes.

Fats Nutrients containing carbon, hydrogen, some oxygen, and sometimes other chemical elements.

Transfatty acid Solidified fat formed by adding hydrogen to monounsaturated and polyunsaturated fats to increase shelf life.

Omega-3 fatty acids Polyunsaturated fatty acids found primarily in cold-water seafood, flaxseed, and flaxseed oil; thought to lower blood cholesterol and triglycerides.

Lipoproteins Lipids covered by proteins, they transport fats in the blood; types are LDL, HDL, and VLDL.

transport fats in the blood. The major forms of lipoproteins are high-density (HDL), low-density (LDL), and very-low-density (VLDL) lipoproteins. Lipoproteins play a large role in developing or in preventing heart disease. High HDL levels have been associated with lower risk for coronary heart disease, while high LDL levels have been linked to increased risk for this disease. HDL is more than 50 percent protein and contains little cholesterol; LDL is approximately 25 percent protein and nearly 50 percent cholesterol. VLDL contains about 50 percent triglycerides and only about 10 percent protein and 20 percent cholesterol.

Derived Fats

Derived fats combine simple and compound fats. **Sterols** are an example. Although sterols contain no fatty acids, they are considered lipids because they do not dissolve in water. The most often mentioned sterol is cholesterol, which is found in many foods or can be manufactured in the body—primarily from saturated fats.

Proteins

Proteins are the main substances the body uses to build and repair tissues such as muscles, blood, internal organs, skin, hair, nails, and bones. They form a part of hormone, antibody, and **enzyme** molecules. Enzymes play a key role in all of the body's processes. Because all enzymes are formed by proteins, this nutrient is necessary for normal functioning. Proteins also help maintain the normal balance of body fluids.

Proteins can be used as a source of energy, too, but only if sufficient carbohydrates are not available. Each gram of protein yields 4 calories of energy (the same as carbohydrates). The main sources of protein are meats and alternatives, milk, and other dairy products. Excess proteins may be converted to glucose or fat or even excreted in the urine.

The human body uses 20 **amino acids** to form different types of protein. Amino acids contain nitrogen, carbon, hydrogen, and oxygen. Of the 20 amino acids, 9 are called "essential amino acids" because the body cannot produce them. The other 11, termed "nonessential amino acids," can be manufactured in the body if food proteins in the diet provide enough nitrogen (see Table 3.2). For the body to function normally, all amino acids must be present in the diet.

Proteins that contain all the essential amino acids, known as "complete" or "higher-quality" protein, are usually of animal origin. If one or more of the essential amino acids is missing, the proteins are termed "incomplete" or "lower-quality" protein. Individuals have to take in enough protein to ensure

Table 3.2	Amino Acids	
Essential Amino Acids*	**Nonessential Amino Acids**
Histidine	Alanine
Isoleucine	Arginine
Leucine	Asparagine
Lysine	Aspartic acid
Methionine	Cysteine
Phenylalanine	Glutamic acid
Threonine	Glutamine
Tryptophan	Glycine
Valine	Proline
	Serine
	Tyrosine

* Must be provided in the diet, because the body cannot manufacture them.

nitrogen for adequate production of amino acids and also to get enough high-quality protein to obtain the essential amino acids.

Protein deficiency is not a problem in the typical U.S. diet. Two glasses of skim milk combined with about 4 ounces of poultry or fish meet the daily protein requirement. Too much animal protein, on the other hand, can cause serious health problems. Some people eat twice as much protein as they need. Protein foods from animal sources often are high in fat, saturated fat, and cholesterol, which can lead to cardiovascular disease and cancer. Too much animal protein also decreases blood enzymes that prevent precancerous cells from developing into tumors.

As mentioned earlier, a well-balanced diet contains a variety of foods from all five basic food groups, including wise selection of foods from animal sources (see also Balancing the Diet, page 56). Based on current nutrition data, meat (poultry and fish included) should be replaced by grains, legumes, vegetables, and fruits as main courses. Meats should be used more for flavoring than for volume. Daily consumption of beef, poultry, or fish should be limited to 3 ounces (about the size of a deck of cards) to 6 ounces.

Vitamins

Vitamins are necessary for normal bodily metabolism, growth, and development. Vitamins are classified into two types based on their solubility: fat-soluble (A, D, E, and K) and water-soluble (B complex and C). The body does not manufacture most vitamins, so these can be obtained only through a well-balanced diet. To decrease loss of vitamins during cooking, natural foods should be

microwaved or steamed rather than boiled in water that is thrown out later.

A few exceptions, such as vitamin A, D, and K, are formed in the body:

Vitamin A is produced from beta-carotene, found mainly in "yellow" foods such as carrots, pumpkin, and sweet potatoes.

Vitamin D is created when ultraviolet light from the sun transforms a compound in the skin called 7-dehydrocholesterol.

Vitamin K is created in the body by intestinal bacteria.

The major functions of vitamins are outlined in Table 3.3.

Sterols Derived fats, of which cholesterol is the best known example.

Proteins Complex organic compounds containing nitrogen and formed by combinations of amino acids; the main substances used in the body to build and repair tissues.

Enzymes Catalysts that facilitate chemical reactions in the body.

Amino acids Chemical compounds that contain nitrogen, carbon, hydrogen, and oxygen; the basic building blocks the body uses to build different types of protein.

Vitamins Organic nutrients essential for normal metabolism, growth, and development of the body.

Table 3.3

Major Functions of Vitamins

Nutrient	Good Sources	Major Functions	Deficiency Symptoms
Vitamin A	Milk, cheese, eggs, liver, yellow and dark green fruits and vegetables	Required for healthy bones, teeth, skin, gums, and hair; maintenance of inner mucous membranes, thus increasing resistance to infection; adequate vision in dim light.	Night blindness; decreased growth; decreased resistance to infection; rough, dry skin
Vitamin D	Fortified milk, cod liver oil, salmon, tuna, egg yolk	Necessary for bones and teeth; needed for calcium and phosphorus absorption.	Rickets (bone softening), fractures, muscle spasms
Vitamin E	Vegetable oils, yellow and green leafy vegetables, margarine, wheat germ, whole grain breads and cereals	Related to oxidation and normal muscle and red blood cell chemistry.	Leg cramps, red blood cell breakdown
Vitamin K	Green leafy vegetables, cauliflower, cabbage, eggs, peas, potatoes	Essential for normal blood clotting.	Hemorrhaging
Vitamin B$_1$ (Thiamin)	Whole grain or enriched bread, lean meats and poultry, fish, liver, pork, poultry, organ meats, legumes, nuts, dried yeast	Assists in proper use of carbohydrates; normal functioning of nervous system; maintenance of good appetite.	Loss of appetite, nausea, confusion, cardiac abnormalities, muscle spasms
Vitamin B$_2$ (Riboflavin)	Eggs, milk, leafy green vegetables, whole grains, lean meats, dried beans and peas	Contributes to energy release from carbohydrates, fats, and proteins; needed for normal growth and development, good vision, and healthy skin.	Cracking of the corners of the mouth, inflammation of the skin, impaired vision.
Vitamin B$_6$ (Pyridoxine)	Vegetables, meats, whole grain cereals, soybeans, peanuts, potatoes	Necessary for protein and fatty acids metabolism and for normal red blood cell formation.	Depression, irritability, muscle spasms, nausea
Vitamin B$_{12}$	Meat, poultry, fish, liver, organ meats, eggs, shellfish, milk, cheese	Required for normal growth, red blood cell formation, nervous system and digestive tract functioning.	Impaired balance, weakness, drop in red blood cell count
Niacin	Liver and organ meats, meat, fish, poultry, whole grains, enriched breads, nuts, green leafy vegetables, and dried beans and peas	Contributes to energy release from carbohydrates, fats, and proteins; normal growth and development; and formation of hormones and nerve-regulating substances.	Confusion, depression, weakness, weight loss
Biotin	Liver, kidney, eggs, yeast, legumes, milk, nuts, dark green vegetables	Essential for carbohydrate metabolism and fatty acid synthesis.	Inflamed skin, muscle pain, depression, weight loss
Folic Acid	Leafy green vegetables, organ meats, whole grains and cereals, dried beans	Needed for cell growth and reproduction and for red blood cell formation.	Decreased resistance to infection
Pantothenic Acid	All natural foods, especially liver, kidney, eggs, nuts, yeast, milk, dried peas and beans, green leafy vegetables	Related to carbohydrate and fat metabolism	Depression, low blood sugar, leg cramps, nausea, headaches
Vitamin C (Ascorbic acid)	Fruits, vegetables	Helps protect against infection; required for formation of collagenous tissue, normal blood vessels, teeth, and bones.	Slow-healing wounds, loose teeth, hemorrhaging, rough scaly skin, irritability

Vitamins C, E, and beta-carotene also function as antioxidants, which are thought to play a key role in preventing chronic diseases. The specific function of these antioxidant nutrients, along with the mineral selenium (also an antioxidant), are discussed under "Antioxidants and Folate," (page 67).

Minerals

Approximately 25 minerals have important roles in body functioning. **Minerals** are contained in all cells, especially those in hard parts of the body (bones, nails, teeth). Minerals are crucial in maintaining water balance and the acid-base balance. They are essential components of respiratory pigments, enzymes, and enzyme systems, and they regulate muscular and nervous tissue impulses, blood clotting, and normal heart rhythm.

The three minerals mentioned most often are calcium, iron, and sodium. Calcium deficiency may result in osteoporosis, and low iron intake can induce iron-deficiency anemia (both are discussed under "Special Nutrient Needs of Women"). High sodium intake may contribute to high blood pressure. The specific functions of some of the most important minerals are given in Table 3.4.

Water

Water is the most important nutrient, involved in almost every vital body process: in digesting and absorbing food, in energy production, in the circulatory process, in body heat regulation, in removing waste products, in building and rebuilding cells, and in transporting other nutrients. Approximately 60 percent of total body weight is water (see Figure 3.5).

Water is contained in almost all foods, but primarily in liquid foods, fruits, and vegetables. Besides the water content obtained from food, every person needs between 8 to 12 glasses of fluids a day. Water loss during the day must be replenished regularly—if they wait for the thirst signal, most people may already have lost too much water. At 2 percent body weight loss within one day, you are dehydrated. At 5 percent, you may become dizzy and disoriented, have trouble with cognitive skills and heart function, and even lose consciousness.

Table 3.4 **Major Functions of Minerals**

Nutrient	Good Sources	Major Functions	Deficiency Symptoms
Calcium	Milk, yogurt, cheese, green leafy vegetables, dried beans, sardines, salmon	Required for strong teeth and bone formation; maintenance of good muscle tone, heartbeat, and nerve function.	Bone pain and fractures, periodontal disease, muscle cramps
Copper	Seafood, meats, beans, nuts, whole grains	Helps with iron absorption and hemoglobin formation; required to synthesize the enzyme cytochrome oxidase.	Anemia (although deficiency is rare in humans)
Iron	Organ meats, lean meats, seafoods, eggs, dried peas and beans, nuts, whole and enriched grains, green leafy vegetables	Major component of hemoglobin; aids in energy utilization.	Nutritional anemia, overall weakness
Phosphorus	Meats, fish, milk, eggs, dried beans and peas, whole grains, processed foods	Required for bone and teeth formation; energy release regulation.	Bone pain and fracture, weight loss, weakness
Zinc	Milk, meat, seafood, whole grains, nuts, eggs, dried beans	Essential component of hormones, insulin, and enzymes; used in normal growth and development.	Loss of appetite, slow-healing wounds, skin problems
Magnesium	Green leafy vegetables, whole grains, nuts, soybeans, seafood, legumes	Needed for bone growth and maintenance; carbohydrate and protein utilization; nerve function; temperature regulation.	Irregular heartbeat, weakness, muscle spasms, sleeplessness
Sodium	Table salt, processed foods, meat	Needed for body fluid regulation; transmission of nerve impulses; heart action.	Rarely seen
Potassium	Legumes, whole grains, bananas, orange juice, dried fruits, potatoes	Required for heart action; bone formation and maintenance; regulation of energy release; acid-base regulation.	Irregular heartbeat, nausea, weakness
Selenium	Seafood, meat, whole grains	Component of enzymes; functions in close association with vitamin E.	Muscle pain, possible heart muscle deterioration, possible hair and nail loss

Figure
3.5

Approximate proportions of nutrients in the human body.

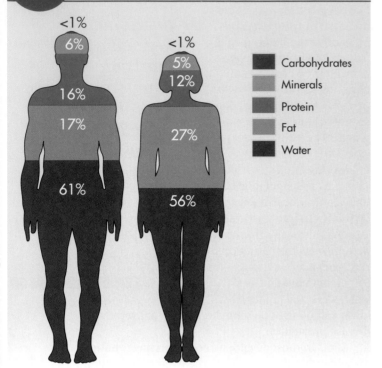

Carbohydrates
Minerals
Protein
Fat
Water

Figure
3.6

Contributions of the energy formation mechanisms during various forms of physical activity.

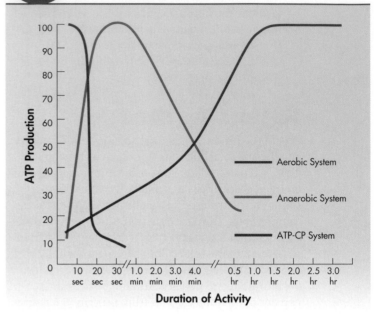

ATP Production

Aerobic System
Anaerobic System
ATP-CP System

10 sec 20 sec 30 sec 1.0 min 2.0 min 3.0 min 4.0 min 0.5 hr 1.0 hr 1.5 hr 2.0 hr 2.5 hr 3.0 hr

Duration of Activity

Energy (ATP) Production

The energy derived from food is not used directly by the cells. It is first transformed into **adenosine triphosphate (ATP)**. The subsequent breakdown of this compound provides the energy used by all energy-requiring processes of the body (also see Figure 3.6). ATP must be recycled continually to sustain life and work. ATP can be resynthesized in three ways:

1. ATP and ATP-CP system. The body stores small amounts of ATP and creatine phosphate (CP). These stores are used during all-out activities such as sprinting, long jumping, and weight lifting. The amount of stored ATP provides energy for just one or two seconds. During brief all-out efforts, ATP is resynthesized from CP, another high-energy phosphate compound. This is referred to as the ATP-CP, or phosphagen, system.

   Depending on the amount of physical training, the concentration of CP stored in cells is sufficient to allow maximum exertion for up to 10 seconds. Once the CP stores are depleted, the person is forced to slow down or rest to allow ATP to form through anaerobic and aerobic pathways.

2. Anaerobic or lactic acid system. During anaerobic exercise that is sustained between 10 and 180 seconds maximum, ATP is replenished from the breakdown of glucose through a series of chemical reactions that do not require oxygen (hence "anaerobic"). In the process, though, **lactic acid** is produced. As lactic acid accumulates, it leads to muscular fatigue.

   Because of the accumulation of lactic acid with high-intensity exercise, the formation of ATP during anaerobic activities is limited to about 3 minutes. A recovery period then is necessary to allow for the elimination of lactic acid. Formation of ATP through the anaerobic system is possible from glucose (carbohydrates) only.

3. Aerobic system. The production of energy during slow-sustained exercise is derived primarily through aerobic metabolism. Glucose (carbohydrates), fatty acids (fat), and oxygen (hence "aerobic") are required to form ATP using this

Minerals Inorganic elements found in the body and in food; essential for normal body functions.

Adenosine triphosphate (ATP) A high-energy chemical compound that the body uses for immediate energy.

Lactic acid End product of anaerobic glycolysis (metabolism).

process and, under steady-state exercise conditions, lactic acid accumulation is minimal.

Because oxygen is required, a person's capacity to utilize oxygen is crucial for successful athletic performance in aerobic events. The higher one's maximal oxygen uptake (VO_{2max}), the greater one's capacity to generate ATP through the aerobic system—and the better the athletic performance.

Balancing the Diet

One of the fundamental ways to enjoy good health and live life to its fullest is through a well-balanced diet. As illustrated in Figure 3.7, the generally recommended guideline states that daily caloric intake should be distributed so that 58 percent of the total calories come from carbohydrates (48 percent complex carbohydrates and 10 percent sugar), less than 30 percent of the total calories from fat (equally divided [10 percent each] among saturated, mono-unsaturated, and polyunsaturated fats), and 12 percent of the total calories from protein (0.8 grams of protein per kilogram of body weight). The diet also must include all of the essential vitamins, minerals, and water. To rate a diet accurately is difficult without a complete nutrient analysis (which will be performed in Lab 3A).

Most health organizations have endorsed the 30 percent fat guideline during the last two decades. More recently, however, nutritionists and preventive medicine specialists are beginning to suggest a daily fat intake lower than the currently recommended 30 percent of total calories. Most scientific studies have shown that a 30 percent-fat diet provides little or no improvement in lowering cholesterol levels.[5] The role of high fat intake in increasing cancer risk is undeniable. An intake of about 20 percent calories from fat is better for overall reduction in risk for cancer.[6] Although the 30 percent guideline is still valid, a gradual change to a lower value might be more beneficial for overall disease prevention.

Diets in most developed countries have changed significantly since the turn of the twentieth century. People in the 1990s eat more fat, fewer carbohydrates, and about the same amount of protein, but fewer

> *Daily caloric intake should be distributed so 58 percent of the total calories come from carbohydrates, less than 30 percent of the total calories come from fat, and 12 percent of the total calories come from protein.*

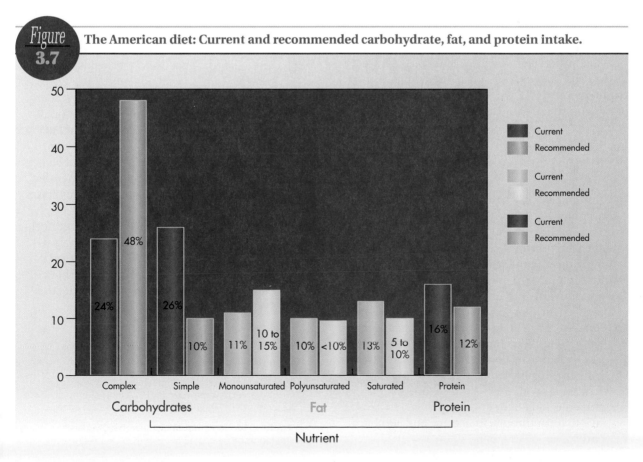

Figure 3.7 The American diet: Current and recommended carbohydrate, fat, and protein intake.

Legend: Current / Recommended

Carbohydrates — Complex: 24% Current, 48% Recommended; Simple: 26% Current, 10% Recommended.
Fat — Monounsaturated: 11% Current, 10 to 15% Recommended; Polyunsaturated: 10% Current, <10% Recommended; Saturated: 13% Current, 5 to 10% Recommended.
Protein: 16% Current, 12% Recommended.

calories. At the same time, people weigh more than they did in 1900, an indication that they are not as physically active as their grandparents were.

Diets also were much healthier at the turn of the twentieth century. In the United States in 1909, carbohydrates accounted for 57 percent of the total daily caloric intake, 67 percent of which were complex carbohydrates. Today, carbohydrate intake has decreased to 51 percent, and complex carbohydrates account for only 24 percent of the daily carbohydrate intake. The proportion of fat has risen from 32 percent to 37 percent. Protein intake has remained unchanged at about 12 percent of the total caloric intake.

Nutrition Standards

Nutritionists use a variety of nutrient standards. The most widely known nutrient standard is the RDA, or Recommended Dietary Allowances. However, this is not the only standard. Others include the Dietary Reference Intakes and the Daily Values on food labels. Each standard has a different purpose and utilization in dietary planning and assessment.

Dietary Reference Intakes

To help people meet dietary guidelines, the National Academy of Sciences has developed a new set of dietary nutrient intakes for healthy people in the United States and Canada, the **Dietary Reference Intakes (DRIs)**. The DRIs are based on a review of the most current research on nutrient needs of healthy people. The DRI reports are written by the Food and Nutrition Board of the Institute of Medicine in cooperation with scientists from Canada. The DRIs are being released in phases: The first, released in 1997, contained revised recommendations for five nutrients important for bone health. The next set was released in 1998 and contained recommendations for eight B-vitamins and choline. In June 2000, recommendations for vitamin C, vitamin E, and selenium were issued.

The general term "DRIs" includes four types of reference values for planning and assessing diets and establishing adequate amounts and maximum safe nutrient intakes in the diet. The type of reference value used for a given nutrient and a specific age/gender group is determined according to available scientific information and the intended use of the dietary standard. The reference values are as follows:

The **Estimated Average Requirement (EAR)** is the amount of nutrient that is estimated to meet the nutrient requirement of half the healthy people in specific age and gender groups. At this nutrient intake level, the upper 50 percent of the people do not have their nutritional requirements met.

The **Recommended Dietary Allowance (RDA)** is the daily amount of a nutrient considered adequate to meet the known nutrient needs of practically all healthy people in the United States. Because the committee must decide what level of intake to recommend for everybody, the RDA is set well above the EAR and covers about 98 percent of the population. Stated another way, the RDA recommendation for any nutrient is well above almost everyone's actual requirement. The RDA could be considered a goal for adequate intake. The process for determining the RDA depends on being able to set an EAR. RDAs are statistically determined from the EAR values. If an EAR cannot be set, no RDA can be established.

When data is insufficient or inadequate to set an EAR, an **Adequate Intake (AI)** value is determined instead of the RDA. The AI value is derived from approximations of observed nutrient intakes by a group or groups of healthy people. The AI value for children and adults is expected to meet or exceed the nutritional requirements of a specific healthy population. Nutrients for which DRIs have been set are presented in Table 3.5.

The **Upper Intake Level (UL)**, which eventually will be available for all nutrients, establishes the highest level of nutrient intake that appears safe for most healthy people and beyond which carries an increased risk of adverse effects. As intakes increase above the UL, so does the risk of adverse effects. In general terms, the optimum nutrient range for healthy eating is between the RDA and the UL. The established ULs are presented in Table 3.6.

Daily Values

In 1993, the Food and Drug Administration (FDA) revised food labeling regulations and introduced the **Daily Values (DVs)**, which are reference values for

Dietary Reference Intakes (DRIs) A general term that describes four types of nutrient standards, which establish adequate amounts and maximum safe nutrient intakes in the diet. These standards are Estimated Average Requirements (EAR), Recommended Dietary Allowances (RDA), Adequate Intakes (AI), and Tolerable Upper Intake Levels (UL).

Estimated Average Requirements (EAR) The amount of a nutrient that meets the dietary needs in half the people.

Recommended Dietary Allowances (RDA) The daily amount of a nutrient (statistically determined from the EARs) considered adequate to meet the known nutrient needs of almost 98 percent of all healthy people in the United States.

Adequate Intakes (AI) The recommended amount of a nutrient intake when sufficient evidence is not available to calculate the EAR and subsequent RDA.

Daily Values (DV) Reference values for nutrients and food components used in food labels.

Table 3.5

Dietary Reference Intakes (DRIs): Recommended Intakes for Individuals

	Recommended Dietary Allowances (RDA)																Adequate Intakes (AI)		
	Calcium (mg)	Vitamin D (mcg)	Thiamin (mg)	Riboflavin (mg)	Niacin (mg NE)	Vitamin B$_6$ (mg)	Folate (mcg DFE)	Vitamin B$_{12}$ (mcg)	Phosphorus (mg)	Magnesium (mg)	Fluoride (mg)	Vitamin A (mcg)	Vitamin C (mg)	Vitamin E (mg)	Selenium (mcg)	Iron (mg)	Pantothenic acid (mg)	Biotin (mg)	Choline (mg)
Males																			
14–18	1300	5	1.2	1.3	16	1.3	400	2.4	1250	410	3	900	75	15	55	11	5.0	25	550
19–30	1000	5	1.2	1.3	16	1.3	400	2.4	700	400	4	900	90	15	55	8	5.0	30	550
31–50	1000	5	1.2	1.3	16	1.3	400	2.4	700	420	4	900	90	15	55	8	5.0	30	550
51–70	1200	10	1.2	1.3	16	1.7	400	2.4	700	420	4	900	90	15	55	8	5.0	30	550
>70	1200	15	1.2	1.3	16	1.7	400	2.4	700	420	4	900	90	15	55	8	5.0	30	550
Females																			
14–18	1300	5	1.0	1.0	14	1.2	400	2.4	1250	360	3	700	65	15	55	15	5.0	25	400
19–30	1000	5	1.1	1.1	14	1.3	400	2.4	700	310	3	700	75	15	55	18	5.0	30	425
31–50	1000	5	1.1	1.1	14	1.3	400	2.4	700	320	3	700	75	15	55	18	5.0	30	425
51–70	1200	10	1.1	1.1	14	1.5	400	2.4	700	320	3	700	75	15	55	8	5.0	30	425
>70	1200	15	1.1	1.1	14	1.5	400	2.4	700	320	3	700	75	15	55	8	5.0	30	425
Pregnancy	*	*	1.4	1.4	18	1.9	600	2.6	*	+40	3	750	85	15	60	27	6.0	30	450
Lactation	*	*	1.5	1.6	17	2.0	500	2.8	*	*	3	1300	120	19	70	10	7.0	35	550

*Values for these nutrients do not change with pregnancy or lactation. Use the value listed for women of comparable age.

Source: Adapted with permission from *Recommended Dietary Allowances*, 10th Edition, and the first two of the *Dietary Reference Intakes* series, National Academy Press. Copyright 1989, 1997, 1998, 1999, 2000, and 2001, respectively, by the National Academy of Sciences. Courtesy of the National Academy Press, Washington, DC.

Table 3.6 Tolerable Upper Intake Levels (UL) of Selected Nutrients for Adults (19–70 years)

Nutrient	UL per Day
Calcium	2.5 gr
Phosphorus	4.0 gr*
Magnesium	350 mg
Vitamin D	50 mcg
Fluoride	10 mg
Niacin	35 mg
Vitamin B$_6$	100 mg
Folate	1000 mcg
Choline	3.5 gr
Vitamin C	2000 mg
Vitamin E	1000 mg
Selenium	400 mcg

*3.5 gr per day for pregnant women 19 years of age and older.

nutrients and food components (such as carbohydrate, fiber and fat) that do not have established RDAs but do have important relationships with health. These values represent dietary intakes to achieve based on a consensus of recommended national standards.

The DVs for use on food labels include fat, saturated fat, and carbohydrate (as a percent of total calories) as well as values for cholesterol, sodium, and potassium (in milligrams) and fiber and protein (in grams). The DVs for total fat, saturated fat, and carbohydrate are expressed as percentages for a 2,000-calorie diet and may therefore require adjustments depending on an individual's total daily caloric needs. For example, on a 2,000-calorie diet, carbohydrate intake should be about 60 percent of total daily calories (300 grams), and fat intake should be limited to less than 30 percent (65 grams) (see Figure 3.8). The vitamin, mineral and protein DVs were adapted from the RDAs but are not the most current recommendations. The DVs are also not as specific for age and gender groups as are the DRIs. Both the DRIs and the DVs apply only to healthy

**Figure
3.8**

Food label with U.S. Recommended Daily Values.

1 Better by Design
How to recognize the new food labels

The new food labels feature a revamped nutrition panel titled "Nutrition Facts," with nutrient listings that reflect current health concerns. Now you'll be able to find information on fat, fiber and other food components fundamental to lowering your risk of cancer and other chronic diseases. Listings for nutrients like thiamin and riboflavin will no longer be required, because Americans generally eat enough of them these days.

2 Size Up the Situation
All serving sizes are created equal

Now you can compare similar products and know that their serving sizes are basically identical. So when you realize how much fat is packed into that carton of double-dutch-chocolate-caramel-chew ice cream you're eyeing, you might opt for low-fat frozen yogurt instead. Serving sizes will also be standardized, so manufacturers can't make nutrition claims for unrealistically small portions. That means a chocolate cake, for example, must be divided into 8 servings sized to satisfy the average person—not 16 servings sized to satisfy the average munchkin.

3 Look Before You Leap
Use the Daily Values

You will find the Daily Values on the bottom half of the "Nutrition Facts" panel. Some represent maximum levels of nutrients that should be consumed each day for a healthful diet (as with fat) while others refer to minimum levels that can be exceeded (as with carbohydrates). They are based on both a 2,000 and 2,500 calorie diet. Your own needs may be more or less, but these figures give you a point from which to compare. For example, the sample label indicates that someone with a 2,000 calorie diet should eat no more than 65 grams of fat per day. This is based on a diet getting 30% of calories as fat. If you normally eat less calories, or want to eat less than 30% of calories as fat, your daily fat consumption will be lower.

4 Rate It Right
Scan the % Daily Values

The % Daily Values make judging the nutritional quality of a food a snap. For instance, you can look at the % Daily Value column and find that a food has 25% of the Daily Value for fiber. This means the product will give you a substantial portion of the recommended amount of fiber for the day. You can also use this column to compare nutrients in similar products. The % Daily Values are based on a 2,000 calorie diet.

5 Trust Adjectives
Descriptors have legal definitions

Terms like "low," "high" and "free" have long been used on food labels. What these words actually mean, however, could vary. Thanks to the new labeling laws, such descriptions must now meet legal definitions. For example, you may be shopping for foods high in vitamin A, which has been linked to lower risk of certain cancers. Under the new label laws, a food described as "high" in a particular nutrient must contain 20% or more of the Daily Value for that nutrient. So if the bottle of juice you're thinking of buying says "high in vitamin A,'" you can now feel confident that it really is a good source of the vitamin.

6 Read Health Claims with Confidence
The nutrient link to disease prevention

You can also expect to see food packages with health claims linking certain nutrients to reduced risk of cancer and other diseases. The federal government has approved three health claims dealing with cancer prevention: a low-fat diet may reduce your risk for cancer; high fiber foods may reduce your risk for cancer; and fruits and vegetables may reduce your risk for cancer. A food may not make such a health claim for one nutrient if it contains other nutrients that undermine its health benefits. A high fiber, but high fat, jelly doughnut cannot carry a health claim!

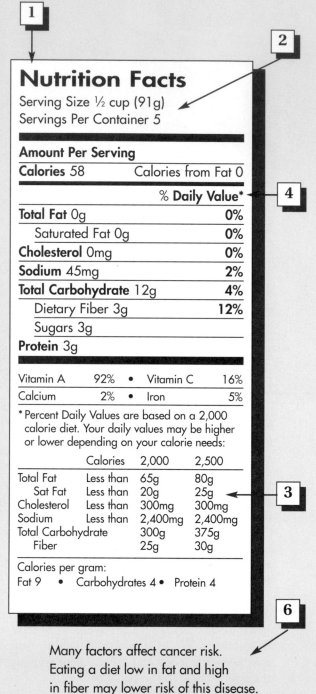

Nutrition Facts

Serving Size ½ cup (91g)
Servings Per Container 5

Amount Per Serving

Calories 58	Calories from Fat 0

% Daily Value*

Total Fat 0g	**0%**
Saturated Fat 0g	**0%**
Cholesterol 0mg	**0%**
Sodium 45mg	**2%**
Total Carbohydrate 12g	**4%**
Dietary Fiber 3g	**12%**
Sugars 3g	
Protein 3g	

Vitamin A	92%	•	Vitamin C	16%
Calcium	2%	•	Iron	5%

* Percent Daily Values are based on a 2,000 calorie diet. Your daily values may be higher or lower depending on your calorie needs:

		Calories	2,000	2,500
Total Fat	Less than		65g	80g
Sat Fat	Less than		20g	25g
Cholesterol	Less than		300mg	300mg
Sodium	Less than		2,400mg	2,400mg
Total Carbohydrate			300g	375g
Fiber			25g	30g

Calories per gram:
Fat 9 • Carbohydrates 4 • Protein 4

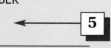

Many factors affect cancer risk. Eating a diet low in fat and high in fiber may lower risk of this disease.

• GOOD SOURCE OF FIBER
• LOWFAT

Reprinted with permission from the American Institute for Cancer Research.

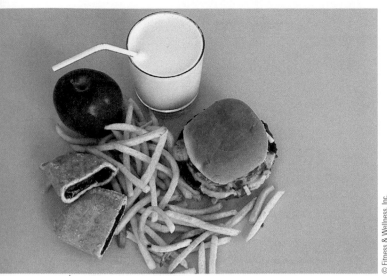

An apple a day will not keep the doctor away if most meals are high in fat content.

adults. They are not intended for people who are ill and may require additional nutrients.

Nutrient Analysis

The first step in evaluating your diet is to conduct a nutrient analysis. This can be quite educational, because most people do not realize how harmful and nonnutritious many common foods are. The analysis covers calories, carbohydrates, fats, cholesterol, and sodium, as well as eight crucial nutrients: protein, calcium, iron, vitamin A, thiamin, riboflavin, niacin, and vitamin C.* If the diet has enough of these eight nutrients, the foods consumed in natural form to provide these nutrients typically contain all the other nutrients the human body needs.

To do the nutrient analysis, keep a 3-day record of everything you eat, using the form in Lab 3A, Figure 3A.1 (make additional copies of this form as needed). At the end of each day, look up the nutrient content for those foods in the list of Nutritive Values of Selected Foods (located in Appendix A). Record this information on the form in Figure 3A.1. (If you do not find a food in Appendix A, the information may be on the food container itself, or you might use the references at the end of Appendix A.)

When you have recorded the nutritive values for each day, add up each column and write the totals at the bottom of the chart. After the third day, fill in your totals on Figure 3A.2 and compute an average for the 3 days. To rate your diet, compare your figures with those in the Recommended Dietary Allowances (RDA)

---

* The following nutrients are also included in the analysis: magnesium, potassium, zinc, vitamin E, folate, phosphorus, and vitamins D_6 and B_{12}.

(Table 3.5). The results give a good indication of areas of strength and deficiency in your current diet.

If you are using the software available with this book when conducting a nutrient analysis, type in the food name and the number of servings based on the standard amounts given in the list of selected foods in Appendix A (see form provided in Figure 3A.3 of Lab 3A or follow the instructions given in the software program).

Some of the most revealing information learned in a nutrient analysis is the source of fat intake in the diet. The average daily fat consumption in the U.S. diet is about 37 percent of the total caloric intake, which increases the risk for chronic diseases such as cardiovascular disease, cancer, diabetes, and obesity. Less than 30 percent of total calories should come from fat.

As illustrated in Figure 3.9, one gram of carbohydrates or of protein supplies the body with 4 calories, and fat provides 9 calories per gram consumed (alcohol yields 7 calories per gram). Therefore, looking at only the total grams consumed for each type of food can be misleading.

For example, a person who eats 160 grams of carbohydrates, 100 grams of fat, and 70 grams of protein has a total intake of 330 grams of food. This indicates that 30 percent of the total grams of food is in the form of fat (100 grams of fat ÷ 330 grams of total food = .30; .30 × 100 = 30 percent). In reality, almost half of that diet is in the form of fat calories.

In the sample diet, 640 calories are derived from carbohydrates (160 grams × 4 calories per gram), 280 calories from protein (70 grams × 4 calories per gram), and 900 calories from fat (100 grams × 9 calories per gram), for a total of 1,820 calories. If 900

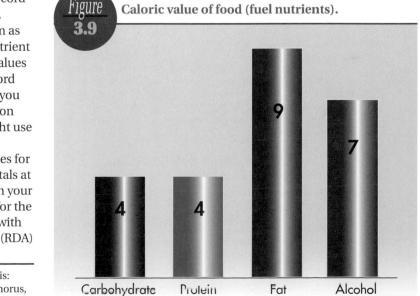

Figure 3.9 Caloric value of food (fuel nutrients).

Carbohydrate — 4
Protein — 4
Fat — 9
Alcohol — 7

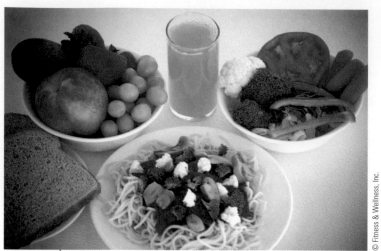

You can restructure your meals so rice, pasta, beans, breads, and vegetables are in the center of the plate; meats are on the side and added primarily for flavoring; fruits are used for desserts; and low- or nonfat milk products are used.

Figure
3.10
Computation for fat content in food.

Nutrition Facts

Serving Size 1 cup (240 ml)
Servings Per Container 4

Amount Per Serving	
Calories 120	Calories from Fat 45

	% Daily Value*
Total Fat 5g	**8%**
Saturated Fat 3g	**15%**
Cholesterol 20mg	**7%**
Sodium 120mg	**5%**
Total Carbohydrate 12g	**4%**
Dietary Fiber 0g	**0%**
Sugars 12g	
Protein 8g	

Vitamin A	10%	Vitamin C	4%
Calcium	30%	Iron	0%

*Percent Daily Values are based on a 2,000 calorie diet. Your daily values may be higher or lower depending on your calorie needs:

	Calories	2,000	2,500
Total Fat	Less than	65g	80g
Sat Fat	Less than	20g	25g
Cholesterol	Less than	300mg	300mg
Sodium	Less than	2,400mg	2,400mg
Total Carbohydrate		300g	375g
Fiber		25g	30g

Calories per gram:
Fat 9 • Carbohydrate 4 • Protein 4

Percent fat calories = (grams of fat × 9) ÷ calories per serving × 100

5 grams of fat × 9 calories per grams of fat = 45 calories from fat

45 calories from fat ÷ 120 calories per serving × 100 = 38% fat

calories are derived from fat, almost half of the total caloric intake is in the form of fat (900 ÷ 1,820 × 100 = 49.5 percent).

Each gram of fat provides 9 calories. When figuring out the percent fat calories of individual foods, you may find Figure 3.10 a useful guideline. Multiply the grams of fat by 9, and divide by the total calories in that particular food (per serving). Then multiply that number by 100 to get the percentage. For example, the food label in Figure 3.10 lists a total of 120 calories and 5 grams of fat, and the equation below shows the fat content to be 38 percent of total calories. This simple guideline can help you decrease the fat in your diet. The fat content of selected foods, given in grams and as a percent of total calories, is presented in Figure 3.11. The percentage of fat is further subdivided into saturated, monounsaturated, polyunsaturated, and other fatty acids.

Beware of products labeled "97 percent fat-free." These products use weight, and not percent of total calories, as a measure of fat. Many of these foods still are in the range of 30 percent fat calories.

Achieving a Balanced Diet

Anyone who has completed a nutrient analysis and has given careful attention to Tables 3.3 (vitamins) and 3.4 (minerals) will probably realize that a well-balanced diet entails eating a variety of foods and reducing daily intake of fats and sweets. The Food Guide Pyramid in Figure 3.1 (page 47) provides simple and sound instructions for nutrition. The pyramid contains five major food groups, along with fats, oils, and sweets (which are to be used sparingly).

The daily recommended number of servings of the five major food groups are as follows:

1. Six to eleven servings of the bread, cereal, rice, and pasta group.
2. Three to five servings of the vegetable group.
3. Two to four servings of the fruit group.

Figure
3.11

Fat content of selected foods.

Food	Calories	Total fat (grams)	% Fat Calories
Avocado/Florida (1)	340	27	71.5
Bacon (3 pieces)	109	9	74.3
Beef/ground/lean/broiled (4 oz)	318	20	56.6
Beef/sirloin (4 oz)	320	21	59.1
Beef/T-bone (4 oz)	338	24	63.9
Butter (1 tbs)	102	11	97.1
Cheese/American (1 oz)	93	7	67.7
Cheese/cheddar (1 oz)	114	9	71.1
Cheese/cottage 4% (1 cup)	216	9	37.5
Cheese/cream (1 oz)	99	10	90.9
Cheese/Parmesan (1 oz)	129	9	62.8
Cheese/Swiss (1 oz)	106	8	67.9
Cheeseburger (1)	305	13	38.4
Chicken/breast/no skin (4 oz)	188	4	19.1
Chicken/thigh/no skin (4 oz)	232	13	50.4
Egg/hard-cooked (1)	77	5	58.4
Frankfurter/beef & pork (1)	182	17	84.1
Halibut/baked (4 oz)	159	3	17.0
Hamburger (1)	255	9	31.8
Ice cream/vanilla (1 cup)	267	15	50.6
Ice milk/vanilla (1 cup)	182	6	29.7
Lamb/lean & fat (4 oz)	293	19	58.4
Margarine (1 tbs)	101	11	98.0
Mayonnaise (1 tbs)	99	11	100.0
Milk 2% (1 cup)	121	5	37.2
Milk/skim (1 cup)	85	.5	5.3
Milk/whole (1 cup)	149	8	48.3
Nuts/cashew/oil roasted (1 oz)	163	14	77.3
Nuts/peanuts/oil roasted (1 oz)	165	14	76.4
Oil/canola (1 tbs)	126	14	100.0
Oil/olive (1 tbs)	124	14	100.0
Salmon/baked (4 oz)	245	12	44.1
Sherbet (1 cup)	266	4	13.5
Shrimp/boiled (3 oz)	85	1	10.6
Tuna/oil/drained (3 oz)	167	7	37.7
Tuna/water/drained (3 oz)	99	1	9.1
Turkey/dark meat/no skin (4 oz)	212	8	34.0
Turkey/light meat/no skin (4 oz)	117	4	30.8

Legend: Saturated fat · Polyunsaturated fat · Monounsaturated fat · Other fatty acids

Percent Fat Calories (axis: 0 10 20 30 40 50 60 70 80 90 100)

4. Two to three servings of the milk, yogurt, and cheese group.
5. Two to three servings of the meat, poultry, fish, dry beans, eggs, and nuts group.

Grains, vegetables, and fruits provide the nutritional base for a healthy diet. Daily fruits and vegetables should include, as a minimum, one good source of **pro-vitamin** A or carotene (apricots, cantaloupe, broccoli, carrots, pumpkin, dark leafy vegetables) and one good source of vitamin C (citrus fruit, kiwi fruit, cantaloupe, strawberries, broccoli, cabbage, cauliflower, green pepper).

In addition to providing nutrients crucial to health, fruits and vegetables are the sole source of **phytochemicals** ("phyto" comes from the Greek word for plant). These compounds, recently discovered by scientists, show promising results in the fight against cancer.

The main function of phytochemicals in plants is to protect them from sunlight. In humans, they seem to have a powerful ability to block the formation of cancerous tumors. Their actions are so diverse that, at almost every stage of cancer, phytochemicals have the ability to block, disrupt, slow down, or even reverse the process. These compounds are not found in pills.

The consistent message is to eat a diet with ample fruits and vegetables. The recommended five to nine servings of fruits and vegetables daily has absolutely no substitute. Science has not yet found a way to allow people to eat a poor diet, pop a few pills, and derive the same benefits.

Milk, poultry, fish, and meats are to be consumed in moderation. Milk and milk products should be low-fat. The recommendation is to consume 3 ounces of poultry, fish, or meat and not to exceed 6 ounces daily. All visible fat and skin should be trimmed off meats and poultry before cooking.

As an aid in balancing your diet, the form in Figure 3B.1 in Lab 3B enables you to record your daily food intake. (This record is much easier to keep than the complete dietary analysis in Lab 3A). Make one copy for each day you wish to record. Whenever you have something to eat, record, in Figure 3B.1, the food and the amount eaten. Do this immediately after each meal so you will be able to keep track of your actual food intake more easily.

If you eat twice the amount of a standard serving, double the number of servings. Evaluate your diet by checking whether you ate the minimum required servings for each food group. If you meet the minimum required servings at the end of each day, you are doing well in balancing your diet.

Rearrange your meals on the plate so rice, pasta, beans, breads, and vegetables are in the center, meats are on the side and are added primarily for

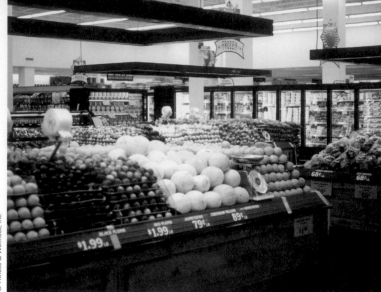

© Fitness & Wellness, Inc.

Most fruits and vegetables contain large amounts of cancer-preventing phytochemicals.

flavoring. Use fruits for dessert. Substitute low-fat or nonfat milk and milk products. These are all strategies to help you enjoy a healthy diet, prevent disease, and improve your overall quality of life.

Vegetarianism

Over 12 million people in the United States follow vegetarian diets. **Vegetarians** rely primarily on foods from the bread, cereal, rice, pasta, and fruit and vegetable groups and avoid most foods from animal sources in the dairy and protein groups. The five basic types of vegetarians are as follows: **Vegans** eat no animal products at all. **Ovovegetarians** allow eggs in the diet. **Lactovegetarians** allow foods from the milk group. **Ovolactovegetarians** include egg and milk products in the diet. **Semivegetarians** do not eat read meat, but do include fish and poultry in addition to milk products and eggs in their diets.

Pro-vitamin A compound that can be converted into a vitamin.

Phytochemicals Chemical compounds thought to prevent and fight cancer; found in large quantities in fruits and vegetables.

Vegetarians Individuals whose diet is of vegetable or plant origin.

Vegans Vegetarians who eat no animal products at all.

Ovovegetarians Vegetarians who allow eggs in their diet.

Lactovegetarians Vegetarians who eat foods from the milk group.

Ovolactovegetarians Vegetarians who include eggs and milk products in their diet.

Semivegetarians Vegetarians who include milk products, eggs, and fish and poultry in the diet.

Vegetarian diets can be healthful and consistent with the Dietary Guidelines for Americans and can meet the DRIs for nutrients. However, vegetarians who do not select their food combinations properly can develop nutritional deficiencies of protein, vitamins, minerals, and even calories. Even greater attention should be paid when planning vegetarian diets for infants and children. Unless carefully planned, a strict plant-based diet will prevent proper growth and development.

Nutrient Concerns

Protein deficiency can be a concern in some vegetarian diets. Vegans in particular must be careful to eat foods that provide a balanced distribution of essential amino acids, such as grain products and legumes. Strict vegans also need a supplement of vitamin B_{12}. This vitamin is not found in plant foods; its only source is animal foods. Deficiency of this vitamin can lead to anemia and nerve damage.

The key to a healthful vegetarian diet is to eat foods that possess complementary proteins. Most plant-based products lack one or more essential amino acids in adequate amounts. For example, both grains and legumes are good protein sources, but neither provides all the essential amino acids. Grains and cereals are low in the amino acid lysine, and legumes lack methionine. Foods from these two groups—such as combinations of tortillas and beans, rice and beans, rice and soybeans, or wheat bread and peanuts—will complement each other and provide all required protein nutrients. These complementary proteins may be consumed over the course of one day, but it is best if they are consumed during the same meal.

Other nutrients likely to be deficient in vegetarian diets—and ways to over come them—are as follows:

- **Vitamin D** can be obtained from moderate sun exposure or by taking a supplement.
- **Riboflavin** can be found in green leafy vegetables, whole grains, and legumes.
- **Calcium** can be obtained from fortified soybean milk or fortified orange juice, calcium-rich tofu, and selected cereals. A calcium supplement is also an option.
- **Iron** can be found in whole grains, dried fruits and nuts, and legumes. To enhance iron absorption, a good source of vitamin C should be consumed with these foods (calcium and iron are the most difficult nutrients to consume in sufficient amounts in a strict vegan diet).
- **Zinc** can be obtained from whole grains, wheat germ, beans, nuts, and seeds.

Most vegetarians today consume dairy products and eggs. A modified version of the Food Guide Pyramid has been prepared for the ovolactovegetarian. All food groups and number of servings remain the same, except that the meat, poultry, fish, dry beans, eggs, and nuts group has been replaced with an eggs, legumes, nuts, and seeds group, and two to four servings are recommended from this group (instead of two to three). Those who are interested in vegetarian diets are encouraged to consult additional resources, because special vegetarian diet planning cannot be covered adequately in a few paragraphs.

Nuts

Consumption of nuts and soy foods, commonly used in vegetarian diets, has received considerable attention in recent years. A few years ago, most people regarded nuts as especially high in fat and calories. Although they are 70 to 90 percent fat, most of it is unsaturated fat. And research indicates that people who eat nuts several times a week have a lower incidence of heart disease. Eating two to three ounces (about one-half cup) of almonds, walnuts, or macadamia nuts a day may decrease high blood cholesterol by about 10 percent. Nuts can even enhance the cholesterol-lowering effects of the Mediterranean diet (discussed in the next section).

Heart-health benefits are attributed not only to the unsaturated fats, but to other nutrients found in nuts, such as vitamin E and folic acid. Nuts are also packed with additional B vitamins, calcium, copper, potassium, magnesium, fiber, and phytochemicals. Many of these nutrients are cancer- and cardioprotective, help lower homocysteine levels, and act as antioxidants (discussed in "Antioxidants and Folate," on page 67).

Nuts do have a drawback: They are still high in calories. A handful of nuts provides as many calories as a piece of cake, so avoid using nuts as a snack. Excessive weight gain is a risk factor for cardiovascular disease. Therefore, nuts are recommended for use *in place of* high-protein foods such as meats, bacon, eggs, or as part of a meal in fruit or vegetable salads, homemade bread, pancakes, casseroles, yogurt, and oatmeal. Peanut butter is also healthier than cheese or some cold cuts in sandwiches.

Soy Products

The increased popularity of soy foods is attributed primarily to Asian research that points to less heart disease, lower cholesterol levels, and fewer hormone-related cancers in people who regularly consume soy foods. The benefits of soy lie in its high protein content and plant chemicals, known as isoflavones, that act as antioxidants and may protect against estrogen-related cancers (breast, ovarian, and endometrial). The compound genistein, one of many phytochemicals in soy, helps to reduce breast cancer

risk, and soy consumption has also been linked to a lower risk for prostate cancer.

Additionally, soy proteins can lower blood cholesterol to a greater extent than would be expected just from its low-fat and high-fiber content. The evidence of heart-protecting benefits from soy foods is so strong that the FDA now allows the following claim on food labels: "25 grams of soy proteins a day, as part of a diet low in saturated fat and cholesterol, may reduce the risk of heart disease." One to two cups of soy milk, one-half cup of tofu, one-and-one-half tablespoons of soy protein isolate, or one-fourth cup of soy flour provide about 10 grams of soy protein. Additional information on the health benefits of soy foods is given in Chapters 12 and 13.

Mediterranean Diet

Much attention has been given recently to the **Mediterranean diet**, because people in that region have notably lower rates of diet-linked diseases and a longer life expectancy. The diet focuses on olive oil, red wine, grains, legumes, vegetables, and fruits, with limited amounts of meat, fish, milk, and cheese. Although it is a semivegetarian diet, up to 40 percent of the total daily caloric intake may come from fat—mostly monounsaturated fat from olive oil. Moderate intake of red wine is included with meals. The dietary

plan also encourages regular physical activity (see Figure 3.12).

Critics of the Mediterranean diet believe that regular wine consumption may lead to alcohol abuse and liver damage. Proponents counter with research that supports a lower risk for heart disease in people who consume one to two alcoholic beverages per day. In terms of heart disease, the Mediterranean diet advocates daily exercise and wine in moderation.

Ethnic Diets

As people migrate, they take their dietary practices with them. Many ethnic diets are healthier than the typical American diet, because they emphasize consumption of complex carbohydrates and limit fat intake. The predominant minority ethnic groups in America are African American, Hispanic American, and Asian American. Unfortunately, ethnic diets quickly become Americanized when they enter the United States. Often, vegetables are cut back and

Mediterranean diet Typical diet of people around the Mediterranean region that focuses on olive oil, red wine, grains, legumes, vegetables, and fruits, with limited amounts of meat, fish, milk, and cheese.

Figure 3.12 Mediterranean Diet Pyramid.

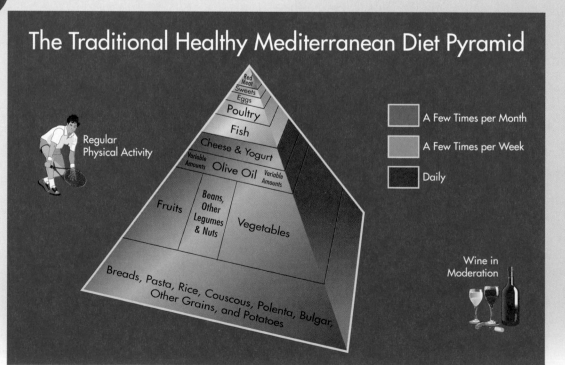

meats and salt are added to these diets to please the American consumer. Ethnic dishes, nonetheless, can be prepared at home. They are easy to make and much healthier if the typical (original) variety of vegetables, corn, rice, spices, and condiments are used. Ethnic dietary plans also encourage daily physical activity and suggest no more than two alcoholic drinks per day.

The African-American diet (soul food) is based on the regional cuisine of the American South. Soul food includes yams, black-eyed peas, okra, and peanuts. The latter were then combined with American foods like corn products and pork. Today, most people view soul food as meat, fried chicken, sweet potatoes, and chitterling.

Hispanic dishes arrived with the conquistadores and evolved through combinations with other ethnic diets and local foods available in Latin America. For example, the Cuban cuisine combined Spanish, Chinese, and native foods; Puerto Rican cuisine developed from Spanish, African, and native products; Mexican diets evolved from Spanish and native food. Corn, beans, squash, chili peppers, avocados, papayas, and fish were primarily used in all these diets. Rice and citrus foods were later added by the colonists. Today a wide variety of foods are used, including red meat; but the staple of the diets still include rice, corn, and beans.

Diets rich in vegetables and using minimal amounts of meat and fat are characteristic in Asian-American diets. The Okinawan diet in Japan, where some of the healthiest and oldest people in the world live, is high in fresh (versus pickled) vegetables, high in fiber, and low in fat and salt. The Chinese cuisine uses more than 200 vegetables, and fat-free sauces and seasoning are used to enhance flavor. The Chinese diet varies somewhat within regions of China. The lowest in fat is that of southern China, with fish, seafood, and stir-fried vegetables used in most meals. Chinese food in American restaurants, however, contains a much higher percentage of fat and protein than the traditional Chinese cuisine.

Table 3.7 provides a list foods to choose from when dining at selected ethnic restaurants.

All healthy diets have similar characteristics. They are high in fruits, vegetables, and grains and low in fat and saturated fat. Low-fat or fat-free dairy products are also used, and portion control is emphasized. The latter is essential in a healthy diet plan, because many people now think that if a food item is labeled "low-fat" or "fat-free," it can be consumed in large quantities. Low-fat or fat-free does not imply calorie-free. Many people who consume low-fat diets increase the amount of food that they eat, which in the long term leads to obesity and its associated health problems.

Table 3.7 Ethnic Eating Guide

	Choose Often	Choose Less Often
Chinese	Beef with broccoli Chinese greens Steamed rice, brown or white Steamed beef with pea pods Stir-fry dishes Teriyaki beef or chicken Wonton soup	Crispy duck Egg rolls Fried rice Kung pao chicken (fried) Peking duck Pork spareribs
Japanese	Chiri nabe (fish stew) Grilled scallops Sushi, Sashimi (raw fish) Teriyaki Yakitori (grilled chicken)	Tempura (fried chicken, shrimp, or vegetables) Tonkatsu (fried pork)
Italian	Cioppino (seafood stew) Minestrone (vegetarian soup) Pasta with marinara sauce Pasta primavera (pasta with vegetables) Steamed clams	Antipasto Cannelloni, ravioli Fettuccini alfredo Garlic bread White clam sauce
Mexican	Beans and rice Black bean/vegetable soup Burritos, bean Chili Enchiladas, bean Fajitas Gazpacho Taco salad Tamales Tortillas, steamed	Chili rellenos Chimichangas Enchiladas, beef or cheese Flautas Guacamole Nachos Quesadillas Tostadas Sour cream (as topping)
Middle Eastern	Tandoori chicken Curry (yogurt-based) Rice pilaf Lentil soup	Falafel Shish kebab
French	Poached salmon Spinach salad Consommé Salad nicoise	Beef Wellington Escargot French onion soup Sauces in general
Soul Food	Baked chicken Baked fish Roasted pork (not smothered or "etouffe") Sauteed okra Baked sweet potato	Fried chicken Fried fish Smothered pork tenderloin Okra in gumbo Sweet potato casserole or pie
Greek	Gyros Pita Lentil soup	Baklava Moussaka

Source: Adapted from P. A. Floyd, S. E. Mimms, and C. Yelding-Howard. *Personal Health: Perspectives & Lifestyles* (Belmont, CA: Wadsworth/Thompson Learning, 1998).

Nutrient Supplementation

Approximately half of all adults in the United States take daily nutrient **supplements**. Nutrient requirements for the body normally can be met by consuming as few as 1,200 calories per day, as long as the diet contains the recommended servings from the five food groups.

Many people consider it necessary to take vitamin supplements. It's true that our bodies cannot retain water-soluble vitamins as long as fat-soluble vitamins. The body excretes excessive intakes readily. Small amounts, however, can be retained for weeks or months in various organs and tissues of the body. Fat-soluble vitamins, on the other hand, are stored in fatty tissue. Therefore, daily intake of these vitamins is not as crucial. Too much vitamin A and vitamin D actually can be detrimental to health.

People should not take **megadoses** of vitamins and minerals. For some nutrients, a dose of five times the RDA taken over several months may create problems. For others, it may not pose any threat to human health. Vitamin and mineral doses should not exceed the ULs. For those nutrients that do not have an established UL, no dosage higher than three times the RDA should be taken.

Iron deficiency (determined through blood testing) is more common in women. Iron supplementation is frequently recommended for women who have heavy menstrual flow. Some pregnant and lactating women also may require supplements. According to 1990 guidelines by the National Academy of Sciences, the average pregnant woman who eats an adequate amount of a variety of foods should take a low dose of iron supplement daily. Women who are pregnant with more than one baby may need additional supplements. Folate supplements also are encouraged prior to and during pregnancy to prevent certain birth defects (see following discussion in "Antioxidants and Folate"). In the above instances, supplements should be taken under a physician's supervision.

Other people who may benefit from supplementation are people with nutrient deficiencies (including low calcium intake), alcoholics and street-drug users who do not have a balanced diet, smokers, vegans (strict vegetarians), individuals on extremely low-calorie diets (less than 1,200 calories per day), older adults who don't eat balanced meals regularly, newborn infants (who are usually given a single dose of vitamin K to prevent abnormal bleeding), and people with disease-related disorders or who are taking medications that interfere with proper nutrient absorption. Although some supplements are encouraged (see discussion that follows), most supplements do not seem to provide additional benefits for healthy people who eat a balanced diet. They do not help people run faster, jump higher, relieve stress, improve sexual prowess, cure a common cold, or boost energy levels.

Antioxidants and Folate

Much research currently is being done to study the effectiveness of **antioxidants** in thwarting several chronic diseases. Although there are probably over 4,000 antioxidants in foods, the four more studied antioxidants are Vitamins C, E, beta-carotene (a precursor to vitamin A), and the mineral selenium (see Table 3.8).

Supplements Tablets, pills, capsules, liquids, or powders that contain vitamins, minerals, amino acids, herbs, or fiber that are taken to increase the intake of these nutrients.

Megadoses For most vitamins, 10 times the RDA or more; for vitamins A and D, 5 and 2 times the RDA, respectively.

Antioxidants Compounds such as vitamins C and E, beta-carotene, and selenium that prevent oxygen from combining with other substances in the body to which it may cause damage.

Table 3.8 Antioxidant Nutrients, Sources, and Functions

Nutrient	Good Sources	Antioxidant Effect
Vitamin C	Citrus fruit, kiwi fruit, cantaloupe, strawberries, broccoli, green or red peppers, cauliflower, cabbage	Appears to inactivate oxygen-free radicals.
Vitamin E	Vegetable oils, yellow and green leafy vegetables, margarine, wheat germ, oatmeal, almonds, whole-grain breads, cereals	Protects lipids from oxidation.
Beta-carotene	Carrots, squash, pumpkin, sweet potatoes, broccoli, green leafy vegetables	Soaks up oxygen-free radicals.
Selenium	Seafood, Brazil nuts, meat, whole grains	Helps prevent damage to cell structures.

Oxygen is used during metabolism to change carbohydrates and fats into energy. During this process, oxygen is transformed into stable forms of water and carbon dioxide. A small amount of oxygen, however, ends up in an unstable form, referred to as **oxygen free radicals**.

A free radical molecule has a normal proton nucleus with a single unpaired electron. Having only one electron makes the free radical extremely reactive, and it looks constantly to pair its electron with one from another molecule. When a free radical steals a second electron from another molecule, that other molecule in turn becomes a free radical. This chain reaction goes on until two free radicals meet to form a stable molecule.

Free radicals attack and damage proteins and lipids, in particular cell membranes and DNA. This damage is thought to contribute to the development of conditions such as cardiovascular disease, cancer, emphysema, cataracts, Parkinson's disease, and premature aging. Solar radiation, cigarette smoke, air pollution, radiation, some drugs, injury or infection, chemicals (such as pesticides), and other environmental factors also seem to encourage the formation of free radicals. Antioxidants are thought to offer protection by absorbing free radicals before they can cause damage and also by interrupting the sequence of reactions once damage has begun, thwarting certain chronic diseases (see Figure 3.13).

The body's own defense systems typically neutralize free radicals so that they don't cause any damage. However, when free radicals are produced faster than the body can neutralize them, they can damage the cells.

Antioxidants are found abundantly in food, especially in fruits and vegetables. Unfortunately, only 9 percent of Americans eat the minimum five daily servings of fruits and vegetables (five to nine is the recommendation).[7]

Many of the benefits of antioxidants are obtained from food sources themselves, and controversy exists as to the benefits of antioxidants taken in supplement form. Many researchers in this area believe that taking antioxidant supplements prevents free-radical damage. In a departure from past recommendations, in 1994 the editorial board of the *University of California at Berkeley Wellness Letter* issued the following antioxidant nutrient supplement guidelines for people who eat at least five daily servings of antioxidant-rich fruits and vegetables:[8]

- 250 to 500 mg of vitamin C
- 200 to 800 IU (**International Units**) of vitamin E
- 10,000 to 25,000 IU of beta-carotene

Supplements should be taken with meals and split in two to three doses per day.[9] Based on these recommendations, however, people who consume nine servings of fresh fruits and vegetables daily could get their daily beta-carotene and vitamin C requirements through the diet. To obtain the recommended guideline for vitamin E through diet alone, however, is practically impossible. Vitamin E, also called tocopherol, is found primarily in oil-rich seeds and vegetable oils. As shown in Table 3.9, vitamin E is not easily found in large quantities in foods typically consumed in the diet. Thus, a daily vitamin E supplement is encouraged.

Antioxidant nutrients often work in conjunction with other nutrients in food that may further enhance their beneficial actions. Because vitamin E is fat-soluble, it should be taken with a meal that has some fat in it. Vitamin C is water-soluble, and the body eliminates it in about 12 hours. For best results, consume vitamin C–rich foods twice a day or divide your vitamin C supplement in half and take it twice a day.

High intake of vitamin E has been linked to reduced risk of heart disease, but may not offer

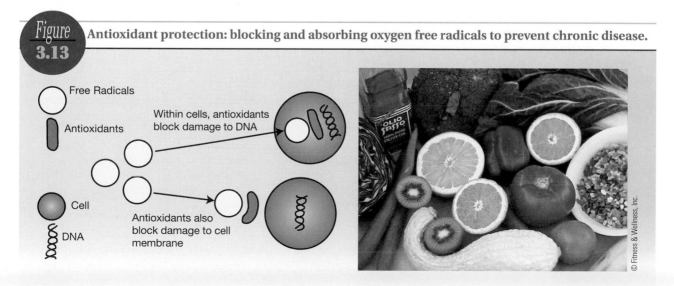

Figure 3.13 Antioxidant protection: blocking and absorbing oxygen free radicals to prevent chronic disease.

Free Radicals

Antioxidants

Cell

DNA

Within cells, antioxidants block damage to DNA

Antioxidants also block damage to cell membrane

© Fitness & Wellness, Inc.

Table 3.9   Antioxidant Content of Selected Foods

Beta-Carotene	IU
Apricot (1 medium)	675
Broccoli (½ cup, frozen)	1,740
Broccoli (½ cup, raw)	680
Cantaloupe (1 cup)	5,160
Carrot (1 medium, raw)	20,255
Green peas (½ cup, frozen)	535
Mango (1 medium)	8,060
Mustard greens (½ cup, frozen)	3,350
Papaya (1 medium)	6,120
Spinach (½ cup, frozen)	7,395
Sweet potato (1 medium, baked)	24,875
Tomato (1 medium)	1,395
Turnip greens (½ cup, boiled)	3,960

Vitamin C	mg
Acerola (1 cup, raw)	1,640
Acerola juice (8 oz)	3,864
Cantaloupe (½ melon, medium)	90
Cranberry juice (8 oz)	90
Grapefruit (½, medium, white)	52
Grapefruit juice (8 oz)	92
Guava (1 medium)	165
Kiwi (1 medium)	75
Lemon juice (8 oz)	110
Orange (1 medium)	66
Orange juice (8 oz)	120
Papaya (1 medium)	85
Pepper (½ cup, red, chopped, raw)	95
Strawberries (1 cup, raw)	88

Vitamin E	IU	mg*
Almond oil (1 tbsp)		5.3
Almonds (1 oz)	10.1	
Canola oil (1 tbsp)		9.0
Cottonseed oil (1 tbsp)		5.2
Hazelnuts (1 oz)	4.4	
Kale (1 cup)	15.0	
Margarine (1 tbsp)		2.0
Peanuts (1 oz)	3.0	
Shrimp (3 oz, boiled)	3.1	
Sunflower seeds (1 oz, dry)	14.2	
Sunflower seed oil (1 tbsp)		6.9
Sweet potato (1 medium, baked)	7.2	
Wheat germ oil (1 tbsp)		20.0

Selenium	mcg
Brazil nuts (1)	100
Bread, whole wheat enriched (1 slice)	15
Beef (3 oz)	33
Cereals (3½ oz)	20
Chicken breast, roasted, no skin (3 oz)	24
Cod, baked (3 oz)	57
Egg, hard boiled (1 large)	15
Fruits (3½ oz)	1
Noodles, enriched, boiled (1 cup)	50
Oatmeal, cooked (1 cup)	23
Red snapper (3 oz)	150
Rice, long grain, cooked (1 cup)	20
Salmon, baked (3 oz)	35
Spaghetti w/meat sauce (1 cup)	36
Tuna, canned, water, drained (3 oz)	68
Turkey breast, roasted, no skin (3 oz)	28
Walnuts, black, chopped (¼ cup)	5
Vegetables (3½ oz)	1

* Vitamin E values for oils are commonly expressed in milligrams (mg). One mg is almost equal to 1 IU (international unit).

additional protection to people who already have the disease.[10] Healthy people who take vitamin E do have fewer heart problems, and the vitamin appears to slow down the progression of plaque (atherosclerosis) in the arteries.[11]

Supplements of vitamin C were recently questioned in the news media because of a single unpublished report that individuals who took over 200 daily mg of this supplement experienced a greater rate of plaque formation in neck arteries. This evidence, however, is preliminary and merely suggestive. Many good studies have shown that vitamin C offers benefits against heart disease, cancer, cataracts, and several other health disorders. Thus, a diet rich in vitamin C and a daily supplement of 250 to 500 mg is recommended.[12] More than 500 daily mg is unnecessary, as research at the National

Institutes of Health showed that the body absorbs very little vitamin C beyond the first 200 mg per serving or dose.[13]

It is better to obtain the daily dose of beta-carotene from food sources rather than supplements.[14] Two separate clinical trials found that beta-carotene supplements offered no protection against heart disease and cancer. One of these studies actually found a higher rate of lung cancer

Oxygen free radicals Substances formed during metabolism that attack and damage proteins and lipids, in particular the cell membrane and DNA, leading to diseases such as heart disease, cancer, and emphysema.

International unit (IU) Measure of nutrients in foods.

and higher mortality rate in smokers who took beta-carotene supplements. For former smokers and nonsmokers, these supplements do not cause any harm, but neither do they offer additional health benefits. Therefore, it is recommended that you "skip the pill and eat the carrot." One medium raw carrot contains about 20,000 IU of beta-carotene (the recommended daily dose).

Adequate intake of the mineral selenium is encouraged. Research indicates that individuals who take 200 micrograms (mcg) of selenium daily decreased their risk of prostate cancer by 63 percent, colorectal cancer by 58 percent, and lung cancer by 46 percent.[15] Data also points to decreased risk of breast, liver, and digestive tract cancers. According to Dr. Edward Giovannucci of the Harvard Medical School, the evidence for the benefits of selenium in reducing prostate cancer risk is so strong that public health officials should recommend that people increase selenium intake now.[16]

Other evidence suggests that taking 100 mcg of selenium supplements daily will increase energy levels, decrease anxiety, and improve immune function.[17] Because selenium may interfere with the body's absorption of vitamin C, the two nutrients should be taken at separate times.[18] Vitamin E supplements, on the other hand, increase the effectiveness of selenium in the body. (See "How and When to Take Supplements" for the most effective ways to take supplements.)

One Brazil nut (unshelled) that you crack yourself provides about 100 mcg of selenium. Shelled nuts found in supermarkets average only about 20 mcg each. Based on the current body of research, a dose of 100 to 200 mcg per day seems to provide the necessary amount of antioxidant for this nutrient. There is no reason to take more than 200 mcg daily—in fact, the UL for selenium has been set at 400 mcg. Too much selenium can damage cells rather than protect them. If you choose to take supplements, take an organic form of selenium from yeast and not selenium selenite. The selenium content of various foods is provided in Table 3.9.

> *There is perhaps no more extensive body of evidence for the cancer-preventing potential of a normal dietary component than there is for selenium.*
>
> —Dr. Gerald Combs, Jr., Cornell University

Folate

Although it is not an antioxidant, 400 mcg of **folate** (a B vitamin) also is recommended for all premenopausal women.[19] Folate helps prevent certain birth defects and seems to offer protection against colon and cervical cancers. Women who might become pregnant should plan on taking a folate supplement, because studies have shown that folate intake (400 mcg per day) during early pregnancy can prevent serious birth defects.

Increasing evidence also indicates that taking 400 mcg of folate along with vitamins B_6 and B_{12} prevents heart attacks by reducing homocysteine levels in the blood (see Chapter 12). High concentrations of homocysteine accelerate the process of plaque formation (atherosclerosis) in the arteries.[20] Five servings of fruits and vegetables per day usually meet the needs for these nutrients. Currently, almost 9 of 10 adults in the United States do not obtain the recommended 400 mcg of folate per day. Because of the critical role of folate in preventing heart disease, some experts recommend a daily vitamin B complex that includes 400 mcg of folate.[21]

Side Effects

Toxic effects from antioxidant supplements are rare when they are taken in the recommended amounts. The daily UL for adults 19 to 70 years of age for

HOW AND WHEN TO TAKE SUPPLEMENTS

Knowing when and how to take nutrient supplements can enhance their potential benefits.

- Take supplements with food.
- Preferably, take vitamin C with other foods that contain this same nutrient.
- Split vitamin C in two or more doses taken throughout the day.
- Do not take vitamin C in combination with selenium. The latter can interfere with absorption of vitamin C.
- Take vitamin E with meals that contain some fat.
- Split vitamin E in two doses when taking more than 400 IU per day.
- Take a vitamin B complex that includes 400 mcg of folate (often found in daily multivitamin complexes). Split the dosage in half and take it twice a day.
- Take some of the vitamin C and the B complex with breakfast. Take vitamin E for breakfast if this meal has some fat in it. Take selenium a couple of hours later with a mid-morning snack. Take vitamin E with lunch if you didn't take it with breakfast. For people taking over 500 mg, the additional vitamin C can be taken with lunch as well. Take the last dose of vitamin C, B complex, and any additional vitamin E with dinner.

vitamin C has been set at 2,000 mg, for vitamin E at 1,000 mg, and for selenium at 400 mcg. Although no UL has been given, up to 50,000 IU of beta-carotene seem safe. If any of the following side effects arise, you should stop supplementation and check with your physician:

- Vitamin E: gastrointestinal disturbances, increase in blood lipids (determined through blood tests)
- Vitamin C: nausea, diarrhea, abdominal cramps, kidney stones, liver problems
- Beta-carotene: (although not harmful) yellow pigmentation of the skin
- Selenium: nausea, vomiting, diarrhea, irritability, fatigue, flu-like symptoms, lesions of the skin and nervous tissue, loss of hair and nails, respiratory failure, liver damage

Substantial supplementation of vitamin E is not recommended for individuals on **anticoagulant** therapy. Vitamin E is an anticoagulant in itself. Therefore, if you are on such therapy, check with your physician. Pregnant women need a physician's approval prior to beta-carotene supplementation. It also may be unsafe if taken with alcohol or by people who drink more than 4 ounces of pure alcohol per day (the equivalent of 8 beers).

Benefits of Foods

Even though you may consider taking some supplements, fruits and vegetables are the richest sources of antioxidants and phytochemicals. Researchers at the U.S. Department of Agriculture compared the antioxidant effects of vitamins C and E with those of various common fruits and vegetables.[22] The results indicated that three-fourths cup of cooked kale (which contains only 11 IU of vitamin E and 76 mg of vitamin C) neutralized as many free radicals as approximately 800 IU of vitamin E or 600 mg of vitamin C. Other excellent sources of antioxidants found by these researchers include blueberries, strawberries, spinach, Brussels sprouts, plums, broccoli, beets, oranges, and grapes. A list of top antioxidant foods is presented in Table 3.10.

Many people who regularly eat foods high in fat content or too many sweets think they need supplementation to balance their diet. This is another fallacy about nutrition. The problem here is not necessarily a lack of vitamins and minerals, but a diet too high in calories, fat, and sodium. Vitamin, mineral, and fiber supplements do not supply all of the nutrients and other beneficial substances present in food and needed for good health. Supplements will provide added health benefits, but by no means do they replace a well-balanced diet.

Wholesome foods contain vitamins, minerals, carbohydrates, fiber, proteins, fats, phytochemicals,

Table 3.10	Top Antioxidant Foods (expressed in ORAC* units per serving)		
Fruits	**ORAC Units**	**Vegetables**	**ORAC Units**
Blueberries, ½ cup	1,750	Kale, 1 cup	1,190
Blackberries, ½ cup	1,470	Beets, 1 cup	570
Prunes, 3	1,460	Red bell peppers, ½ cup	530
Plums, 2	1,250	Brussel sprouts, ½ cup	430
Strawberries, ½ cup	1,170	Corn, ½ cup	420
Raisins, ¼ cup	1,030	Spinach, 1 cup	380
Raspberries, ½ cup	760	Onions, ½ cup	360
Orange, ½ cup	680	Broccoli, ½ cup	320
Red grapes, ½ cup	590	Eggplant, ½ cup	160
Cherries, ½ cup	520	Alfalfa sprouts, ½ cup	150

*ORAC = oxygen radical absorbance capacity

Source: Adapted from USDA, Agricultural Research Service, *Food & Nutrition Research Briefs*, April 1999 (downloaded from www.ars.usda.gov/is/np/fnrb).

and other substances not yet discovered. Researchers do not know if the protective effects are caused by the antioxidants alone, in combination with other nutrients (such as phytochemicals), or by some other nutrients in food that have not been investigated yet. Many nutrients work in **synergy**, enhancing chemical processes in the body. Supplementation will not offset poor eating habits. Pills are no substitute for common sense.

If you think your diet is not balanced, you first need to conduct a nutrient analysis (as in Lab 3A) to determine which nutrients you lack in sufficient amounts. Eat more of them, as well as foods that are high in antioxidants and phytochemicals. Following a nutrient assessment, a **registered dietician** can help you decide what supplement(s) might be necessary. If you take supplements in pill form, look for products that meet the USP (U.S. Pharmacopoeia) disintegration standards on the bottle. The USP symbol suggests that the supplement should completely dissolve in 45 minutes or less. Supplements that do not dissolve, of course, cannot get into the bloodstream.

Folate One of the B vitamins.

Anticoagulant Any substance that inhibits blood clotting.

Synergy A reaction in which the result is greater than the sum of its two parts.

Registered dietician (RD) A person with a college degree in dietetics who meets all certification and continuing education requirements by the American Dietetic Association or Dietitians of Canada.

Functional Foods

Functional foods are any food or food ingredient that offers specific health benefits beyond those supplied by the traditional nutrients it contains. Many functional foods come in their natural form. A tomato for example, is a functional food because it contains the phytochemical lycopene, thought to reduce prostate cancer risk. Other examples of functional foods are kale, broccoli, blueberries, red grapes, and green tea.

The term "functional food," however, has been used primarily as a marketing tool by the food industry to attract the consumer. Unlike fortified foods, which have been modified to help prevent nutrient deficiencies, functional foods are being created by the food industry by adding ingredients aimed at treating or preventing symptoms or disease. With such "functional foods," the added ingredient(s) is often *not* typically found in the particular food item in its natural form, but it is added to allow manufacturers to make appealing health claims.

In most cases only one extra ingredient is added (a vitamin, mineral, phytochemical, or herb). An example is calcium added to orange juice to make the claim that this particular brand offers protection against osteoporosis. Thus, food manufacturers now offer cholesterol-lowering margarines (enhanced with plant stanol), cancer-protective (lycopene-fortified) ketchup, memory-boosting (ginkgo-added) candy, calcium-fortified chips, and kava-kava–containing corn chips (to enhance relaxation).

The use of some functional foods, however, may undermine good nutrition. Margarines may contain saturated fats or partially hydrogenated oils. Regular ketchup consumption on top of large orders of fries adds many calories and fat to the diet. Sweets are also high in calories and sugar. Chips are high in calories, salt, and fat. In all of these cases, the consumer would be better off taking the specific ingredient in a supplement form rather than consuming the "functional food" with its extra calories, sugar, salt, and/or fat.

Functional foods can provide added benefits if used in conjunction with a healthful diet. You may use nutrient-dense functional foods in your overall wellness plan as an adjunct to health-promoting strategies and treatments.[23]

Genetically Modified Foods

A genetically modified organism (GMO) is one whose DNA (or basic genetic material) is manipulated to obtain certain results. This is done by inserting genes with desirable traits from one plant, animal, or microorganism, into another one to either introduce new traits or enhance existing ones.

Crops are genetically modified to make them more resistant to disease and extreme environmental conditions (such as heat and frost), require less fertilizers and pesticides, last longer, and improve their nutrient content and taste. Such crops could help save billions of dollars in more productive crops and help feed the hungry in developing countries around the world.

Concerns over the safety of genetically modified (GM) foods have created heated public debates in Europe and to a lesser extent in the United States, although the issue is now receiving more attention. The concern is that genetic modifications create "transgenic" organisms that have not previously existed and that have potentially unpredictable effects on the environment and on humans. Concerns exist that GM foods may cause illness or allergies in humans, cross-pollination may destroy other plants, or create "superweeds" with herbicide-resistant genes.

Genetically modified crops were first introduced in the United States in 1996. This technology is moving forward so rapidly that the USDA has already approved more than 50 GM crops. In 1999, about 25 percent of the U.S. cropland produced GM foods. About 60 percent of our soybeans and 35 percent of corn came from GM crops.

Total avoidance of GM foods is difficult, because over 60 percent of processed foods on the market today contain GM organisms.[24] For people who do not wish to consume GM foods, organic foods are an option because organic trade organizations do not certify foods with genetic modifications. Produce bought at the local farmers' market may also be an

---

HEALTH CLAIMS APPROVED BY THE FDA THAT LINK FOODS AND DISEASE PREVENTION

- Calcium-rich foods and reduced risk of osteoporosis
- Low-sodium foods and reduced risk of high blood pressure
- Low-fat diet and reduced risk of cancer
- A diet low in saturated fat and cholesterol and reduced risk of heart disease
- High-fiber foods and reduced risk of cancer
- Soluble fiber in fruits, vegetables, and grains and reduced risk of heart disease
- Soluble fiber in oats and psyllium seed husk and reduced risk of heart disease
- Fruit- and vegetable-rich diet and reduced risk of cancer
- Folate-rich foods and reduced risk of neural tube defects
- Less sugar and reduced risk of dental caries

option, because small farmers are less likely to use this new technology.

At this point, there is no evidence that indicates that GM foods are harmful—but no compelling evidence guarantees that they are safe, either. Many questions remain and much research is required in this field. As a consumer, you need to continue educating yourself as more evidence becomes available in the next few years. ⌐NOT TESTING↓

Nutrition for Athletes

The two main fuels that supply energy for physical activity are glucose (sugar) and fat (fatty acids). The body uses amino acids, derived from proteins, as an energy substrate when glucose is low, such as during fasting, prolonged aerobic exercise, or a low-carbohydrate diet.

Glucose is derived from foods high in carbohydrates such as breads, cereals, grains, pasta, beans, fruits, vegetables, and sweets in general. Glucose is stored as glycogen in muscles and the liver. Fatty acids (discussed on page 51) are the product of the breakdown of fats. Unlike glucose, an almost unlimited supply of fatty acids, stored as fat in the body, can be used during exercise.

During resting conditions, fat supplies about two-thirds of the energy to sustain the body's vital processes. During exercise, the body uses both glucose (glycogen) and fat in combination to supply the energy demands. The proportion of fat to glucose changes with the intensity of exercise. When a person is exercising below 60 percent of his or her maximal work capacity, fat is used as the primary energy substrate. As the intensity of exercise increases, so does the percentage of glucose utilization—up to 100 percent during maximal work that can only be sustained for 2 to 3 minutes.

In general, athletes do not require special supplementation or any other special type of diet. Unless the diet is deficient in basic nutrients, no special, secret, or magic diet will help people perform better or develop faster as a result of what they eat. As long as the diet is balanced—that is, based on a large variety of nutrients from all basic food groups—athletes do not require additional supplements (other than the antioxidant recommendations made under "Antioxidants and Folate"). Even in strength training and body building, protein in excess of 20 percent of total daily caloric intake is not necessary.

The main difference between sensible diet for a sedentary person and a highly active individual is in the total number of calories required daily and the amount of carbohydrate intake needed during prolonged physical activity. People in training consume more calories because of their greater energy expenditure—which is required as a result of intense physical training.

Carbohydrate Loading

On a regular diet, the body is able to store between 1,500 and 2,000 calories in the form of glycogen. About 75 percent of this glycogen is stored in muscle tissue. This amount, however, can be increased greatly through **carbohydrate loading**.

A regular diet should be altered during several days of heavy aerobic training or when a person is going to participate in a long-distance event of more than 90 minutes (for example, marathon, triathlon, or road cycling). For events shorter than 90 minutes, carbohydrate loading does not seem to enhance performance.

During prolonged exercise, glycogen is broken down into glucose, which then is readily available to the muscles for energy production. In comparison to fat, glucose frequently is referred to as the "high-octane fuel," because it provides about 6 percent more energy per unit of oxygen consumed.

Heavy training over several consecutive days leads to depletion of glycogen faster than it can be replaced through the diet. Glycogen depletion with heavy training is common in athletes. Signs of depletion include chronic fatigue, difficulty in maintaining accustomed exercise intensity, and lower performance.

On consecutive days of exhaustive physical training (this means several hours daily), a carbohydrate-rich diet—70 percent of total daily caloric intake or 8 grams of carbohydrate per kilogram of body weight—is recommended. This diet often restores glycogen levels in 24 hours. Along with the high-carbohydrate diet, a day of rest often is needed to allow the muscles to recover from glycogen depletion following days of intense training. For people who exercise less than an hour a day, a 60 percent carbohydrate diet or 6 grams of carbohydrate per 2.2 pounds (1 kilogram) of body weight is enough to replenish glycogen stores.

Carbohydrate loading is necessary only for endurance events that last longer than 90 minutes.

Following an exhaustive workout, eating a combination of carbohydrates and protein (such as a tuna sandwich) within 30 minutes of exercise seems to speed up glycogen storage even more. Protein intake increases insulin activity, thereby enhancing

Carbohydrate loading Increasing intake of carbohydrates during heavy aerobic training or prior to aerobic endurance events that last longer than 90 minutes.

glycogen replenishment. A 70 percent carbohydrate intake then should be maintained throughout the rest of the day.

By following a special diet/exercise regimen 5 days before a long-distance event, highly (aerobically) trained individuals are capable of storing two to three times the amount of glycogen found in the average person. Athletic performance may be enhanced for long-distance events of more than 90 minutes by eating a regular balanced diet along with intensive physical training the fifth and fourth days before the event, followed by a diet high in carbohydrates (about 70 percent) and a gradual decrease in training intensity over the last 3 days before the event.

The amount of glycogen stored as a result of a carbohydrate-rich diet does not seem to be affected by the proportion of complex and simple carbohydrates. Intake of simple carbohydrates (sugars) can be raised while on a 70 percent carbohydrate diet, as long as 48 percent of the total calories is derived from complex carbohydrates. The latter provide more nutrients and fiber, making them a better choice for a healthier diet.

On the day of the long-distance event, carbohydrates are still the recommended choice of substrate. As a rule of thumb, athletes should consume 1 gram of carbohydrate for each 2.2 pounds of body weight 1 hour prior to exercise (that is, if you weigh 160 pounds, you should consume $160/2.2 = 72$ grams). The amount of carbohydrate can be increased to 2, 3, or 4 grams per 2.2 pounds of weight 2, 3, or 4 hours, respectively, before exercise.

During the long-distance event, researchers recommend that 30 to 60 grams of carbohydrates (120 to 240 calories) be consumed every hour. This is best accomplished by drinking 8 ounces of a 6 to 8 percent-carbohydrate sports drink every 15 minutes. This also lessens the chance of dehydration during exercise, which hinders performance and endangers health. The percentage of the carbohydrate drink is determined by dividing the amount of carbohydrate (in grams) by the amount of fluid (in ml), and multiplying by 100. For example, 18 grams of carbohydrate in 240 ml (8 oz) of fluid yields a drink at 7.5 percent ($18 \div 240 \times 100$).

Creatine Supplementation

Creatine is an organic compound obtained in the diet primarily from meat and fish. In the human body, creatine combines with inorganic phosphate and forms the high-energy compound **creatine phosphate (CP)**. CP is then used to resynthesize ATP during short bursts of all-out physical activity. Individuals on a normal mixed diet consume an average of 1 gram of creatine per day. Each day, 1 additional gram is synthesized from various amino acids. One pound of meat or fish provides approximately 2 grams of creatine.

Creatine supplementation has become popular in recent years among individuals who want to increase muscle mass and improve athletic performance. Creatine monohydrate—a white, tasteless powder that is mixed with fluids prior to ingestion—is the form most popular among people who use the supplement. Supplementation can result in an approximate 20 percent increase in the amount of creatine that is stored in muscles. Most of this creatine binds to phosphate to form CP, while 30 to 40 percent remains as free creatine in the muscle. Increased creatine storage is believed to enable individuals to train more intensely, thus build more muscle mass; and enhance performance in all-out activities of very short duration.

There are two phases to creatine supplementation: the loading phase and the maintenance phase. During the loading phase, the person consumes between 20 and 25 grams (one teaspoonful is about 5 grams) of creatine per day for 5 to 6 days, divided into 4 or 5 dosages of 5 grams each throughout the day (this amount represents the equivalent of consuming 10 or more pounds of meat per day). Research also suggests that the amount of creatine stored in muscle is enhanced by taking creatine in combination with a high-carbohydrate food. Once the loading phase is complete, 2 grams per day appear to be sufficient to maintain the increased muscle stores.

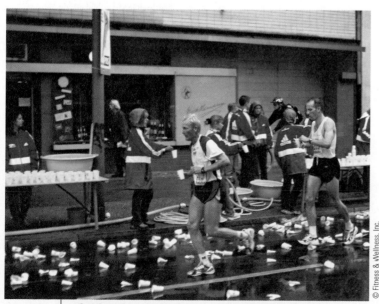

Fluid and carbohydrate replenishment during exercise are essential when participating in long-distance aerobic endurance events, such as a marathon or a triathlon.

To date, no serious side effects have been documented in people who take up to 25 grams of creatine per day for 5 days. Stomach distress and cramping has been reported only in rare instances. The 2 grams taken per day during the maintenance phase is only slightly above the average intake in our daily diet. Long-term effects of creatine supplementation on health, however, have not been established.

A frequently documented result following 5 to 6 days of creatine loading is an increase of 2 to 3 pounds in body weight. This increase appears to be related to increased water retention necessary to maintain the additional creatine stored in muscles. Some data, however, suggests that the increase in stored water and CP stimulates protein synthesis, thus leading to an increase in lean body mass.

The benefits of elevated creatine stores may be limited to high-intensity/short-duration activities like sprinting, strength training (weight lifting), and sprint cycling. Supplementation is most beneficial during exercise training itself, rather than as an aid to enhance athletic performance a few days before competition. The availability of extra creatine in muscles may help individuals train at a higher intensity, thus enhancing the physiological adaptations to training and subsequent athletic performance.

Enhanced creatine stores do *not* benefit athletes competing in aerobic endurance events, because CP is not used in energy production for long-distance events. In fact, the additional weight can be detrimental in long-distance running and swimming events, because the athlete must expend more energy to carry the extra weight during competition.

Amino Acid Supplements

A myth regarding athletic performance is that protein (amino acid) supplements will increase muscle mass. The claims and safety of these products have not been proven scientifically. The RDA for protein is .8 grams per kilogram of body weight.

Most athletes, including weight lifters and body builders, increase their caloric intake automatically during intense training. As caloric intake increases, so does the intake of protein, often approaching 2 or more grams per kilogram of body weight. This amount is more than enough to build and repair muscle tissue. Typically, athletes in strength training consume between 3 and 4 grams per kilogram of body weight. In response, supplement manufacturers have created expensive "free-amino acid supplements."

People who buy costly free-amino acid supplements are led to believe that they contribute to the development of muscle mass. However, the human body cannot distinguish between amino acids obtained from food or through supplements. Excess protein is either used for energy or turned into fat. With amino acid supplements, each capsule provides up to 500 milligrams of amino acids and no additional nutrients. In contrast, 3 ounces of meat or fish provide more than 20,000 milligrams of amino acids, along with other essential nutrients such as iron, niacin, and thiamin. The benefits of natural foods to health and budget are clear.

Proponents of free-amino acid supplements further claim that only a small amount of amino acids in food is absorbed and that free-amino acids are absorbed more readily than protein food. Neither claim is correct. The human body absorbs and utilizes between 85 and 99 percent of all protein from food intake. The body handles whole, natural proteins better than single amino acids predigested in the laboratory setting.

Amino acid supplementation can even be dangerous: Supplementation of a group of chemically similar amino acids often prevents the absorption of other amino acids, potentially causing critical imbalances and toxicities. Long-term risks associated with amino acid supplementation have not been determined.

The advertised rate of absorption provides no additional benefit, because building muscle takes hours, not minutes. Muscle overload through heavy training, not supplementation, builds muscle. Expensive protein supplements benefit only those who sell them.

Special Nutrient Needs of Women

Three considerations specific to women are bone health, hormone replacement therapy beginning at menopause, and iron supplementation to offset the iron lost through menstruation.

Bone Health and Osteoporosis

In **osteoporosis**, bones—primarily of the hip, wrist, and spine—become so weak and brittle that they fracture readily. The process begins slowly in the third

---

Creatine An organic compound derived from meat, fish, and amino acids that combines with inorganic phosphate to form creatine phosphate.

Creatine phosphate (CP) A high-energy compound that is used by the cells to resynthesize ATP during all-out activities of very short duration.

Osteoporosis Softening, deterioration, or loss of bone mass.

and fourth decades of life. Women are especially susceptible after menopause because of the accompanying loss of **estrogen**, which increases the rate at which bone mass is broken down.

Approximately 20 million women in the United States have osteoporosis, and about 1.5 million fractures are attributed to this condition each year. Of women who have hip fractures, half die within 6 months and the other half do not return to independent living. Based on current trends, a 50-year-old woman in the United States has at least a 40 percent probability of a future fracture because of osteoporosis. According to Dr. Barbara Drinkwater, a leading researcher in this area, "Shocking as these figures are, they cannot adequately convey the pain and deterioration in the quality of life of women who suffer the crippling effects of osteoporotic fractures."[25]

Although osteoporosis is viewed primarily as a women's disease, more than 30 percent of all men will be affected by age 75. About 100,000 of the yearly 300,000 hip fractures in the United States occur in men. Although the genetic component is strong, osteoporosis is preventable. Maximizing bone density at a young age and subsequently decreasing the rate of bone loss later in life are critical in preventing osteoporosis. Normal hormone levels (estrogen for women, testosterone at a later age for men), adequate calcium intake, and physical activity cannot be overemphasized. All three factors are crucial to prevent osteoporosis. The absence of any one of these three factors leads to bone loss for which the other two factors never completely compensate. Smoking, excessive use of alcohol, and corticosteroid drugs also accelerate the rate of bone loss in both women and men. Figure 3.14 depicts these variables.

Estrogen is the most important factor in preventing osteoporosis in women.

Bone health begins at a young age. Some experts have called osteoporosis a "pediatric disease." Bone density can be promoted early in life by making sure the diet has sufficient calcium and participating in weight-bearing activities. Although the RDA for calcium is between 1,000 and 1,300 mg per day, leading researchers in this area recommend even higher intakes (see Table 3.11). Although these recommended daily intakes can be met easily through diet alone, some experts recommend calcium supplements even for children before puberty. Table 3.12 provides a list of selected foods along with their calcium content. Along with adequate calcium intake, 400 to 800 IU of vitamin D daily are recommended for optimal calcium absorption.

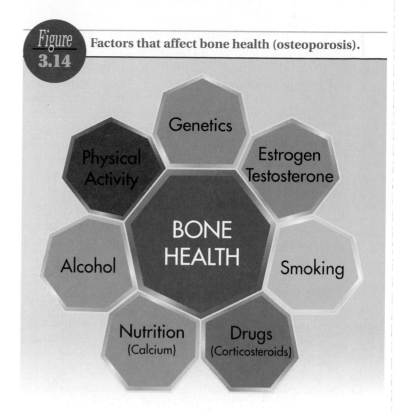

Figure 3.14 Factors that affect bone health (osteoporosis).

Table 3.11 Recommended Daily Calcium Intake

Age	Amount (gr)
1–5	800
6–10	800–1,200
11–24	1,200–1,500
25–50 Women	1,000
25–64 Men	1,000
PMW* on HRT**	1,000
PMW not on HRT	1,500
> 65	1,200–1,500

*PMW = Post-menopausal women
**HRT = Hormone replacement therapy

High protein intake also may affect the body's absorption of calcium. The more protein eaten, the higher the calcium content in the urine (that is, the more calcium excreted). This might be the reason why countries with a high protein intake, including the United States, also have the highest rates of osteoporosis.

Exercise seems to play a key role in preventing osteoporosis by decreasing the rate of bone loss following menopause. Active people are able to maintain bone density much more effectively than

Table 3.12 Low-Fat Calcium-Rich Foods

Food	Amount	Calcium (mg)	Calories
Beans, red kidney, cooked	1 cup	70	218
Beet, greens, cooked	½ cup	82	19
Bok choy (Chinese cabbage)	1 cup	158	20
Broccoli, cooked, drained	1 cup	72	44
Burrito, bean (no cheese)	1	57	225
Cottage cheese, 2% low-fat	½ cup	78	103
Ice milk (vanilla)	½ cup	102	100
Instant breakfast, nonfat milk	1 cup	407	216
Kale, cooked, drained	1 cup	94	36
Milk, nonfat, powdered	1 tbs	52	15
Milk, skim	1 cup	296	88
Oatmeal, instant, fortified, plain	½ cup	109	70
Okra, cooked, drained	1/2 cup	74	23
Orange juice, fortified	1 cup	300	110
Soy milk, fortified, fat free	1 cup	400	110
Spinach, raw	1 cup	56	12
Turnip greens, cooked	1 cup	197	29
Tofu (some types)	½ cup	138	76
Yogurt, fruit	1 cup	372	250
Yogurt, low-fat, plain	1 cup	448	155

their inactive counterparts. A combination of weight-bearing exercises, such as walking or jogging and weight training, is especially helpful. The benefits of exercise go beyond maintaining bone density. Exercise strengthens muscles, ligaments, and tendons—all of which provide support to the bones (skeleton). Exercise also improves balance and coordination, which can help prevent falls and injuries.

Current studies indicate that people who are active have denser bone mineral than inactive people do. Similar to other benefits of participating in exercise, there is no such thing as "bone in the bank." To have good bone health, people need to participate in a regular lifetime exercise program.

Prevailing research also tells us that estrogen is the most important factor in preventing bone loss. Lumbar bone density in women who have always had regular menstrual cycles exceeds that of women with a history of **oligomenorrhea** and **amenorrhea** interspersed with regular cycles. Furthermore, the lumbar density of these two groups of women is higher than that of women who have never had regular menstrual cycles.

As a baseline test, women should get a bone density test at menopause. Following menopause, every woman should consider some type of therapy to prevent bone loss. The various therapy modalities

available should be discussed with a physician. Although regular weight-bearing exercise and plenty of calcium in the diet can slow bone loss, osteoporosis can be stopped only through traditional hormone replacement therapy (HRT), such as estrogen and calcitonin, or other more recent nonhormonal modalities.[26]

Estrogen Replacement Therapy

Estrogen replacement therapy (ERT) is the most common treatment to prevent bone loss following menopause. ERT also may produce a slight increase in bone mass density. Women on ERT do not lose bone mineral density at the rate of women who are not using this therapy. Neither exercise nor calcium supplementation will offset the damaging effects of lower estrogen levels.

For instance, athletes with amenorrhea (who have lower estrogen levels) have lower bone mineral density than even nonathletes with normal estrogen levels. One study showed that amenorrheic athletes at age 25 have the bones of a 52-year-old woman.[27] Other research showed four amenorrheic athletes with a bone density equivalent to that of 70- to 80-year-old women.[28] Over the last few years, it has become clear that sedentary women with normal estrogen levels have better bone mineral density than active amenorrheic athletes. Many experts believe the best predictor of bone mineral content is the history of menstrual regularity.

Many women stop taking estrogen within a year because of unpleasant side effects that include headaches, breast tenderness, bleeding, and fluid retention. To obtain the benefits of ERT on bone mass retention, however, estrogen must be taken over the long term. ERT also reduces the risk of cardiovascular disease. Although the evidence is inconclusive, ERT may increase the risk of breast and endometrial cancer.

A second treatment modality to prevent bone loss is Miacalcin, a synthetic form of the hormone calcitonin. Calcitonin is a thyroid hormone that helps maintain the body's delicate balance of calcium by taking calcium from the blood and depositing it in the bones. Miacalcin is recommended for women who refuse, cannot use, or do not tolerate ERT. Though it is effective in preventing bone loss, it does not help much in rebuilding bone; therefore, Miacalcin therapy should be started soon after

Estrogen Female sex hormone; essential for bone formation and conservation of bone density.

Oligomenorrhea Irregular menstrual cycles.

Amenorrhea Cessation of regular menstrual flow.

menopause. The drug seems to have no side effects. It is available in injectable and nasal spray forms.

Fosamax (alendronate), a promising non-hormonal drug, has been approved by the FDA for the treatment of osteoporosis.[29] Studies of menopausal women younger than age 60 showed that Fosamax therapy not only prevented bone loss but actually helped increase bone mass by about 6 percent. Fosamax is recommended for women who have osteoporosis already and who cannot or will not take estrogen. Fosamax is used primarily for bone health and does not provide benefits to the cardiovascular system. Although the research is limited, this drug seems to be safe and effective. Like estrogen, it must be taken for the rest of a woman's life.

New treatment modalities being developed to prevent bone loss are the selective estrogen receptor modulators (SERMs). Unlike ERT, these compounds have a positive effect on blood lipids, and pose no risk to breast and uterine tissue. SERMs, however, do not help increase bone density. Examples of SERMs currently used to prevent osteoporosis are evista, tamoxifen, and raloxifene.

Adequate Iron Intake

Iron is a key element of **hemoglobin** in blood. The RDA of iron for adult women is 15 mg per day (10 mg for men). According to a survey by the U.S. Department of Agriculture, 19- to 50-year-old women in the United States consumed only 60 percent of the RDA for iron. People who do not have enough iron in the body can develop iron-deficiency anemia, in which the concentration of hemoglobin in the red blood cells is lower than it should be.

Physically active women may also have a greater-than-average need for iron. Heavy training creates a demand for iron that is higher than the recommended intake because small amounts of iron are lost through sweat, urine, and stools. Mechanical trauma, caused by the pounding of the feet on the pavement during extensive jogging, may also lead to destruction of iron-containing red blood cells.

A large percentage of female endurance athletes are reported to have iron deficiency. The blood **ferritin** levels of women who participate in intense physical training should be checked frequently.

The rates of iron absorption and iron loss vary from person to person. In most cases, though, people can get enough iron by eating more iron-rich foods such as beans, peas, green leafy vegetables, enriched grain products, egg yolk, fish, and lean meats. Although organ meats, such as liver, are especially good sources, they also are high in cholesterol. A list of foods high in iron is given in Table 3.13.

Dietary Guidelines for Americans

In 2000 the Scientific Committee of the U.S. Department of Health and Human Services and the U.S. Department of Agriculture on diet and health issued the fifth edition of the Dietary Guidelines for healthy American adults and children. These guidelines—based on the available scientific research on nutrition and health and current dietary habits—can potentially reduce the risk of developing certain chronic diseases. The committee issued three goals that include 10 guidelines. These goals, listed here,

Table 3.13 Iron-Rich Foods

Food	Amount	Iron (mg)	Calories	Cholesterol	% Calories From Fat
Beans, red kidney, cooked	1 cup	3.2	218	0	4
Beef, ground lean (21% fat)	3 oz	2.1	237	86	57
Beef, sirloin, lean only	3 oz	2.9	171	76	36
Beef, liver, fried	3 oz	5.3	184	409	33
Beet, greens, cooked	½ cup	1.4	19	0	—
Broccoli, cooked, drained	1 cup	1.3	44	0	—
Burrito, bean (no cheese)	1	2.3	225	2	28
Egg, hard-cooked	1	.7	77	212	58
Farina (Cream of Wheat), cooked	½ cup	5.2	65	0	—
Instant breakfast, nonfat milk	1 cup	4.8	216	9	4
Peas, frozen, cooked, drained	½ cup	1.3	62	0	—
Shrimp, boiled	3 oz	2.7	87	172	10
Spinach, raw	1 cup	1.5	12	0	—
Vegetables, mixed, cooked	1 cup	1.5	108	0	—

have been defined as the ABC's for your health and that of your family.[30]

Goal 1: Aim for Fitness

- Aim for a healthy weight.
- Be physically active each day.

Following these two guidelines will help keep you and your family healthy and fit. Healthy eating and regular physical activity enable people of all ages to work productively, enjoy life, and feel their best. They also help children grow, develop, and do well in school.

Balance the food you eat with physical activity to maintain or improve your weight. Excessive body weight increases the risk for heart disease, stroke, diabetes, high blood pressure, and certain cancers. Many people gain weight as adults, and this can be avoided. To maintain body weight, you need to balance food intake with the amount of calories your body uses. Ensuing chapters present extensive information on weight management and exercise programs to help you balance your energy requirements according to your personal needs.

Goal 2: Build a Healthy Base

- Let the Food Pyramid guide your food choices.
- Choose a variety of grains daily, especially whole grains.
- Choose a variety of fruits and vegetables daily.
- Keep food safe to eat.

Following these four guidelines builds a base for healthy eating. Eat a variety of foods. No single food can provide all of the necessary nutrients and other beneficial substances in the amounts the body needs. Let the Food Guide Pyramid guide you so that you get the nutrients your body needs each day.

Make grains, fruits, and vegetables the foundation of your meals. They contain ample vitamins, minerals, complex carbohydrates, and other substances important to good health and have been shown to reduce your risk of certain chronic diseases. Most of your daily calories should come from these food products.

Within each food group, choose a variety of foods. Food items vary, and each item provides different combinations of nutrients and other substances needed for good health. Be flexible and adventurous—try new choices from these three groups in place of some less-nutritious or higher calorie foods you usually eat. Whatever you eat, always take steps to keep your food safe to eat.

DIETARY GUIDELINES FOR AMERICANS

Aim for Fitness . . .

- Aim for a healthy weight.
- Be physically active each day.

Build a Healthy Base . . .

- Let the Food Pyramid guide your food choices.
- Choose a variety of grains daily, especially whole grains.
- Choose a variety of fruits and vegetables daily.
- Keep food safe to eat.

Choose Sensibly . . .

- Choose a diet that is low in saturated fat and cholesterol and moderate in total fat.
- Choose beverages and foods to moderate your intake of sugars.
- Choose and prepare foods with less salt.
- If you drink alcoholic beverages, do so in moderation.

Goal 3: Choose Sensibly

- Choose a diet that is low in saturated fat and cholesterol and moderate in total fat.
- Choose beverages and foods to moderate your intake of sugars.
- Choose and prepare foods with less salt.
- If you drink alcoholic beverages, do so in moderation.

These four guidelines help you make sensible choices that promote health and reduce the risk of certain chronic diseases. You can enjoy all foods as part of a healthy diet, as long as you don't overdo it on fat (especially saturated fat), sugars, salt, and alcohol. Read labels to identify foods that are higher in saturated fats, sugars, and salt (sodium).

Choose a diet low in fat, saturated fat, and cholesterol. Reduce fat intake to 30 percent or (preferably) less of total calories. Reduce saturated fatty acid intake to less than 10 percent of total calories and intake of cholesterol to no more than 300 mg daily. Intake of fat and cholesterol can be lowered by substituting fish, poultry without skin, lean meats, and low-fat or nonfat dairy products for fatty meats and whole-milk dairy products; by

---

Hemoglobin Protein–iron compound in red blood cells that transports oxygen in the blood.

Ferritin Iron stored in the body.

choosing more vegetables, fruits, cereals, and legumes; and by limiting oils, fats, egg yolks, and fried and other fatty foods.

Choose a diet moderate in sugars. Excessive intake of sugar and starch can contribute to weight gain and tooth decay. This guideline advises against frequent and large consumption of food items and snacks high in sugar, which provide unnecessary calories and few nutrients. The more often that high-sugar foods are consumed, and the longer before brushing the teeth following their consumption, the greater the risk for tooth decay.

Choose a diet moderate in salt and sodium. Daily intake of salt (sodium chloride) should be 6 grams or less. This amount equals the 2,400 mg of sodium listed in the Daily Value of the food label. Sodium intake can be decreased by limiting the use of salt in cooking and not adding it to food at the table. Salty, highly processed, salt-preserved, and salt-pickled foods (such as bacon, olives, pickles, and lunch meats) should be consumed sparingly.

If you drink alcoholic beverages, do so in moderation. Alcoholic beverages provide calories but few or no nutrients. Moderate drinking has been linked to lower risk for coronary heart disease in some people. Excessive alcohol consumption leads to increased risk for heart disease, stroke, high blood pressure, certain cancers, cirrhosis of the liver, inflammation of the pancreas, brain damage, birth defects, accidents, violence, suicides, and malnutrition. Consumption should be limited to no more than one daily drink for women and two for men. In general, a 12-ounce bottle of beer, a 4-ounce glass of wine, and a 1.5-ounce shot of 80 proof liquor all contain the same amount of alcohol. Pregnant women should avoid alcoholic beverages altogether.

Proper Nutrition: A Lifetime Prescription for Healthy Living

The three factors that do the most for health, longevity, and quality of life are proper nutrition, a sound exercise program, and quitting (or never starting) smoking. Achieving and maintaining a balanced diet is not as difficult as most people would think. If parents did a better job of teaching and reinforcing proper nutrition habits in early youth, the current

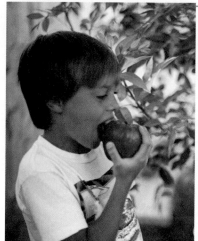

Positive nutrition habits should be taught and reinforced in early youth.

© Fitness & Wellness, Inc.

magnitude of nutrition-related health problems would be much smaller. Although treatment of obesity is important, we should place far greater emphasis on preventing obesity in youth and adults in the first place.

Children tend to eat the way their parents do. If parents adopt a healthy diet, children most likely will follow. The difficult part for most people is retraining themselves to follow a lifetime healthy nutrition plan—a diet that includes lots of grains, legumes, fruits, vegetables, and low-fat dairy products, with moderate use of animal protein, junk food, sodium, and alcohol.

In spite of the ample scientific evidence linking poor dietary habits to early disease and mortality rates, many people remain precontemplators: They are not willing to change their eating patterns. Even when faced with obesity, elevated blood lipids, hypertension, and other nutrition-related conditions, people do not change. The motivating factor to change one's eating habits seems to be a major health breakdown, such as a heart attack, a stroke, or cancer. By this time the damage has been done already. In many cases it is irreversible and, for some, fatal.

An ounce of prevention is worth a pound of cure. The sooner you implement the dietary guidelines presented in this chapter, the better your chances of preventing chronic diseases and reaching a higher state of wellness.

Web Interactive

- Dietary Guidelines from the Food and Nutrition Information Center. This site is very interesting, as it not only features the 2000 American Dietary guidelines, but also has links to historical dietary guidelines (since 1894) and dietary guidelines from 20 countries.

  http://www.nal.usda.gov/fnic/dga/index.html

- Five a Day Program. This excellent site, sponsored by the National Cancer Institute describes the national program to increase the consumption of fruits and vegetables. The site also features delicious low fat, low cholesterol recipes using fruits and vegetables.

  http://dccps.nci.nih.gov/5aday

- Dietary Supplements. Information from the Food and Drug Administration Center for Food Safety and Applied Nutrition.

  http://vm.cfsan.fda.gov/~dms/supplmnt.html

- CyberDiet's Eating Out Guidelines. Information on healthy food selections from the following cuisines: USA, France, India, Mexico, Italy, Thailand, Japan, China, and Greece.

  http://www.CyberDiet.com/foodfact/eatguide.html

Interactive Sites:

- The Cyberkitchen. This very interactive site, sponsored by Shape Up America, will show you how to balance your dietary intake with your physical activity to maintain healthy weight. You provide personal information regarding your age, gender, height, weight, and activity level and the Cyberkitchen provides you with a healthy diet plan to meet your goals (weight loss or weight gain). It's fun and educational.

  http://www.shapeup.org/kitchen/frameset1.htm

- Nutrition Quizzes. Take the vitamin quiz, safe food quiz, rate your diet quiz, or the "Fat or Fiction" Nutrition Action Fat Quiz. These tests are sponsored by the Center for Science in the Public Interest.

  http://www.cspinet.org/quiz

- The Interactive Food Guide Pyramid. Click on the different components of the Food Guide Pyramid to learn how to incorporate the proper nutrients into your daily diet.

  http://www.nal.usda.gov:8001/py/pmap.htm

- Fast Food Finder. You can select from a variety of fast food items from a variety of chain restaurants to discover the food's calories, fat content, cholesterol, sodium, and more. You can also preview selected books on nutrition.

  http://www.olen.com/food

- Ask the Dietitian. Have your many questions on nutrition answered by a registered dietitian. Some of the topics covered include fast food, vitamins, food supplements, diets, sports nutrition, children's nutrition, fiber and constipation, junk foods, food safety, food fallacies, drug-nutrient interactions, and others. There is a link providing tips on how to spot nutrition quackery.

  http://www.dietitian.com

Notes

1. *Surgeon General's Report on Nutrition and Health: Summary and Recommendations* (DHHS [PHS] Publication no. 88-50211) (Washington, DC: U.S. Government Printing Office, 1988).

2. E. B. Rimm, A. Ascherio, E. Giovannucci, D. Spiegelman, M. J. Stampfer, and W. C. Willett, "Vegetable, Fruit, and Cereal Fiber Intake and Risk of Coronary Heart Disease Among Men," *Journal of the American Medical Association* 275 (1996): 447–451.

3. "The Facts About Fats," *Consumer Reports on Health* (Boulder, CO: The Editors, March, 1997).

4. A. H. Lichtenstein, L. M. Ausman, S. M. Jalbert, and E. J. Schaefer, "Effects of Different Forms of Dietary Hydrogenated Fats on Serum Lipoprotein Cholesterol Levels," *The New England Journal of Medicine* 340 (1999): 1933–1940.

5. R. J. Barnard, "Effects of Lifestyle Modification on Serum Lipids," *Archives of Internal Medicine* 151 (1991): 1389–1394.

6. J. H. Weisburger and G. M. Williams, "Causes of Cancer," in *Textbook of Clinical Oncology*, edited by G. P. Murphy, W. Lawrence, Jr., and R.E. Lenhard, Sr. (Atlanta: American Cancer Society, 1995).

7. "Vitamin Report," *University of California at Berkeley Wellness Letter* (Palm Coast, FL: The Editors, October 1994).

8. "Antioxidants: Never Too Late," *University of California at Berkeley Wellness Letter* (Palm Coast, FL: The Editors, August 1994).

9. S. Kalish, "The Free Radical Radical: Kenneth Cooper, M.D., on Antioxidants and the Dangers of Hard Running," *Running Times* (March 1995): 16–17.

10. S. Yusunf et al., "Vitamin E Supplementation and Cardiovascular Events in High-Risk Patients," *The New England Journal of Medicine* 342 (2000): 154–160.

11. "Vitamin E: Have We Jumped the Gun?" *Tufts University Health & Nutrition Letter* (Palm Coast, FL, The Editors, January 2000).

12. "Vitamin C: We Still Take It, and So Should You," *University of California at Berkeley Wellness Letter* (Palm Coast, FL: The Editors, May 2000).

Continued

Notes (continued)

13. "Megadoses of Vitamin C," *Consumer Reports on Health* (Boulder, CO: The Editors, February 2000).

14. "Beta Carotene Pills: Should You Take Them?" *University of California at Berkeley Wellness Letter* 12, no. 7 (1996): 1–2.

15. L. C. Clark et al., "Effects of Selenium Supplementation for Cancer Prevention in Patients with Carcinoma of the Skin: A Randomized Controlled Trial," *Journal of the American Medical Association* 276 (1996): 1957–1963.

16. "Does This Mineral Prevent Cancer?" *University of California at Berkeley Wellness Letter* 16, no. 9 (2000): 1–2.

17. J. Carper, "Selenium: A Cancer Knockout?" *USA Weekend* (October 2–4, 1996): 8.

18. A. Weil, "Dr. Andrew Weil's Surprising Secrets of Optimum Health," *Bottom Line/Personal Health* 18, no. 13 (1997): 9–10.

19. See note 7.

20. C. J. Boushey, S. A. A. Beresford, G. S. Omenn, and A. G. Motulsky, "A Quantitative Assessment of Plasma Homocysteine as a Risk Factor for Vascular Disease," *Journal of the American Medical Association* 274 (1995): 1049–1057.

21. W. Castelli, "Smart Heart Strategies: Best Ways to Beat Heart Disease," *Bottom Line/Personal Health* 19, no. 4 (1998): 1–3.

22. "The Antioxidant All-Stars," *University of California at Berkeley Wellness Letter* (March 1997).

23. C. M. Hasler, "How to Use the 'New 'Functional Foods,' What Works . . . What Doesn't Work," *Bottom Line/Personal Health* (April 2000).

24. "Genetically Modified Foods: What You Should Know," *Self-Healing* (June 2000).

25. Pacific Medical Center, *Nutrition, Exercise, and Bone Health* (Seattle: PMC, 1990).

26. "Preventing Osteoporosis," *Health News* 4, no. 3 (1998): 1–2.

27. B. L. Drinkwater, "Osteoporosis and the Female Masters Athlete," in *Sports Medicine for the Mature Athlete*, ed. J. R. Sutton and R. M. Brock (Carmel, IN: Benchmark Press, 1986): 353–359.

28. K. H. Myburgh, L. K. Bachrach, B. Lewis, K. Kent, and R. Marcus, "Low Bone Mineral Density at Axial and Appendicular Sites in Amenorrheic Athletes," *Medicine and Science in Sports and Exercise* 25, no. 11 (1993): 1197–1202.

29. "Will this Drug Prevent Osteoporosis?" *University of California at Berkeley Wellness Letter* 14, no. 9 (1998): 1–2.

30. U.S. Department of Health and Human Services, Department of Agriculture. *Nutrition and Your Health: Dietary Guidelines for Americans*. Home and Garden Bulletin No. 232, (Washington, DC: DHHS, 2000).

Suggested Readings

Coleman, E. *Eating for Endurance*. Palo Alto, CA: Bull Publishing, 1997.

Drinkwater, B. L. "Does Physical Activity Play a Role in Preventing Osteoporosis?" *Research Quarterly for Exercise and Sport* 65 (1994): 197–206.

Hoeger, W. W. K., and S. A. Hoeger. *Lifetime Physical Fitness and Wellness*. Belmont, CA: Wadsworth/ Thompson Learning, 1999.

McArdle, W. D., F. I. Katch, and V. L. Katch. *Sports & Exercise Nutrition*. Baltimore: Lippincott Williams & Wilkins, 1999.

National Academy of Sciences, Institute of Medicine. *Dietary Reference Intakes*. Washington, DC: National Academy Press, 1998.

National Academy of Sciences, Institute of Medicine. *Eat for Life: The Food and Nutrition Board's Guide to Reducing Your Risk of Chronic Disease*. Edited by C. E. Woteki and P. R. Thomas. Washington, DC: National Academy Press, 1992.

Volek, J. S. "Creatine Supplementation and Its Possible Role in Improving Physical Performance." *ACSM's Health & Fitness Journal* 1, no. 4, (1997): 23–29.

Whitney, E. N., and S. R. Rolfes. *Understanding Nutrition*. St. Paul: West Publishing, 1996.

Wardlaw, G. M. *Contemporary Nutrition: Issues and Insights*. Boston: McGraw Hill, 2000.

Williams, M. H., R. B. Kreider, and J. D. Branch. *Creatine: The Power Supplement*. Champaign, IL: Human Kinetics, 1999.

Wynder, E. L., J. H. Weisburger, and S. K. Ng. "Nutrition: The Need to Define 'Optimal' Intake as a Basis for Public Policy Decisions." *American Journal of Public Health* 82 (1992): 346–350.

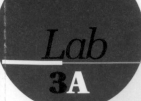

Lab 3A

NUTRIENT ANALYSIS

Name:

Date:

Grade:

Instructor:

Course:

Section:

Necessary Lab Equipment

List of "Nutritive Value of Selected Foods," Appendix A. An IBM-PC or Macintosh computer, if the computer software for use with this book is used. Otherwise, only a small calculator is needed.

Objective

To evaluate your present diet using the Recommended Dietary Allowances (RDA).

Instructions

To conduct the following nutritional analysis, you need a record of all foods eaten during a 3-day period (use the list of "Nutritive Value of Selected Foods" given in Appendix A). Record this information prior to this lab session in the forms provided in Figure 3A.1 of this lab. After recording the nutritive values for each day, add up the values in each column and record the totals at the bottom of the form. During your lab, proceed to compute an average for the 3 days. The percentages for carbohydrates, fat, saturated fat, and the protein requirements can be computed by using the instructions at the bottom of Figure 3A.2. The results can then be compared against the Recommended Dietary Allowances.

The analysis can be simplified by using the computer software for this lab. Up to 7 days may be analyzed when using the software, and Figure 3A.3 should be used instead of 3A.1. Further, you have to record only the amount of servings eaten for each food (.5 for half a serving, 2 for twice the standard serving, and so forth).

Figure 3A.1   Daily nutrient intake.

Date: _____

Foods	Amount	Calories	Protein (gm)	Fat (total gm)	Sat. Fat (gm)	Cholesterol (mg)	Carbohydrates (gm)	Calcium (mg)	Iron (mg)	Sodium (mg)	Vit. A (IU)	Vit. B_1 (mg)	Vit. B_2 (mg)	Niacin (mg)	Vit. C (mg)
Totals															

Figure 3A.2 Daily nutrient intake.

Day	Calories	Protein (gm)	Fat (gm)	Sat. Fat (gm)	Chol-esterol (mg)	Carbo-hydrates (gm)	Calcium (mg)	Iron (mg)	Sodium (mg)	Vit. A (µg RE)	Thiamin Vit. B_1 (mg)	Riboflavin Vit. B_2 (mg)	Niacin (mg)	Vit. C (mg)
One														
Two														
Three														
Totals														
Average[a]														
Percentages[b]														

Recommended Dietary Allowances*

	Calories	Protein	Fat	Sat. Fat	Chol-esterol (mg)	Carbo-hydrates	Calcium (mg)	Iron (mg)	Sodium (mg)	Vit. A (µg RE)	Thiamin Vit. B_1 (mg)	Riboflavin Vit. B_2 (mg)	Niacin (mg)	Vit. C (mg)
Men 14–18 yrs.	See below[c]	See below[d]	<30%[e]	<10%[e]	<300[e]	>58%[e]	1,300	12	2,400[e]	1,000	1.2	1.3	16	75
19–30 yrs.			<30%[e]	<10%[e]	<300[e]	>58%[e]	1,000	10	2,400[e]	1,000	1.2	1.3	16	90
31–50 yrs.			<30%[e]	<10%[e]	<300[e]	>58%[e]	1,000	10	2,400[e]	1,000	1.2	1.3	16	90
51+ yrs.			<30%[e]	<10%[e]	<300[e]	>58%[e]	1,200	10	2,400[e]	1,000	1.2	1.3	16	90
Women 14–18 yrs.			<30%[e]	<10%[e]	<300[e]	>58%[e]	1,300	15	2,400[e]	800	1.0	1.0	14	65
19–30 yrs.			<30%[e]	<10%[e]	<300[e]	>58%[e]	1,000	15	2,400[e]	800	1.1	1.1	14	75
31–50 yrs.			<30%[e]	<10%[e]	<300[e]	>58%[e]	1,000	15	2,400[e]	800	1.1	1.1	14	75
51+ yrs.			<30%[e]	<10%[e]	<300[e]	>58%[e]	1,200	10	2,400[e]	800	1.1	1.1	14	75
Pregnant			<30%[e]	<10%[e]	<300[e]	>58%[e]	1,200	30	2,400[e]	800	1.4	1.4	18	75
Lactating			<30%[e]	<10%[e]	<300[e]	>58%[e]	1,200	15	2,400[e]	1,300	1.5	1.5	17	95

[a]Divide totals by 3 or number of days assessed.

[b]Percentages: Protein and carbohydrates = multiply average by 4, divide by average calories, and multiply by 100.
Fat and saturated fat = multiply average by 9, divide by average calories, and multiply by 100.

[c]Use Table 5.2 (Page 125) for all categories.

[d]Protein intake should be .8 grams per kilogram of body weight. Pregnant women should consume an additional 15 grams of daily protein, and lactating women should have an extra 20 grams.

[e]Based on recommendations by nutrition experts.

Source: Adapted from *Recommended Dietary Allowances*, © 1989, by the National Academy of Sciences, National Academy Press, Washington, DC.

Figure 3A.3   **Daily nutrient intake form for computer software use.**

Name: _____   Date: _____

Gender: ☐ Male   ☐ Female   ☐ Pregnant   ☐ Nursing

Activity: ☐ Sedentary   ☐ Lightly active   ☐ Moderately active   ☐ Very active   ☐ Extremely active

Height: _____ ft _____ in   Weight: _____ lbs   Age _____

Student ID #: _____   Instructor's Name: _____

Class Days: _____   Class Times: _____

No.	Item	Amount
1		
2		
3		
4		
5		
6		
7		
8		
9		
10		
11		
12		
13		
14		
15		
16		
17		
18		
19		
20		
21		
22		
23		
24		
25		
26		
27		
28		
29		
30		
31		

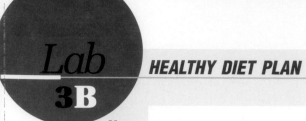

HEALTHY DIET PLAN

Homework Assignment

Name: _____   Date: _____   Grade: _____

Instructor: _____   Course: _____   Section: _____

Assignment

This laboratory experience should be carried out as a homework assignment to be completed over the next 7 days.

Objective

To meet the minimum daily required servings of the basic food groups and monitor total daily fat intake.

Lab Resources

"Food Guide Pyramid" (Figure 3.1, page 47) and list of "Nutritive Value of Selected Foods" (Appendix A).

I. Instructions

Keep a 7-day record of your food consumption using the Food Guide Pyramid and the form given in Figure 3B.1 (make additional copies of this form as needed—at least 3 days are recommended). Whenever you have something to eat, record the food from the Nutritive Value of Selected Foods list contained in Appendix A, the number of calories, grams of fat, and the servings in the corresponding spaces provided for each food group. If a food item is not listed in the Nutritive Value of Selected Foods list, the information can be obtained from the food container itself.

Record all information immediately after each meal, because it will be easier to keep track of foods and amounts eaten. If twice the amount of a particular serving is eaten, the calories and grams of fat must be doubled and two servings should be recorded under the respective food group.

At the end of the day, evaluate the diet by checking whether the minimum required servings for each food group were met, and by the total amount of fat consumed. If you meet the required servings, you are well on your way to achieving a well-balanced diet. In addition, fat intake should not exceed 30 percent of the total daily caloric consumption. If you are on a diet, you may want to reduce fat intake to less than 20 percent of total daily calories (see Table 5.4, page 127)

II. Nutrition Stage of Change

Using Figure 2.3 (page 40) and Table 2.3 (page 41) identify your current stage of change for nutrition (healthy diet):

_____

III. What I Learned and What I Can Do to Improve My Nutrition:

Based on the nutrient analysis conducted in Lab 3A and your daily diet analysis conducted in this lab, explain what these experiences have taught you and list specific changes and strategies that you can use to improve your present nutrition habits. Use an extra blank sheet of paper as needed.

I have learned the following about myself/my current diet: _____

_____

_____

Specific changes I plan to make: _____

_____

_____

Strategies I will use: _____

_____

_____

Daily diet record form.

Name:

No.	Food*	Amount	Calories	Fat (gm)	Food Groups (servings)				
					Bread, Cereal, Rice, and Pasta	Vegetable	Fruit	Milk, Yogurt, and Cheese	Meat, Poultry, Fish, Dry Beans, Eggs, and Nuts
1									
2									
3									
4									
5									
6									
7									
8									
9									
10									
11									
12									
13									
14									
15									
16									
17									
18									
19									
20									
21									
22									
23									
24									
25									
26									
27									
28									
29									
30									
Totals									
Recommended Amount*			**	***	6-11	3-5	2-4	2-3	2-3
Deficiencies*									

*See "List of Nutritive Value of Selected Foods" in Appendix A.

**Compute using Table 5.1, page 115.

***Multiply the recommended amount of calories by .30 (30%) and divide by 9 to obtain the recommended amount of grams of fat (if on a diet, multiply by .20 or .10—see Table 5.4, page 127).

Chapter 4

Body Composition Assessment

Objectives

- Define body composition and understand its relationship to recommended body weight assessment.

- Identify the difference between essential and storage fat.

- Explain various techniques used to assess body composition.

- Be able to assess body composition using the skinfold thickness technique.

- Be able to assess body composition using the girth measurements technique.

- Understand the importance of waist-to-hip ratio and body mass index (BMI).

- Be able to determine recommended weight according to recommended percent body fat values.

Body composition consists of fat and nonfat components. The fat component is usually called fat mass or **percent body fat**. The nonfat component is termed **lean body mass**.

For many years people relied on simple height/weight charts to determine their recommended body weight. We know, however, that these tables can be highly inaccurate and fail to identify critical fat values associated with higher risk for disease. The proper way to determine recommended weight is to find out what percent of total body weight is fat and what amount is lean tissue—in other words, to determine body composition.

Once the fat percentage is known, **recommended body weight** can be calculated from recommended body fat. Recommended body weight, also called "healthy weight," implies the absence of any medical condition that would improve with weight loss and a fat distribution pattern that is not associated with higher risk for illness.

> *To determine whether people are truly overweight or falsely at recommended body weight, body composition must be established.*

Although various techniques for determining percent body fat were developed several years ago, many people still are unaware of these procedures and continue to depend on height/weight charts to find out their recommended body weight. Unfortunately, the standard height/weight tables, first published in 1912, were based on average weights (including shoes and clothing) for men and women who obtained life insurance policies between 1888 and 1905: a notably unrepresentative population. The recommended body weight on these tables is obtained according to sex, height, and frame size. Because no scientific guidelines are given to determine frame size, most people choose their frame size based on the column in which the weight comes closest to their own!

To determine whether people are truly **overweight** or falsely at recommended body weight, body composition must be established. **Obesity** is an excess of body fat. If body weight is the only criterion, an individual may easily appear overweight according to height/weight charts, yet not have too much body fat. Football players, body builders, weight lifters, and other athletes with large muscle size are typical examples. Some athletes who appear to be 20 or 30 pounds overweight really have little body fat.

The inaccuracy of height/weight charts was illustrated clearly when a young man who weighed about 225 pounds applied to join a city police force, but was turned down without having been granted an interview. The reason? He was "too fat," according to the height/weight charts. When this young man's body composition later was assessed at a preventive medicine clinic, he was shocked to find that only 5 percent of his total body weight was in the form of fat—considerably lower than the recommended standard. In the words of the technical director of the clinic, "The only way this fellow could come down to the chart's target weight would have been through surgical removal of a large amount of his muscle tissue."

At the other end of the spectrum, some people who weigh very little (and may be viewed as skinny or underweight) can actually be classified as obese because of their high body fat content. People who weigh as little as 100 pounds but are more than 35 percent fat (about one-third of their total body weight) are not uncommon. These cases are found more readily in the sedentary population and among people who are always dieting. Physical inactivity and a constant negative caloric balance both lead to a loss in lean body mass (see Chapter 5). These examples illustrate that body weight alone clearly does not tell the whole story.

Essential and Storage Fat

Total fat in the human body is classified into two types: essential fat and storage fat. **Essential fat** is needed for normal physiological function. Without it, human health deteriorates. This type of fat is found within tissues such as muscles, nerve cells, bone marrow, intestines, heart, liver, and lungs. This essential fat constitutes about 3 percent of the total weight in men and 12 percent in women (see Figure 4.1). The percentage is higher in women because it includes sex-specific fat, such as that found in the breast tissue, the uterus, and other sex-related fat deposits.

Storage fat is the fat stored in adipose tissue, mostly just beneath the skin (subcutaneous fat) and around major organs in the body. This fat serves three basic functions:

1. As an insulator to retain body heat.
2. As energy substrate for metabolism.
3. As padding against physical trauma to the body.

The amount of storage fat does not differ between men and women, except that men tend to store fat around the waist and women around the hips and thighs.

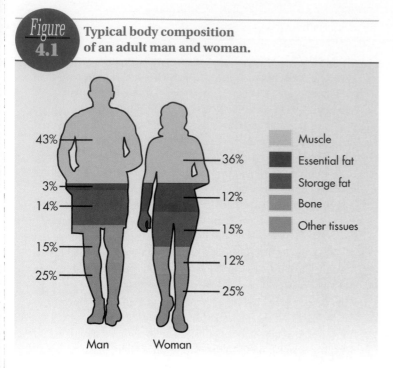

Figure 4.1 Typical body composition of an adult man and woman.

Man: 43%, 3%, 14%, 15%, 25%

Woman: 36%, 12%, 15%, 12%, 25%

Legend:
- Muscle
- Essential fat
- Storage fat
- Bone
- Other tissues

Man   Woman

Techniques to Assess Body Composition

Body composition can be assessed through several procedures. The most common techniques are: (a) hydrostatic or underwater weighing, (b) skinfold thickness, (c) girth measurements, (d) bioelectrical impedance, and (e) air displacement. Because these procedures yield only estimates of body fat, each technique may yield slightly different values. Therefore, when assessing changes in body composition, the same technique should be used for pre- and post-test comparisons.

More sophisticated techniques to assess body composition are presently available, but the equipment is costly and not readily accessible to the general population. These procedures are used primarily in research and medical facilities. In addition to lean tissue and body fat, some of these newer methods also provide information on total body water and bone mass. Among these techniques are magnetic resonance imaging (MRI), dual energy X-ray absorptiometry (DEXA), computed tomography (CT), and total body electrical conductivity (TOBEC). In terms of predicting percent body fat, they do not appear to be more accurate than hydrostatic weighing.

Hydrostatic Weighing

Hydrostatic weighing has been used for decades as the "standard" for determining body composition

in exercise laboratories. In essence, a person's "regular" weight is compared to a weight taken underwater. Because fat is more buoyant than lean tissue, comparing the two weights can be used to determine a person's percent of fat. Almost all other techniques are validated against hydrostatic weighing. It is the most accurate technique if it is done properly and if the individual is able to perform the test adequately. The procedure requires a considerable amount of time, skill, space, and equipment and must be administered by a well-trained technician.

This technique has several drawbacks: Because each individual assessment can take as long as 30 minutes, hydrostatic weighing is not feasible when testing a lot of people. Furthermore, the person's residual lung volume (amount of air left in the lungs following complete forceful exhalation) should be measured before testing. If residual volume cannot be measured, as is the case in many laboratories and health/fitness centers, it must be estimated using the predicting equations—which may decrease the accuracy of hydrostatic weighing. Also, the requirement of being completely underwater makes hydrostatic weighing difficult to administer to **aquaphobic** people.

As described in Figure 4.2 and in Lab 4A, for each reading, the person has to (a) force out all of the air in the lungs, (b) lean forward and completely submerge in a sitting position for about 5 to 10 seconds (long enough to take a reading on the scale), and (c) remain as calm as possible (chair

---

Body composition The fat and nonfat components of the human body; important in assessing recommended body weight.

Percent body fat Proportional amount of fat in the body based on the person's total weight; includes both essential and storage fat.

Lean body mass Body weight without body fat.

Recommended body weight Body weight at which there seems to be no harm to human health; healthy weight.

Overweight An excess amount of weight against a given standard, such as height or recommended percent body fat.

Obesity An excessive accumulation of body fat, usually at least 30 percent above recommended body weight.

Essential fat Minimal amount of body fat needed for normal physiological functions; constitutes about 3 percent of total weight in men and 12 percent in women.

Storage fat Body fat in excess of essential fat; stored in adipose tissue.

Hydrostatic weighing Underwater technique to assess body composition; considered the most accurate of the body composition assessment techniques.

Aquaphobic Having a fear of water.

Figure 4.2   Hydrostatic weighing procedure.

A small tank or pool, an autopsy scale, and a submersible chair are needed. The scale should measure up to about 10 kilograms (kg) and should be readable to the nearest .01 kilogram. The chair is suspended from the scale and submerged in a tank of water or pool measuring at least 5 × 5 × 5 feet. A swimming pool can be used in place of the tank.

The procedure for the technician is

1. Ask the person to be weighed to fast for approximately 6 to 8 hours and to have a bladder and bowel movement prior to underwater weighing.

2. Measure the individual's residual lung volume (RV, or amount of air left in the lungs following complete exhalation). If no equipment (spirometer) is available to measure the residual volume, estimate it using the following predicting equations* (to convert inches to centimeters, multiply inches by 2.54):

Men: RV = [(0.027 × height in centimeters) + (0.017 × age)] − 3.447

Women: RV = [(0.032 × height in centimeters) + (0.009 × age)] − 3.9

3. Have the person remove all jewelry prior to weighing. Weigh the person on land in a swimsuit and subtract the weight of the suit. Convert the weight from pounds to kilograms (divide pounds by 2.2046).

4. Record the water temperature in the tank in degrees Centigrade. Use that temperature to obtain the water density factor provided below, which is required in the formula to compute body density.

Temp (°C)	Water Density (gr/ml)	Temp (°C)	Water Density (gr/ml)
28	0.99626	35	0.99406
29	0.99595	36	0.99371
30	0.99567	37	0.99336
31	0.99537	38	0.99299
32	0.99505	39	0.99262
33	0.99473	40	0.99224
34	0.99440		

5. After the person is dressed in the swimsuit, have him or her enter the tank and completely wipe off all air clinging to the skin. Have the person sit in the chair with the water at chin level (raise or lower the chair as needed). Make sure the water and scale remain as still as possible during the entire procedure, because this allows for a more accurate reading. (During underwater weighing, you can decrease scale movement by holding and slowly releasing the neck of the scale until the subject is floating freely in the water.)

6. Place a clip on the person's nose and have him or her forcefully exhale all of the air out of the lungs. The individual then totally submerges underwater. Make sure that all the air is exhaled from the lungs prior to submerging. Record the reading on the scale. Repeat this procedure 8 to 10 times, because practice and experience increases the accuracy of the underwater weight. Use the average of the three heaviest underwater weights as the gross underwater weight.

7. Because tare weight (the weight of the chair and chain or rope used to suspend the chair) accounts for part of the gross underwater weight, subtract this weight to obtain the person's net underwater weight. To determine tare weight, place a clothespin on the chain or rope at the water level when the person is submerged completely. After the person comes out of the water, lower the chair into the water to the pin level. Now record tare weight. Determine the net underwater weight by subtracting the tare weight from the gross underwater weight.

8. Compute body density and percent fat using the following equations:

$$\text{Body density} = \frac{BW}{\dfrac{BW - UW}{WD} - RV - .1}$$

$$\text{Percent fat**} = \frac{495}{BD} - 450$$

WHERE:

BW = body weight in kg

UW = net underwater weight

WD = water density (determined by water temperature)

RV = residual volume

BD = body density

A sample computation for body fat assessment according to hydrostatic weighing is provided in Lab 4A.

---

* From: H. L. Goldman and M. R. Becklake, "Respiratory Function Tests: Normal Values at Medium Altitudes and the Prediction of Normal Results," in *American Review of Tuberculosis* 79 (1959): 457–467.

** From W. E. Siri, *Body Composition from Fluid Spaces and Density*, (Berkeley, CA: University of California, Donner Laboratory of Medical Physics, March 19, 1956).

---

movement makes reading the scale difficult). This procedure has to be repeated 8 to 10 times.

Forcing all of the air out of the lungs is not easy for everyone, but is important for an accurate reading: Leaving additional air (beyond residual volume) in the lungs makes a person more buoyant. Because fat is less dense than water, overweight individuals weigh less in water. Additional air in the lungs makes a person lighter in water, yielding a false higher body fat percentage.

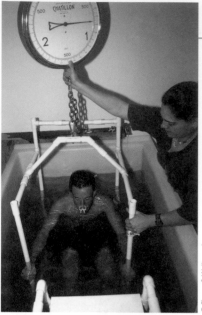

Hydrostatic weighing technique.

Because of the cost, time, and complexity of hydrostatic weighing, most health and fitness programs prefer **anthropometric measurement techniques**, which correlate quite well with hydrostatic weighing. These techniques, primarily skinfold thickness and girth measurements, allow quick, simple, and inexpensive estimates of body composition.

Skinfold Thickness

Assessing body composition using **skinfold thickness** is based on the principle that approximately half of the body's fatty tissue is directly beneath the skin. Valid and reliable measurements of this tissue give a good indication of percent body fat.

The skinfold test is done with the aid of pressure calipers. Several sites must be measured to reflect the total percentage of fat: triceps, suprailium, and thigh skinfolds for women; and chest, abdomen, and thigh for men (see Figure 4.3). All measurements should be taken on the right side of the body.

Even with the skinfold technique, training is necessary to obtain accurate measurements. Additionally, different technicians may produce slightly different measurements of the same person. Therefore, the same technician should take pre- and post-test measurements.

Figure 4.3 Anatomical landmarks for skinfold measurements.

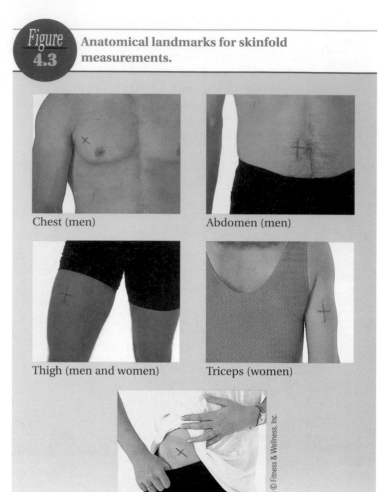

Chest (men)

Abdomen (men)

Thigh (men and women)

Triceps (women)

Suprailium (women)

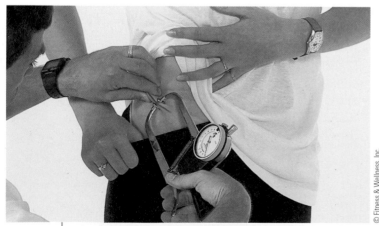

Skinfold thickness technique.

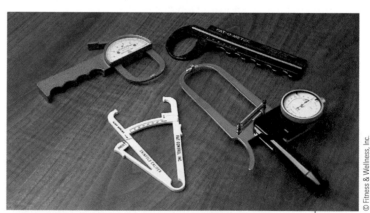

Various types of skinfold calipers used to assess skinfold thickness.

Anthropometric techniques Measurement of body girths at different sites.

Skinfold thickness Technique to assess body composition by measuring a double thickness of skin at specific body sites.

Measurements should be done at the same time of the day—preferably in the morning, because changes in water hydration from activity and exercise can affect skinfold girth. The procedure is given in Figure 4.4. If skinfold calipers are available to you, you may assess your percent body fat with the help of your instructor or an experienced technician (also see Lab 4B). Then locate the percent fat estimates on the appropriate Table 4.1, 4.2, or 4.3.

Figure 4.4 Procedure for body fat assessment using skinfold thickness technique.

1. Select the proper anatomical sites. For men, use chest, abdomen, and thigh skinfolds. For women, use triceps, suprailium, and thigh skinfolds. Take all measurements on the right side of the body with the person standing. The correct anatomical landmarks for skinfolds are

   Chest: a diagonal fold halfway between the shoulder crease and the nipple.

   Abdomen: a vertical fold taken about one inch to the right of the umbilicus.

   Triceps: a vertical fold on the back of the upper arm, halfway between the shoulder and the elbow.

   Thigh: a vertical fold on the front of the thigh, midway between the knee and the hip.

   Suprailium: a diagonal fold above the crest of the ilium (on the side of the hip).

2. Measure each site by grasping a double thickness of skin firmly with the thumb and forefinger, pulling the fold slightly away from the muscular tissue. Hold the calipers perpendicular to the fold and take the measurement ½ inch below the finger hold. Measure each site three times and read the values to the nearest .1 to .5 mm. Record the average of the two closest readings as the final value. Take the readings without delay to avoid excessive compression of the skinfold. Releasing and refolding the skinfold is required between readings.

3. When doing pre- and post-assessments, conduct the measurement at the same time of day. The best time is early in the morning to avoid hydration changes resulting from activity or exercise.

4. Obtain percent fat by adding the three skinfold measurements and looking up the respective values on Table 4.1 for women, Table 4.2 for men under age 40, and Table 4.3 for men over 40.

For example, if the skinfold measurements for an 18-year-old female are (a) triceps = 16, (b) suprailium = 4, and (c) thigh = 30 (total = 50), the percent body fat is 20.6%

Table 4.1 Skinfold Thickness Technique: Percent Fat Estimates for Women Calculated from Triceps, Suprailium, and Thigh

Sum of 3 Skinfolds	Age at Last Birthday								
	22 or Under	23 to 27	28 to 32	33 to 37	38 to 42	43 to 47	48 to 52	53 to 57	58 and Over
23– 25	9.7	9.9	10.2	10.4	10.7	10.9	11.2	11.4	11.7
26– 28	11.0	11.2	11.5	11.7	12.0	12.3	12.5	12.7	13.0
29– 31	12.3	12.5	12.8	13.0	13.3	13.5	13.8	14.0	14.3
32– 34	13.6	13.8	14.0	14.3	14.5	14.8	15.0	15.3	15.5
35– 37	14.8	15.0	15.3	15.5	15.8	16.0	16.3	16.5	16.8
38– 40	16.0	16.3	16.5	16.7	17.0	17.2	17.5	17.7	18.0
41– 43	17.2	17.4	17.7	17.9	18.2	18.4	18.7	18.9	19.2
44– 46	18.3	18.6	18.8	19.1	19.3	19.6	19.8	20.1	20.3
47– 49	19.5	19.7	20.0	20.2	20.5	20.7	21.0	21.2	21.5
50– 52	20.6	20.8	21.1	21.3	21.6	21.8	22.1	22.3	22.6
53– 55	21.7	21.9	22.1	22.4	22.6	22.9	23.1	23.4	23.6
56– 58	22.7	23.0	23.2	23.4	23.7	23.9	24.2	24.4	24.7
59– 61	23.7	24.0	24.2	24.5	24.7	25.0	25.2	25.5	25.7
62– 64	24.7	25.0	25.2	25.5	25.7	26.0	26.2	26.4	26.7
65– 67	25.7	25.9	26.2	26.4	26.7	26.9	27.2	27.4	27.7
68– 70	26.6	26.9	27.1	27.4	27.6	27.9	28.1	28.4	28.6
71– 73	27.5	27.8	28.0	28.3	28.5	28.8	29.0	29.3	29.5
74– 76	28.4	28.7	28.9	29.2	29.4	29.7	29.9	30.2	30.4
77– 79	29.3	29.5	29.8	30.0	30.3	30.5	30.8	31.0	31.3
80– 82	30.1	30.4	30.6	30.9	31.1	31.4	31.6	31.9	32.1
83– 85	30.9	31.2	31.4	31.7	31.9	32.2	32.4	32.7	32.9
86– 88	31.7	32.0	32.2	32.5	32.7	32.9	33.2	33.4	33.7
89– 91	32.5	32.7	33.0	33.2	33.5	33.7	33.9	34.2	34.4
92– 94	33.2	33.4	33.7	33.9	34.2	34.4	34.7	34.9	35.2
95– 97	33.9	34.1	34.4	34.6	34.9	35.1	35.4	35.6	35.9
98–100	34.6	34.8	35.1	35.3	35.5	35.8	36.0	36.3	36.5
101–103	35.2	35.4	35.7	35.9	36.2	36.4	36.7	36.9	37.2
104–106	35.8	36.1	36.3	36.6	36.8	37.1	37.3	37.5	37.8
107–109	36.4	36.7	36.9	37.1	37.4	37.6	37.9	38.1	38.4
110–112	37.0	37.2	37.5	37.7	38.0	38.2	38.5	38.7	38.9
113–115	37.5	37.8	38.0	38.2	38.5	38.7	39.0	39.2	39.5
116–118	38.0	38.3	38.5	38.8	39.0	39.3	39.5	39.7	40.0
119–121	38.5	38.7	39.0	39.2	39.5	39.7	40.0	40.2	40.5
122–124	39.0	39.2	39.4	39.7	39.9	40.2	40.4	40.7	40.9
125–127	39.4	39.6	39.9	40.1	40.4	40.6	40.9	41.1	41.4
128–130	39.8	40.0	40.3	40.5	40.8	41.0	41.3	41.5	41.8

Body density is calculated based on the generalized equation for predicting body density of women developed by A. S. Jackson, M. L. Pollock, and A. Ward and published in *Medicine and Science in Sports and Exercise* 12 (1980): 175–182. Percent body fat is determined from the calculated body density using the Siri formula.

Table 4.2 — Skinfold Thickness Technique: Percent Fat Estimates for Men Under 40 Calculated from Chest, Abdomen, and Thigh

Sum of 3 Skinfolds	Age at Last Birthday							
	19 or Under	20 to 22	23 to 25	26 to 28	29 to 31	32 to 34	35 to 37	38 to 40
8– 10	.9	1.3	1.6	2.0	2.3	2.7	3.0	3.3
11– 13	1.9	2.3	2.6	3.0	3.3	3.7	4.0	4.3
14– 16	2.9	3.3	3.6	3.9	4.3	4.6	5.0	5.3
17– 19	3.9	4.2	4.6	4.9	5.3	5.6	6.0	6.3
20– 22	4.8	5.2	5.5	5.9	6.2	6.6	6.9	7.3
23– 25	5.8	6.2	6.5	6.8	7.2	7.5	7.9	8.2
26– 28	6.8	7.1	7.5	7.8	8.1	8.5	8.8	9.2
29– 31	7.7	8.0	8.4	8.7	9.1	9.4	9.8	10.1
32– 34	8.6	9.0	9.3	9.7	10.0	10.4	10.7	11.1
35– 37	9.5	9.9	10.2	10.6	10.9	11.3	11.6	12.0
38– 40	10.5	10.8	11.2	11.5	11.8	12.2	12.5	12.9
41– 43	11.4	11.7	12.1	12.4	12.7	13.1	13.4	13.8
44– 46	12.2	12.6	12.9	13.3	13.6	14.0	14.3	14.7
47– 49	13.1	13.5	13.8	14.2	14.5	14.9	15.2	15.5
50– 52	14.0	14.3	14.7	15.0	15.4	15.7	16.1	16.4
53– 55	14.8	15.2	15.5	15.9	16.2	16.6	16.9	17.3
56– 58	15.7	16.0	16.4	16.7	17.1	17.4	17.8	18.1
59– 61	16.5	16.9	17.2	17.6	17.9	18.3	18.6	19.0
62– 64	17.4	17.7	18.1	18.4	18.8	19.1	19.4	19.8
65– 67	18.2	18.5	18.9	19.2	19.6	19.9	20.3	20.6
68– 70	19.0	19.3	19.7	20.0	20.4	20.7	21.1	21.4
71– 73	19.8	20.1	20.5	20.8	21.2	21.5	21.9	22.2
74– 76	20.6	20.9	21.3	21.6	22.0	22.2	22.7	23.0
77– 79	21.4	21.7	22.1	22.4	22.8	23.1	23.4	23.8
80– 82	22.1	22.5	22.8	23.2	23.5	23.9	24.2	24.6
83– 85	22.9	23.2	23.6	23.9	24.3	24.6	25.0	25.3
86– 88	23.6	24.0	24.3	24.7	25.0	25.4	25.7	26.1
89– 91	24.4	24.7	25.1	25.4	25.8	26.1	26.5	26.8
92– 94	25.1	25.5	25.8	26.2	26.5	26.9	27.2	27.5
95– 97	25.8	26.2	26.5	26.9	27.2	27.6	27.9	28.3
98–100	26.6	26.9	27.3	27.6	27.9	28.3	28.6	29.0
101–103	27.3	27.6	28.0	28.3	28.6	29.0	29.3	29.7
104–106	27.9	28.3	28.6	29.0	29.3	29.7	30.0	30.4
107–109	28.6	29.0	29.3	29.7	30.0	30.4	30.7	31.1
110–112	29.3	29.6	30.0	30.3	30.7	31.0	31.4	31.7
113–115	30.0	30.3	30.7	31.0	31.3	31.7	32.0	32.4
116–118	30.6	31.0	31.3	31.6	32.0	32.3	32.7	33.0
119–121	31.3	31.6	32.0	32.3	32.6	33.0	33.3	33.7
122–124	31.9	32.2	32.6	32.9	33.3	33.6	34.0	34.3
125–127	32.5	32.9	33.2	33.5	33.9	34.2	34.6	34.9
128–130	33.1	33.5	33.8	34.2	34.5	34.9	35.2	35.5

Body density is calculated based on the generalized equation for predicting body density of men developed by A. S. Jackson and M. L. Pollock and published in the *British Journal of Nutrition* 40 (1978): 497–504. Percent body fat is determined from the calculated body density using the Siri formula.

Table 4.3 — Skinfold Thickness Technique: Percent Fat Estimates for Men Over 40 Calculated from Chest, Abdomen, and Thigh

Sum of 3 Skinfolds	Age at Last Birthday							
	41 to 43	44 to 46	47 to 49	50 to 52	53 to 55	56 to 58	59 to 61	62 and Over
8– 10	3.7	4.0	4.4	4.7	5.1	5.4	5.8	6.1
11– 13	4.7	5.0	5.4	5.7	6.1	6.4	6.8	7.1
14– 16	5.7	6.0	6.4	6.7	7.1	7.4	7.8	8.1
17– 19	6.7	7.0	7.4	7.7	8.1	8.4	8.7	9.1
20– 22	7.6	8.0	8.3	8.7	9.0	9.4	9.7	10.1
23– 25	8.6	8.9	9.3	9.6	10.0	10.3	10.7	11.0
26– 28	9.5	9.9	10.2	10.6	10.9	11.3	11.6	12.0
29– 31	10.5	10.8	11.2	11.5	11.9	12.2	12.6	12.9
32– 34	11.4	11.8	12.1	12.4	12.8	13.1	13.5	13.8
35– 37	12.3	12.7	13.0	13.4	13.7	14.1	14.4	14.8
38– 40	13.2	13.6	13.9	14.3	14.6	15.0	15.3	15.7
41– 43	14.1	14.5	14.8	15.2	15.5	15.9	16.2	16.6
44– 46	15.0	15.4	15.7	16.1	16.4	16.8	17.1	17.5
47– 49	15.9	16.2	16.6	16.9	17.3	17.6	18.0	18.3
50– 52	16.8	17.1	17.5	17.8	18.2	18.5	18.8	19.2
53– 55	17.6	18.0	18.3	18.7	19.0	19.4	19.7	20.1
56– 58	18.5	18.8	19.2	19.5	19.9	20.2	20.6	20.9
59– 61	19.3	19.7	20.0	20.4	20.7	21.0	21.4	21.7
62– 64	20.1	20.5	20.8	21.2	21.5	21.9	22.2	22.6
65– 67	21.0	21.3	21.7	22.0	22.4	22.7	23.0	23.4
68– 70	21.8	22.1	22.5	22.8	23.2	23.5	23.9	24.2
71– 73	22.6	22.9	23.3	23.6	24.0	24.3	24.7	25.0
74– 76	23.4	23.7	24.1	24.4	24.8	25.1	25.4	25.8
77– 79	24.1	24.5	24.8	25.2	25.5	25.9	26.2	26.6
80– 82	24.9	25.3	25.6	26.0	26.3	26.6	27.0	27.3
83– 85	25.7	26.0	26.4	26.7	27.1	27.4	27.8	28.1
86– 88	26.4	26.8	27.1	27.5	27.8	28.2	28.5	28.9
89– 91	27.2	27.5	27.9	28.2	28.6	28.9	29.2	29.6
92– 94	27.9	28.2	28.6	28.9	29.3	29.6	30.0	30.3
95– 97	28.6	29.0	29.3	29.7	30.0	30.4	30.7	31.1
98–100	29.3	29.7	30.0	30.4	30.7	31.1	31.4	31.8
101–103	30.0	30.4	30.7	31.1	31.4	31.8	32.1	32.5
104–106	30.7	31.1	31.4	31.8	32.1	32.5	32.8	33.2
107–109	31.4	31.8	32.1	32.4	32.8	33.1	33.5	33.8
110–112	32.1	32.4	32.8	33.1	33.5	33.8	34.2	34.5
113–115	32.7	33.1	33.4	33.8	34.1	34.5	34.8	35.2
116–118	33.4	33.7	34.1	34.4	34.8	35.1	35.5	35.8
119–121	34.0	34.4	34.7	35.1	35.4	35.8	36.1	36.5
122–124	34.7	35.0	35.4	35.7	36.1	36.4	36.7	37.1
125–127	35.3	35.6	36.0	36.3	36.7	37.0	37.4	37.7
128–130	35.9	36.2	36.6	36.9	37.3	37.6	38.0	38.5

Body density is calculated based on the generalized equation for predicting body density of men developed by A. S. Jackson and M. L. Pollock and published in the *British Journal of Nutrition* 40 (1978): 497–504. Percent body fat is determined from the calculated body density using the Siri formula.

Girth Measurements

A simpler method to determine body fat is by measuring circumferences (**girth measurements**) at various body sites. This technique requires only a standard measuring tape. Good accuracy can be achieved with little practice. The limitation is that it may not be valid for athletic individuals (men or women) who participate actively in strenuous physical activity or for people who can be classified visually as thin or obese.

The required procedure for girth measurements is given in Figure 4.5; conversion constants are in Tables 4.4 and 4.5. Measurements for women are the upper arm, hip, and wrist; for men, the waist and wrist.

Girth measurements Technique to assess body composition by measuring circumferences at specific body sites.

Figure 4.5 Procedure for body fat assessment according to girth measurements.

Girth Measurements for Women*

1. Using a regular tape measure, determine the following girth measurements in centimeters (cm):

   Upper arm: Take the measure halfway between the shoulder and the elbow.
   Hip: Measure at the point of largest circumference.
   Wrist: Take the girth in front of the bones where the wrist bends.

2. Obtain the person's age.
3. Using Table 4.4, find the subject's age, girth measurement for each site in the left column below, then look up the constant values for each. These values will allow you to derive body density (BD) by substituting the constants in the following formula:

   $BD = A - B - C + D$

4. Using the derived body density, calculate percent body fat (%F) according to the following equation:

   $\%F = (495 \div BD) - 450**$

Example: Jane is 20 years old, and the following girth measurements were taken: biceps = 27 cm, hip = 99.5 cm, wrist = 15.4 cm.

Data	Constant
Upper arm = 27 cm	A = 1.0813
Age = 20	B = .0102
Hip = 99.5 cm	C = .1206
Wrist = 15.4 cm	D = .0971

$BD = A - B - C + D$
$BD = 1.0813 - .0102 - .1206 + .0971 = 1.0476$
$\%F = (495 \div BD) - 450$
$\%F = (495 \div 1.0476) - 450 = 22.5$

Girth Measurements for Men***

1. Using a regular tape measure, determine the following girth measurements in inches (the men's measurements are taken in inches, as opposed to centimeters for women):

   Waist: Measure at the umbilicus (belly button).
   Wrist: Measure in front of the bones where the wrist bends.

2. Subtract the wrist from the waist measurement.
3. Obtain the weight of the subject in pounds.
4. Look up the percent body fat (%F) in Table 4.5 by using the difference obtained in number 2 above and the person's body weight.

Example: John weighs 160 pounds, and his waist and wrist girth measurements are 36.5 and 7.5 inches, respectively.

Waist girth = 36.5 inches
Wrist girth = 7.5 inches
Difference = 29.0 inches
Body weight = 160.0 lbs.
%F = 22

---

* From R. B. Lambson, "Generalized Body Density Prediction Equations for Women Using Simple Anthropometric Measurements." Unpublished doctoral dissertation, Brigham Young University, Provo, UT, August 1987. Reproduced by permission.

** From W. E. Siri, *Body Composition from Fluid Spaces and Density*. (Berkeley, CA: University of California, Donner Laboratory of Medical Physics, 1956).

*** From A. G. Fisher and P. E. Allsen, *Jogging*, Dubuque, IA: Wm. C. Brown, 1987. This table was developed according to "Generalized Body Composition Equation for Men Using Simple Measurement Techniques," by K. W. Penrouse, A. G Nelson, and A G. Fisher, *Medicine and Science in Sports and Exercise* 17, no. 2 (1985): 189. © American College of Sports Medicine 1985.

Table 4.4

Girth Measurement Technique:
Conversion Constants to Calculate Body Density for Women

Upper Arm (cm)	Constant A	Age	Constant B	Hip (cm)	Constant C	Hip (cm)	Constant C	Wrist (cm)	Constant D
20.5	1.0966	17	.0086	79	.0957	114.5	.1388	13.0	.0819
21	1.0954	18	.0091	79.5	.0963	115	.1394	13.2	.0832
21.5	1.0942	19	.0096	80	.0970	115.5	.1400	13.4	.0845
22	1.0930	20	.0102	80.5	.0976	116	.1406	13.6	.0857
22.5	1.0919	21	.0107	81	.0982	116.5	.1412	13.8	.0870
23	1.0907	22	.0112	81.5	.0988	117	.1418	14.0	.0882
23.5	1.0895	23	.0117	82	.0994	117.5	.1424	14.2	.0895
24	1.0883	24	.0122	82.5	.1000	118	.1430	14.4	.0908
24.5	1.0871	25	.0127	83	.1006	118.5	.1436	14.6	.0920
25	1.0860	26	.0132	83.5	.1012	119	.1442	14.8	.0933
25.5	1.0848	27	.0137	84	.1018	119.5	.1448	15.0	.0946
26	1.0836	28	.0142	84.5	.1024	120	.1454	15.2	.0958
26.5	1.0824	29	.0147	85	.1030	120.5	.1460	15.4	.0971
27	1.0813	30	.0152	85.5	.1036	121	.1466	15.6	.0983
27.5	1.0801	31	.0157	86	.1042	121.5	.1472	15.8	.0996
28	1.0789	32	.0162	86.5	.1048	122	.1479	16.0	.1009
28.5	1.0777	33	.0168	87	.1054	122.5	.1485	16.2	.1021
29	1.0775	34	.0173	87.5	.1060	123	.1491	16.4	.1034
29.5	1.0754	35	.0178	88	.1066	123.5	.1497	16.6	.1046
30	1.0742	36	.0183	88.5	.1072	124	.1503	16.8	.1059
30.5	1.0730	37	.0188	89	.1079	124.5	.1509	17.0	.1072
31	1.0718	38	.0193	89.5	.1085	125	.1515	17.2	.1084
31.5	1.0707	39	.0198	90	.1091	125.5	.1521	17.4	.1097
32	1.0695	40	.0203	90.5	.1097	126	.1527	17.6	.1109
32.5	1.0683	41	.0208	91	.1103	126.5	.1533	17.8	.1122
33	1.0671	42	.0213	91.5	.1109	127	.1539	18.0	.1135
33.5	1.0666	43	.0218	92	.1115	127.5	.1545	18.2	.1147
34	1.0648	44	.0223	92.5	.1121	128	.1551	18.4	.1160
34.5	1.0636	45	.0228	93	.1127	128.5	.1558	18.6	.1172
35	1.0624	46	.0234	93.5	.1133	129	.1563		
35.5	1.0612	47	.0239	94	.1139	129.5	.1569		
36	1.0601	48	.0244	94.5	.1145	130	.1575		
36.5	1.0589	49	.0249	95	.1151	130.5	.1581		
37	1.0577	50	.0254	95.5	.1157	131	.1587		
37.5	1.0565	51	.0259	96	.1163	131.5	.1593		
38	1.0554	52	.0264	96.5	.1169	132	.1600		
38.5	1.0542	53	.0269	97	.1176	132.5	.1606		
39	1.0530	54	.0274	97.5	.1182	133	.1612		
39.5	1.0518	55	.0279	98	.1188	133.5	.1618		
40	1.0506	56	.0284	98.5	.1194	134	.1624		
40.5	1.0495	57	.0289	99	.1200	134.5	.1630		
41	1.0483	58	.0294	99.5	.1206	135	.1636		
41.5	1.0471	59	.0300	100	.1212	135.5	.1642		
42	1.0459	60	.0305	100.5	.1218	136	.1648		
42.5	1.0448	61	.0310	101	.1224	136.5	.1654		
43	1.0434	62	.0315	101.5	.1230	137	.1660		
43.5	1.0424	63	.0320	102	.1236	137.5	.1666		
44	1.0412	64	.0325	102.5	.1242	138	.1672		
		65	.0330	103	.1248	138.5	.1678		
		66	.0335	103.5	.1254	139	.1685		
		67	.0340	104	.1260	139.5	.1691		
		68	.0345	104.5	.1266	140	.1697		
		69	.0350	105	.1272	140.5	.1703		

(continued)

Table 4.4 (Continued)

Upper Arm (cm)	Constant A	Age	Constant B	Hip (cm)	Constant C	Hip (cm)	Constant C	Wrist (cm)	Constant D
		70	.0355	105.5	.1278	141	.1709		
		71	.0360	106	.1285	141.5	.1715		
		72	.0366	106.5	.1291	142	.1721		
		73	.0371	107	.1297	142.5	.1728		
		74	.0376	107.5	.1303	143	.1733		
		75	.0381	108	.1309	143.5	.1739		
				108.5	.1315	144	.1745		
				109	.1321	144.5	.1751		
				109.5	.1327	145	.1757		
				110	.1333	145.5	.1763		
				110.5	.1339	146	.1769		
				111	.1345	146.5	.1775		
				111.5	.1351	147	.1781		
				112	.1357	147.5	.1787		
				112.5	.1363	148	.1794		
				113	.1369	148.5	.1800		
				113.5	.1375	149	.1806		
				114	.1382	149.5	.1812		
						150	.1818		

Bioelectrical Impedance

The **bioelectrical impedance** technique is much simpler to administer, but it does require costly equipment. In this technique, the individual is hooked up to a machine and several sensors are applied to the skin. A weak (totally painless) electrical current is then run through the body to analyze body composition (body fat, lean body mass, and body water). The technique is based on the principle that fat tissue is a less efficient conductor of an electrical current than lean tissue is. The easier the conductance, the leaner the individual.

The accuracy of equations used to estimate percent body fat with this technique is still questionable. More research is required before it approaches the accuracy of hydrostatic weighing, skinfold thickness, or girth measurement techniques. Following all manufacturer's instructions will ensure the most accurate result.

An advantage of bioelectrical impedance is that the results are highly reproducible. Unlike other techniques in which experienced technicians are necessary to obtain valid results, almost anyone can administer a bioelectrical impedance assessment. And, although the test results may not be completely accurate, this instrument is valuable in assessing changes in body composition over time.

Air Displacement

Air displacement is a relatively new technique that holds considerable promise. With this technique, an individual sits inside a small chamber, commercially known as the **Bod Pod**. Body volume is determined by subtracting the air volume with the person inside the chamber from the volume of the empty chamber. The amount of air in the person's lungs is also taken into consideration when determining the actual body volume. Body density and percent body fat are then calculated from the obtained body volume.

Initial research has shown that this technique compares very favorably with hydrostatic weighing, and it is less cumbersome to administer—the procedure takes only about 5 minutes. Additional

Bioelectrical impedance Technique to assess body composition by running a weak electrical current through the body.

Air displacement Technique to assess body composition by calculating the body volume from the air displaced by an individual sitting inside a small chamber.

Bod Pod Commercial name of the equipment used for the assessment of body composition through the air displacement technique.

Table 4.5

Girth Measurement Technique: Estimated Percent Body Fat for Men

Waist Minus Wrist Girth Measurement (inches)

Body Weight (pounds)	22	22.5	23	23.5	24	24.5	25	25.5	26	26.5	27	27.5	28	28.5	29	29.5	30	30.5	31	31.5	32	32.5	33	33.5	34	34.5	35	35.5	36	36.5	37	37.5	38	38.5	39	39.5	40	40.5	41	41.5	42	42.5	43	43.5	44	44.5	45	45.5	46	46.5	47	47.5	48	48.5	49	49.5	50
120	4	6	8	10	12	14	16	18	20	21	23	25	27	29	31	33	35	37	39	41	43	45	47	49	50	52	54	56	58																												
125	4	6	7	9	11	13	15	17	19	20	22	24	26	28	30	32	33	35	37	39	41	43	45	46	48	50	52	54	56	58																										
130	3	5	7	9	11	12	14	16	18	20	21	23	25	27	28	30	32	33	35	37	39	41	43	44	46	48	50	52	53	55	57																								
135	3	5	7	8	10	12	14	15	17	19	20	22	24	26	27	29	31	32	34	36	38	39	41	43	44	46	48	50	51	53	55	56																						
140	3	5	6	8	10	12	13	15	17	18	20	21	23	25	26	28	29	31	33	34	36	38	39	41	43	44	46	48	49	51	53	54	56																				
145	3	4	6	8	9	11	13	15	16	18	20	21	23	24	26	28	29	31	32	34	36	38	39	41	43	44	46	47	49	51	52	54	55																				
150	2	4	6	7	9	11	13	14	16	18	19	21	22	24	26	27	29	30	32	33	35	37	38	40	41	43	45	46	48	50	51	53	55																			
155	2	4	5	7	9	11	12	14	16	17	19	20	22	24	25	27	28	30	31	33	35	36	38	39	41	43	44	46	48	49	51	52	53	55																		
160	2	4	5	7	8	10	12	14	15	17	18	20	22	23	25	26	28	29	31	32	34	36	37	39	40	42	44	45	47	48	50	52	53																		
165	2	4	5	6	8	10	11	13	15	16	18	19	21	22	24	26	27	29	30	32	33	35	37	38	40	41	43	44	46	48	49	51	52	54																	
170	2	3	5	6	8	9	11	13	14	16	17	19	20	22	23	25	26	28	30	31	33	34	36	37	39	40	42	44	45	47	48	50	52	53																
175	2	3	4	6	7	9	11	12	14	15	17	18	20	21	23	24	26	27	29	30	32	34	35	37	38	40	41	43	45	46	48	49	51	52	53															
180	3	3	4	5	7	9	10	12	14	15	17	18	20	21	23	24	26	27	29	30	31	33	34	36	37	39	40	42	44	45	47	48	50	51	53															
185	3	3	4	5	7	8	10	11	13	14	16	18	19	21	22	24	25	27	28	30	31	33	34	35	37	38	40	41	43	44	46	47	49	50	51	53													
190	2	3	4	5	6	8	9	11	12	14	15	17	18	20	21	23	24	26	27	29	30	32	33	35	36	37	39	40	42	43	45	46	48	49	50	51	52												
195	2	3	4	5	6	8	9	10	12	13	15	16	18	19	21	22	24	25	27	28	29	31	32	34	35	37	38	39	41	42	44	45	47	48	49	50	51	52											
200	2	3	4	5	6	7	9	10	12	13	14	16	17	19	20	22	23	24	26	27	29	30	31	33	34	35	37	38	40	41	43	44	45	46	48	49	50	51	52										
205	2	3	4	5	6	7	8	10	11	12	14	15	17	18	19	21	22	24	25	26	28	29	31	32	33	35	36	37	39	40	42	43	44	45	47	48	49	50	51	52									
210	2	3	3	5	6	7	8	9	11	12	13	15	16	17	19	20	22	23	24	26	27	28	30	31	32	34	35	36	38	39	40	42	43	44	45	47	48	49	50	51	52								
215	2	3	3	4	5	7	8	9	10	12	13	14	16	17	18	20	21	22	24	25	26	28	29	30	32	33	34	36	37	38	40	41	42	43	44	46	47	48	49	50	51	52							
220		2	3	4	5	6	7	8	10	11	12	13	15	16	17	18	20	21	22	24	25	26	28	29	30	31	33	34	35	36	38	39	40	41	43	44	45	46	47	48	49	50	51						
225		2	3	4	5	6	7	8	9	10	12	13	14	15	16	18	19	20	21	23	24	25	26	28	29	30	31	33	34	35	36	37	39	40	41	42	43	44	46	47	48	49	50	51					
230		2	3	4	5	6	7	8	9	10	11	12	13	15	16	17	18	19	21	22	23	24	25	27	28	29	30	31	33	34	35	36	37	38	40	41	42	43	44	45	46	47	48	50	51				
235		2	3	4	5	6	7	8	9	10	11	12	13	14	15	16	18	19	20	21	22	23	25	26	27	28	29	30	31	33	34	35	36	37	38	39	41	42	43	44	45	46	47	48	49	50			
240		2	3	4	5	6	7	8	9	10	11	12	13	14	15	16	17	18	19	20	22	23	24	25	26	27	28	29	30	32	33	34	35	36	37	38	39	40	41	42	43	44	45	46	47	48	50		
245		2	3	4	5	6	6	7	8	9	10	11	12	13	14	15	16	17	18	19	21	22	23	24	25	26	27	28	29	30	31	32	33	34	35	37	38	39	40	41	42	43	44	45	46	47	48	50	
250		2	3	4	4	5	6	7	8	9	10	11	12	13	14	15	16	17	18	19	20	21	22	23	24	25	26	27	28	30	31	32	33	34	35	36	37	38	39	40	41	42	43	44	45	46	47	48	50
255		2	3	3	4	5	6	7	8	9	10	11	12	12	13	14	15	16	17	18	19	20	21	22	23	24	25	26	27	28	29	30	31	32	33	34	35	36	37	38	39	40	41	42	43	44	45	46	47
260	2	2	3	3	4	5	6	7	8	9	10	11	11	12	13	14	15	16	17	18	19	20	21	22	23	24	25	26	27	28	29	30	31	32	33	34	35	36	37	38	39	40	41	42	43	44	45	46	47	48	49	50					
265		2	2	3	4	5	6	7	8	9	9	10	11	12	13	14	15	16	17	18	19	20	21	22	23	24	25	26	26	27	28	29	30	31	32	33	34	35	36	37	38	39	40	41	42	43	44	45	46	47	48	49					
270		2	2	3	4	5	5	6	7	8	9	10	11	12	13	13	14	15	16	17	18	19	20	21	22	23	24	25	26	27	28	29	30	31	32	33	34	35	36	37	37	38	39	40	41	42	43	44	45	46	47	48					
275		2	2	3	4	4	5	6	7	8	9	10	11	12	12	13	14	15	16	17	18	19	20	21	21	22	23	24	25	26	27	28	29	30	31	32	33	34	35	36	37	38	39	40	41	42	43	44	45	46	46	47					
280		2	2	3	3	4	5	6	7	8	8	9	10	11	12	13	14	15	16	17	17	18	19	20	21	22	23	24	24	25	26	27	28	29	30	31	32	33	34	35	36	37	38	38	39	40	41	42	43	44	45	46					
285		2	2	3	3	4	5	6	7	7	8	9	10	11	12	13	14	14	15	16	17	18	19	20	21	21	22	23	24	25	26	27	28	29	30	31	31	32	33	34	35	36	37	38	38	39	40	41	42	43	44	45					
290		2	2	3	3	4	5	6	6	7	8	9	10	11	12	12	13	14	15	16	17	18	19	19	20	21	22	23	24	25	26	27	27	28	29	30	31	32	33	34	35	36	36	37	38	39	40	41	42	42	43	44					
295		2	2	3	3	4	5	5	6	7	8	9	10	11	11	12	13	14	15	16	17	17	18	19	20	21	22	23	24	24	25	26	27	28	29	30	31	31	32	33	34	35	36	37	38	38	39	40	41	42	43	43					
300		2	2	3	3	4	5	5	6	7	8	9	9	10	11	12	13	14	15	15	16	17	18	19	20	21	21	22	23	24	25	26	26	27	28	29	30	31	32	32	33	34	35	36	37	37	38	39	40	41	42	43					

research is needed, however, to determine its accuracy among different age groups, ethnic backgrounds, and athletic populations. Administering this assessment is a relatively easy procedure, but because of the high cost of the equipment, the Bod Pod is not readily available in fitness centers and exercise laboratories.

Waist-to-Hip Ratio

Scientific evidence suggests that the way people store fat affects their risk for disease. Some individuals tend to store fat in the abdominal area (which produces the "apple" shape). Others store it mainly around the hips and thighs (in gluteal and femoral fat, which creates the "pear" shape).

Statistics show that obese individuals with a lot of abdominal fat are clearly at higher risk for coronary heart disease, congestive heart failure, hypertension, Type II diabetes (also called "adult-onset" or "non-insulin–dependent" diabetes), and strokes than are obese people with similar amounts of total body fat stored primarily in the hips and thighs. Evidence also indicates that, among individuals with a lot of abdominal fat, those whose fat deposits are located around internal organs (visceral fat) have an even greater risk for disease than those with fat mainly just beneath the skin (subcutaneous fat).[1]

Because of the higher risk for disease in individuals who tend to store a lot of fat in the abdominal area (versus in the hips and thighs), a **waist-to-hip ratio** test was designed to estimate this risk. The waist measurement is taken at the point of smallest circumference, and the hip measurement is taken at the point of greatest circumference. The waist measurement is then divided by the hip measurement.

The waist-to-hip ratio differentiates the "apples" from the "pears." Most men are apples, and most women are pears. The panel recommends that men need to lose weight if the waist-to-hip ratio is 1.0 or higher (that is, if the waist is even slightly larger than the hips). Women need to lose weight if the ratio is .85 or higher (see Table 4.6).

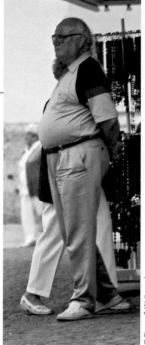

Individuals who accumulate body fat around the midsection are at greater risk for disease than those who accumulate body fat in other areas.

© Fitness & Wellness, Inc.

More conservative estimates indicate that the risk starts to increase when the ratio exceeds .95 and .80 for men and women, respectively. For example, the waist-to-hip ratio for a man with a 40-inch waist and a 38-inch hip would be 1.05 (40 ÷ 38)—which may indicate higher risk for disease.

Body Mass Index

Another technique to determine thinness and excessive fatness is the **body mass index (BMI),** which incorporates height and weight to estimate critical fat values at which the risk for disease increases.

BMI is calculated by either (1) dividing the weight in kilograms by the square of the height in meters or (2) multiplying body weight in pounds by 705 and dividing this figure by the square of the height in inches. For example, the BMI for an individual who weighs 172 pounds (78 kg) and is 67 inches (1.7 m) tall would be 27 [78 ÷ $(1.7)^2$] or [172 × 705 ÷ $(67)^2$]. You can also look up your BMI in Table 4.7 according to your height and weight; then see Table 4.8 for the resultant disease risk.

According to BMI, the lowest risk for chronic disease is in the 22-to-25 range.[2] Individuals are classified as overweight if their indexes lie between 25 and 30. BMIs above 30 are defined as obese; those below 20 as **underweight**. As compared with individuals with a BMI below 25, mortality rates are up to 25 percent higher for people with a BMI between 25 and 30, and 50 to 100 percent higher for those with a BMI above 30.[3] Approximately 20 percent of U.S. adults have a body BMI of 30 or more.

BMI is a useful tool to screen the general population, but its one weakness (similar to the original height/weight charts) is that it fails to differentiate fat from lean body mass or note where most of the fat is located (the waist-to-hip ratio). Using BMI, athletes with a large amount of muscle

Table 4.6	Disease Risk According to Waist-to-Hip Ratio		
Waist-to-Hip Ratio			
Men	**Women**		**Disease Risk**
≤0.95	≤0.80		Very Low
0.96–0.99	0.81–0.84		Low
>1.00	≥0.85		High

Table 4.7 Disease Risk According to Body Mass Index (BMI)

Determine your BMI by looking up the number where your weight and height intersect on the table. According to your results, look up your disease risk in Table 4.8.

Height	Weight																												
	110	115	120	125	130	135	140	145	150	155	160	165	170	175	180	185	190	195	200	205	210	215	220	225	230	235	240	245	250
5'0"	21	22	23	24	25	26	27	28	29	30	31	32	33	34	35	36	37	38	39	40	41	42	43	44	45	46	47	48	49
5'1"	21	22	23	24	25	26	26	27	28	29	30	31	32	33	34	35	36	37	38	39	40	41	42	43	43	44	45	46	47
5'2"	20	21	22	23	24	25	26	27	27	28	29	30	31	32	33	34	35	36	37	37	38	39	40	41	42	43	44	45	46
5'3"	19	20	21	22	23	24	25	26	27	27	28	29	30	31	32	33	34	35	35	36	37	38	39	40	41	42	43	43	44
5'4"	19	20	21	21	22	23	24	25	26	27	27	28	29	30	31	32	33	33	34	35	36	37	38	39	39	40	41	42	43
5'5"	18	19	20	21	22	22	23	24	25	26	27	27	28	29	30	31	32	32	33	34	35	36	37	37	38	39	40	41	42
5'6"	18	19	19	20	21	22	23	23	24	25	26	27	27	28	29	30	31	31	32	33	34	35	36	36	37	38	39	40	40
5'7"	17	18	19	20	20	21	22	23	23	24	25	26	27	27	28	29	30	31	31	32	33	34	34	35	36	37	38	38	39
5'8"	17	17	18	19	20	21	21	22	23	24	24	25	26	27	27	28	29	30	30	31	32	33	33	34	35	36	36	37	38
5'9"	16	17	18	18	19	20	21	21	22	23	24	24	25	26	27	27	28	29	30	30	31	32	32	33	34	35	35	36	37
5'10"	16	17	17	18	19	19	20	21	22	22	23	24	24	25	26	27	27	28	29	29	30	31	32	32	33	34	34	35	36
5'11"	15	16	17	17	18	19	20	20	21	22	22	23	24	24	25	26	26	27	28	29	29	30	31	31	32	33	33	34	35
6'0"	15	16	16	17	18	18	19	20	20	21	22	22	23	24	24	25	26	26	27	28	28	29	30	31	31	32	33	33	34
6'1"	15	15	16	16	17	18	18	19	20	20	21	22	22	23	24	24	25	26	26	27	28	28	29	30	30	31	32	32	33
6'2"	14	15	15	16	17	17	18	19	19	20	21	21	22	22	23	24	24	25	26	26	27	28	28	29	30	30	31	31	32
6'3"	14	14	15	16	16	17	17	18	19	19	20	21	21	22	22	23	24	24	25	26	26	27	27	28	29	29	30	31	31
6'4"	13	14	15	15	16	16	17	18	18	19	19	20	21	21	22	23	23	24	24	25	26	26	27	27	28	29	29	30	30

Table 4.8 Disease Risk According to Body Mass Index (BMI)

BMI	Disease Risk	Classification
<20.00	Moderate to Very High	Underweight
20.00 to 21.99	Low	Acceptable
22.00 to 24.99	Very Low	
25.00 to 26.99	Low	Overweight
27.00 to 29.99	Moderate	
30.00 to 39.99	High	Obese
≥40.00	Very High	

Determining Recommended Body Weight

After finding out your percent body fat, you can determine your current body composition classification by consulting Table 4.9, which presents percentages of fat according to both the health fitness and the high physical fitness standards (see Fitness Standards: Health Fitness Versus Physical Fitness, page 12).

For example, the recommended health fitness fat percentage for a 20-year-old female is 28 percent or less. The health fitness standard is established at the point at which there seems to be no harm to health in terms of percent body fat. A high physical mass (such as body builders and football players) can easily fall in the moderate- or even high-risk categories. Therefore, body composition and waist-to-hip ratios are better procedures to determine health risk and recommended body weight.

Waist-to-hip ratio A measurement to assess potential risk for disease based on distribution of body fat.

Body mass index (BMI) Ratio of weight to height used to determine thinness and fatness.

Underweight Extremely low body weight.

Table 4.9	Body Composition Classification According to Percent Body Fat

MEN

Age	Excellent	Good	Moderate	Overweight	Significantly Overweight
≤19	12.0	12.1–17.0	17.1–22.0	22.1–27.0	≥27.1
20–29	13.0	13.1–18.0	18.1–23.0	23.1–28.0	≥28.1
30–39	14.0	14.1–19.0	19.1–24.0	24.1–29.0	≥29.1
40–49	15.0	15.1–20.0	20.1–25.0	25.1–30.0	≥ 30.1
≥50	16.0	16.1–21.0	21.1–26.0	26.1–31.0	≥31.1

WOMEN

Age	Excellent	Good	Moderate	Overweight	Significantly Overweight
≤19	17.0	17.1–22.0	22.1–27.0	27.1–32.0	≥32.1
20–29	18.0	18.1–23.0	23.1–28.0	28.1–33.0	≥33.1
30–39	19.0	19.1–24.0	24.1–29.0	29.1–34.0	≥34.1
40–49	20.0	20.1–25.0	25.1–30.0	30.1–35.0	≥35.1
≥50	21.0	21.1–26.0	26.1–31.0	31.1–36.0	≥36.1

☐ High physical fitness standard

☐ Health fitness standard

decreases with age, one extra percentage point is allowed for every additional decade of life.

Your recommended body weight is computed based on the selected health or high fitness fat percentage for your age and sex. Your decision to select a "desired" fat percentage should be based on your current percent body fat and your personal health/fitness objectives. Following are steps to compute your own recommended body weight:

1. **Determine the pounds of body weight that are fat (FW)** by multiplying your body weight (BW) by the current percent fat (%F) expressed in decimal form (FW = BW × %F).
2. **Determine lean body mass (LBM)** by subtracting the weight in fat from the total body weight (LBM = BW − FW). (Anything that is not fat must be part of the lean component.)
3. Select a desired body fat percentage (DFP) based on the health or high fitness standards given in Table 4.9.
4. **Compute recommended body weight (RBW)** according to the formula RBW = LBM ÷ (1.0 − DFP).

As an example of these computations, a 19-year-old female who weighs 160 pounds and is 30 percent fat would like to know what her recommended body weight would be at 22 percent:

Sex: female
Age: 19
BW: 160 lbs
%F: 30% (.30 in decimal form)

1. FW = BW × %F
    FW = 160 × .30 = 48 lbs
2. LBM = BW − FW
    LBM = 160 − 48 = 112 lbs

3. DFP: 22% (.22 in decimal form)
4. RBW = LBM ÷ (1.0 − DFP)
    RBW = 112 ÷ (1.0 − .22)
    RBW = 112 ÷ .78 = 143.6 lbs

fitness range for this same woman would be between 18 and 23 percent.

The high physical fitness standard does not mean you cannot be somewhat below this number. Many highly trained male athletes are as low as 3 percent, and some female distance runners have been measured at 6 percent body fat (which may not be healthy).

Although people generally agree that the mortality rate is higher for obese people, some evidence indicates that the same is true for underweight people. "Underweight" and "thin" do not necessarily mean the same thing. The body fat of a healthy thin person is around the high physical fitness standard, whereas an underweight person has extremely low body fat, even to the point of compromising the essential fat.

The lower limits for people to maintain good health seem to be 3 percent essential fat for men and 12 percent for women. Below these percentages, normal physiological functions can be seriously impaired. Some experts point out that a little storage fat (in addition to the essential fat) is better than none at all. As a result, the health and high fitness standards for percent fat in Table 4.9 are set higher than the minimum essential fat requirements, at a point beneficial to optimal health and well-being. Finally, because lean tissue

In Labs 4A and 4B, you will have the opportunity to determine your own body composition, recommended body weight, and disease risk according to waist-to-hip ratio and BMI. A second column is provided in both labs for a follow-up assessment at a future date.

Other than hydrostatic weighing, skinfold thickness seems to be the most practical and valid technique to estimate body fat. If skinfold calipers are available, use this technique to assess your percent body fat. If calipers are not available, estimate your percent fat according to the girth measurements technique or another technique available to you. You may also wish to use several techniques and compare the results.

Importance of Regular Body Composition Assessment

Children in the United States do not start with a weight problem. Although a small group struggles with weight throughout life, most are not overweight when they reach age 20.

Current trends indicate that, starting at age 25, the average person in the United States gains 1 pound of weight per year. Thus, by age 65, the average American will have gained 40 pounds. Because of the typical reduction in physical activity in our society, however, each year the average person also loses a half a pound of lean tissue. Therefore, this span of 40 years has produced an actual fat gain of 60 pounds accompanied by a 20-pound loss of lean body mass[4] (see Figure 4.6). These changes cannot be detected unless body composition is assessed periodically.

If you are on a diet/exercise program, you should repeat your percent body fat assessment and recommended weight computations about once a month. This is important because lean body mass is affected by weight reduction programs and amount of physical activity. As lean body mass changes, so will your recommended body weight. To make valid comparisons, the same technique should be used for both pre- and post-program assessments.

Changes in body composition resulting from a weight control/exercise program were illustrated in a co-ed aerobic dance course taught during a 6-week summer term. Students participated in a 60-minute aerobics routine four times a week. On the first and last days of class, several physiological parameters, including body composition, were assessed. Students also were given information on diet and nutrition, but they followed their own dietary program.

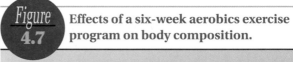

Starting at age 25, the average U.S. adult gains 1.5 pounds of body fat per year.

At the end of the 6 weeks, the average weight loss for the entire class was 3 pounds (see Figure 4.7). But, because body composition was assessed, class members were surprised to find that the average fat loss was actually 6 pounds, accompanied by a 3-pound increase in lean body mass.

When dieting, have your body composition reassessed periodically because of the effects of negative caloric balance on lean body mass. As discussed in Chapter 5, dieting does decrease lean body mass. This loss of lean body mass can be offset or eliminated by combining a sensible diet with physical exercise.

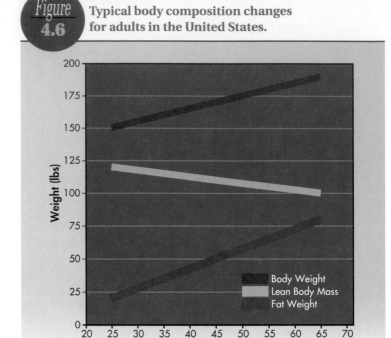

Figure 4.6 Typical body composition changes for adults in the United States.

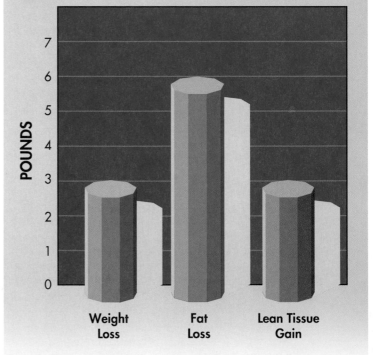

Figure 4.7 Effects of a six-week aerobics exercise program on body composition.

Web Interactive

- Body Mass Index. A comprehensive site from Shape Up, America describing body mass measurements, including a chart.

  http://www.shapeup.org/bmi/index.html

- Body Composition Tests from the American Heart Association. This site describes the importance of waist-to-hip ratio and body mass index as two types of body composition measurements. The site contains tables for adult measurements on each of these two types of measurements.

  http://www.justmove.org/myfitness/lowarticles/lowframes. cfm?Target=bodycomp.html

- Body Composition and Somatype. This site features a table listing male and female % body fat ranges, body fat myths and truths, and specific activities to help achieve proper body composition.

  http://www.worldguide.com/Fitness/med.html

- Skinfold caliper measurements. This site describes how and where to take these measurements, as well as the equations used to determine body fat.

  http://www.solid.net/lowcarb/lylemcd/skinfold.htm

- Bioelectric impedance analysis in body composition measurement. This technical paper from the National Library of Medicine features useful information and a wealth of references.

  http://www.nlm.nih.gov/pubs/cbm/bioellmp.html

Interactive Sites:

- Measuring Your Percentage of Body Fat. This site features a wellness link, nutrition information, a virtual gym, and enables you to determine your exercise efficiency by calculating your body mass index and your target heart rate.

  http://www.fitnesslink.com/exercise/bodyfat.shtml

- Home Body Fat Test: Calculate your approximate percent body fat, by answering three simple questions pertaining to your age, gender, and weight in pounds (or kilograms). This site also contains information about body composition as discussed by Covert Bailey, a noted fitness expert.

  http://www.healthcentral.com/cooltools/CT_Fitness/ bodyfat1.cfm

- Calculate Your BMI, using your height and weight. BMI stands for "Body Mass Index," a ratio between weight and height. It is a mathematical formula that correlates with body fat. BMI is a better predictor of disease risk than body weight alone. This site also features tools to calculate your ideal weight and your target heart rate.

  http://www.drkoop.com/wellness/weight_loss/#

Notes

1. C. Bouchard, G. A. Bray, and V. S. Hubbard, "Basic and Clinical Aspects of Regional Fat Distribution," *American Journal of Clinical Nutrition* 52 (1990): 946–950.

2. E. E. Calle, M. J. Thun, J. M. Petrelli, C. Rodriguez, and C. W. Heath, "Body-Mass Index and Mortality in a Prospective Cohort of U.S. Adults," *The New England Journal of Medicine* 341 (1999): 1097–1105.

3. K. M. Flegal, M. D. Carrol, R. J. Kuczmarski, and C. L. Johnson, "Overweight and Obesity in the United States: Prevalence and Trends, 1960–1994," *International Journal of Obesity and Related Metabolic Disorders* 22 (1998): 39–47.

4. J. H. Wilmore, "Exercise and Weight Control: Myths, Misconceptions, and Quackery," (lecture given at annual meeting of American College of Sports Medicine, Indianapolis, June 1994).

Suggested Readings

Bouchard, C., and F. E. Johnson, eds. *Fat Distribution During Growth and Later Health Outcomes.* New York: Alan R. Liss, 1988.

Bouchard, C., G. A. Bray, and V. S. Hubbard. "Basic and Clinical Aspects of Regional Fat Distribution." *American Journal of Clinical Nutrition* 52 (1990): 946–950.

Bray, G. A. "Pathophysiology of Obesity." *American Journal of Clinical Nutrition* 55 (1992): 488S–494S.

Hoeger, W. W. K., and S. A. Hoeger. *Lifetime Physical Fitness and Wellness.* Belmont, CA: Wadsworth/Thompson Learning, 1999.

Jackson, A. S., and M. L. Pollock. "Generalized Equations for Predicting Body Density of Men." *British Journal of Nutrition* 40 (1978): 497–504.

Jackson, A. S., M. L. Pollock, and A. Ward. "Generalized Equations for Predicting Body Density of Women." *Medicine and Science in Sports and Exercise* 3 (1980): 175–182.

Lambson, R. B. "Generalized Body Density Prediction Equations for Women Using Simple Anthropometric Measurements." Unpublished doctoral dissertation, Brigham Young University, Provo, UT, August 1987.

Penrouse, K. W., A. G. Nelson, and A. G. Fisher. "Generalized Body Composition Equation for Men Using Simple Measurement Techniques." *Medicine and Science in Sports and Exercise* 17, no. 2 (1985): 189.

Siri, W. E. "Body Composition from Fluid Spaces and Density." Berkeley, CA: Donner Laboratory of Medical Physics, University of California, 1956.

Stensland, S. H., and S. Margolis. "Simplifying the Calculation of Body Mass Index for Quick Reference." *Journal of the American Dietetic Association* 90 (1990): 856.

HYDROSTATIC WEIGHING FOR BODY COMPOSITION ASSESSMENT

Name: Date: Grade:

Instructor: Course: Section:

Necessary Lab Equipment

Hydrostatic or underwater weighing tank and residual volume spirometer (if no spirometer is available, predicting equations can be used to determine this volume — see Figure 4.1, page 93).

Objective

To determine body density and percent body fat.

Lab Preparation

Bring a swimsuit and towel to this lab. A 6- to 8-hour fast and bladder and bowel movements are recommended prior to underwater weighing.

Instructions

Follow the procedure outlined in Figure 4.1. If time is a factor, assess only the body composition of one or two participants in the course and compute the results using the form provided below. A sample of the computations is provided on the back of this page.

I. Hydrostatic Weighing

Name: Age: Weight: lbs

Height: inches $\times$ 2.54 =   cm   Water temperature: °C   Water density (WD):   gr/ml

Residual volume (RV):   lt   See Figure 4.1.

Body weight (BW) in kg = weight in pounds ÷ 2.2046

BW in kg =   ÷ 2.2046 =   kg

Gross underwater weights:

   1.   kg   2.   kg   3.   kg   4.   kg   5.   kg

   6.   kg   7.   kg   8.   kg   9.   kg   10.   kg

Average of three heaviest underwater weights (AUW):   kg

Tare weight (TW):   kg

Net underwater weight (UW) = AUW − TW

Net underwater weight (UW) =   −   =   kg

Body density (BD):

$$BD = \frac{BW}{\dfrac{BW - UW}{WD} - RV - .1} \qquad\qquad BD = \frac{\underline{}}{\dfrac{}{} - - .1} = $$

Percent body fat (%Fat):

$$\%Fat = \frac{495}{BD} - 450 = \frac{495}{} - 450 = \% \qquad \textbf{Follow-up} \text{ percent body fat: } \%$$

Figure 4A.1 Sample computation for percent body fat according to hydrostatic weighing.

Name: Jane Doe   Age: 20   Weight: 148.5 lbs

Height: 67 inches × 2.54 = 170.2 cm   Water temperature: 33 °C   Water density (WD): .99473 gr/ml

Residual volume (RV): 1.37 lt   See Figure 4.1.

Body weight (BW) in kg = weight in pounds ÷ 2.2046

BW in kg = 148.5 ÷ 2.2046 = 67.36 kg

Gross underwater weights:

1. 6.15 kg   2. 6.12 kg   3. 6.24 kg   4. 6.26 kg   5. 6.21 kg

6. 6.29 kg   7. 6.27 kg   8. 6.28 kg   9.   kg   10.   kg

Average of three heaviest underwater weights (AUW): 6.28 kg

Tare weight (TW): 5.154 kg

Net underwater weight (UW) = AUW − TW

Net underwater weight (UW) = 6.28 − 5.154 = 1.126 kg

Body density (BD):

$$BD = \cfrac{BW}{\cfrac{BW - UW}{WD} - RV - .1}$$

$$BD = \cfrac{67.36}{\cfrac{67.34 - 1.126}{.99473} - 1.37 - .1} = 1.0344$$

Percent body fat (%Fat):

$$\%Fat = \frac{495}{BD} - 450 = \frac{495}{1.0344} - 450 = 28.5\ \%$$ **Follow-up** percent body fat: %

II. What I Learned from the underwater weighing procedure.

Describe the experience of being weighed underwater. Do you feel that the results of the test were accurate?

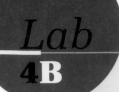

Lab 4B

BODY COMPOSITION ASSESSMENT, DISEASE RISK ASSESSMENT, AND RECOMMENDED BODY WEIGHT DETERMINATION

Name: _____   Date: _____   Grade: _____

Instructor: _____   Course: _____   Section: _____

Necessary Lab Equipment
Skinfold calipers and standard measuring tapes.

Objective
To assess percent body fat using skinfold thickness or girth measurements, disease risk according to waist-to-hip ratio and body mass index, and recommended body weight.

Instructions
If skinfold calipers are available, use the skinfold thickness technique to assess your percent body fat (see Figure 4.4, page 96). If calipers are unavailable, estimate the percent fat according to the girth measurements technique (see Figure 4.5, page 98). You may wish to use both techniques and compare the results. Next, compute your recommended body weight according to your current percent body fat and the recommended percent body fat guidelines provided in Table 4.9, page 104. Determine also your waist-to-hip ratio, body mass index, and recommended weight using the guidelines provided in this lab.

I. Percent Body Fat According to Skinfold Thickness

Men

Chest (mm): _____

Abdomen (mm): _____

Thigh (mm): _____

Total (mm): _____

% Fat: _____

Women

Triceps (mm): _____

Suprailium (mm): _____

Thigh (mm): _____

Total (mm): _____

% Fat: _____

Follow-up

% Fat _____ %

II. Percent Fat According to Girth Measurements

Men

Waist (inches): _____

Wrist (inches): _____

Difference: _____

Body Weight: _____

% Fat: _____

Women

Upper Arm (cm): _____   Constant A = _____

Age: _____   Constant B = _____

Hip (cm): _____   Constant C = _____

Wrist (cm): _____   Constant D = _____

BD* = A − B − C + D

BD = _____ − _____ − _____ + _____ = _____

% Fat = (495 ÷ BD) − 450 = (495 ÷ _____) − 450 = _____

*Body density

Follow-up

% Fat _____ %

III. Disease Risk According to Waist-to-Hip Ratio and Body Mass Index

Waist-to-Hip Ratio

Waist (inches): _____

Hip (inches): _____

Ratio (waist − hip: _____

Disease Risk: _____

Follow-up

_____

_____

_____

Recommended Standards

Waist-to-Hip Ratio		
Men	Women	Disease Risk
≤ 0.95	≤ 0.80	Very Low
0.96–0.99	0.81–0.84	Low
≥ 1.00	≥ 0.85	High

Body Mass Index

Weight: [____] lbs [____] kg

Height: [____] inches [____] meters

BMI = Weight (lbs) × 705 ÷ Height (in) ÷ Height (in)

BMI = [____] (lbs) × 705 ÷ [____] (in) ÷ [____] (in)

BMI = Weight (kg) ÷ Height (m) ÷ Height (m)

BMI = [____] (kg) ÷ [____] (m) ÷ [____] (m)

Disease Risk: [____]

Follow-up BMI = [____]   Disease Risk: [____]

Recommended Standards

BMI	Disease Risk	Classification
<20.00	Moderate to Very High	Underweight
20.00 to 21.99	Low	Acceptable
22.00 to 24.99	Very Low	
25.00 to 26.99	Low	Overweight
27.00 to 29.99	Moderate	
30.00 to 39.99	High	Obese
≥40.00	Very High	

IV. Recommended Body Weight Determination

A. Body weight (BW): [____]

B. Current %F*: [____] %

C. Fat weight (FW) = BW × %F

   FW = [____] × [____] = [____]

D. Lean body mass (LBM) = BW − FW = [____] − [____] = [____]

E. Age: [____]

F. Desired fat percent (DFP − see Table 4.9, page 104): [____] %

G. Recommended body weight (RBW) = LBM ÷ (1.0 − DFP*)

   RBW = [____] ÷ (1.0 − [____]) = [____]

   *Express percentages in decimal form (for example, 25% = .25)

Follow Up

A. BW: [____]

B. %F: [____] %

C. FW: [____]

D. LBM: [____]

E. Age: [____]

F. DFP: [____] %

G. RBW: [____]

V. Body Composition Conclusions and Goals

Briefly state your feelings about your body composition results and your recommended body weight. Do you plan to reduce percent body fat and increase lean body mass? Write the goal(s) you want to achieve by the end of the term and indicate how you plan to achieve them.

Chapter 5

Principles of Weight Management

■ Objectives

- Understand the health consequences of obesity.

- Learn about fad diets and other myths and fallacies regarding weight control.

- Become familiar with eating disorders and their associated medical problems and behavior patterns; understand the need for professional help in treating these conditions.

- Become familiar with the physiology of weight loss, including setpoint theory and the effects of diet on basal metabolic rate.

- Recognize the role of a lifetime exercise program as the key to a successful weight loss and maintenance program.

- Learn how to implement a physiologically sound weight reduction and weight maintenance program.

- Learn behavior modification techniques that help a person adhere to a lifetime weight maintenance program.

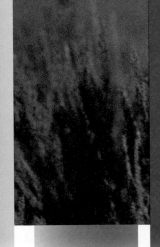

Two terms commonly used to describe the condition of weighing more than recommended are "overweight" and "obesity." Obesity levels are the point at which excess body fat can lead to serious health problems. Obesity is a health hazard of epidemic proportions in most developed countries around the world. According to the World Health Organization, an estimated 35 percent of the adult population in industrialized nations is obese. Obesity has been defined as a body mass index (BMI) of 30 or higher.

A 1999 study estimated that, in the United States, 63 percent of men and 55 percent of women are overweight (with a BMI greater than 25) and 21 percent of men and 27 percent of women are obese (see Figure 5.1).[1] An estimated 97 million people are overweight and 30 million are obese.[2] Between 1960 and 1994, the overall (men and women combined) prevalence of adult obesity increased from about 13 percent to 22.5 percent. Most of this increase occurred in the 1990s.[3] In the last decade alone, the average weight of American adults increased by about 15 pounds. The prevalence of obesity is even higher in ethnic groups, especially African Americans and Hispanic Americans.

About 44 percent of all women and 29 percent of all men are on a diet at any given moment.[4] People spend about $40 billion yearly attempting to lose weight. More than $10 billion goes to memberships in weight reduction centers and another $30 billion to diet food sales. Furthermore, according to the National Institutes of Health, the total cost attributable to obesity-related disease is approximately $100 billion per year.

> *The lack of exercise, not the weight problem itself, may cause many of the health risks associated with obesity.*

As the second leading cause of preventable death in the United States, overweight and obesity have been associated with several serious health problems and account for 15 to 20 percent of the annual mortality rate. About 300,000 deaths each year are caused by excessive body weight. In 1998, the American Heart Association identified obesity as one of the six major risk factors for coronary heart disease. Obesity also is a risk factor for hypertension, congestive heart failure, high blood lipids, atherosclerosis, stroke, thromboembolitic disease, varicose veins, Type II diabetes, osteoarthritis, gallbladder disease, sleep apnea, respiratory problems, ruptured intervertebral discs, and for endometrial, breast, prostate, and colon cancers. Furthermore, it is implicated in psychological maladjustment and a higher accidental death rate.

Percentage of the adult population that is obese (BMI ≥ 30) and overweight (BMI = 25 to 29.9) in the United States.

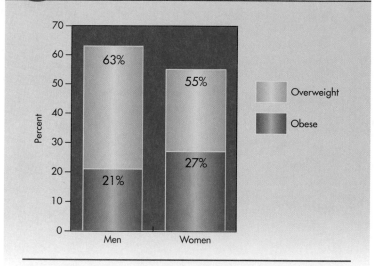

Source: A. Must et al., "The Disease Burden Associated with Overweight and Obesity," *Journal of the American Medical Association* 282 (1999): 1523–1529.

Overweight and **obesity** are not the same thing. Many overweight people (that is, people who weigh 10 to 20 pounds over the recommended weight) are not obese. Although research findings from studies are inconsistent, the health consequences of a few extra pounds of body fat might be exaggerated and may apply primarily to severely overweight individuals.

Data from the Aerobics Research Institute in Dallas confirm that, as body fat increases, so do blood cholesterol and triglycerides. The study also showed that the higher the fitness level, the lower the mortality rate, regardless of body weight.[5] This finding is significant because obese men who were fit had a lower risk of death than unfit men of average weight and as low as fit men of average weight. Thus, at least partially, lack of physical activity and not the weight problem itself may be the cause of premature death in some obese people.

Although the premature mortality of obese men in the study who became active decreased regardless of whether they lost weight, few obese men in the study were fit. This pattern holds true in life. Most obese people either don't or can't exercise because of functional limitations when they attempt to participate in traditional fitness activities such as jogging, walking, and cycling. Those who do exercise tend to lose weight.

A few pounds of excess weight may not be harmful to most people, but this is not always the case. People with excessive body fat who have diabetes and other cardiovascular risk factors (elevated blood lipids, high blood pressure, physical inactivity,

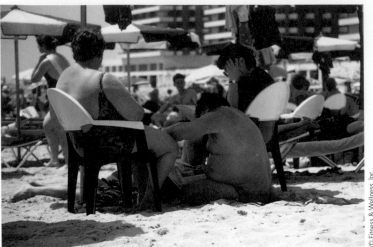

Obesity is a health hazard of epidemic proportions in developed countries.

and poor eating habits) benefit from weight loss. Even a modest reduction of 5 to 10 percent can reduce high blood pressure and total cholesterol levels. People who have a few extra pounds of weight but who otherwise are healthy and physically active, exercise regularly, and eat a healthy diet may not be at greater risk for early death.

Recommended body composition is a primary objective to achieve overall physical fitness and enhanced quality of life. Individuals at recommended body weight are able to participate in a wide variety of moderate-to-vigorous activities without functional limitations. These people have the freedom to enjoy most of life's recreational activities to their fullest potential. Excessive body weight does not afford an individual the fitness level to enjoy vigorous lifetime activities such as basketball, soccer, racquetball, surfing, mountain cycling, or mountain climbing. Maintaining high fitness and recommended body weight gives a person a degree of independence throughout life that most people in developed nations no longer enjoy.

Scientific evidence also recognizes problems with being underweight. Although the social pressure to be thin has declined slightly in recent years, the pressure to attain model-like thinness is still with us and contributes to the gradual increase in the number of people who develop eating disorders (anorexia nervosa and bulimia, discussed later in this chapter).

Extreme weight loss can lead to medical conditions such as heart damage, gastrointestinal problems, shrinkage of internal organs, immune system abnormalities, disorders of the reproductive system, loss of muscle tissue, damage to the nervous system, and even death. About 14 percent of people in the United States are underweight.

Tolerable Weight

Many people want to lose weight so they will look better. That's a noteworthy goal. The problem, however, is that they have a distorted image of what they would really look like if they were to reduce to what they think is their ideal weight. Hereditary factors play a big role, and only a small fraction of the population has the genes for a "perfect body."

When people set their own target weight, they should be realistic. Attaining the "Excellent" percent of body fat shown in Table 4.9 (page 104) is extremely difficult for some. It is even more difficult to maintain, unless the person makes a commitment to a vigorous lifetime exercise program and permanent dietary changes. Few people are willing to do that. The "Moderate" percent body fat category may be more realistic for many people.

A question you should ask yourself is: Am I happy with my weight? Part of enjoying a higher quality of life is being happy with yourself. If you are not, you either need to do something about it or learn to live with it.

If your percent of body fat is higher than those in the Moderate category of Table 4.9, you should try to come down and stay in this category, for health reasons. This is the category that seems to pose no detriment to health.

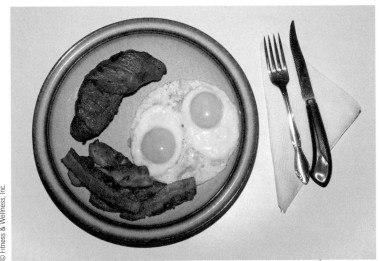

Low-carbohydrate/high-protein diets create nutritional deficiencies and contribute to the development of cardiovascular disease, cancer, and osteoporosis.

Overweight Excess weight according to a given standard, such as height or recommended percent body fat; less than obese.

Obesity A chronic disease characterized by excessive body fat in relation to lean body mass.

If you are in the Moderate category but would like to reduce your percent of body fat further, you need to ask yourself a second question: How badly do I want it? Do I want it badly enough to implement lifetime exercise and dietary changes? If you are not willing to change, you should stop worrying about your weight and deem the Moderate category "tolerable" for you.

The Weight Loss Dilemma

Yo-yo dieting carries as great a health risk as being overweight and remaining overweight in the first place. Epidemiological data show that frequent fluctuations in weight (up or down) markedly increase the risk of dying of cardiovascular disease.

Based on the findings that constant losses and regains can be hazardous to health, quick-fix diets should be replaced by a slow but permanent weight loss program (as described under "Losing Weight the Sound and Sensible Way"). Individuals reap the benefits of recommended body weight when they get to that weight and stay there throughout life.

Unfortunately, only about 10 percent of all people who begin a traditional weight loss program without exercise are able to lose the desired weight. Worse, only 5 in 100 are able to keep the weight off. The body is highly resistant to permanent weight changes through caloric restrictions alone.

Traditional diets have failed because few of them incorporate lifetime changes in food selection and exercise as fundamental to successful weight loss. When the diet stops, weight gain begins. The $40-billion diet industry tries to capitalize on the idea that weight can be lost quickly without considering the consequences of fast weight loss or the importance of lifetime behavioral changes to ensure proper weight loss and maintenance.

In addition, various studies indicate that most people, especially obese people, underestimate their energy intake. Those who try to lose weight but apparently fail to do so are often described as "diet-resistant." One study found that, while on a "diet," a group of obese individuals with a self-reported history of diet resistance underreported their average daily caloric intake by almost 50 percent (1,028 self-reported versus 2,081 actual calories—see Figure 5.2).[6] These individuals also overestimated their amount of daily physical activity by about 25 percent (1,022 self-reported versus 771 actual calories). These differences represent an additional 1,304 calories of energy per day unaccounted for by the subjects in the study. The findings indicate that failing to lose weight often is related to misreports of actual food intake and level of physical activity.

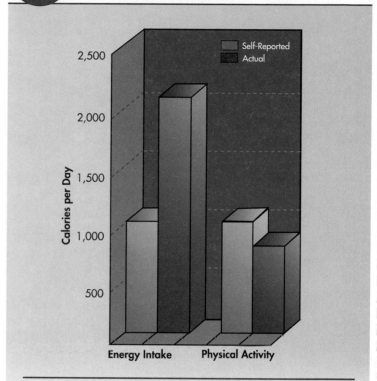

Figure 5.2 Differences between self-reported and actual daily caloric intake and exercise in obese individuals attempting to lose weight.

Source: S. W. Lichtman et al., "Discrepancy Between Self-Reported and Actual Caloric Intake and Exercise in Obese Subjects" *New England Journal of Medicine* 327 (1992): 1893–1898.

The Diet Craze

Capitalizing on hopes that the latest diet to hit the market will really work this time, fad diets continue to appeal to people of all shapes and sizes. These diets may work for awhile, but their success is usually short-lived. These diets deceive people and claim that dieters will lose weight by following all instructions. Most fad diets are very low in calories and deprive the body of certain nutrients, generating a metabolic imbalance. Under these conditions, a lot of the weight lost is in the form of water and protein, and not fat.

On a crash diet, close to half the weight loss is in lean (protein) tissue. When the body uses protein instead of a combination of fats and carbohydrates as a source of energy, weight is lost as much as 10 times faster. This is because a gram of protein produces half the amount of energy that fat does. In the case of muscle protein, one-fifth of protein is mixed with four-fifths water. Therefore, each pound of muscle yields only one-tenth the amount of energy of a pound of fat. As a result, most of the weight lost is in the form of water, which on the scale, of course, looks good.

The largest diet craze in the market today are the low-carbohydrate diet plans. Although small variations exist among them, in general, "low-carb" diets limit the intake of carbohydrate-rich foods like bread, potatoes, rice, pasta, cereals, crackers, juices, sodas, sweets (candy, cake, cookies), and even fruits and vegetables. Dieters are allowed to eat all the protein-rich foods they desire, including steak, ham, chicken, fish, bacon, eggs, nuts, cheese, tofu, high-fat salad dressings, butter, and small amounts of a few fruits and vegetables. Examples of these diets are the Atkins Diet, The Zone, Protein Power, the Scarsdale Diet, The Carb Addict's Diet, and Sugar Busters.

> *When I get calls about the latest diet fad, I imagine a trick birthday cake candle that keeps lighting up and we have to keep blowing it out.*
>
> —Dr. Kelly Brownell, Yale University

During digestion, carbohydrates are converted into glucose, a basic fuel used by every cell in the body. As blood glucose rises, insulin is released from the pancreas. Insulin is a hormone that facilitates the entry of glucose into the cells, thus lowering the glucose level in the bloodstream.

Not all carbohydrates cause a similar rise in blood glucose. The rise in glucose is based on the speed of digestion, which depends on a number of factors, including the size of the food particles. Small-particle carbohydrates break down rapidly and cause a quick, sharp rise in blood glucose. Thus, to gauge a food's effect on blood glucose, carbohydrates are classified by the **glycemic index**.

A high glycemic index signifies a quick rise in blood glucose. At the top of the 100-point scale is glucose itself. This index is not directly related to simple and complex carbohydrates, and the glycemic values are not always what one might expect. Rather, the index is based on the actual laboratory-measured speed of absorption. Processed foods generally have a high glycemic index, whereas high-fiber foods tend to have a lower index (see Table 5.1).

The body functions best when blood sugar remains at a constant level. Although this is best accomplished with low–glycemic index foods, elimination of all high–glycemic index foods from the diet is not necessary (foods with a high glycemic index are useful to replenish depleted glycogen stores following prolonged or exhaustive exercise). Combining high- with low-glycemic index items or with some fat and protein brings the average index down. Regular consumption of high-glycemic foods, nonetheless, can increase the risk of cardiovascular disease, especially in people at risk for diabetes.

Table 5.1	**Glycemic Index of Selected Foods**		
Food Item	**Index**	**Food Item**	**Index**
Glucose	100	Muesli	56
Carrots	92	Peas	51
Honey	87	White pasta	50
Baked potatoes	85	Oatmeal	59
White rice	72	Whole-wheat pasta	42
White bread	69	Oranges	40
Whole-wheat bread	69	Apples	39
Bananas	62	Low-fat yogurt	33
Boiled potatoes	62	Fructose	20
Corn	59	Peanuts	13

Proponents of low-carb diets indicate that if a person eats fewer carbohydrates and more protein, the pancreas will produce less insulin, and as insulin drops, the body will turn to its own fat deposits for energy. There is no scientific proof, however, that high levels of insulin lead to weight gain. None of the authors of these diets have published any studies that validate their claims. Yet, these authors base their diets on the faulty premise that high insulin leads to obesity. In fact, we know the opposite to be true—excessive body fat causes insulin levels to rise, thus increasing the risk for developing diabetes.

Low-carb diets are contrary to the nutrition advice of most national leading health organizations (who recommend a diet low in animal fat and saturated fat and high in complex carbohydrates). Without fruits, vegetables, and grains, high-protein diets lack many vitamins, minerals, and fiber—all dietary factors that protect against an array of ailments and diseases. The major risk associated with low-carb diets is an increased risk of heart disease because high-protein foods are also high in fat content. A low carbohydrate intake also produces a loss of vitamin B, calcium, and potassium. Potential bone loss can further accentuate the risk for osteoporosis. Weakness, nausea, bad breath, constipation, irritability, lightheadedness, and fatigue are side effects commonly associated with these diets. Long-term adherence to a high-protein diet can also increase the risk of certain types of cancer.

Yo-yo dieting Constantly losing and gaining weight.

Glycemic index An index that is used to rate the plasma glucose response of carbohydrate-containing foods with the response produced by the same amount of carbohydrate from a standard source, usually glucose or white bread.

In addition to the low-carb diets, "combo-diets" such as the Schwarzbein and Suzanne Sommers diets are also popular of late. The Schwarzbein diet claims that eating proteins and nonstarchy carbohydrates together will keep the food from being stored as fat. The Suzanne Sommers diet doesn't allow you to eat proteins within 3 hours of carbohydrates, and if fruits are eaten, the dieter must wait at least 20 minutes before eating other carbohydrate foods. Both of these diets allow consumption of high-protein/high-fat food items, which increases risk for heart disease.

Other diets allow only certain specialized foods. If people would realize that no magic foods will provide all of the necessary nutrients, that a person has to eat a variety of foods to be well-nourished, the diet industry would not be as successful. Most of these diets create a nutritional deficiency, which at times may be fatal.

The reason many of these diets succeed is because a large number of foods are restricted on the diet, thus people tend to eat less food overall. With the extraordinary variety of foods available to us, it is unrealistic to think that people will adhere to these diets for very long. People eventually get tired of eating the same thing day in and day out and start eating less, thus leading to weight loss. If they happen to achieve the lower weight but do not make permanent dietary changes, they regain the weight quickly once they go back to their previous eating habits.

A few diets recommend exercise along with caloric restrictions—the best method for weight reduction, of course. People who adhere to these programs will succeed, so the diet has achieved its purpose. Unfortunately, if the people do not change their food selection and activity level permanently, they gain back the weight once they discontinue dieting and exercise.

Also, let's not forget that we eat for reasons other than to lose weight—we eat for pleasure and for health. Healthy eating along with regular physical activity are two of the most essential components of a wellness lifestyle, and they provide the best weight management program available today.

Eating Disorders

Anorexia nervosa and bulimia nervosa are physical and emotional conditions thought to stem from some combination of individual, family, and social pressures. These disorders are characterized by an intense fear of becoming fat that does not disappear even when losing extreme amounts of weight. Anorexia nervosa and bulimia nervosa are increasing steadily in most industrialized nations where society encourages low-calorie diets and thinness.

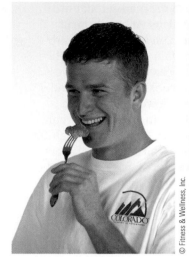
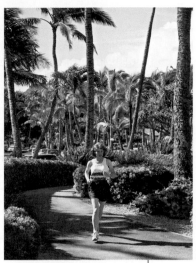

Achieving and maintaining a high physical fitness percent body fat standard requires a lifetime commitment to regular physical activity and proper nutrition.

Anorexia Nervosa

Approximately 19 of every 20 individuals with **anorexia nervosa** are young women. An estimated 1 percent of the female population in the United States is anorexic. Anorexic individuals seem to fear weight gain more than death from starvation. Furthermore, they have a distorted image of their body and think of themselves as being fat even when they are emaciated.

Although a genetic predisposition may contribute to the syndrome, the anorexic person often comes from a mother-dominated home, with possible drug addictions in the family. The syndrome may emerge following a stressful life event and uncertainty about one's ability to cope efficiently.

The female role in society is changing rapidly, and women seem to be especially susceptible. Life experiences such as gaining weight, starting the menstrual period, beginning college, losing a boyfriend, having poor self-esteem, being socially rejected, starting a professional career, or becoming a wife or a mother can trigger the syndrome.

These individuals typically begin a diet and at first feel in control and happy about the weight loss, even if they are not overweight. To speed the weight loss, they frequently combine extreme dieting with exhaustive exercise and overuse of laxatives and diuretics.

Anorexics commonly develop obsessive and compulsive behaviors and emphatically deny their condition. They are preoccupied with food, meal planning, and grocery shopping, and they have unusual eating habits. As they lose weight and their health begins to deteriorate, anorexics feel weak and

tired. They might realize they have a problem, but they will not stop the starvation and will refuse to consider the behavior abnormal.

Once anorexics have lost a lot of weight and malnutrition sets in, physical changes become more visible. Typical changes are amenorrhea (stopping menstruation), digestive problems, extreme sensitivity to cold, hair and skin problems, fluid and electrolyte abnormalities (which may lead to an irregular heartbeat and sudden stopping of the heart), injuries to nerves and tendons, abnormalities of immune function, anemia, growth of fine body hair, mental confusion, inability to concentrate, lethargy, depression, dry skin, lower skin and body temperature, and osteoporosis.

> *Anorexic individuals seem to fear weight gain more than death from starvation.*

Diagnostic criteria for anorexia nervosa are[7]

■ Refusal to maintain body weight over a minimal normal weight for age and height (weight loss leading to maintenance of body weight less than 85 percent of that expected or failure to make expected weight gain during periods of growth, leading to body weight less than 85 percent of that expected).

■ Intense fear of gaining weight or becoming fat, even though underweight.

■ Disturbance in the way in which one perceives one's own body weight, size, or shape, undue influences of body weight or shape on self-evaluation, or denial of the seriousness of the current low body weight.

■ In postmenarcheal females, amenorrhea (absence of at least three consecutive menstrual cycles). (A woman is considered to have amenorrhea if her periods occur only following estrogen therapy.)

Many of the changes induced by anorexia nervosa can be reversed. Treatment almost always requires professional help, and the sooner it is started, the better the chances for reversibility and cure. Therapy consists of a combination of medical and psychological techniques to restore proper nutrition, prevent medical complications, and modify the environment or events that triggered the syndrome. Anorexics seldom overcome the problem by themselves. They strongly deny their condition. They are able to hide it and deceive friends and relatives. In their behavior, many of them meet all of the characteristics of anorexia nervosa, but it goes undetected because both thinness and dieting are socially acceptable. Only a well-trained clinician is able to diagnose anorexia nervosa.

Bulimia Nervosa

Bulimia nervosa is more prevalent than anorexia nervosa. For many years it was thought to be a variant of anorexia nervosa, but now it is identified as a separate condition. It afflicts mainly young people. As many as 1 in every 5 women on college campuses may be bulimic, according to some estimates. Bulimia nervosa also is more prevalent than anorexia nervosa in males, although bulimia is still much more prevalent in females.

Bulimics usually are healthy-looking people, well-educated, and near recommended body weight. They seem to enjoy food and often socialize around it. In actuality, they are emotionally insecure, rely on others, and lack self-confidence and self-esteem. Recommended weight and food are abnormally important to them.

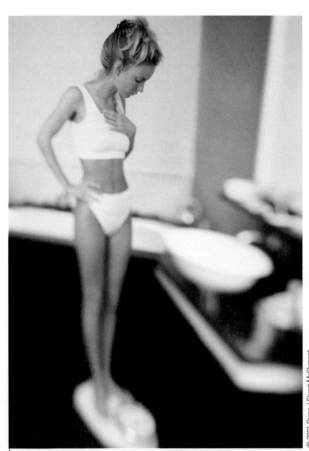

Society's unrealistic view of what constitutes recommended weight and "ideal" body image contributes to the development of eating disorders.

© 2001 Stone / Stuart McClymont

Anorexia nervosa An eating disorder characterized by self-imposed starvation to lose and maintain very low body weight.

Bulimia nervosa An eating disorder characterized by a pattern of binge eating and purging in an attempt to lose weight and maintain low body weight.

The binge-purge cycle usually occurs in stages. As a result of stressful life events or the simple compulsion to eat, bulimics periodically engage in binge eating that may last an hour or longer. With some apprehension, bulimics anticipate and plan the cycle. Next they feel an urgency to begin, followed by large and uncontrollable food consumption during which they may eat several thousand calories (up to 10,000 calories in extreme cases). After a short period of relief and satisfaction, feelings of deep guilt, shame, and intense fear of gaining weight ensue. Purging seems to be an easy answer, because the bingeing cycle can continue without fear of gaining weight.

> *The sooner treatment for eating disorders is initiated, the better the chances for recovery.*

The diagnostic criteria for bulimia nervosa are[8]

- Recurrent episodes of binge eating. An episode of binge eating is characterized by both of the following:
    1. Eating, in a discrete period of time (for example, within any 2-hour period), an amount of food that is definitely more than most people would eat during a similar period and under similar circumstances.
    2. A sense of lack of control over eating during the episode (a feeling that one cannot stop eating or control what or how much one is eating).
- Recurring inappropriate compensatory behaviors to prevent weight gain, such as self-induced vomiting; misuse of laxatives, diuretics, enemas, or other medications; fasting; or excessive exercise.
- The binge eating and inappropriate compensatory behaviors both occur, on average, at least twice a week for 3 months.
- Self-evaluation is unduly influenced by body shape and weight.
- The binge eating causes marked distress.

The most typical form of purging is self-induced vomiting. Bulimics, too, frequently ingest strong laxatives and emetics. Near-fasting diets and strenuous bouts of exercise are common. Medical problems associated with bulimia nervosa include cardiac arrhythmias, amenorrhea, kidney and bladder damage, ulcers, colitis, tearing of the esophagus or stomach, tooth erosion, gum damage, and general muscular weakness.

Unlike anorexics, bulimics realize their behavior is abnormal and feel great shame about it. Fearing social rejection, they pursue the binge-purge cycle in secrecy and at unusual hours of the day.

Bulimia nervosa can be treated successfully when the person realizes that this destructive behavior is not the solution to life's problems. A change in attitude can prevent permanent damage or death.

Treatment for anorexia nervosa and bulimia nervosa is available on most school campuses through the school's counseling center or the health center. Local hospitals also offer treatment for these conditions. Many communities have support groups, frequently led by professional personnel and usually free of charge.

Physiology of Weight Loss

Only a few years ago the principles governing a weight loss and maintenance program seemed to be clear, but now we know the final answers are not in yet. Traditional concepts related to weight control have centered on three assumptions: (a) that balancing food intake against output allows a person to achieve recommended weight, (b) that all fat people just eat too much, and (c) that the human body doesn't care how much (or little) fat it stores. Although these statements contain some truth, they still are open to much debate and research. We now know that the causes of obesity are complex, including a combination of genetics, behavior, and lifestyle factors.

Energy-Balancing Equation

The principle embodied in the **energy-balancing equation** is simple: If daily energy requirements could be determined accurately, caloric intake could be balanced against output. This is not always the case, though, because genetic and lifestyle-related individual differences determine the number of calories required to maintain or lose body weight.

Table 5.2 (page 125) offers some general guidelines for estimating daily caloric intake according to lifestyle patterns. This is only an estimated figure and (as discussed under "Losing Weight the Sound and Sensible Way") it serves only as a starting point from which individual adjustments have to be made.

One pound of fat represents 3,500 calories. Assuming that a person's basic daily caloric expenditure is 2,500 calories, if this person were to decrease intake by 500 calories per day, it should result in a loss of one pound of fat in 7 days ($500 \times 7 = 3,500$). But research has shown—and many people have experienced—that even when dieters carefully balance caloric input against caloric output, weight loss does not always happen as predicted. Furthermore, two people with similar measured caloric intake and output seldom lose weight at the same rate.

The most common explanation of individual differences in weight loss and weight gain has been the variation in human metabolism from one person to another. We are all familiar with people

who can eat "all day long" and not gain an ounce of weight, whereas others cannot even "dream about food" without gaining weight. Because experts did not believe that human metabolism alone could account for such extreme differences, they developed several theories that might better explain these individual variations.

Setpoint Theory

Results of several research studies point toward a **weight-regulating mechanism (WRM)** that has a **setpoint** for controlling both appetite and the amount of fat stored. Setpoint is hypothesized to work like a thermostat for body fat, maintaining fairly constant body weight, because it "knows" at all times the exact amount of adipose tissue stored in the fat cells. Some people have high settings; others have low settings.

If body weight decreases (as in dieting), the setpoint senses this change and triggers the WRM to increase the person's appetite or make the body conserve energy to maintain the "set" weight. The opposite also may be true. Some people have a hard time gaining weight. In this case, the WRM decreases appetite or causes the body to waste energy to maintain the lower weight.

Setpoint and Caloric Input

Every person has his or her own certain body fat percentage (as established by the setpoint) that the body attempts to maintain. The genetic instinct to survive tells the body that fat storage is vital, and therefore it sets an acceptable fat level. This level may remain somewhat constant or may climb gradually because of poor lifestyle habits.

For instance, under strict calorie reduction, the body may make extreme metabolic adjustments in an effort to maintain its setpoint for fat. The **basal metabolic rate**, the lowest level of caloric intake necessary to sustain life, may drop dramatically when operating under a consistent negative caloric balance, and that person's weight loss may plateau for days or even weeks. A low metabolic rate compounds a person's problems in maintaining recommended body weight.

These findings were substantiated by research conducted at Rockefeller University in New York.[9] The authors showed that the body resists maintaining altered weight. Obese and lifetime non-obese individuals were used in the investigation. Following a 10 percent weight loss, in an attempt to regain the lost weight, the body compensated by burning up to 15 percent fewer calories than expected for the new reduced weight (after accounting for the 10 percent loss). The effects were similar in the obese and non-obese participants. These results imply that

after a 10 percent weight loss, a person would have to eat less or exercise more to account for the estimated difference of about 200 to 300 calories.

In this same study, when the participants were allowed to increase their weight to 10 percent above their "normal" body (pre-weight loss) weight, the body burned 10 to 15 percent more calories than expected—the body's attempt to waste energy and maintain the pre-set weight. This is another indication that the body is highly resistant to weight changes unless additional lifestyle changes are incorporated to ensure successful weight management. (These methods will be discussed under "Losing Weight the Sound and Sensible Way".)

Dietary restriction alone will not lower the setpoint, even though the person may lose weight and fat. When the dieter goes back to the normal or even below-normal caloric intake (at which the weight may have been stable for a long time), he or she quickly regains the fat loss as the body strives to regain a comfortable fat store.

Let's use a practical illustration. A person would like to lose some body fat and assumes that his or her current, stable body weight has been reached at an average daily caloric intake of 1,800 calories (no weight gain or loss occurs at this daily intake). In an attempt to lose weight rapidly, this person now goes on a strict low-calorie diet, or even worse, a near-fasting diet. Immediately the body activates its survival mechanism and readjusts its metabolism to a lower caloric balance. After a few weeks of dieting at fewer than 400 to 600 calories per day, the body becomes able to maintain its normal functions at 1,000 calories per day.

Having lost the desired weight, the person terminates the diet, but realizes that the original intake of 1,800 calories per day will have to be lower to maintain the new lower weight. To adjust to the new lower body weight, the person restricts intake to about 1,500 calories per day. The individual is surprised to find that, even at this lower daily intake (300 fewer calories), weight comes back at a rate of 1 pound every 1 to 2 weeks. After the diet is over,

Energy-balancing equation A principle holding that as long as caloric input equals caloric output, the person will not gain or lose weight. If caloric intake exceeds output, the person gains weight; when output exceeds input, the person loses weight.

Weight-regulating mechanism (WRM) A feature of the hypothalamus of the brain that controls how much the body should weigh.

Setpoint Weight control theory that the body has an established weight and strongly attempts to maintain that weight.

Basal metabolic rate (BMR) The lowest level of oxygen consumption necessary to sustain life.

this new lowered metabolic rate may take several months to kick back up to its normal level.

From this explanation, individuals clearly should not go on very low-calorie diets. Not only will this slow down resting metabolic rate, but it will also deprive the body of basic daily nutrients required for normal function.

Daily caloric intakes of 1,200 to 1,500 calories provide the necessary nutrients if they are distributed properly over the five basic food groups (meeting the daily required servings from each group). Of course, the individual will have to learn which foods meet the requirements and yet are low in fat and sugar.

Under no circumstances should a person go on a diet that calls for less than 1,200 calories for women or 1,500 calories for men. Weight (fat) is gained over months and years, not overnight. Likewise, weight loss should be gradual, not abrupt.

A second way in which the setpoint may work is by keeping track of the nutrients and calories consumed daily. It is thought that the body, like a cash register, records the daily food intake and that the brain will not feel satisfied until the calories and nutrients have been "registered."

This setpoint for calories and nutrients seems to operate even when people participate in moderately intense exercise. Some evidence suggests that people do not become hungrier with moderate physical activity. Therefore, people can choose to lose weight either by going hungry or by stepping up their daily physical activity. Burning more calories through physical activity helps to lower body fat.

Lowering the Setpoint

The most common question regarding the setpoint is how it can be lowered so the body will feel comfortable at a reduced fat percentage. These factors seem to affect the setpoint directly by lowering the fat thermostat:

1. Aerobic exercise.
2. A diet high in complex carbohydrates.
3. Nicotine.
4. Amphetamines.

The last two are more destructive than the extra fat weight, so they are not reasonable alternatives (as far as the extra strain on the heart is concerned, smoking one pack of cigarettes per day is said to be the equivalent of carrying 50 to 75 pounds of excess body fat).

On the other hand, a diet high in fats and refined carbohydrates, near-fasting diets, and perhaps even artificial sweeteners seem to raise the setpoint. Therefore, the only practical and sensible way to lower the setpoint and lose fat weight is a combination of aerobic exercise and a diet high in complex carbohydrates and low in fat.

Because of the effects of proper food management on the body's setpoint, many nutritionists believe the total number of calories should not be the main concern in a weight-control program. Rather, it should be the source of those calories. In this regard, most of the successful dieter's effort is spent in re-forming eating habits, increasing the intake of complex carbohydrates and high-fiber foods, and decreasing the consumption of refined carbohydrates (sugars) and fats. In most cases, this change in eating habits will bring about a decrease in total daily caloric intake. Because 1 gram of carbohydrates provides only 4 calories, as opposed to 9 calories per gram of fat, you could eat twice the volume of food (by weight) when substituting carbohydrates for fat.

In 1996 the Food and Drug Administration (FDA) approved a new fat substitute, **olestra,** for use in "savory snacks." According to the *University of California at Berkeley Wellness Letter*, consumers should "just say no" to olestra and not buy products that contain this fat substitute.[10]

Olestra can cause diarrhea and cramping, and it can deplete the body of fat-soluble vitamins, including A, D, E, and K. Vitamin E is a strong antioxidant, and low levels of vitamin K pose a risk for people with bleeding disorders and those on blood-thinning medication. In addition, potential cancer-causing changes in liver cells have been found in animal studies of olestra. Although the fat and caloric content of olestra-containing foods is lower than that of foods cooked with natural fats, consuming snacks using this fat substitute not only can pose a risk to good health but also will reinforce unhealthy eating habits.

A "diet" is no longer viewed as a temporary tool to aid in weight loss but, instead, as a permanent change in eating behaviors to ensure weight management and better health. The role of increased physical activity also must be considered, because successful weight loss, maintenance, and recommended body composition seldom are attained without a moderate reduction in caloric intake combined with a regular exercise program.

Diet and Metabolism

Fat can be lost by selecting the proper foods, exercising, or restricting calories. When a person tries to lose weight by dietary restrictions alone, lean body mass (muscle protein, along with vital organ protein) always decreases. The amount of lean body mass lost depends entirely on caloric limitation.

When people go on a near-fasting diet, up to half of the weight loss is lean body mass and the other half is actual fat loss (see Figure 5.3).[11] When diet is combined with exercise, close to 100 percent

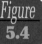

Figure 5.3

Effects of three forms of diet on fat loss.

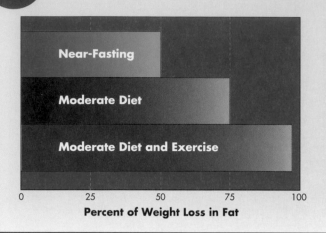

Adapted from R. J. Shephard, *Alive Man: The Physiology of Physical Activity.*
(Springfield, IL: Charles C Thomas, 1975): 484–488.

of the weight loss is in the form of fat, and lean tissue actually may increase. Loss of lean body mass is never good, because it weakens the organs and muscles and slows down metabolism. Large losses in lean tissue can cause disturbances in heart function and damage to other organs. Equally important is not to overindulge (binge) following a very low-calorie diet. This may cause changes in metabolic rate and electrolyte balance, which could trigger fatal cardiac arrhythmias.

Contrary to some beliefs, aging is not the main reason for the lower metabolic rate. It is not so much that metabolism slows down as that people slow down. As people age, they tend to rely more on the amenities of life (remote controls, cellular telephones, intercoms, single-level homes, riding lawn-mowers) that lull a person into sedentary living.

Basal metabolism is related directly to lean body weight. The more lean tissue, the higher the metabolic rate. As a consequence of sedentary living and less physical activity, the lean component decreases and fat tissue increases. The human body requires a certain amount of oxygen per pound of lean body mass. Given that fat is considered metabolically inert from the point of view of caloric use, the lean tissue uses most of the oxygen, even at rest. As muscle and organ mass (lean body mass) decreases, so do the energy requirements at rest.

Reductions in lean body mass are common in aging people (primarily because of physical inactivity) and those on severely restricted diets. The loss of lean body mass also may account for a lower metabolic rate and the longer time it takes to kick back up.

Diets with caloric intakes below 1,200 to 1,500 calories cannot guarantee the retention of lean body mass. Even at this intake level, some loss is inevitable, unless the diet is combined with exercise. Despite the claims of many diets that they do not alter the lean component, the simple truth is that, regardless of what nutrients may be added to the diet, severe caloric restrictions always prompt the loss of lean tissue. Too many people go on low-calorie diets constantly. Every time they do, the metabolic rate slows down as more lean tissue is lost.

People in their 40s and older who weigh the same as they did when they were 20 tend to think they are at recommended body weight. During this span of 20 years or more, they may have dieted many times without participating in an exercise program. They regain the weight shortly after they terminate each diet, and most of that gain is in fat. Maybe at age 20 they weighed 150 pounds, of which only 15 percent was fat. Now at age 40, even though they still weigh 150 pounds, they might be 30 percent fat (see Figure 5.4). At recommended body weight, they wonder why they are eating very little and still having trouble staying at that weight.

Olestra Fat substitute made from sugar and fatty acids; provides no calories to the body because it passes through the digestive system without being absorbed.

Figure 5.4

Effects of frequent dieting without exercise on body weight, percent body fat, and lean body mass.

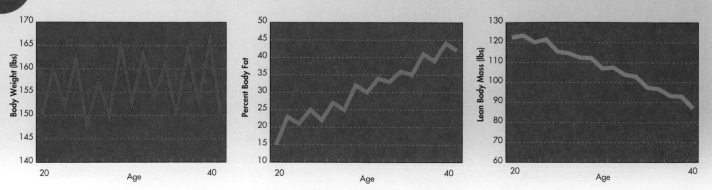

Exercise: The Key to Weight Loss and Weight Maintenance

A more effective way to tilt the energy-balancing equation in your favor is by burning calories through physical activity. Exercise also seems to exert control over how much a person weighs.

Starting at age 25, the typical American gains 1 pound of weight per year. This weight gain represents a simple energy surplus of under 10 calories per day. In most cases, the additional weight accumulated in middle age comes from people becoming less physically active, and not as a result of increased caloric intake. Dr. Jack Wilmore, a leading exercise physiologist and expert weight management researcher, stated:

> Physical inactivity is certainly a major, if not the primary, cause of obesity in the United States today. A certain minimal level of activity might be necessary for us to accurately balance our caloric intake to our caloric expenditure. With too little activity, we appear to lose the fine control we normally have to maintain this incredible balance. This fine balance amounts to less than 10 calories per day, or the equivalent of one potato chip.[12]

Exercise is crucial to losing weight and maintaining weight. Not only will exercise maintain lean tissue, but advocates of the setpoint theory say that exercise resets the fat thermostat to a new, lower level. This change may be rapid, or it may take time. A few overweight individuals have exercised faithfully almost daily, 60 minutes at a time, for a whole year before seeing significant weight change. People with a "sticky" setpoint have to be patient and persistent.

If a person is trying to lose weight, a combination of aerobic and strength-training exercises works best. Aerobic exercise is the best to offset the setpoint, and the continuity and duration of these types of activities cause many calories to be burned in the process. The role of aerobic exercise in successful lifetime weight management cannot be overestimated. Strength training is critical in helping raise the basal metabolic rate.

As illustrated in Figure 5.5, greater weight loss is achieved by combining a diet with an aerobic exercise program.[13] Of even greater significance, only the individuals who participated in an 18-month post-diet aerobic exercise program were able to keep the weight off. Those who discontinued exercise regained weight. Furthermore, of those who initiated or resumed exercise during the 18-month follow-up, all were able to lose weight again. Individuals who only dieted and did not exercise regained 60 percent and 92 percent of their weight loss at the 6- and 18-month follow-ups, respectively.

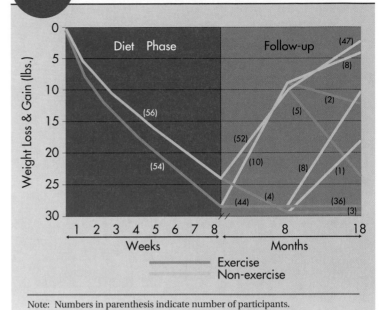

Figure 5.5 Aerobic exercise and weight loss and maintenance in moderately obese individuals.

Note: Numbers in parenthesis indicate number of participants.

Source: K. N. Pavlou, S. Krey, and W. P. Steffe, "Exercise as an Adjunct to Weight Loss and Maintenance in Moderately Obese Subjects," *American Journal of Clinical Nutrition* 49 (1989): 1115–1123.

Weight loss might be more rapid when aerobic exercise is combined with a strength-training program. Each additional pound of muscle tissue can raise the basal metabolic rate by about 35 calories per day.[14] Thus, an individual who adds 5 pounds of muscle tissue as a result of strength training increases the basal metabolic rate by 175 calories per day (35×5), which equals 63,875 calories per year (175×365) or the equivalent of 18.25 pounds of fat ($63,875 \div 3,500$).

Strength training is suggested especially for people who think they are at their recommended body weight, yet their body fat percentage is higher than recommended. The number of calories burned during a typical hour-long strength-training session is much less than during an hour of aerobic exercise. Because of the high intensity of strength training, the person needs frequent rest intervals to recover from each set of exercise. The average person actually lifts weights only 10 to 12 minutes during each hour of exercise. In the long run, however, the person enjoys the benefits of gains in lean tissue. Guidelines for developing aerobic and strength-training programs are given in Chapters 7 and 8.

Although size (inches) and percent body fat both decrease when sedentary individuals begin an exercise program, body weight often remains the same or may even increase during the first couple of weeks of the program. Exercise helps to increase

muscle tissue, connective tissue, blood volume (as much as 500 ml, or the equivalent of 1 pound, following the first week of aerobic exercise), enzymes and other structures within the cell, and glycogen (which binds water). All of these changes lead to a higher functional capacity of the human body. With exercise, most of the weight loss becomes apparent after a few weeks of training, after the lean component has stabilized.

Although we know that a negative caloric balance of 3,500 calories does not always result in a loss of exactly 1 pound of fat, the role of exercise in achieving a negative balance by burning additional calories is significant in weight reduction and maintenance programs. Sadly, some individuals claim that the number of calories burned during exercise is hardly worth the effort. They think that cutting their daily intake by some 300 calories is easier than participating in some sort of exercise that would burn the same amount of calories. The problem is that the willpower to cut those 300 calories lasts only a few weeks, and then the person goes right back to the old eating patterns.

If a person gets into the habit of exercising regularly, say 3 times a week, jogging 3 miles per exercise session (about 300 calories burned), this represents 900 calories in one week, about 3,600 calories in one month, or 46,800 calories per year. This minimal amount of exercise represents as many as 13.5 extra pounds of fat in one year, 27 in two, and so on.

We tend to forget that our weight creeps up gradually over the years, not just overnight. Hardly worth the effort? And we have not even taken into consideration the increase in lean tissue, possible resetting of the setpoint, benefits to the cardiovascular system, and, most important, the improved quality of life. The fundamental reasons for overfatness and obesity, few could argue, are sedentary living and lack of physical activity.

In terms of preventing disease, many of the health benefits people try to achieve by losing weight are reaped through exercise alone, even without weight loss. Exercise offers protection against premature morbidity and mortality for everyone, including people who already have risk factors for disease (see Chapter 12). The lack of exercise, not the weight problem itself, may be the cause of many of the health risks associated with obesity.

Low-Intensity Versus High-Intensity Exercise for Weight Loss

Some individuals promote low-intensity exercise over high-intensity for weight loss purposes. As compared to high intensity, a greater proportion of calories burned during low-intensity exercise are derived from fat. The lower the intensity of exercise, the higher the percentage of fat utilization as an energy source. In theory, if you are trying to lose fat, this principle makes sense, but in reality it is misleading. The bottom line when you are trying to lose weight is to burn more calories. When your daily caloric expenditure exceeds your intake, weight is lost. The more calories you burn, the more fat is lost.

During low-intensity exercise, up to 50 percent of the calories burned may be derived from fat (the other 50 percent from glucose [carbohydrates]). With intense exercise, only 30 to 40 percent of the caloric expenditure comes from fat. Overall, however, you can burn twice as many (or more) calories during high-intensity exercise, and, subsequently more fat as well.

Let's look at a practical illustration. If you exercise for 30 minutes at a moderate intensity and burn 200 calories, about 100 of those calories (50 percent) would come from fat. If you exercise at high intensity during those same 30 minutes, you may burn 400 calories—with 120 to 160 of the calories (30 to 40 percent) coming from fat. Thus, if you exercised at a low intensity, you would have to do so twice as long to burn the same number of calories. Another benefit is that the metabolic rate remains at a higher level longer after high-intensity exercise, so you continue to burn more calories following exercise.

Moreover, high-intensity exercise by itself appears to trigger greater fat loss than low-intensity exercise. Research conducted at Laval University in Quebec, Canada, showed that subjects who performed a high-intensity intermittent-training program lost more body fat than participants in a low- to moderate-intensity continuous aerobic endurance group.[15] Even more surprisingly, this finding occurred despite the fact that the high-intensity group burned fewer total calories per exercise session. The results support the notion that vigorous exercise is more conducive to weight loss than low- to moderate-intensity exercise.

Before you start high-intensity exercise sessions, a word of caution is in order. Be sure that it is medically safe for you to participate in such activities and that you build up gradually to that level. If you are cleared to participate in high-intensity exercise, do not attempt to do too much too quickly, because you may suffer injuries and discouragement. You must allow your body a proper conditioning period of 8 to 12 weeks, or even longer for people with a moderate-to-serious weight problem. High intensity also does not mean high impact. High-impact activities are the most common cause of exercise-related injuries. Additional information on these topics is presented in Chapter 7.

The previous discussion on high- versus low-intensity exercise does not mean that low intensity is not effective. Low-intensity exercise provides substantial health benefits, and people who initiate exercise programs are more willing to participate and stay with low-intensity programs. Low-intensity exercise does promote weight loss, but it is not as effective. You will need to exercise longer to obtain the same results.

Healthy Weight Gain

"Skinny" people, too, should realize that the only healthy way to gain weight is through exercise (mainly strength-training exercises) and a slight increase in caloric intake. Attempting to gain weight just by overeating will raise the fat component and not the lean component—which is not the path to better health. Exercise is the best solution to weight (fat) reduction and weight (lean) gain alike.

A strength-training program such as the one outlined in Chapter 8 is the best approach to add body weight. The training program should include at least two exercises of three sets for each major body part. Each set should consist of about 10 repetitions maximum.

Even though the metabolic cost of synthesizing a pound of muscle tissue is still unclear, consuming an estimated 500 additional calories daily, including 15 grams of protein above the RDA, is the recommendation to gain an average of 1 pound of muscle tissue per week. Based on the typical American diet, the extra 15 grams of protein are not necessary. Each day, the average person in the United States already consumes 30 to 60 grams of protein above the RDA. The extra 500 calories should be primarily in the form of complex carbohydrates. If the higher caloric intake is not accompanied by a strength-training program, the increase in body weight will be in the form of fat, not muscle tissue.

Weight-Loss Myths

Cellulite and **spot reducing** are mythical concepts. **Cellulite** is nothing but enlarged fat cells that bulge out from accumulated body fat.

Doing several sets of daily sit-ups will not get rid of fat in the midsection of the body. When fat comes off, it does so throughout the entire body, not just the exercised area. The greatest proportion of fat may come off the biggest fat deposits, but the caloric output of a few sets of sit-ups has practically no effect on reducing total body fat. A person has to exercise much longer to really see results.

Other touted means toward quick weight loss—rubberized sweatsuits, steam baths, mechanical vibrators—are misleading. When a person wears a

sweatsuit or steps into a sauna, the weight lost is not fat, but merely a significant amount of water. Sure, it looks nice when you step on the scale immediately afterward, but this represents a false loss of weight. As soon as you replace body fluids, you gain back the weight quickly.

Wearing rubberized sweatsuits not only hastens the rate of body fluid loss—fluid that is vital during prolonged exercise—but it raises core temperature at the same time. This combination puts a person in danger of dehydration, which impairs cellular function and, in extreme cases, can even cause death.

Similarly, mechanical vibrators are worthless in a weight-control program. Vibrating belts and turning rollers may feel good, but they require no effort whatsoever. Fat cannot be shaken off. It is lost primarily by burning it in muscle tissue.

Losing Weight the Sound and Sensible Way

Dieting never has been fun and never will be. People who are overweight and are serious about losing weight, however, have to include regular exercise in their life along with proper food management and a sensible reduction in caloric intake.

Some precautions are in order, because excessive body fat is a risk factor for cardiovascular disease. Depending on the extent of the weight problem, a medical examination and possibly a stress ECG (see "Abnormal Electrocardiograms" in Chapter 12) may be a good idea before undertaking the exercise program. A physician should be consulted in this regard.

Significantly overweight individuals also may have to choose activities in which they will not have to support their own body weight but that still will be effective in burning calories. Injuries to joints and muscles are common in overweight individuals who participate in weight-bearing exercises such as walking, jogging, and aerobics.

Swimming may not be a good weight-loss exercise either. More body fat makes a person more buoyant, and most people are not at the skill level to swim fast enough to get the best training effect. They tend to just float along, limiting the number of calories burned as well as the benefits to the cardio-respiratory system.

Some better alternatives are riding a bicycle (either road or stationary), walking in a shallow pool, doing water aerobics, or running in place in deep water (treading water). The latter forms of water exercise are gaining popularity and have proven to be effective in reducing weight without the fear of injuries.

How long should each exercise session last? To develop and maintain cardiorespiratory fitness, 20

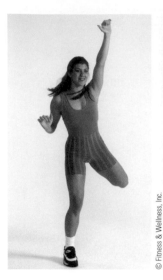

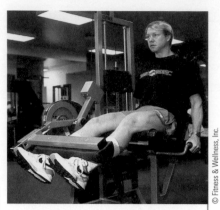

Regular participation in a lifetime exercise program is the key to successful weight management.

2. Developing new behaviors takes time, and some people have trouble changing and adjusting to new eating habits.
3. Many individuals are in such poor physical condition that they take a long time to increase their activity level enough to offset the setpoint and burn enough calories to aid in loss of body fat.
4. Some dieters have difficulty succeeding unless they can count calories.
5. A few people simply will not alter their food selection. For those who will not (which will still increase the risk for chronic diseases), a large increase in physical activity, a negative caloric balance, or a combination of the two is the only solution to lose weight successfully.

You can estimate your daily caloric requirement by consulting Tables 5.2 and 5.3 and completing Lab 5A. Given that this is only an estimated value, individual adjustments related to many of the factors discussed in this chapter may be necessary to establish a more precise value. Nevertheless, the estimated value does offer a beginning guideline for weight control or reduction.

The average daily caloric requirement without exercise is based on typical lifestyle patterns, total body weight, and gender. Individuals who hold jobs that require heavy manual labor burn more calories during the day than those who have sedentary jobs (such as working behind a desk). To find your

to 30 minutes of exercise at the recommended target rate, 3 to 5 times per week, is suggested (see Chapter 7). For weight-loss purposes, many experts recommend exercising at least 45 minutes at a time, 5 to 6 times a week.

A person should not try to do too much too fast. Unconditioned beginners should start with about 15 minutes of aerobic exercise 3 times a week, gradually increasing the duration by approximately 5 minutes per week and the frequency by 1 day per week during the next 3 to 4 weeks.

One final benefit of long-duration exercise for weight control is that it allows fat to be burned more efficiently. Carbohydrates and fats are both sources of energy. When the glucose levels begin to drop during prolonged exercise, more fat is used as energy substrate.

Equally important is that fat-burning enzymes increase with aerobic training. Fat is lost primarily by burning it in muscle. Therefore, as the concentration of the enzymes increases, so does the ability to burn fat.

In addition to exercise and adequate food management, sensible adjustments in caloric intake are recommended. Most research finds that a negative caloric balance is required to lose weight. Perhaps the only exception is with people who are eating too few calories. A nutrient analysis (see Chapter 3) often reveals that faithful dieters are not consuming enough calories. These people actually need to increase their daily caloric intake (and combine that with an exercise program) to get their metabolism to kick back up to a normal level.

The reasons for prescribing a lower caloric figure to lose weight are as follows:

1. Most people underestimate their caloric intake and are eating more than they should be eating.

Table 5.2	Average Caloric Requirement Per Pound of Body Weight Based on Lifestyle Patterns and Gender

	Calories Per Pound	
	Men	Women*
Sedentary — limited physical activity	13.0	12.0
Moderate physical activity	15.0	13.5
Hard labor — strenuous physical effort	17.0	15.0

* Pregnant or lactating women add 3 calories to these values.

Spot reducing Fallacious theory that exercising a specific body part will result in significant fat reduction in that area.

Cellulite Term frequently used in reference to fat deposits that "bulge out"; these deposits are nothing but enlarged fat cells from excessive accumulation of body fat.

Table
5.3

Caloric Expenditure of Selected Physical Activities

Activity*	Cal/lb/min	Activity*	Cal/lb/min	Activity*	Cal/lb/min
Aero-belt Exercise		Dance		Stairmaster	
Aero-belt jogging/6 mph	0.098	Moderate	0.030	Moderate	0.070
Aero-belt Step-aerobics/8"	0.105	Vigorous	0.055	Vigorous	0.090
Aero-belt walking/4 mph	0.073	Golf	0.030	Stationary Cycling	
Aerobics		Gymnastics		Moderate	0.055
Moderate	0.065	Light	0.030	Vigorous	0.070
Vigorous	0.095	Heavy	0.056	Strength Training	0.050
Step aerobics	0.070	Handball	0.064	Swimming (crawl)	
Archery	0.030	Hiking	0.040	20 yds/min	0.031
Badminton		Judo/Karate	0.086	25 yds/min	0.040
Recreation	0.038	Racquetball	0.065	45 yds/min	0.057
Competition	0.065	Rope Jumping	0.060	50 yds/min	0.070
Baseball	0.031	Rowing (vigorous)	0.090	Table Tennis	0.030
Basketball		Running (on a level surface)		Tennis	
Moderate	0.046	11.0 min/mile	0.070	Moderate	0.045
Competition	0.063	8.5 min/mile	0.090	Competition	0.064
Bowling	0.030	7.0 min/mile	0.102	Volleyball	0.030
Calisthenics	0.033	6.0 min/mile	0.114	Walking	
Cycling (on a level surface)		Deep water**	0.100	4.5 mph	0.045
5.5 mph	0.033	Skating (moderate)	0.038	Shallow pool	0.090
10.0 mph	0.050	Skiing		Water Aerobics	
13.0 mph	0.071	Downhill	0.060	Moderate	0.050
		Level (5 mph)	0.078	Vigorous	0.070
		Soccer	0.059	Wrestling	0.085

*Values are for actual time engaged in the activity.　　　　　　　**Treading water

Adapted from:
P. E. Allsen, J. M. Harrison, and B. Vance. *Fitness for Life: An Individualized Approach* (Dubuque, IA: Wm. C. Brown, 1989).
C. A. Bucher and W. E. Prentice, *Fitness for College and Life* (St. Louis: Times Mirror/Mosby College Publishing, 1989).
C. F. Consolazio, R. E. Johnson, and L. J. Pecora. *Physiological Measurements of Metabolic Functions in Man* (New York: McGraw-Hill, 1963).
R. V. Hockey, *Physical Fitness: The Pathway to Healthful Living* (St. Louis: Times Mirror/Mosby College Publishing, 1989).
W. W. K. Hoeger, et al. Research conducted at Boise State University, 1986–1993.

activity level, refer to Table 5.2 and rate yourself accordingly. The number given in Table 5.2 is per pound of body weight, so you multiply your current weight by that number. For example, the typical caloric requirement to maintain body weight for a moderately active male who weighs 160 pounds is 2,400 calories (160 lbs × 15 cal/lb).

To determine the average number of calories you burn daily as a result of exercise, figure out the total number of minutes you exercise weekly, then figure the daily average exercise time. For instance, a person cycling at 13 miles per hour 5 times a week, 30 minutes each time, exercises 150 minutes per week (5 × 30). The average daily exercise time is therefore 21 minutes (150 ÷ 7, rounded off to the lowest unit).

Next, from Table 5.3, find the energy expenditure for the activity (or activities) chosen for the exercise program. In the case of cycling (13 miles per hour), the expenditure is .071 calories per pound of body weight per minute of activity (cal/lb/min). With a body weight of 160 pounds, this man would burn 11.4 calories each minute (body weight × .071, or 160 × .071). In 21 minutes he burns approximately 240 calories (21 × 11.4).

Now you can obtain the estimated total caloric requirement, with exercise, needed to maintain body weight. To do this, add the typical daily requirement (without exercise) obtained from Table 5.2 and the average calories burned through exercise. In our example, it is 2,640 calories (2,400 + 240).

If a negative caloric balance is recommended to lose weight, this person has to consume fewer than 2,640 calories daily to achieve the objective. Because of the many factors that play a role in weight control, this 2,640-calorie value is only an estimated

daily requirement. Furthermore, we cannot predict that you will lose exactly 1 pound of fat in 1 week if you cut your daily intake by 500 calories (500 × 7 = 3,500 calories, or the equivalent of 1 pound of fat).

The estimated daily caloric figure is only a target guideline for weight control. Periodic readjustments are necessary because individuals differ, and the estimated daily cost changes as you lose weight and modify your exercise habits.

To determine the target caloric intake to lose weight, multiply your current weight by 5 and subtract this amount from the total caloric requirement (2,640 in our example) with exercise. For our moderately active male example, this would mean 1,840 calories per day to lose weight (160 × 5 = 800 and 2,640 − 800 = 1,840 calories).

This final caloric intake to lose weight should never be below 1,200 calories for women and 1,500 for men. If distributed properly over the various food groups, these figures are the lowest caloric intakes that provide the necessary nutrients the body needs. In terms of percentages of total calories, the daily distribution should be approximately 60 percent carbohydrates (mostly complex carbohydrates), less than 30 percent fat, and about 12 percent protein.

Many experts believe a person can take off weight more efficiently by reducing the amount of daily fat intake to 10 to 20 percent of the total daily caloric intake. Because 1 gram of fat supplies more than twice the amount of calories that carbohydrates and protein do, the general tendency when someone eats less fat is to consume fewer calories.

Further, it takes only 3 to 5 percent of ingested calories to store fat as fat, whereas it takes approximately 25 percent of ingested calories to convert carbohydrates to fat. Other research indicates that if people eat the same number of calories as carbohydrate or fat, those on the fat diet will store more fat. Successful weight-loss programs allow only small amounts of fat in the diet.

Many people have trouble adhering to a 10- to 20-percent fat-calorie diet. During weight loss periods, however, you are strongly

© Fitness & Wellness, Inc.

The establishment of healthy eating patterns starts at a young age.

encouraged to do so. Start with a 20 percent fat-calorie diet. Refer to Table 5.4 to aid you in determining the grams of fat at 10 percent, 20 percent, and 30 percent of the total calories for selected energy intakes. Also, use the form provided in Lab 3B to monitor your daily fat intake.

The time of day when food is consumed also may play a part in weight reduction. A study conducted at the Aerobics Research Institute in Dallas, Texas, indicated that when a person is on a diet, weight is lost most effectively if the person consumes most of the calories before 1:00 P.M. and not during the evening meal. The institute recommends that, when a person is attempting to lose weight, intake should consist of a minimum of 25 percent of the total daily calories for breakfast, 50 percent for lunch, and 25 percent or less at dinner.

Other experts have reported that, if most of the daily calories are consumed during one meal, the body may perceive that something is wrong and will slow down the metabolism so it can store more calories in the form of fat. Also, eating most of the calories during one meal causes a person to go hungry the rest of the day, making it more difficult to adhere to the diet.

Consuming most of the calories earlier in the day seems helpful in losing weight and also in managing atherosclerosis. The time of day when

Table 5.4 Grams of Fat at 10, 20, and 30% of Total Calories for Selected Energy Intakes

Caloric Intake	Grams of Fat		
	10%	20%	30%
1,200	13	27	40
1,300	14	29	43
1,400	16	31	47
1,500	17	33	50
1,600	18	36	53
1,700	19	38	57
1,800	20	40	60
1,900	21	42	63
2,000	22	44	67
2,100	23	47	70
2,200	24	49	73
2,300	26	51	77
2,400	27	53	80
2,500	28	56	83
2,600	29	58	87
2,700	30	60	90
2,800	31	62	93
2,900	32	64	97
3,000	33	67	100

most of the fats and cholesterol are consumed can influence blood lipids and coronary heart disease. Peak digestion time following a heavy meal is about 7 hours after that meal. If most lipids are consumed during the evening meal, digestion peaks while the person is sound asleep, when the metabolism is at its lowest rate. Consequently, the body may not metabolize fats and cholesterol as well, leading to a higher blood lipid count and increasing the risk for atherosclerosis and coronary heart disease.

Monitoring Your Diet With Daily Food Logs

To help you monitor and adhere to your diet plan, you may use the daily food logs provided in Lab 5B. Before using any of these forms, make a master copy for your files so you can make future copies as needed. Guidelines are provided for 1,200-, 1,500-, 1,800-, and 2,000-calorie diet plans. These plans have been developed based on the Food Guide Pyramid and the Dietary Guidelines for Americans to meet the Recommended Dietary Allowances.[16] The objective is to meet (not exceed) the number of servings allowed for each diet plan. Each time you eat a serving of a certain food, record it in the appropriate box.

To lose weight, you should use the diet plan that most closely approximates your target caloric intake. The plan is based on the following caloric allowances for each food group:

- Bread, cereal, rice, and pasta group: 80 calories per serving.
- Fruit group: 60 calories per serving.
- Vegetable group: 25 calories per serving.
- Milk, yogurt, and cheese group (use low-fat products): 120 calories per serving.
- Meat, poultry, fish, dry beans, eggs, and nuts group: Use low-fat (300 calories per serving) frozen entrees or an equivalent amount if you prepare your own main dish (see discussion below).

As you start your diet plan, pay particular attention to food serving sizes. To find out what counts as one serving, refer to the Food Guide Pyramid (see Figure 3.1, page 47). Take care with cup and glass sizes. A standard cup is 8 ounces, and

most glasses nowadays contain between 12 and 16 ounces. If you drink 12 ounces of fruit juice, in essence you are getting two servings of fruit because a standard serving is 3/4 cup of juice.

Read food labels carefully to compare the caloric value of the serving listed on the label with the caloric guidelines provided above. Here are some examples:

- One slice of standard white bread has about 80 calories. A plain bagel may have 200 to 350 calories. Although it is low in fat, a 350-calorie bagel is equivalent to almost 4 servings in the bread, cereal, rice, and pasta group.
- The standard serving size listed on the food label for most cereals is 1 cup. As you read the nutrition information, however, you find that for the same cup of cereal, one type of cereal has 120 calories whereas another cereal has 200 calories. Because a standard serving in the bread, cereal, rice and pasta group is 80 calories, the first cereal would be 1½ servings and the second one 2½ servings.
- A medium-size fruit usually is considered 1 serving. Large fruits could provide as many as 3 servings.
- In the milk, yogurt, and cheese groups, 1 serving represents 120 calories. A cup of whole milk has about 160 calories, whereas a cup of skim milk contains 88 calories. A cup of whole milk, therefore, would provide 1⅓ servings in this food group.

To be more accurate with caloric intake and to simplify meal preparation, use commercially prepared low-fat frozen entrees as the main dish for lunch and dinner meals (only one entree per meal for the 1,200-calorie diet plan—see Lab 5B). Look for entrees that provide about 300 calories and no more than 6 grams of fat per entree. These two entrees can be used as selections for the meat, poultry, fish, dry beans, eggs, and nuts group and will provide most of the daily protein requirement for the body. Along with each entree, supplement the meal with some of your servings from the other food groups. This diet plan has been used successfully in weight-loss research programs.[17] If you choose not to use these low-fat entrees, prepare a similar meal using 3 ounces (cooked) of lean meat, poultry, or fish with additional vegetables, rice, or pasta, which will provide 300 calories with fewer than 6 grams of fat per dish.

In your daily logs, be sure to record the precise amount in each serving. If you choose to do so, you can run a computerized nutrient analysis to verify your caloric intake and food distribution pattern (percent of total calories from carbohydrate, fat, and protein).

Behavior Modification and Adherence to a Weight Management Program

Achieving and maintaining recommended body composition is by no means impossible, but it does require desire and commitment. If weight management is to become a priority in life, people must realize that they have to transform their behavior to some extent.

Modifying old habits and developing new, positive behaviors take time. Individuals have applied the following management techniques to change detrimental behavior successfully and adhere to a positive lifetime weight-control program. In developing a retraining program, people are not expected to incorporate all of the strategies listed, but should note the ones that apply to them. The form provided in Lab 5C will allow you to evaluate and monitor your own weight management behaviors.

■ Make a commitment to change. The first necessary ingredient is the desire to modify your behavior. You need to stop precontemplating and contemplating change and get going! The reasons for change must be more compelling than those for continuing your present lifestyle patterns. You must accept that you have a problem and decide by yourself whether you really want to change. If you are sincerely committed, the chances for success are enhanced already.

The desire to lose weight must become more important than the desire to overeat or not exercise.

■ Set realistic goals. Most people with a weight problem would like the pounds to melt away, failing to realize that the weight problem developed over several years. A sound weight reduction and maintenance program can be accomplished only by establishing new lifetime eating and exercise habits, both of which take time to develop. In setting a realistic long-term goal, short-term objectives also should be planned. The long-term goal may be to decrease body fat to 20 percent of total body weight. The short-term objective may be a 1 percent decrease in body fat each month. Objectives like these allow for regular evaluation and help maintain motivation and renewed commitment to attain the long-term goal.

■ Incorporate exercise into the program. Choosing enjoyable activities, places, times, equipment, and people to work with helps a person adhere to an exercise program. Details on developing a complete exercise program are given in Chapters 7, 8, and 9.

■ Differentiate hunger and appetite. Hunger is the actual physical need for food. Appetite is a desire for food, usually triggered by factors such as stress, habit, boredom, depression, availability of food, or just the thought of food itself. People should eat only when they have a physical need. In this regard, developing and sticking to a regular meal pattern help control hunger.

■ Eat less fat. Each gram of fat provides 9 calories, and protein and carbohydrates provide only 4. In essence, you can eat more food on a low-fat diet because you consume fewer calories with each meal.

■ Pay attention to calories. Some people think that because a certain food is low in fat, they can eat as much as they want. Entire boxes of fat-free cookies and bags of pretzels have been consumed under this pretense. A homemade chocolate-chip cookie may have 100 calories, whereas a low-fat one may have 50. Simple math will tell you that eating one homemade cookie is better than eating a half dozen low-fat ones. When reading food labels, don't just look at the fat content, but pay attention to calories as well.

■ Cut unnecessary items from your diet. Many people regularly drink a 140-calorie can of soda pop (or more) each day. Substituting a glass of water would cut 51,100 (140 × 365) calories yearly from the diet—the equivalent of 14.6 (51,000 ÷ 3,500) pounds of fat.

■ Add foods to your diet that reduce cravings.[18] Many people have a biological imbalance of insulin. Insulin helps the body use and conserve energy. Some people produce so much insulin that their bodies can't use it all. This imbalance leads to an overpowering craving for carbohydrates. As they eat more carbohydrates, even more insulin is released. Foods that reduce cravings include eggs, red meat, fish, poultry, cheese, tofu, oils, fats, and nonstarchy vegetables such as lettuce, green beans, peppers, asparagus, broccoli, mushrooms, and Brussels sprouts. If you watch your portion sizes, eating foods that reduce cravings at regular meals and for snacks helps to decrease the intense desire for carbohydrates, prevent overeating, and aid with weight loss.

■ Avoid automatic eating. Many people associate certain daily activities with eating. For example, people may eat while cooking, watching television, or reading. Most of the time the foods consumed in these situations lack nutritional value or are high in sugar and fat.

- Stay busy. People tend to eat more when they sit around and do nothing. Occupying the mind and body with activities not associated with eating helps take away the desire to eat. Some options are walking; cycling; playing sports; gardening; sewing; or visiting a library, a museum, or a park. To break the routine of life, you might develop other skills and interests or try something new and exciting.
- Plan meals ahead of time. Sensible shopping is necessary to accomplish this objective. Always shop on a full stomach, because hungry shoppers tend to buy unhealthy foods impulsively—and then snack on the way home. The shopping list should include whole-grain breads and cereals, fruits and vegetables, low-fat milk and dairy products, lean meats, fish, and poultry.
- Cook wisely.
  - Use less fat and fewer refined foods in food preparation.
  - Trim all visible fat from meats and remove skin from poultry before cooking.
  - Skim the fat off gravies and soups.
  - Bake, broil, boil, or steam instead of frying.
  - Sparingly use butter, cream, mayonnaise, and salad dressings.
  - Avoid coconut oil, palm oil, and cocoa butter.
  - Prepare plenty of foods that contain fiber.
  - Include whole-grain breads and cereals, vegetables, and legumes in most meals.
  - Eat fruits for dessert.
  - Stay away from soda pop, fruit juices, and fruit-flavored drinks.
  - In addition to using less sugar, cut down on other refined carbohydrates such as corn syrup, malt sugar, dextrose, and fructose.
  - Drink plenty of water—at least six glasses a day.

- Do not serve more food than you should eat. Measure the food in portions, and keep serving dishes away from the table. In this way you will eat less, have a harder time getting seconds, and have less appetite because the food is not visible. People should not be forced to eat when they are satisfied (including children after they already have had a healthy, nutritious serving).
- Try "junior size" instead of "super size." Use smaller plates, bowls, cups, and glasses. Try eating half as much food as you commonly eat. Over the years, the sizes of dishes and glasses have gotten bigger. Consequently, people serve and eat a lot more food than they need. If you use a smaller plate, it will look like more food and you'll tend to eat less. Watch for portion sizes at restaurants as well. Plate and portion sizes at restaurants now are so large that people overeat and still end up with leftovers to take home. Similarly, the original bottle of Coca-Cola contained 6.5 ounces. Machines now routinely dispense 20-ounce bottles, and convenience stores sell 64-ounce "buckets" of soda pop (about 750 calories). Supersized foods create supersized people.

Supersized foods create supersized people.

- Eat out infrequently. Research indicates that the more often people of all ages eat out, the more body fat they have. People who eat out 6 or more times per week consume an average of about 300 extra calories per day and 30 percent more fat than those who eat out less often.
- Eat slowly and at the table only. Eating is one of the pleasures of life, and we need to take time to enjoy it. Eating on the run is not good because

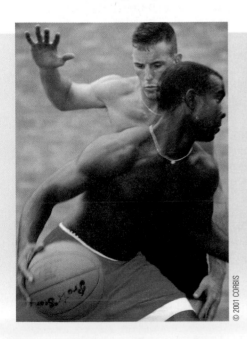

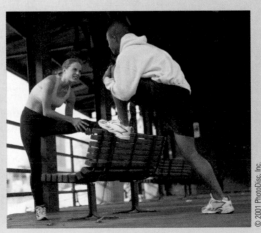

Exercising with other people and in different places helps maintain exercise adherence.

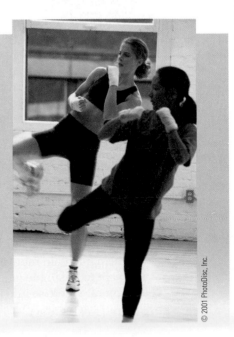

the body doesn't have enough time to "register" nutritive and caloric consumption, and people overeat before the body perceives the fullness signal. Eating at the table also forces people to take time out to eat, and it deters snacking between meals, primarily because of the extra time and effort required to sit down and eat. When people are done eating, they should not sit around the table but, rather, clean up and put away the food to avoid snacking.

- Avoid social binges. Social gatherings tend to entice self-defeating behavior. Visual imagery might help before attending social gatherings. Plan ahead and visualize yourself there. Do not feel pressured to eat or drink and don't rationalize in these situations. Choose low-calorie foods and entertain yourself with other activities such as dancing and talking.

- Do not raid the refrigerator or the cookie jar. In these tempting situations, take control. Stop and think. Do not bring high-calorie, high-sugar, or high-fat foods into the house. If they are there already, store them where they are hard to get to or see. If they are out of sight or not readily available, the temptation is less. Keeping food in places such as the garage and basement discourages people from taking the time and effort to get them. By no means should you have to eliminate treats entirely, but all things should be done in moderation.

- Avoid evening food raids. Most people with weight problems do really well during the day but then "lose it" at night. Excessive snacking following the evening meal is a common pitfall. Stay busy after your evening meal. Go for a short walk and get to bed earlier. In most cases the intense desire for food that you get during the evening hours disappears following a good night's rest.

- Practice stress-management techniques (more on stress in Chapter 11). Many people snack and increase food consumption in stressful situations. Eating is not a stress-releasing activity and, instead, can aggravate the problem if weight control is an issue.

- Get support. People who receive support from friends, relatives, and formal support groups are much more likely to lose and maintain weight loss than those without such support. The more support you receive, the better off you will be.

- Monitor changes and reward accomplishments. Feedback on fat loss and lean tissue gain is a reward in itself. Awareness of changes in body composition also helps reinforce new behaviors. Being able to exercise without interruption for 15, 20, 30, or 60 minutes; swimming a certain distance; running a mile—all these accomplishments deserve recognition. Meeting objectives calls for rewards that are not related to eating: new clothing, a tennis racquet, a bicycle, exercise shoes, or something else that is special and you would not have acquired otherwise.

- Prepare for slips. Most people will slip and occasionally splurge. If that happens, do not despair and give up. Reevaluate and continue with your efforts. An occasional slip will not make much difference in the long run.

- Think positive. Avoid negative thoughts about how difficult changing past behaviors might be. Instead, think of the benefits you will reap, such as feeling, looking, and functioning better, plus enjoying better health and improving the quality of life. Avoid negative environments and people who will not be supportive.

In Conclusion

There is no simple and quick way to take off excess body fat and keep it off for good. Weight management is accomplished by making a lifetime commitment to physical activity and proper food selection. When taking part in a weight (fat) reduction program, people also have to decrease their caloric intake moderately and implement strategies to modify unhealthy eating behaviors.

During the process, relapses into past negative behaviors are almost inevitable. The three most common reasons for relapse are the following:

1. Stress-related factors (such as major life changes, depression, job changes, illness).
2. Social reasons (entertaining, eating out, business travel).
3. Self-enticing behaviors (placing yourself in a situation to see how much you can get away with ("One small taste won't hurt," leading to "I'll eat just one slice," and finally, "I haven't done well, so I might as well eat some more").

Making mistakes is human and does not necessarily mean failure. Failure comes to those who give up and do not use previous experiences to build upon and, in turn, develop skills that will prevent self-defeating behaviors in the future. Where there's a will, there's a way, and those who persist will reap the rewards.

Web Interactive

- Weight Management: This site describes how to select a safe weight loss plan, combining exercise and healthy diet, including the FDA diet plan.

  http://www.wellweb.com/nutri/weight_management.htm

- Weight Control Information Network. This comprehensive site, sponsored by the National Institutes of Health, features health education information, as well as publications and information on clinical trials.

  http://www.niddk.nih.gov/health/nutrit/win.htm

- Eating Disorders: Don't Let Time Run Out Before You Get Help. A visually appealing site from the American Family Physician journal that describes the signs and symptoms of anorexia and bulimia, body image and improving self-esteem, treatment, and how to help a friend who has an eating disorder.

  http://health4teens.org/eating

- Eating Disorders. This award-winning site by Mental Health Net features links describing symptoms, possible causes, consequences, treatment, online resources, organizations, online support, and research.

  http://eatingdisorders.mentalhelp.net

Interactive Sites:

- The Shape Up America Nutrition Center is designed to help you understand nutritional requirements for active people. The Daily Calorie Goal is an interactive assessment that will give you an estimate of the number of calories you need daily at your current level of activity to maintain your weight. You will also find out the percentage of protein, carbohydrate, and fat calories you should have in your diet to maximize your workout. To learn how these percentages translate to foods, you can also visit the Food Guide Pyramid link and even test your knowledge by taking the Food Guide Pyramid quiz.

  http://www.shapeup.org/fitness/nutrition/fset3.htm

- Calculate Your Basal Metabolic Rate using the kCal-culator©. This site is sponsored by the University of Minnesota.

  http://www.agricola.umn.edu/nutritiontools/kcalculator.cfm

Notes

1. A. Must et al., "The Disease Burden Associated with Overweight and Obesity," *Journal of the American Medical Association* 282 (1999): 1523–1529.

2. National Institutes of Health, *Clinical Guidelines on the Identification, Evaluation, and Treatment of Overweight and Obesity in Adults*, NIH Publication No. 98-4083 (Washington, DC: NIH, 1998).

3. K. M. Flegal, M. D. Carrol, R. J. Kuczmarski, and C. L. Johnson, "Overweight and Obesity in the United States: Prevalence and Trends, 1960–1994," *International Journal of Obesity and Related Metabolic Disorders* 22 (1998): 39–47.

4. Serdula et al., "Prevalence of Attempting Weight Loss and Strategies for Controlling Weight," *Journal of the American Medical Association* 282 (1999): 1353–1358.

5. C. E. Barlow, H. W. Kohl, III, L. W. Gibbons, and S. N. Blair, "Physical Fitness, Mortality, and Obesity," *International Journal of Obesity* 19 (1996): S41–44.

6. Dr. Steven Lichtman and associates, "Discrepancy Between Self-Reported and Actual Caloric Intake and Exercise in Obese Subjects," *New England Journal of Medicine* 327 (1992): 1893–1898.

7. American Psychiatric Association, *Diagnostic and Statistical Manual of Mental Disorders* (Washington, DC: APA, 1994).

8. See note 7.

9. R. L. Leibel, M. Rosenbaum, and J. Hirsh, "Changes in Energy Expenditure Resulting from Altered Body Weight," *New England Journal of Medicine* 332(1995): 621–628.

10. "Olestra: Just Say No," *University of California at Berkeley Wellness Letter* (Palm Coast, FL: The Editors, February 1996).

11. R. J. Shepard, *Alive Man: The Physiology of Physical Activity* (Springfield, IL: Charles C Thomas, 1975): 484–488.

12. J. H. Wilmore, "Exercise, Obesity, and Weight Control," *Physical Activity and Fitness Research Digest* (Washington DC: President's Council on Physical Fitness & Sports, 1994).

13. K. N. Pavlou, S. Krey, and W. P. Steffe, "Exercise as an Adjunct to Weight Loss and Maintenance in Moderately Obese Subjects," *American Journal of Clinical Nutrition* 49 (1989): 1115–1123.

14. W. W. Campbell, M. C. Crim, V. R. Young, and W. J. Evans, "Increased Energy Requirements and Changes in Body Composition with Resistance Training in Older Adults," *American Journal of Clinical Nutrition* 60 (1994): 167–175.

15. A. Tremblay, J. A. Simoneau, and C. Bouchard. "Impact of Exercise Intensity on Body Fatness and Skeletal Muscle Metabolism." *Metabolism* 43 (1994): 814–818.

16. U.S. Department of Health and Human Services: Department of Agriculture. *Nutrition and Your Health: Dietary Guidelines for Americans.* Home and Garden Bulletin 232, 2000.

    U.S. Department of Agriculture, Human Nutrition Information Service, *The Food Guide Pyramid*, Home and Garden Bulletin 252 (Dec. 1992).

    National Academy Press, Food and Nutrition Board, *Recommended Dietary Allowances*, (Washington DC: National Academy Press, 1989).

17. W. W. K. Hoeger, C. Harris, E. M. Long, and D. R. Hopkins, "Four-Week Supplementation With a Natural Dietary Compound Produces Favorable Changes in Body Composition," *Advances in Therapy* 15, no. 5 (1998): 305–313.

    W. W. K. Hoeger, C. Harris, E. M. Long, R. L. Kjorstad, M. Welch, T. L. Hafner, D. R. Hopkins, "Dietary Supplementation with Chromium Picolinate/L-Carnitine Complex in Combination with Diet and Exercise Enhances Body Composition," *Journal of the American Nutraceutical Association* 2, no. 2 (1999): 40–45.

18. R. Heller and R. Heller, "How The Weight-Loss Scientists Lost Their Weight: You Can, Too," *Bottom Line/Personal* 18, no. 11 (1997): 9–10.

Suggested Readings

American Diabetes Association and American Dietetic Association. *Exchange Lists for Meal Planning.* Chicago: American Dietetic Association and American Diabetes Association, 1995.

Bouchard, C., et al. *Physical Activity, Fitness, and Health.* Champaign, IL: Human Kinetics, 1994.

Bray, G. "The Nutrient Balance Approach to Obesity." *Nutrition Today* 28 (May/June 1993): 13–18.

Broeder, C. E., K. A. Burrhus, L. S. Svanevick, and J. H. Wilmore. "The Effects of Either High-Intensity Resistance or Endurance Training on Resting Metabolic Rate." *American Journal of Clinical Nutrition* 55 (1992): 802–810.

Broeder, C. E., et al. "The Metabolic Consequences of Low and Moderate Intensity Exercise With or Without Feeding in Lean and Borderline Obese Males." *International Journal of Obesity* 15 (1990): 95–104.

Brownell, K. *The Learn Program for Weight Control.* Dallas: American Health Publishing, 1997.

Clark, N. "How to Gain Weight Healthfully." *Physician and Sportsmedicine* 19 (1991): 53.

Clarkson, P. M. "Nutritional Supplements for Weight Gain." Gatorade Sports Science Institute: *Sports Science Exchange* 11 (1998): 68.

Clarkson, P. M. "The Skinny on Weight Loss Supplements and Drugs: Winning the War Against Fat." *ACSM's Health and Fitness Journal*, (1998): 18.

Kassirer, J. P., and M. Angell. "Losing Weight—An Ill-fated New Year's Resolution." *New England Journal of Medicine* 338 (1998): 52–54.

Mokdad, A. H., et al. "The Spread of the Obesity Epidemic in the United States, 1991–1998." *Journal of the American Medical Association* 282 (1999): 1519–1522.

National Institutes of Health. *Clinical Guidelines on the Identification, Evaluation, and Treatment of Overweight and Obesity in Adults.* NIH Publication No. 98-4083. Washington, DC: NIH, 1998.

Parr, R. B., and L. Capozzi. "Counseling Patients About Physical Activity." *Journal of the American Academy of Physician Assistants* 10 (1997): 45–49.

Prentice, A., et al. "Effects of Weight Cycling on Body Composition." *American Journal of Clinical Nutrition* 56 (1992): 209S–216S.

Robison, J., et al. "Obesity, Weight Loss, and Health." *Journal of the American Dietetic Association* 93 (1993): 445–449.

Rolls, B., and D. Shide. "The Influence of Dietary Fat on Food Intake and Body Weight." *Nutrition Reviews* 50 (1992): 283–290.

Rosenbaum, M., R. L. Leibel, and J. Hirsh. "Obesity." *New England Journal of Medicine* 337 (1997): 396–406.

Sjüdin, A. M., et al. "The Influence of Physical Activity on BMR." *Medicine and Science in Sports and Exercise* 28 (1996): 85–91.

Stefanick, M. "Exercise and Weight Control." *Exercise and Sport Sciences Review* 21 (1993): 363–396.

Stunkard, A. J., et al. "An Adoption Study of Human Obesity." *New England Journal of Medicine* 314 (1986): 193–198.

Wadden, T. A., T. B. Van Itallie, and G. L. Blackburn. "Responsible and Irresponsible Use of Very-Low-Calorie Diets in the Treatment of Obesity." *Journal of the American Medical Association* 263 (1990): 83–85.

Wilmore, J. "Exercise, Obesity, and Weight Control." *Physical Activity and Fitness Research Digest* 1 (May, 1994): 1–8.

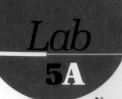

Lab 5A

ESTIMATION OF DAILY CALORIC REQUIREMENT, STAGE OF CHANGE, AND EXERCISE PROGRAM SELECTION

Name: _____ Date: _____ Grade: _____

Instructor: _____ Course: _____ Section: _____

Necessary Lab Equipment
Tables 5.1 and 5.2.

Objective
To estimate your daily caloric requirement for weight maintenance or reduction and to select fitness activities for your exercise program.

Instructions
Complete all of the sections provided in this lab.

I. Computation Form for Daily Caloric Requirement

A. Current body weight in pounds .... _____

B. Caloric requirement per pound of body weight (use Table 5.2) .... _____

C. Typical daily caloric requirement without exercise to maintain body weight (A × B) ... _____

D. Selected physical activity (e.g., jogging)[a] .... _____

E. Number of exercise sessions per week .... _____

F. Duration of exercise session (in minutes) .... _____

G. Total weekly exercise time in minutes (E × F) .... _____

H. Average daily exercise time in minutes (G ÷ 7) .... _____

I. Caloric expenditure per pound per minute (cal/lb/min) of physical activity (use Table 5.3) ... _____

J. Total calories burned per minute of physical activity (A × I) .... _____

K. Average daily calories burned as a result of the exercise program (H × J) .... _____

L. Total daily caloric requirement with exercise to maintain body weight (C + K) .... _____

M. Number of calories to subtract from daily requirement to achieve a negative caloric balance (multiply current body weight by 5) .... _____

N. Target caloric intake to lose weight (L − M)[b] .... _____

---

[a] If more than one physical activity is selected, you will need to estimate the average daily calories burned as a result of each additional activity (steps D through K) and add all of these figures to L above.

[b] This figure should never be below 1,200 calories for women or 1,500 calories for men. See Lab 5B for the 1,200-, 1,500-, 1,800-, and 2,000-calorie-diet plans.

II. Stage of Change

1. Using Figure 2.3 (page 40) and Table 2.3 (page 41), identify your current stage of change regarding **recommended body weight**: _____

2. How much weight do you want to lose? _____ Is it a realistic goal? _____

3. Based on the processes and techniques of change discussed in Chapter 2, indicate what you can do to help yourself implement a weight management program.

_____

_____

III. Exercise Program Selection

1. How much effort are you willing to put into reaching your weight loss goal?

_____

_____

_____

_____

2. Indicate your feelings about participating in an exercise program.

_____

_____

_____

_____

3. Will you commit to participate in a combined aerobic and strength-training program?[c]   Yes ☐   No ☐

   If your answer is "Yes," proceed to the next question; if you answered "No," please review Chapters 3, 4, and 5 again and read Chapters 6, 7, 8, and 9.

4. List aerobic activities you enjoy or may enjoy doing.

_____

_____

5. Select one or two aerobic activities in which you will participate regularly.

[_____]   [_____]

6. List facilities available to you where you can carry out the aerobic and strength-training programs.

_____

_____

_____

7. Indicate days and times you will set aside for your aerobic and strength-training program (5 to 6 days per week should be devoted to aerobic exercise and 1 to 3 nonconsecutive days per week to strength training).

Monday: [_____]

Tuesday: [_____]

Wednesday: [_____]

Thursday: [_____]

Friday: [_____]

Saturday: [_____]

Sunday: A complete day of rest once a week is recommended to allow your body to fully recover from exercise.

---

[c] Flexibility programs are necessary for injury prevention, adequate fitness, and good health but do not help with weight loss. Stretching exercises can be conducted regularly during the cool-down phase of your aerobic and strength-training programs (see Chapter 8).

CALORIE-RESTRICTED DIET PLANS

Name: _____   Date: _____   Grade: _____

Instructor: _____   Course: _____   Section: _____

Necessary Lab Equipment
None required.

Objective
To help you implement a calorie-restricted diet plan according to your target caloric intake obtained in Lab 5A.

Lab Preparation
Read Chapter 5 prior to this lab and make additional copies (as needed) of your selected diet plan.

1,200 Calorie Diet Plan

Instructions:

The objective of the diet plan is to meet (not exceed) the number of servings allowed for the food groups listed. Each time that you eat a particular food, record it in the space provided for each group along with the amount you ate. Refer to the Food Guide Pyramid to find out what counts as one serving for each group listed (see Figure 3.1, page 47). Instead of the meat, poultry, fish, dry beans, eggs, and nuts group, you are allowed to have a commercially available low-fat frozen entree for your main meal (this entree should provide no more than 300 calories and less than 6 grams of fat). You can make additional copies of this form as needed.

Bread, Cereal, Rice, Pasta Group (80 calories/serving): 6 servings

1. _____
2. _____
3. _____
4. _____
5. _____
6. _____

Vegetable Group (25 calories/serving): 3 servings

1. _____
2. _____
3. _____

Fruit Group (60 calories/serving): 2 servings

1. _____
2. _____

Milk Group (120 calories/serving, use low-fat milk and milk products): 2 servings

1. _____
2. _____

Low-fat Frozen Entree (300 calories and less than 6 grams of fat): 1 serving

1. _____

1,500 Calorie Diet Plan

Instructions:

The objective of the diet plan is to meet (not exceed) the number of servings allowed for the food groups listed. Each time that you eat a particular food, record it in the space provided for each group along with the amount you ate. Refer to the Food Guide Pyramid to find out what counts as one serving for each group listed (see Figure 3.1, page 47). Instead of the meat, poultry, fish, dry beans, eggs, and nuts group, you are allowed to have two commercially available low-fat frozen entrees for your main meal (these entrees should provide no more than 300 calories and less than 6 grams of fat). You can make additional copies of this form as needed.

Bread, Cereal, Rice, Pasta Group (80 calories/serving): 6 servings

1.
2.
3.
4.
5.
6.

Vegetable Group (25 calories/serving): 3 servings

1.
2.
3.

Fruit Group (60 calories/serving): 2 servings

1.
2.

Milk Group (120 calories/serving, use low-fat milk and milk products): 2 servings

1.
2.

Two Low-fat Frozen Entrees (300 calories and less than 6 grams of fat): 2 servings

1.
2.

1,800 Calorie Diet Plan

Instructions:

The objective of the diet plan is to meet (not exceed) the number of servings allowed for the food groups listed. Each time that you eat a particular food, record it in the space provided for each group along with the amount you ate. Refer to the Food Guide Pyramid to find out what counts as one serving for each group listed (see Figure 3.1, page 47). Instead of the meat, poultry, fish, dry beans, eggs, and nuts group, you are allowed to have two commercially available low-fat frozen entrees for your main meal (these entrees should provide no more than 300 calories and less than 6 grams of fat). You can make additional copies of this form as needed.

Bread, Cereal, Rice, Pasta Group (80 calories/serving): 8 servings

1

2

3

4

5

6

7

8

Vegetable Group (25 calories/serving): 5 servings

1

2

3

4

5

Fruit Group (60 calories/serving): 3 servings

1

2

3

Milk Group (120 calories/serving, use low-fat milk and milk products): 2 servings

1

2

Two Low-fat Frozen Entrees (300 calories and less than 6 grams of fat): 2 servings

1

2

2,000 Calorie Diet Plan

Instructions:

The objective of the diet plan is to meet (not exceed) the number of servings allowed for the food groups listed. Each time that you eat a particular food, record it in the space provided for each group along with the amount you ate. Refer to the Food Guide Pyramid to find out what counts as one serving for each group listed (see Figure 3.1, page 47). Instead of the meat, poultry, fish, dry beans, eggs, and nuts group, you are allowed to have two commercially available low-fat frozen entrees for your main meal (these entrees should provide no more than 300 calories and less than 6 grams of fat). You can make additional copies of this form as needed.

Bread, Cereal, Rice, Pasta Group (80 calories/serving): 10 servings

1
2
3
4
5
6
7
8
9
10

Vegetable Group (25 calories/serving): 5 servings

1
2
3
4
5

Fruit Group (60 calories/serving): 4 servings

1
2
3
4

Milk Group (120 calories/serving, use low-fat milk and milk products): 2 servings

1
2

Two Low-fat Frozen Entrees (300 calories and less than 6 grams of fat): 2 servings

1
2

Lab
5C

Name: _____ Date: _____ Grade: _____

Instructor: _____ Course: _____ Section: _____

Necessary Lab Equipment
None.

Lab Preparation
Read Chapters 2, 3, 4, and 5 prior to this lab.

Objective
To prepare and monitor behavioral changes for weight management.

I. Please answer all of the following:

1. State your own feelings regarding your current body weight, your target body composition, and a completion date for this goal.

   _____
   _____
   _____
   _____
   _____

2. Do you have an eating disorder? If so, express your feelings about it. Can your instructor help you find professional advice so that you can work toward resolving this problem?

   _____
   _____
   _____
   _____
   _____

3. Is your present diet adequate according to the nutrient analysis?   Yes [ ]   No [ ]

4. State dietary changes necessary to achieve a balanced diet and/or to lose weight (increase or decrease caloric intake, decrease fat intake, increase intake of complex carbohydrates, etc.). List specific foods that will help you improve in areas where you may have deficiencies and food items to avoid or consume in moderation to help you achieve better nutrition.

   Changes to make: _____
   _____

   Foods that will help: _____
   _____

   Foods to avoid: _____
   _____

II. Behavior Modification Progress Form

Instructions: Read the section on tips for behavior modification and adherence to a weight management program (pp. 129–131). On a weekly or bi-weekly basis, go through the list of strategies and provide a "Yes" or "No" answer to each statement. If you are able to answer "Yes" to most questions, you have been successful in implementing positive weight management behaviors. (Make additional copies of this page as needed.)

Strategy Date						
1. I have made a commitment to change.						
2. I set realistic goals.						
3. I exercise regularly.						
4. I have healthy eating patterns.						
5. I exercise control over my appetite.						
6. I am consuming less fat in my diet.						
7. I pay attention to the number of calories in food.						
8. I have eliminated unnecessary food items from my diet.						
9. I use craving-reducing foods in my diet.						
10. I avoid automatic eating.						
11. I stay busy.						
12. I plan meals ahead of time.						
13. I cook wisely.						
14. I do not serve more food than I should eat.						
15. I use portion control in my diet.						
16. I eat slowly and at the table only.						
17. I avoid social binges.						
18. I avoid food raids.						
19. I do not eat out more than once per week. When I do, I eat low-fat meals.						
20. I practice stress management.						
21. I have a strong support group.						
22. I monitor behavior changes.						
23. I prepare for lapses/relapses.						
24. I reward my accomplishments.						
25. I think positive.						

Chapter 6

Cardiorespiratory Endurance Assessment

Exercise is the closest thing we'll ever get to the miracle pill that everyone is seeking. It brings weight loss, appetite control, improved mood and self-esteem, an energy kick, and longer life by decreasing the risk of heart disease, diabetes, stroke, osteoporosis, and chronic disabilities.[1]

◼ Objectives

- ◼ Define cardiorespiratory endurance and understand the benefits of cardiorespiratory endurance training.

- ◼ Understand the importance of adequate cardiorespiratory endurance in maintaining good health and well-being.

- ◼ Define aerobic and anaerobic exercise.

- ◼ Be able to assess cardiorespiratory fitness through six different test protocols (1.5-Mile Run Test, 1.0-Mile Walk Test, Step Test, Astrand-Ryhming Test, 12-Minute Swim Test, and the University of Houston Non-Exercise Test).

- ◼ Learn to interpret cardiorespiratory endurance assessment test results according to health fitness and physical fitness standards.

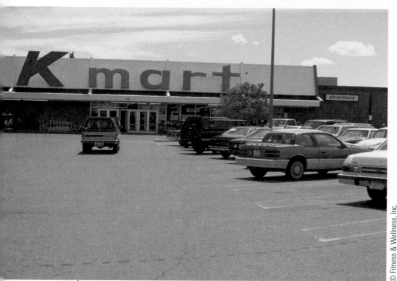

The epitome of physical inactivity is driving around a parking lot for several minutes in search of a parking spot 20 yards closer to the store's entrance.

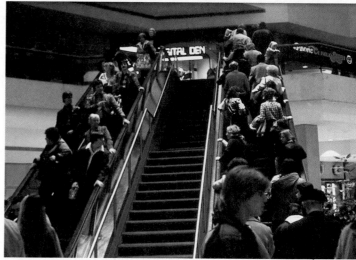

Advances in modern technology have almost completely eliminated the need for physical activity, significantly enhancing the deterioration rate of the human body.

The most important component of physical fitness and best indicator of overall health—**cardiorespiratory endurance**—is being eroded by our lifestyle.

> *Modern-day commodities have reduced the amount of daily physical activity, thus enhancing the deterioration rate of the human body.*

Physical activity is no longer a natural part of our existence. Current technological developments have driven most people in developed countries into sedentary lifestyles. For instance, to go to a store only a couple of blocks away, most people drive their automobiles and then spend several minutes driving around the parking lot to find a spot 20 yards closer to the store's entrance. They do not even have to carry out the groceries any more: A youngster working at the store usually takes them out in a cart and places them in the vehicle.

Similarly, during a visit to a multilevel shopping mall, almost everyone chooses to ride the escalators instead of taking the stairs (which tend to be inaccessible). Automobiles, elevators, escalators, telephones, intercoms, remote controls, electric garage door openers—all are modern-day commodities that minimize the amount of movement and effort required of the human body.

One of the most harmful effects of modern-day technology is an increase in chronic conditions related to a lack of physical activity. These include hypertension, heart disease, chronic low-back pain, and obesity. They are referred to as **hypokinetic diseases**. The term "hypo" means low or little, and "kinetic" implies motion. Lack of adequate physical activity is a fact of modern life that most people can avoid no longer. If we want to enjoy modern-day commodities and still expect to live life to its fullest, however, we must adopt a personalized lifetime exercise program as a part of daily living.

Cardiorespiratory endurance is a measure of how efficiently our bodies work. As a person breathes, part of the oxygen in the air is taken up in the lungs and transported in the blood to the heart. The heart then is responsible for pumping the oxygenated blood through the circulatory system to all organs and tissues of the body. At the cellular level, oxygen is used to convert food substrates, primarily carbohydrates and fats, into energy necessary to conduct body functions and maintain constant internal equilibrium. During physical exertion,

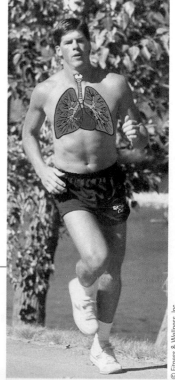

Cardiorespiratory endurance refers to the ability of the lungs, heart, and blood vessels to deliver adequate amounts of oxygen to the cells to meet the demands of prolonged physical activity.

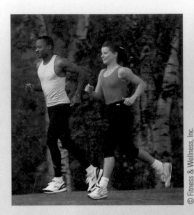
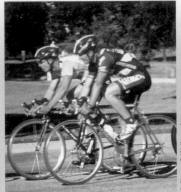
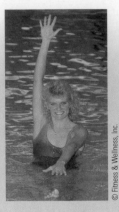

AEROBIC ACTIVITIES

ANAEROBIC ACTIVITIES

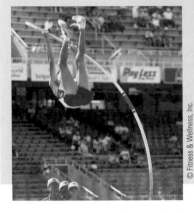
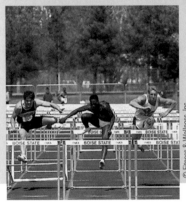
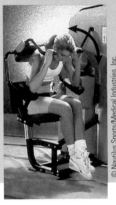

more energy is needed to perform the activity. As a result, the heart, lungs, and blood vessels have to deliver more oxygen to the cells to supply the required energy.

During prolonged exercise, an individual with a high level of cardiorespiratory endurance is able to deliver the required amount of oxygen to the tissues with relative ease. The cardiorespiratory system of a person with a low level of endurance has to work much harder, because the heart has to pump more often to supply the same amount of oxygen to the tissues and, consequently, fatigues faster. Hence, a higher capacity to deliver and utilize oxygen (oxygen uptake or VO_2) indicates a more efficient cardiorespiratory system.

Aerobic and Anaerobic Exercise

Cardiorespiratory endurance activities often are called **aerobic** exercises. Examples of cardiorespiratory or aerobic exercises are walking, jogging, swimming, cycling, cross-country skiing, water aerobics, rope skipping, and aerobics.

In contrast, the intensity of **anaerobic** exercise is so high that oxygen cannot be delivered and utilized to produce energy. Because energy production is limited in the absence of oxygen, these activities can be carried out for only short periods—

2 to 3 minutes. The higher the intensity of the activity, the shorter the duration.

Activities such as the 100-, 200-, and 400-meter races in track and field; the 100-meter race in swimming; gymnastics routines; and strength training are good examples of anaerobic activities. Anaerobic activities do not contribute much to development of the cardiorespiratory system. Only aerobic activities will help increase cardiorespiratory endurance. The basic guidelines for cardiorespiratory exercise prescription are set forth in Chapter 7.

> *Good cardiorespiratory or aerobic fitness implies an efficient system to deliver and utilize oxygen.*

Cardiorespiratory endurance The ability of the lungs, heart, and blood vessels to deliver adequate amounts of oxygen to the cells to meet the demands of prolonged physical activity.

Hypokinetic diseases Diseases related to a lack of physical activity.

Aerobic Exercise that requires oxygen to produce the necessary energy (ATP) to carry out the activity.

Anaerobic Exercise that does not require oxygen to produce the necessary energy (ATP) to carry out the activity.

Benefits of Aerobic Training

Everyone who participates in a cardiorespiratory or aerobic exercise program can expect a number of beneficial physiological adaptations from training. Among them are the following:

1. A higher **maximal oxygen uptake**. The amount of oxygen the body is able to use during physical activity increases significantly. This allows the individual to exercise longer and more intensely before becoming fatigued. Depending on the initial fitness level, maximal oxygen uptake may increase as much as 30% (although higher increases have been reported in people with very low initial levels of fitness).

2. An increase in the oxygen-carrying capacity of the blood. As a result of training, the red blood cell count goes up. Red blood cells contain hemoglobin, which transports oxygen in the blood.

3. A decrease in resting heart rate and an increase in cardiac muscle strength. During resting conditions, the heart ejects between 5 and 6 liters of blood per minute (a liter is slightly larger than a quart). This amount of blood, also referred to as **cardiac output**, meets the body's energy demands in the resting state.

   Like any other muscle, the heart responds to training by increasing in strength and size. As the heart gets stronger, the muscle can produce a more forceful contraction, which causes the heart to eject more blood with each beat. This **stroke volume** yields a lower heart rate. The lower heart rate also allows the heart to rest longer between beats. Average resting and maximal cardiac outputs, stroke volumes, and heart rates for sedentary, trained, and highly trained (elite) individuals are shown in Table 6.1.

   Resting heart rates frequently decrease by 10 to 20 beats per minute (bpm) after only 6 to 8 weeks of training. A reduction of 20 bpm saves the heart about 10,483,200 beats per year. The average heart beats between 70 and 80 bpm. As seen in the table, resting heart rates in highly trained athletes are often around 45 bpm.

4. A lower heart rate at given **workloads**. When compared with untrained individuals, a trained person has a lower heart rate response to a given task. This is because of the greater efficiency of the cardiorespiratory system. Individuals also are surprised to find that, following several weeks of training, a given workload (let's say a 10-minute mile) elicits a much lower heart rate response compared with the response when training first started.

5. An increase in the number and size of the **mitochondria**. All energy necessary for cell function is produced in the mito-chondria. As their size and numbers increase, so does the potential to produce energy for muscular work.

> *If the benefits of exercise could be packaged in a pill, it would be the most widely prescribed drug in the world.*

6. An increase in the number of functional **capillaries**. Capillaries allow for the exchange of oxygen and carbon dioxide between the blood and the cells. As more vessels open up, more gas exchange can take place, delaying the onset of fatigue during prolonged exercise. This increase in capillaries also speeds up the rate at which waste products of cell metabolism can be removed. Increased capillarization also is seen in the heart, which enhances the oxygen delivery capacity to the heart muscle itself.

7. A faster **recovery time**. Trained individuals recover more rapidly after exercising. A fit system is able to restore more quickly any internal equilibrium disrupted during exercise.

Table 6.1 Average Resting and Maximal Cardiac Output, Stroke Volume, and Heart Rate for Sedentary, Trained, and Highly Trained Males (cardiac output and stroke volume in women are about 5 to 10 percent lower than in men)

	Resting			Maximal		
	Cardiac Output (l/min)	Stroke Volume (ml)	Heart Rate (bpm)	Cardiac Output l/min	Stroke Volume (ml)	Heart Rate (bpm)
Sedentary	5–6	68	74	20	100	200
Trained	5–6	90	56	30	150	200
Highly Trained	5–6	110	45	35	175	200

8. Lower blood pressure and blood lipids. A regular aerobic exercise program leads to lower blood pressure and fats (such as cholesterol and triglycerides), all of which have been linked to the formation of atherosclerotic plaque, which obstructs the arteries. This decreases the risk of coronary heart disease (see Chapter 12). High blood pressure is also a leading risk factor for strokes.

9. An increase in fat-burning enzymes. The role of fat-burning enzymes is significant because fat is lost primarily by burning it in muscle. As the concentration of the enzymes increases, so does the ability to burn fat.

Assessment of Cardiorespiratory Endurance

The level of cardiorespiratory endurance, cardiorespiratory fitness, or aerobic capacity is determined by the maximal amount of oxygen the human body is able to utilize per minute of physical activity. This value can be expressed in liters per minute (l/min) or milliliters per kilogram per minute (ml/kg/min). The relative value in ml/kg/min is used most often because it considers total body mass (weight). When comparing two individuals with the same absolute value, the one with the lesser body mass will have a higher relative value, indicating that more oxygen is available to each kilogram (2.2 pounds) of body weight. Because all tissues and organs of the body need oxygen to function, higher oxygen consumption indicates a more efficient cardiorespiratory system.

The most precise way to determine maximal oxygen uptake (VO_{2max}) is through gas analysis. This is done by using a metabolic cart through which the amount of oxygen consumption can be measured directly. This type of equipment is not available in most health/fitness centers. Therefore, several alternative methods of estimating maximal oxygen uptake using limited equipment have been developed.

Even though most cardiorespiratory endurance tests probably are safe to administer to apparently healthy individuals (those with no major coronary risk factors or symptoms), the American College of Sports Medicine recommends that a physician be present for all maximal exercise tests on apparently healthy men over age 40 and women over age 50. A maximal test is any test that requires the participant's all-out or nearly all-out effort. For submaximal exercise tests, a physician should be present when testing higher risk/symptomatic individuals or people with illness, regardless of the participant's current age.

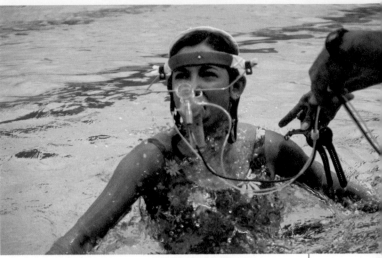

© Fitness & Wellness, Inc.

Maximal oxygen uptake (VO_{2max}, or cardiorespiratory fitness) is determined through direct gas analysis.

Five exercise tests used to assess cardiorespiratory fitness are introduced in this chapter: 1.5-Mile Run Test, 1.0-Mile Walk Test, Step Test, Astrand-Ryhming Test, and 12-Minute Swim Test.

These multiple tests are provided so that you may choose one test depending on time, equipment, and individual physical limitations. For example, people who can't jog or walk could take the bike or swim test. You may perform more than one of these tests, but because these are different tests, and they estimate maximal oxygen uptake, they will not necessarily yield the same results. Therefore, to make valid comparisons, you should take the same test when doing pre- and post-assessments. You may record the results of your test(s) in Lab 6A.

A sixth test, the University of Houston Non-Exercise Test, also is presented, at the end of this

Maximal oxygen uptake (VO_{2max}) Maximum amount of oxygen the body is able to utilize per minute of physical activity, commonly expressed in ml/kg/min. The best indicator of cardiorespiratory or aerobic fitness.

Cardiac output Amount of blood pumped by the heart in one minute.

Stroke volume Amount of blood pumped by the heart in one beat.

Workload Load placed on the body during physical activity, which determines the intensity of exercise.

Mitochondria Structures within the cells where energy transformations take place.

Capillaries Smallest blood vessels carrying oxygenated blood to body tissues.

Recovery time Amount of time the body takes to return to resting levels after exercise.

chapter (Figure 6.6). This non-exercise test is a valuable tool for making initial estimates of maximal oxygen uptake, hopefully to motivate people to exercise. The test is also valuable for mass screening, because the required information is collected through a self-reported method.

1.5-Mile Run Test

The 1.5-Mile Run Test is used most frequently to predict cardiorespiratory fitness according to the time the person takes to run or walk a 1.5-mile course (see Figure 6.1). Maximal oxygen uptake is estimated based on the time the person takes to cover the distance (see Table 6.2).

The only equipment necessary to conduct this test is a stopwatch and a track or premeasured 1.5-mile course. This perhaps is the easiest test to administer, but a note of caution is in order when conducting the test. As the objective is to cover the distance in the shortest time, it is considered a maximal exercise test. The 1.5-Mile Run Test should be limited to conditioned individuals who have been cleared for exercise. The test is not recommended for unconditioned beginners, men over age 40, and women over age 50 without proper medical

<table>
<tr><th colspan="2">Table 6.2</th><th colspan="4">Estimated Maximal Oxygen Uptake (VO$_{2max}$) for the 1.5-Mile Run Test</th></tr>
<tr><th>Time</th><th>VO$_{2max}$ (ml/kg/min)</th><th></th><th>Time</th><th>VO$_{2max}$ (ml/kg/min)</th></tr>
<tr><td>6:10</td><td>80.0</td><td></td><td>12:40</td><td>39.8</td></tr>
<tr><td>6:20</td><td>79.0</td><td></td><td>12:50</td><td>39.2</td></tr>
<tr><td>6:30</td><td>77.9</td><td></td><td>13:00</td><td>38.6</td></tr>
<tr><td>6:40</td><td>76.7</td><td></td><td>13:10</td><td>38.1</td></tr>
<tr><td>6:50</td><td>75.5</td><td></td><td>13:20</td><td>37.8</td></tr>
<tr><td>7:00</td><td>74.0</td><td></td><td>13:30</td><td>37.2</td></tr>
<tr><td>7:10</td><td>72.6</td><td></td><td>13:40</td><td>36.8</td></tr>
<tr><td>7:20</td><td>71.3</td><td></td><td>13:50</td><td>36.3</td></tr>
<tr><td>7:30</td><td>69.9</td><td></td><td>14:00</td><td>35.9</td></tr>
<tr><td>7:40</td><td>68.3</td><td></td><td>14:10</td><td>35.5</td></tr>
<tr><td>7:50</td><td>66.8</td><td></td><td>14:20</td><td>35.1</td></tr>
<tr><td>8:00</td><td>65.2</td><td></td><td>14:30</td><td>34.7</td></tr>
<tr><td>8:10</td><td>63.9</td><td></td><td>14:40</td><td>34.3</td></tr>
<tr><td>8:20</td><td>62.5</td><td></td><td>14:50</td><td>34.0</td></tr>
<tr><td>8:30</td><td>61.2</td><td></td><td>15:00</td><td>33.6</td></tr>
<tr><td>8:40</td><td>60.2</td><td></td><td>15:10</td><td>33.1</td></tr>
<tr><td>8:50</td><td>59.1</td><td></td><td>15:20</td><td>32.7</td></tr>
<tr><td>9:00</td><td>58.1</td><td></td><td>15:30</td><td>32.2</td></tr>
<tr><td>9:10</td><td>56.9</td><td></td><td>15:40</td><td>31.8</td></tr>
<tr><td>9:20</td><td>55.9</td><td></td><td>15:50</td><td>31.4</td></tr>
<tr><td>9:30</td><td>54.7</td><td></td><td>16:00</td><td>30.9</td></tr>
<tr><td>9:40</td><td>53.5</td><td></td><td>16:10</td><td>30.5</td></tr>
<tr><td>9:50</td><td>52.3</td><td></td><td>16:20</td><td>30.2</td></tr>
<tr><td>10:00</td><td>51.1</td><td></td><td>16:30</td><td>29.8</td></tr>
<tr><td>10:10</td><td>50.4</td><td></td><td>16:40</td><td>29.5</td></tr>
<tr><td>10:20</td><td>49.5</td><td></td><td>16:50</td><td>29.1</td></tr>
<tr><td>10:30</td><td>48.6</td><td></td><td>17:00</td><td>28.9</td></tr>
<tr><td>10:40</td><td>48.0</td><td></td><td>17:10</td><td>28.5</td></tr>
<tr><td>10:50</td><td>47.4</td><td></td><td>17:20</td><td>28.3</td></tr>
<tr><td>11:00</td><td>46.6</td><td></td><td>17:30</td><td>28.0</td></tr>
<tr><td>11:10</td><td>45.8</td><td></td><td>17:40</td><td>27.7</td></tr>
<tr><td>11:20</td><td>45.1</td><td></td><td>17:50</td><td>27.4</td></tr>
<tr><td>11:30</td><td>44.4</td><td></td><td>18:00</td><td>27.1</td></tr>
<tr><td>11:40</td><td>43.7</td><td></td><td>18:10</td><td>26.8</td></tr>
<tr><td>11:50</td><td>43.2</td><td></td><td>18:20</td><td>26.6</td></tr>
<tr><td>12:00</td><td>42.3</td><td></td><td>18:30</td><td>26.3</td></tr>
<tr><td>12:10</td><td>41.7</td><td></td><td>18:40</td><td>26.0</td></tr>
<tr><td>12:20</td><td>41.0</td><td></td><td>18:50</td><td>25.7</td></tr>
<tr><td>12:30</td><td>40.4</td><td></td><td>19:00</td><td>25.4</td></tr>
</table>

Source: Adapted from K. H. Cooper, "A Means of Assessing Maximal Oxygen Intake," *Journal of the American Medical Association*, 203 (1968): 201–204; M. L. Pollock, J. H. Wilmore, and S. M. Fox III, *Health and Fitness Through Physical Activity*, (New York: John Wiley & Sons, 1978); and J. H. Wilmore and D. L. Costill, *Training for Sport and Activity* (Dubuque, IA: Wm. C. Brown Publishers, 1988).

Figure 6.1 Procedure for the 1.5-Mile Run Test.

1. Make sure you qualify for this test. This test is contraindicated for unconditioned beginners, individuals with symptoms of heart disease, and those with known heart disease or risk factors.
2. Select the testing site. Find a school track (each lap is one-fourth of a mile) or a premeasured 1.5-mile course.
3. Have a stopwatch available to determine your time.
4. Conduct a few warm-up exercises prior to the test. Do some stretching exercises, some walking, and slow jogging.
5. Initiate the test and try to cover the distance in the fastest time possible (walking or jogging). Time yourself during the run to see how fast you have covered the distance. If any unusual symptoms arise during the test, do not continue. Stop immediately and retake the test after another 6 weeks of aerobic training.
6. At the end of the test, cool down by walking or jogging slowly for another 3 to 5 minutes. Do not sit or lie down after the test.
7. According to your performance time, look up your estimated maximal oxygen uptake(VO$_{2max}$) in Table 6.2.

Example: A 20-year-old female runs the 1.5-mile course in 12 minutes and 40 seconds. Table 6.2 shows a VO$_{2max}$ of 39.8 ml/kg/min for a time of 12:40. According to Table 6.8, this VO$_{2max}$ would place her in the "good" cardiorespiratory fitness category.

clearance, symptomatic individuals, and those with known disease or coronary heart disease risk factors. A program of at least 6 weeks of aerobic training is recommended before unconditioned individuals take this test.

1.0-Mile Walk Test

This test can be used by individuals who are unable to run because of low fitness levels or injuries. All that is required is a brisk 1-mile walk that will elicit an exercise heart rate of at least 120 beats per minute at the end of the test.

You will need to know how to take your heart rate by counting your pulse. This can be done by gently placing the middle and index fingers over the radial artery on the wrist (inside the wrist on the side of the thumb) or over the carotid artery in the neck just below the jaw, next to the voice box. The thumb should not be used to check the pulse as it has a strong pulse of it's own that can make you miscount. When checking the carotid pulse, do not press too hard because it may cause a reflex action that slows the heart. Some exercise leaders recommend that when you check the pulse over the carotid artery, the hand on the same side of the neck (left hand over left carotid artery) be used to avoid excessive pressure on the artery. With minimum experience, however, you can be accurate using either hand as long as only gentle pressure is applied. If available, heart rate monitors can be used to increase the accuracy of heart rate assessment.

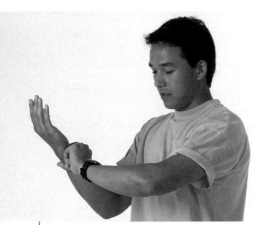

| Pulse taken at the radial artery.

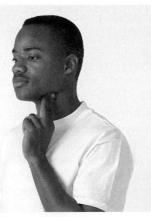

| Pulse taken at the carotid artery.

Maximal oxygen uptake is estimated according to a prediction equation that requires the following data: 1.0-mile walk time, exercise heart rate at the end of the walk, gender, and body weight in pounds. The procedure for this test and the equation are given in Figure 6.2.

Figure 6.2 Procedure for the 1.0-Mile Walk Test.

1. Select the testing site. Use a 440-yard track (4 laps to a mile) or a premeasured 1.0-mile course.
2. Determine your body weight in pounds prior to the test.
3. Have a stopwatch available to determine total walking time and exercise heart rate.
4. Walk the 1.0-mile course at a brisk pace (the exercise heart rate at the end of the test should be above 120 beats per minute).
5. At the end of the 1.0-mile walk, check your walking time and immediately count your pulse for 10 seconds. Multiply the 10-second pulse count by 6 to obtain the exercise heart rate in beats per minute.
6. Convert the walking time from minutes and seconds to minute units. Because each minute has 60 seconds, divide the seconds by 60 to obtain the fraction of a minute. For instance, a walking time of 12 minutes and 15 seconds would equal 12 + (15 ÷ 60), or 12.25 minutes.
7. To obtain the estimated maximal oxygen uptake (VO_{2max}) in ml/kg/min, plug your values in the following equation:
   $VO_{2max} = 88.768 - (0.0957 \times W) + (8.892 \times G) - (1.4537 \times T) - (0.1194 \times HR)$

WHERE:

W = Weight in pounds

G = Gender (use 0 for women and 1 for men)

T = Total time for the one-mile walk in minutes (see item 6 above)

HR = Exercise heart rate in beats per minute at the end of the 1.0-mile walk

Example: A 19-year-old female who weighs 140 pounds completed the 1.0-mile walk in 14 minutes 39 seconds and with an exercise heart rate of 148 beats per minute. The estimated VO_{2max} would be:

W = 140 lbs

G = 0 (female gender = 0)

T = 14:39 = 14 + (39 ÷ 60) = 14.65 min

HR = 148 bpm

VO_{2max} = 88.768 − (0.0957 × 140) + (8.892 × 0) − (1.4537 × 14.65) − (0.1194 × 148)

VO_{2max} = 36.4 ml/kg/min

Source: F. A. Dolgener, L. D. Hensley, J. J. Marsh, and J. K. Fjelstul, "Validation of the Rockport Fitness Walking Test in College Males and Females," *Research Quarterly for Exercise and Sport* 65 (1994): 152–158.

© Fitness & Wellness, Inc.

Step Test

The Step Test requires little time and equipment and can be administered to almost anyone, as a submaximal workload is used to estimate maximal oxygen uptake. Symptomatic and diseased individuals should not take this test. Significantly overweight individuals and those with joint problems in the lower extremities may have difficulty performing the test.

The actual test takes only 3 minutes. A 15-second recovery heart rate is taken between 5 and 20 seconds following the test (see Figure 6.3 and Table 6.3). The equipment required consists of a bench or gymnasium bleacher 16¼ inches high, a stopwatch, and a metronome.

You also will need to know how to take your heart rate by counting your pulse (explained under

Figure 6.3 Procedure for the Step Test.

1. Conduct the test with a bench or gymnasium bleacher 16¼ inches high.
2. Perform the stepping cycle to a four-step cadence (up-up-down-down). Men should perform 24 complete step-ups per minute, regulated with a metronome set at 96 beats per minute. Women perform 22 step-ups per minute, or 88 beats per minute on the metronome.
3. Allow a brief practice period of 5 to 10 seconds to familiarize yourself with the stepping cadence.
4. Begin the test and perform the step-ups for exactly 3 minutes.
5. Upon completing the 3 minutes, remain standing and take your heart rate for a 15-second interval from 5 to 20 seconds into recovery. Convert recovery heart rate to beats per minute (multiply 15-second heart rate by 4).
6. Maximal oxygen uptake (VO_{2max}) in ml/kg/min is estimated according to the following equations:
   Men:
   $$VO_{2max} = 111.33 - (0.42 \times \text{recovery heart rate in bpm})$$
   Women:
   $$VO_{2max} = 65.81 - (0.1847 \times \text{recovery heart rate in bpm})$$

Example: The recovery 15-second heart rate for a male following the 3-minute step test is found to be 39 beats. VO_{2max} is estimated as follows:
   15-second heart rate = 39 beats
   Minute heart rate = 39 × 4 = 156 bpm
$VO_{2max} = 111.33 - (0.42 \times 156) = 45.81$ ml/kg/min
VO_{2max} also can be obtained according to recovery heart rates in Table 6.3.

From W. D. McArdle et al., *Exercise Physiology: Energy, Nutrition, and Human Performance* (Philadelphia: Lea & Febiger, 1986).

Table 6.3 Predicted Maximal Oxygen Uptake (VO_{2max}) for the Step Test

15-Sec Heart Rate	Heart Rate (bpm)	VO_{2max} (ml/kg/min) Men	VO_{2max} (ml/kg/min) Women
30	120	60.9	43.6
31	124	59.3	42.9
32	128	57.6	42.2
33	132	55.9	41.4
34	136	54.2	40.7
35	140	52.5	40.0
36	144	50.9	39.2
37	148	49.2	38.5
38	152	47.5	37.7
39	156	45.8	37.0
40	160	44.1	36.3
41	164	42.5	35.5
42	168	40.8	34.8
43	172	39.1	34.0
44	176	37.4	33.3
45	180	35.7	32.6
46	184	34.1	31.8
47	188	32.4	31.1
48	192	30.7	30.3
49	196	29.0	29.6
50	200	27.3	28.9

the 1.0-Mile Walk Test). By teaching people to take their own heart rate, a large group of people can be tested at once, using gymnasium bleachers.

Astrand-Ryhming Test

Because of its simplicity and practicality, the Astrand-Ryhming is one of the most popular tests used to estimate maximal oxygen uptake in the laboratory setting. The test is conducted on a bicycle ergometer, and, similar to the Step Test, it requires only submaximal workloads and little time to administer.

The cautions given for the Step Test also apply to the Astrand-Ryhming Test. Nevertheless, because the participant does not have to support his or her own body weight while riding the bicycle, overweight individuals and those with limited joint problems in the lower extremities can take this test.

The bicycle ergometer to be used for this test should allow for the regulation of workloads (see the test procedure in Figure 6.4). Besides the bicycle ergometer, a stopwatch and an additional technician to monitor the heart rate are needed to conduct the test.

The heart rate is taken every minute for 6 minutes. At the end of the test, the heart rate should be in the range given for each workload in Table 6.5 (generally between 120 and 170 beats per minute). (Tables 6.4 and 6.6 contain conversion and correction factors for this test.)

Figure
6.4

Procedure for the Astrand-Rhyming Test.

1. Adjust the bike seat so the knees are almost completely extended as the foot goes through the bottom of the pedaling cycle.
2. During the test, keep the speed constant at 50 revolutions per minute. Test duration is 6 minutes.
3. Select the appropriate workload for the bike based on age, weight, health, and estimated fitness level. For unconditioned individuals: women, use 300 kpm (kilopounds per meter) or 450 kpm; men, 300 kpm or 600 kpm. Conditioned adults: women, 450 kpm or 600 kpm; men, 600 kpm or 900 kpm.*
4. Ride the bike for 6 minutes and check the heart rate every minute, during the last 10 seconds of each minute. Determine heart rate by recording the time it takes to count 30 pulse beats and then converting to beats per minute using Table 6.4.
5. Average the final two heart rates (5th and 6th minutes). If these two heart rates are not within 5 beats per minute of each other, continue the test for another few minutes until this is accomplished. If the heart rate continues to climb significantly after the 6th minute, stop the test and rest for 15 to 20 minutes. You may then retest, preferably at a lower workload. The final average heart rate should also fall between the ranges given for each workload in Table 6.5 (men: 300 kpm = 120 to 140 beats per minute; 600 kpm = 120 to 170 beats per minute).
6. Based on the average heart rate of the final 2 minutes and your workload, look up the maximal oxygen uptake (VO_{2max}) in Table 6.5 (for example: men: 600 kpm and average heart rate = 145, VO_{2max} = 2.4 liters/minute).
7. Correct VO_{2max} using the correction factors found in Table 6.6 (if VO_{2max} = 2.4 and age 35, correction factor = .870. Multiply 2.4 × .870 and final corrected VO_{2max} = 2.09 liters/minute).
8. To obtain VO_{2max} in ml/kg/min, multiply the VO_{2max} by 1,000 (to convert liters to milliliters) and divide by body weight in kilograms (to obtain kilograms, divide your body weight in pounds by 2.2046).

Example: Corrected VO_{2max} = 2.09 liters/minute
Body weight = 132 pounds or 60 kilograms (132 ÷ 2.2046 = 60)

$$VO_{2max} \text{ in ml/kg/min} = \frac{2.09 \times 1,000}{60} = 39.8 \text{ ml/kg/min}$$

2,090 divided by 60 = 34.8 ml/kg/min

* On the Monarch bicycle ergometer, at a speed of 50 revolutions per minute, a load of 1 kp = 300 kpm, 1.5 kp = 450, 2 kp = 600 kpm, and so forth, with increases of 150 kpm to each half kp.

Table
6.4

Conversion of Time for 30 Pulse Beats to Pulse Rate Per Minute

Sec.	bpm	Sec.	bpm	Sec.	bpm	Sec.	bpm	Sec.	bpm	Sec.	bpm	Sec.	bpm
22.0	82	20.0	90	18.0	100	16.0	113	14.0	129	12.0	150	10.0	180
21.9	82	19.9	90	17.9	101	15.9	113	13.9	129	11.9	151	9.9	182
21.8	83	19.8	91	17.8	101	15.8	114	13.8	130	11.8	153	9.8	184
21.7	83	19.7	91	17.7	102	15.7	115	13.7	131	11.7	154	9.7	186
21.6	83	19.6	92	17.6	102	15.6	115	13.6	132	11.6	155	9.6	188
21.5	84	19.5	92	17.5	103	15.5	116	13.5	133	11.5	157	9.5	189
21.4	84	19.4	93	17.4	103	15.4	117	13.4	134	11.4	158	9.4	191
21.3	85	19.3	93	17.3	104	15.3	118	13.3	135	11.3	159	9.3	194
21.2	85	19.2	94	17.2	105	15.2	118	13.2	136	11.2	161	9.2	196
21.1	85	19.1	94	17.1	105	15.1	119	13.1	137	11.1	162	9.1	198
21.0	86	19.0	95	17.0	106	15.0	120	13.0	138	11.0	164	9.0	200
20.9	86	18.9	95	16.9	107	14.9	121	12.9	140	10.9	165	8.9	202
20.8	87	18.8	96	16.8	107	14.8	122	12.8	141	10.8	167	8.8	205
20.7	87	18.7	96	16.7	108	14.7	122	12.7	142	10.7	168	8.7	207
20.6	87	18.6	97	16.6	108	14.6	123	12.6	143	10.6	170	8.6	209
20.5	88	18.5	97	16.5	109	14.5	124	12.5	144	10.5	171	8.5	212
20.4	88	18.4	98	16.4	110	14.4	125	12.4	145	10.4	173	8.4	214
20.3	89	18.3	98	16.3	110	14.3	126	12.3	146	10.3	175	8.3	217
20.2	89	18.2	99	16.2	111	14.2	127	12.2	148	10.2	176	8.2	220
20.1	90	18.1	99	16.1	112	14.1	128	12.1	149	10.1	178		

Table 6.5

Maximal Oxygen Uptake (VO_{2max}) Estimates in liters per minute (l/min) for the Astrand-Ryhming Test

Heart Rate	Men Workload 300	600	900	1200	1500	Women Workload 300	450	600	750	900
120	2.2	3.4	4.8			2.6	3.4	4.1	4.8	
121	2.2	3.4	4.7			2.5	3.3	4.0	4.8	
122	2.2	3.4	4.6			2.5	3.2	3.9	4.7	
123	2.1	3.4	4.6			2.4	3.1	3.9	4.6	
124	2.1	3.3	4.5	6.0		2.4	3.1	3.8	4.5	
125	2.0	3.2	4.4	5.9		2.3	3.0	3.7	4.4	
126	2.0	3.2	4.4	5.8		2.3	3.0	3.6	4.3	
127	2.0	3.1	4.3	5.7		2.2	2.9	3.5	4.2	
128	2.0	3.1	4.2	5.6		2.2	2.8	3.5	4.2	4.8
129	1.9	3.0	4.2	5.6		2.2	2.8	3.4	4.1	4.8
130	1.9	3.0	4.1	5.5		2.1	2.7	3.4	4.0	4.7
131	1.9	2.9	4.0	5.4		2.1	2.7	3.4	4.0	4.6
132	1.8	2.9	4.0	5.3		2.0	2.7	3.3	3.9	4.5
133	1.8	2.8	3.9	5.3		2.0	2.6	3.2	3.8	4.4
134	1.8	2.8	3.9	5.2		2.0	2.6	3.2	3.8	4.4
135	1.7	2.8	3.8	5.1		2.0	2.6	3.1	3.7	4.3
136	1.7	2.7	3.8	5.0		1.9	2.5	3.1	3.6	4.2
137	1.7	2.7	3.7	5.0		1.9	2.5	3.0	3.6	4.2
138	1.6	2.7	3.7	4.9		1.8	2.4	3.0	3.5	4.1
139	1.6	2.6	3.6	4.8		1.8	2.4	2.9	3.5	4.0
140	1.6	2.6	3.6	4.8	6.0	1.8	2.4	2.8	3.4	4.0
141		2.6	3.5	4.7	5.9	1.8	2.3	2.8	3.4	3.9
142		2.5	3.5	4.6	5.8	1.7	2.3	2.8	3.3	3.9
143		2.5	3.4	4.6	5.7	1.7	2.2	2.7	3.3	3.8
144		2.5	3.4	4.5	5.7	1.7	2.2	2.7	3.2	3.8
145		2.4	3.4	4.5	5.6	1.6	2.2	2.7	3.2	3.7
146		2.4	3.3	4.4	5.6	1.6	2.2	2.6	3.2	3.7
147		2.4	3.3	4.4	5.5	1.6	2.1	2.6	3.1	3.6
148		2.4	3.2	4.3	5.4	1.6	2.1	2.6	3.1	3.6
149		2.3	3.2	4.3	5.4		2.1	2.6	3.0	3.5
150		2.3	3.2	4.2	5.3		2.0	2.5	3.0	3.5
151		2.3	3.1	4.2	5.2		2.0	2.5	3.0	3.4
152		2.3	3.1	4.1	5.2		2.0	2.5	2.9	3.4
153		2.2	3.0	4.1	5.1		2.0	2.4	2.9	3.3
154		2.2	3.0	4.0	5.1		2.0	2.4	2.8	3.3
155		2.2	3.0	4.0	5.0		1.9	2.4	2.8	3.2
156		2.2	2.9	4.0	5.0		1.9	2.3	2.8	3.2
157		2.1	2.9	3.9	4.9		1.9	2.3	2.7	3.2
158		2.1	2.9	3.9	4.9		1.8	2.3	2.7	3.1
159		2.1	2.8	3.8	4.8		1.8	2.2	2.7	3.1
160		2.1	2.8	3.8	4.8		1.8	2.2	2.6	3.0
161		2.0	2.8	3.7	4.7		1.8	2.2	2.6	3.0
162		2.0	2.8	3.7	4.6		1.8	2.2	2.6	3.0
163		2.0	2.8	3.7	4.6		1.7	2.2	2.6	2.9
164		2.0	2.7	3.6	4.5		1.7	2.1	2.5	2.9
165		2.0	2.7	3.6	4.5		1.7	2.1	2.5	2.9
166		1.9	2.7	3.6	4.5		1.7	2.1	2.5	2.8
167		1.9	2.6	3.5	4.4		1.6	2.1	2.4	2.8
168		1.9	2.6	3.5	4.4		1.6	2.0	2.4	2.8
169		1.9	2.6	3.5	4.3		1.6	2.0	2.4	2.8
170		1.8	2.6	3.4	4.3		1.6	2.0	2.4	2.7

From Astrand, I. *Acta Physiologica Scandinavica* 49(1960). Supplementum 169:45-60.

Table 6.6

Age-Based Correction Factors for Maximal Oxygen Uptake for the Astrand-Ryhming Test

Age	Correction Factor	Age	Correction Factor
14	1.11	40	.830
15	1.10	41	.820
16	1.09	42	.810
17	1.08	43	.800
18	1.07	44	.790
19	1.06	45	.780
20	1.05	46	.774
21	1.04	47	.768
22	1.03	48	.762
23	1.02	49	.756
24	1.01	50	.750
25	1.00	51	.742
26	.987	52	.734
27	.974	53	.726
28	.961	54	.718
29	.948	55	.710
30	.935	56	.704
31	.922	57	.698
32	.909	58	.692
33	.896	59	.686
34	.883	60	.680
35	.870	61	.674
36	.862	62	.668
37	.854	63	.662
38	.846	64	.656
39	.838	65	.650

Adapted from Astrand, I. *Acta Physiologica Scandinavica* 49(1960). Supplementum 169:45-60.

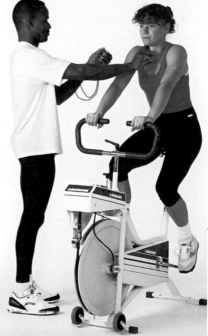

Monitoring heart rate on the carotid artery during the Astrand-Ryhming Test.

© Fitness & Wellness, Inc.

If you administer the test to older people, good judgment is essential. Low workloads should be used, because if the higher heart rates are reached (around 150 to 170 bpm), these individuals could be working near or at their maximal capacity, making it an unsafe test without adequate medical supervision. When choosing workloads for older people, be sure that final exercise heart rates do not exceed 130 to 140 bpm.

12-Minute Swim Test

Similar to the 1.5-Mile Run test, the 12-Minute Swim Test is considered a maximal exercise test, and the same precautions apply. The objective is to swim as far as possible during the 12-minute test.

A swimming test (Figure 6.5) is practical only for those who are planning to take part in a swimming program. Unlike land-based tests, predicting maximal oxygen uptake through a swimming test is difficult. Differences in skill level, swimming conditioning, and body composition greatly affect the energy requirements (oxygen uptake) of swimming.

A skilled swimmer is able to swim more efficiently and expend much less energy than an unskilled swimmer. Improper breathing patterns cause premature fatigue. Overweight individuals are more buoyant in the water, and the larger surface area (body size) produces greater friction against movement in the water medium—both affect test results.

Lack of specific, appropriate conditioning affects swimming test results as well. A skilled but unconditioned swimmer who is in good cardiorespiratory shape because of a regular jogging program will not perform as effectively in a swimming test. Swimming conditioning is important for adequate performance on this test.

Because of these limitations, maximal oxygen uptake cannot be estimated for a swimming test and the fitness categories given in Table 6.7 are only estimated ratings. This test should be limited to

Table 6.7	Fitness Categories for 12-Minute Swim Test

Distance (yards)	Fitness Category
≥700	Excellent
500–700	Good
400–500	Average
200–400	Fair
≤200	Poor

Adapted from K. H. Cooper, *The Aerobics Program for Total Well-Being* (New York: Bantam Books, 1982).

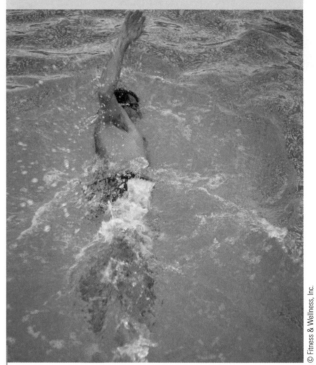
© Fitness & Wellness, Inc.

Only those with swimming skill and proper conditioning should take the 12-minute swim test.

people who cannot perform any of the other tests and whose primary aerobic exercise will be a swimming program. Unskilled and unconditioned swimmers can expect lower cardiorespiratory fitness ratings than those obtained with a land-based test.

University of Houston Non-Exercise Test

The University of Houston Non-Exercise Test (N-Ex) is a way to estimate maximal oxygen uptake that does not involve any form of exercise testing. This protocol can be used as an initial estimate of maximal oxygen uptake and for mass screening purposes. The information for this test is collected through self-reports.

Figure 6.5	Procedure for the 12-Minute Swim Test.

1. Enlist a friend to time the test. The only other requisites are a stopwatch and a swimming pool. Do not attempt to do this test in an unsupervised pool.
2. Warm up by swimming slowly and doing a few stretching exercises before taking the test.
3. Start the test and swim as many laps as possible in 12 minutes. Pace yourself throughout the test and do not swim to the point of complete exhaustion.
4. After completing the test, cool down by swimming another 2 or 3 minutes at a slower pace.
5. Determine the total distance you swam during the test and look up your fitness category in Table 6.7.

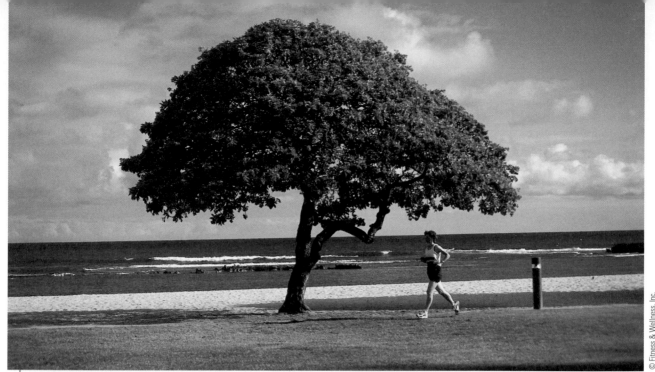

Aerobic fitness leads to better health and a higher quality of life.

This N-Ex test is especially useful when testing individuals who are taking high blood pressure medication. Hypertensive medication lowers the heart rate. Therefore, tests based on heart rate (walk test, step test, and Astrand-Ryhming) cannot be used with these people. Maximal exercise tests (1.5-Mile Run) also are not to be administered to hypertensive people. The N-Ex equations to predict maximal oxygen uptake have a high degree of accuracy with men on anti-hypertensive medication.

> *Good cardio-respiratory fitness leads to better health, improved quality of life, and increased longevity.*

The N-Ex test is based on research findings in exercise physiology indicating that maximal oxygen uptake is related negatively to age and body composition but related positively to exercise habits. Based on these variables, multiple regression equations were developed to estimate maximal oxygen uptake in ml/kg/min. The procedure for the Houston Non-Exercise Test is outlined in Figures 6.6 and 6.7. The test is suitable for men and women alike.

Interpreting Your Maximal Oxygen Uptake Results

After obtaining your maximal oxygen uptake, you can determine your current level of cardiorespiratory fitness by consulting Table 6.8. Locate the maximal oxygen uptake in your age category, and on the top

Figure 6.6 Physical Activity Rating (PAR) for the University of Houston Non-Exercise Test.

Use the number (0–7) that best describes your general physical activity rating (PAR) for the previous month:

I. Do not participate regularly in programmed recreation sport or physical activity.

0   Avoid walking or exertion, e.g., always use elevator, drive whenever possible instead of walking.

1   Walk for pleasure, routinely use stairs, occasionally exercise sufficiently to cause heavy breathing or perspiration.

II. Participate regularly in recreation or work requiring modest physical activity, such as golf, horseback riding, calisthenics, gymnastics, table tennis, bowling, weight lifting, yard work.

2   10 to 60 minutes per week.

3   Over one hour per week.

III. Participate regularly in heavy physical exercise such as running or jogging, swimming, cycling, rowing, skipping rope, running in place or engaging in vigorous aerobic activity type exercise such as tennis, basketball, or handball.

4   Run less than one mile per week or spend less than 30 minutes per week in comparable physical activity.

5   Run 1 to 5 miles per week or spend 30 to 60 minutes per week in comparable physical activity.

6   Run 5 to 10 miles per week or spend 1 to 3 hours per week in comparable physical activity.

7   Run over 10 miles per week or spend over 3 hours per week in comparable physical activity.

Figure 6.7 Procedure for the University of Houston Non-Exercise Test.

Multiple regression equations have been developed to estimate maximal oxygen uptake in ml/kg/min according to physical activity rating (PAR—see Figure 6.6), age (A), and percent body fat (%Fat) or body mass index (BMI). The first equation uses percent body fat determined through skinfolds (N-Ex %Fat). The procedure to determine percent body fat through skinfolds is outlined in Figure 4.4 (page 96). The second equation uses body mass index (N-Ex BMI). The computation of body mass index is explained in Chapter 4, page 102. The N-Ex %Fat equation is slightly more accurate than the N-Ex BMI equation. The physical activity rating code provided in Figure 6.6 is used for a global self-rating of physical activity. The subject uses the code to rate his or her physical activity during the past month. The selected number is a global rating of the subject's exercise habits. This value is used in the equation. The regression equations are as follows:

N-Ex %Fat Model

Men $VO_{2max} = 56.370 - (.289 \times A) - (.552 \times \%Fat) + (1.589 \times PAR)$

Women $VO_{2max} = 50.513 - (.289 \times A) - (.552 \times \%Fat) + (1.589 \times PAR)$

N-Ex BMI Model (BMI = Weight in pounds $\times$ 705 $\div$ Height in inches $\div$ Height in inches)

Men $VO_{2max} = 67.350 - (.381 \times A) - (.754 \times BMI) + (1.951 \times PAR)$

Women $VO_{2max} = 56.363 - (.381 \times A) - (.754 \times BMI) + (1.951 \times PAR)$

Examples

The N-Ex %fat model is illustrated with a 40-year-old man with 17% body fat and an activity rating of 6. Estimated VO_{2max} for the man would be

$VO_{2max} = 56.37 - (.289 \times 40) - (.552 \times 17) + (1.589 \times 6)$

$VO_{2max} = 45.0$ ml/kg/min

The N-Ex BMI for a 30-year-old woman who weighs 130 pounds, is 64 inches tall, and has a physical activity rating of 5 would be:

BMI = Weight in pounds $\times$ 705 $\div$ Height in inches $\div$ Height in inches [or weight in kilograms $\times$ (height in meters)^2]

BMI = $130 \times 705 \div 64 \div 64 = 22.38$

$VO_{2max} = 56.363 - (.381 \times 30) - (.754 \times 22.38) + (1.951 \times 5)$

$VO_{2max} = 37.8$ ml/kg/min

University of Houston Non-Exercise Test reproduced with permission from R. M. Ross and A. S. Jackson, Exercise Concepts, Calculations, & Computer Applications. Camel, IN: Benchmark Press, Inc., (1990): 108–110.

row you will find your present level of cardiorespiratory fitness. For example, a 19-year-old male with a maximal oxygen uptake of 35 ml/kg/min would be classified in the average cardiorespiratory fitness category. After you initiate your personal cardio-respiratory exercise program (see Chapter 7), you may wish to retest yourself periodically to evaluate your progress. (Table 6.8 also shows ratings according to health versus physical fitness standards, discussed in Chapter 1, page 12.)

Table 6.8 Cardiorespiratory Fitness Classification According to Maximal Oxygen Uptake (VO_{2max})

Gender	Age	FITNESS CLASSIFICATION (based on VO_{2max} in ml/kg/min)				
		Poor	Fair	Average	Good	Excellent
Men	≤29	≤24.9	25–33.9	34–43.9	44–52.9	≥53
	30–39	≤22.9	23–30.9	31–41.9	42–49.9	≥50
	40–49	≤19.9	20–26.9	27–38.9	39–44.9	≥45
	50–59	≤17.9	18–24.9	25–37.9	38–42.9	≥43
	60–69	≤15.9	16–22.9	23–35.9	36–40.9	≥41
Women	≤29	≤23.9	24–30.9	31–38.9	39–48.9	≥49
	30–39	≤19.9	20–27.9	28–36.9	37–44.9	≥45
	40–49	≤16.9	17–24.9	25–34.9	35–41.9	≥42
	50–59	≤14.9	15–21.9	22–33.9	34–39.9	≥40
	60–69	≤12.9	13–20.9	21–32.9	33–36.9	≥37

■ High physical fitness standard   □ Health fitness standard

Resting Heart Rate and Blood Pressure Assessment

You will learn in Lab 6B how to determine your heart rate and blood pressure. As mentioned previously, heart rate can be obtained by counting your pulse either on the wrist using the radial artery or in the neck using the carotid artery.

Resting Heart Rate

You may count your pulse for 30 seconds and multiply by 2 or take it for a full minute. The heart rate usually is at its lowest point (resting heart rate) late in the evening after you have been sitting quietly for about half an hour watching a relaxing TV show or reading in bed, or early in the morning just before you get out of bed.

Unless you have a pathological condition, a lower resting heart rate indicates a stronger heart. To adapt to cardiorespiratory or aerobic exercise, the heart enlarges and the muscle gets stronger. A bigger and stronger heart can pump more blood with fewer strokes.

Resting heart rate ratings are given in Table 6.9. Although resting heart rate decreases with training, the extent of **bradycardia** depends not only on the amount of training but also on genetic factors. Although most highly trained athletes have a resting heart rate around 40 beats per minute, occasionally, an athlete exhibits a resting heart rate in the 60s or 70s—even during peak training months of the season. For most individuals, however, the resting heart rate decreases as the level of cardiorespiratory endurance increases.

Resting Blood Pressure

Blood pressure is assessed using a **sphygmomanometer** and a stethoscope. A cuff of the appropriate size must be used to get accurate readings. Size is determined by the width of the inflatable bladder, which should be about 40% of the circumference of the midpoint of the arm.

Blood pressure usually is measured while the subject is in the sitting position, with the forearm and the manometer at the same level as the heart. At first, the pressure is recorded from each arm, and after that from the arm with the highest reading.

The cuff should be applied approximately an inch above the antecubital space (natural crease of the elbow), with the center of the bladder directly over the medial (inner) surface of the arm. The stethoscope head should be applied firmly, but with little pressure, over the brachial artery in the antecubital space. The subject's arm should be flexed slightly and placed on a flat surface.

The person recording the blood pressure inflates the bladder while feeling the radial pulse to about 30 to 40 mm Hg above the point at which the pulse disappears. The cuff should not be over-inflated, because this may cause blood vessel spasm, resulting in higher blood pressure readings. The pressure should then be released at a rate of 2 to 4 mm Hg per second.

As the pressure is released, the recorder listens for the heartbeat and watches the mercury manometer, noting (1) the point at which the pulse becomes audible (**systolic pressure**) and (2) the point at which the sound of the pulse disappears (**diastolic pressure**). The recordings should be expressed as systolic over diastolic pressure—for example, 124/80.

If you take more than one reading, allow the bladder to deflate completely and wait at least one minute before making the next recording. The recorder should also note whether the pressure was recorded from the left or the right arm. Resting blood pressure risk levels are given in Table 6.10.

In some cases the pulse sounds do not disappear abruptly, but simply become less intense (point of muffling sounds) and still can be heard at a

Table 6.9	Resting Heart Rate Ratings
Heart Rate (beats/minute)	**Rating**
≤59	Excellent
60–69	Good
70–79	Average
80–89	Fair
≥90	Poor

Table 6.10	Resting Blood Pressure Risk Levels	
Systolic (in mm Hg)	**Diastolic (in mm Hg)**	**Risk for Cardiovascular Diseases**
≤120	≤80	Very Low
121–130	81–85	Low
131–140	86–90	Moderate
141–150	91–100	High
≥151	≥101	Very High

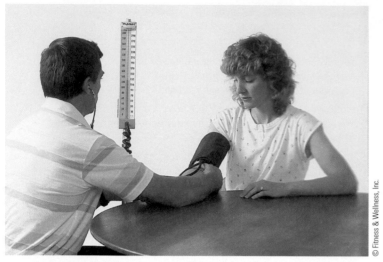

lower pressure (50 or 40 mm Hg)—perhaps all the way down to 0 mm Hg. In this situation, the diastolic pressure is recorded at the point of a clear, definite change in the loudness of the sound (also referred to as "fourth phase"), and at complete disappearance of the sound ("fifth phase") (for example, 120/78/60 or 120/82/0).

When measuring resting heart rate and blood pressure, ask different people to take several readings at different times of the day, to establish the real values. A single reading may not be an accurate value because of the various factors that can affect blood pressure.

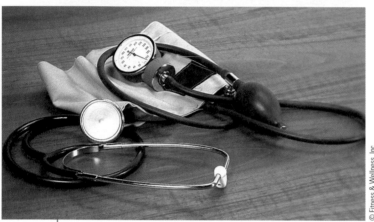

Blood pressure can be measured with a stethoscope and a mercury gravity manometer or an aneroid blood pressure gauge.

Bradycardia Slower heart rate than normal.

Sphygmomanometer Inflatable bladder contained within a cuff and a mercury gravity manometer (or aneroid manometer) from which the pressure is read.

Systolic blood pressure Pressure exerted by blood against walls of arteries during forceful contraction (systole) of the heart.

Diastolic blood pressure Pressure exerted by the blood against the walls of the arteries during the relaxation phase (diastole) of the heart.

Web Interactive

- American Council of Exercise Cardiovascular Fitness Facts. This site features information about a variety of cardio-vascular forms of exercise, including walking, running, jumping rope, swimming, spinning, cross-training, interval training, and others.

  http://www.acefitness.org/fitfacts/fitfacts_list.cfm#1

- Improving Cardiovascular Health In African Americans. This document written by the National Heart, Lung, and Blood Institute provides information on the value of cardio-vascular exercise to improving health.

  http://www.nhlbi.nih.gov/health/public/heart/other/chdblack/energize.htm

- The Cooper Institute for Aerobics Research. The Cooper Institute for Aerobics Research, founded on June 22, 1970 by Kenneth H. Cooper, M.D., M.P.H, has become widely acclaimed as one of the leaders in preventive medicine research and education. As a nonprofit research

organization, the Cooper Institute is dedicated to advancing the understanding of the relationship between living habits and health and to providing leadership in implementing these concepts to enhance the physical and emotional well-being of individuals.

http://www.cooperinst.org

Interactive Sites:

- Check Your Physical Activity and Heart IQ. This site, sponsored by the National Heart, Lung, and Blood Institute, provides a true-false quiz to allow you to assess what you know about how physical activity affects your heart. The answers provided will uncover exercise myths and give you information on ways to improve your heart health.

  http://www.nhlbi.nih.gov/health/public/heart/obesity/pa_iq_ab.htm

Notes

1. H. Atkinson, "Exercise for Longer Life: The Physician's Perspective," *HealthNews* 7:3 (1997): 3.

Suggested Readings

American College of Sports Medicine. *Guidelines for Exercise Testing and Prescription*. Philadelphia: Lea & Febiger, 2000.

Hoeger, W. W. K., and S. A. Hoeger. *Lifetime Fitness & Wellness: A Personalized Program*. Belmont, CA: Wadsworth/Thompson Learning, 2000.

McArdle, W. D., F. I. Katch, and V. L. Katch. *Essentials of Exercise Physiology*. Philadelphia: Lippincott Williams & Wilkins, 2000.

Wilmore, J. H., and D. L. Costill. *Physiology of Sport and Exercise*. Champaign, IL: Human Kinetics, 1999.

CARDIORESPIRATORY ENDURANCE ASSESSMENT

Name: _____   Date: _____   Grade: _____

Instructor: _____   Course: _____   Section: _____

Necessary Lab Equipment

1.5-Mile Run: School track or premeasured course and a stopwatch.

1.0-Mile Walk Test: School track or premeasured course and a stopwatch.

Step Test: A bench or gymnasium bleachers 16¼ inches high, a metronome, and a stopwatch.

Astrand-Ryhming Test: A bicycle ergometer that allows for regulation of workloads in kilopounds per meter (or watts) and a stopwatch.

12-Minute Swim Test: Swimming pool and a stopwatch.

Objective

To estimate maximal oxygen uptake (VO_{2max}) and cardiorespiratory endurance classification.

Lab Preparation

Wear appropriate exercise clothing including jogging shoes and a swimsuit if required. Be prepared to take the 1.0-Mile Walk Test, the Step Test, the Astrand-Ryhming Test, the 1.5-Mile Run Test, and/or the 12-Minute Swim Test. If more than one test will be conducted, perform them in the order just listed and allow at least 15 minutes between tests. Avoid vigorous physical activity 24 hours prior to this lab.

I. 1.5-Mile Run Test

1.5-Mile Run Time: _____ min and _____ sec VO_{2max} (see Table 6.2, page 148): _____ ml/kg/min

Cardiorespiratory Fitness Classification (Table 6.8, page 155): _____

II. 1.0-Mile Walk Test

Weight (W) = _____ lbs   Gender (G) = _____ (female = 0, male = 1)   Time = _____ min and _____ sec

Heart Rate (HR) = _____ bpm

Time in minutes (T) = min + (sec ÷ 60) or T = _____ + (_____ ÷ 60) = _____ min

VO_{2max} = 88.768 − (0.0957 × W) + (8.892 × G) − (1.4537 × T) − (0.1194 × HR)

VO_{2max} = 88.768 − (0.0957 × _____) + (8.892 × _____) − (1.4537 × _____) − (0.1194 × _____)

VO_{2max} = 88.768 − (_____) + (_____) − (_____) − (_____) = ml/kg/min

Cardiorespiratory Fitness Classification (Table 6.8, page 155): _____

III. Step Test

15 second recovery heart rate: _____ beats VO_{2max} (Table 6.3, page 150): _____ ml/kg/min

Cardiorespiratory Fitness Classification (Table 6.8, page 155): _____

IV. Astrand-Ryhming Test

Weight (W) = [   ] lbs   Weight (BW) in kilograms = (W ÷ 2.2046) = [   ] kg   Workload = [   ] kpm

Exercise Heart Rates	30-second pulse count	Heart Rate (bpm) (from Table 6.4, page 151)		30-second pulse count	Heart Rate (bpm) (from Table 6.4, page 151)
First minute:			Fourth minute:		
Second minute:			Fifth minute:		
Third minute:			Sixth minute:		

Average heart rate for the fifth and sixth minutes = [   ] bpm

VO_{2max} in l/min (Table 6.5, page 152) = [   ] l/min   Correction factor (from Table 6.6, page 152) = [   ]

Corrected VO_{2max} = VO_{2max} in l/min × correction factor = [   ] × [   ] = [   ] l/min

VO_{2max} in ml/kg/min = corrected VO_{2max} in l/min × 1000 ÷ BW in kg = [   ] × 1000 ÷ [   ] = [   ] ml/kg/min

Cardiorespiratory Fitness Classification (Table 6.8, page 155): [   ]

V. 12-Minute Swim Test

Distance swum in 12 minutes: [   ] yards

Cardiorespiratory Fitness Classification (Table 6.7, page 153): [   ]

VI. University of Houston Non-Exercise Test (See sample computation in Figure 6.7, page 155)

Age (A) = [   ]   Physical Activity Rating (PAR) (see Figure 6.6, page 154) = [   ]

Percent Fat (N-Ex % Fat) Model

Men VO_{2max} = 56.370 − (.289 × A) − (.552 × %Fat) + (1.589 × PAR)

Women VO_{2max} = 50.513 − (.289 × A) − (.552 × %Fat) + (1.589 × PAR)

VO_{2max} = [   ] − (.289 × [   ]) − (.552 × [   ]) + (1.589 × [   ]) = [   ] ml/kg/min

Body Mass Index (N-Ex BMI) Model

BMI = Weight in pounds × 705 ÷ Height in inches ÷ Height in inches

BMI = [   ] × 705 ÷ [   ] ÷ [   ] = [   ]

Men VO_{2max} = 67.350 − (.381 × A) − (.754 × BMI) + (1.951 × PAR)

Women VO_{2max} = 56.363 − (.381 × A) − (.754 × BMI) + (1.951 × PAR)

VO_{2max} = [   ] − (.381 × [   ]) − (.754 × [   ]) + (1.951 × [   ]) = [   ] ml/kg/min

Cardiorespiratory Fitness Classification (Table 6.8, page 155): [   ]

VII. What I Learned and Where I Go From Here:

Briefly interpret the results of your cardiorespiratory endurance test(s). Indicate the cardiorespiratory fitness classification you would like to achieve by the end of the term and explain how you are planning to achieve this goal.

_____

_____

_____

_____

_____

_____

Lab 6B

RESTING HEART RATE AND BLOOD PRESSURE ASSESSMENT

Name: _____   Date: _____   Grade: _____

Instructor: _____   Course: _____   Section: _____

Necessary Lab Equipment
Stopwatches, stethoscopes, and blood pressure sphygmomanometers.

Objective
To determine resting heart rate and blood pressure.

Preparation
The instructions to determine heart rate and blood pressure are given on pages 155–157. Many factors can affect heart rate and blood pressure. Factors such as excitement, nervousness, stress, food, smoking, pain, temperature, and physical exertion all can alter heart rate and blood pressure significantly. Therefore, whenever possible, readings should be taken in a quiet, comfortable room following a few minutes of rest in the recording position. Avoid any form of exercise several hours prior to the assessment. Wear exercise clothing, including a shirt with short or loose-fitting sleeves to allow for placement of the blood pressure cuff around the upper arm.

I. Resting Heart Rate and Blood Pressure

Determine your resting heart rate and blood pressure in the right and left arms while sitting comfortably in a chair.

Resting Heart Rate: _____ bpm   Rating (see Table 6.9, page 156): _____

Blood Pressure:	Right Arm	Risk Level (from Table 6.10, page 156)	Left Arm	Risk Level (from Table 6.10, page 156)
Systolic				
Diastolic				

II. Standing, Walking, Jogging Heart Rate and Blood Pressure

Have one individual measure your heart rate and another individual your blood pressure immediately after standing for one minute, after walking for one minute, and after jogging in place for one minute. For blood pressure assessment use the arm that showed the highest reading in the sitting position (in Part I, above).

Activity	Heart Rate (bpm)	Systolic/Diastolic Blood Pressure (mm Hg)
Standing		/
Walking		/
Jogging		/

III. Effects of Aerobic Activity on Resting Heart Rate

Using your actual resting heart rate (RHR) from Part I of this lab, compute the total number of times your heart beats each day and each year:

A. Beats per day = RHR (bpm) × 60 (min per hour) × 24 (hours per day) = _____ × 60 × 24 = _____ beats per day

B. Beats per year = heart rate in beats per day (use item A) × 365 = _____ × 365 = _____ beats per year

If your RHR dropped 20 bpm through an aerobic exercise program, determine the number of beats that your heart would save each year at that lower RHR:

C. Beats per day = RHR (use your current RHR) − 20 × 60 × 24 = (_____ − 20) × 60 × 24 = _____ beats per day

D. Beats per year = heart rate in beats per day (use item C) × 365 = _____ × 365 = _____ beats per year

E. Number of beats saved per year (B − D) = _____ − _____ = _____ beats saved per year

Assuming that you will reach the average U.S. life expectancy of 80 years for women or 73 for men, determine the additional number of "heart rate life years" available to you if your RHR was 20 bpm lower:

F. Years of life ahead = 80 or 73 − current age = _____ − _____ = _____ years

G. Number of beats saved during the next _____ (use item F) years of life (E × F) = _____ (E) × _____ (F)

= _____ beats saved.

H. Number of heart rate life years based on the lower RHR = _____ (G) ÷ _____ (D) = _____ years

IV. Mean Blood Pressure Computation

During a normal resting contraction/relaxation cycle of the heart, the heart spends more time in the relaxation (diastolic) phase than in the contraction (systolic) phase. Accordingly, mean blood pressure (MBP) cannot be computed by taking an average of the systolic (SBP) and diastolic (DBP) blood pressures. The following equations are, therefore, used to determine MBP:

$MBP = DBP + ⅓ PP$ Where PP = pulse pressure or the difference between the systolic and diastolic pressures.

A. Compute your MBP using your own blood pressure results:

PP = _____ (systolic) − _____ (diastolic) = _____ mm Hg

$MBP = $ _____ $(DBP) + \dfrac{\text{_____ (PP)}}{3} = $ _____ mm Hg

B. Determine the MBP for a person with a BP of 130/80 and a second person with a BP of 120/90.

130/80	120/90

Which subject has the lower MBP? _____

V. What I Learned

Draw conclusions based on your observed resting and activity heart rates and blood pressures. Discuss the importance of a lower resting heart rate to your health and comment on the effects of a higher systolic versus diastolic blood pressure on the mean arterial blood pressure.

_____

_____

_____

_____

_____

_____

Principles of Cardiorespiratory Exercise Prescription

*No drug in current or prospective use
holds as much promise for sustained health
as a lifetime program of physical exercise.*[1]

Objectives

- Determine readiness to start an exercise program.

- Learn the principles that govern cardiorespiratory exercise prescription: intensity, mode, duration, and frequency.

- Identify some popular cardiorespiratory activities and their specific benefits.

- Learn concepts for preventing and treating injuries.

- Learn some ways to foster adherence to exercise.

- Describe the relationship between fitness and aging.

- Learn to predict oxygen uptake and caloric expenditure from exercise heart rate.

Cardiorespiratory endurance is the single most important component of health-related physical fitness. The exception occurs among older adults, for whom muscular strength is particularly important. A person does need a certain amount of muscular strength and flexibility to engage in normal daily activities. Nevertheless, one can get by without a lot of strength and flexibility, but cannot do without a good cardiorespiratory system.

Aerobic exercise is especially important in preventing coronary heart disease. A poorly conditioned heart, which has to pump more often just to keep a person alive, is subject to more wear and tear than a well-conditioned heart. In situations that place strenuous demands on the heart, such as doing yard work, lifting heavy objects or weights, or running to catch a bus, the unconditioned heart may not be able to sustain the strain. Regular participation in cardiorespiratory endurance activities also helps a person achieve and maintain recommended body weight, the fourth component of health-related physical fitness (shown in Figure 1.9, page 11).

> *Cardiorespiratory endurance is the most important component of health-related physical fitness.*

Readiness for Exercise

Before proceeding with the principles of exercise prescription, you should ask yourself if you are willing to give exercise a try. A low percentage of the U.S. population is truly committed to exercise. Further, surveys indicate that more than half of the people who start exercising drop out during the first 3 to 6 months of the program.[2] Sports psychologists are trying to find out why some people exercise habitually and many do not. All of the benefits of exercise cannot help unless people commit to a lifetime program of physical activity.

The first step is to answer the question: Am I ready to start an exercise program? The information provided in Lab 7A can help you answer this question. You are evaluated in four categories: mastery (self-control), attitude, health, and commitment. The higher you score in any category—mastery, for example—the more important that reason is for you to exercise.

Scores can vary from 4 to 16. A score of 12 and above is a strong indicator that that factor is important to you, whereas 8 and below is low. If you score 12 or more points in each category, your chances of initiating and sticking to an exercise program are good. If you do not score at least 12 points each in any three categories, your chances of succeeding at exercise may be slim. You need to be better

informed about the benefits of exercise, and a retraining process may be helpful. More tips on how you can become committed to exercise are provided in the section "Getting Started and Adhering to a Lifetime Exercise Program" (page 184).

Next, you will have to decide positively that you will try. Also using Lab 7A, you can list the advantages and disadvantages of incorporating exercise into your lifestyle. Your list may include things such as the following:

- It will make me feel better.
- I will lose weight.
- I will have more energy.
- It will lower my risk for chronic diseases.

Your list of disadvantages might include the following:

- I don't want to take the time.
- I'm too out of shape.
- There's no good place to exercise.
- I don't have the willpower to do it.

When the reasons for exercise outweigh the reasons for not exercising, it will become easier to try. In Lab 7A you will also determine your stage of change for aerobic exercise. Using the information learned in Chapter 2, you can outline specific processes and techniques for change.

> *If you are not exercising regularly, are you willing to stop contemplating and give exercise a try?*

Guidelines for Cardiorespiratory Exercise Prescription

All too often, individuals who exercise regularly and then take a cardiorespiratory endurance test are surprised to find that their maximal oxygen uptake is not as good as they think it is. Although these individuals may be exercising regularly, they most likely are not following the basic principles of cardiorespiratory exercise prescription. Therefore, they do not reap significant improvements in cardiorespiratory endurance. Only about 15 percent of adults in the United States exercise at the intensity and frequency required to meet minimum recommendations of the American College of Sports Medicine (ACSM) for the improvement and maintenance of cardiorespiratory fitness.[3]

To develop the cardiorespiratory system, the heart muscle has to be overloaded—like any other muscle in the human body. Just as the biceps muscle in the upper arm is developed through

strength-training exercises, the heart muscle has to be exercised to increase in size, strength, and efficiency. To better understand how the cardiorespiratory system can be developed, we have to be familiar with four variables of exercise: intensity, mode, duration, and frequency.[4]

First, however, you should be aware that the ACSM recommends that a medical exam and a diagnostic exercise stress test be administered prior to **vigorous exercise** by apparently healthy men over age 40 and women over age 50.[5] ACSM has defined vigorous exercise as an exercise **intensity** above 60 percent of maximal capacity. For people initiating an exercise program, this intensity is the equivalent of exercise that provides a "substantial challenge" to the participant or one that cannot be maintained for 20 continuous minutes.

Intensity of Exercise

When trying to develop the cardiorespiratory system, many people often ignore intensity of exercise. For muscles to develop, they have to be overloaded to a given point. The training stimulus to develop the biceps muscle, for example, can be accomplished with arm curl-up exercises with increasing weights. Likewise, the cardiorespiratory system is stimulated by making the heart pump faster for a specified period.

Cardiorespiratory development occurs when the heart is working between 40 and 85 percent of heart rate reserve (see the section below on calculating intensity).[6] Individuals who are not fit should use a 40 to 50 percent training intensity. Active and fit people can train at higher intensities. Increases in maximal oxygen uptake (VO_{2max}) are accelerated when the heart is working closer to 85 percent of **heart rate reserve (HRR)**. For this reason, many experts prescribe exercise between 60 and 85 percent. Intensity of exercise can be calculated easily, and training can be monitored by checking your pulse.

To determine the intensity of exercise or cardiorespiratory training zone according to heart rate reserve, follow these steps:

1. Estimate your **maximal heart rate (MHR)** according to the following formula:

   MHR = 220 minus age (220 − age)

2. Check your **resting heart rate (RHR)** some time after you have been sitting quietly for 15 to 20 minutes. You may take your pulse for 30 seconds and multiply by 2, or take it for a full minute. As explained in Chapter 6, you can check your pulse on the wrist, by placing two or three fingers over the radial artery or in the neck, using the carotid artery.

3. Determine the heart rate reserve (HRR) by subtracting the resting heart rate from the maximal heart rate (HRR = MHR − RHR).

4. Calculate the training intensities (TI) at 40, 50, 60, and 85 percent. Multiply the heart rate reserve by the respective .40, .50, .60, and .85, and then add the resting heart rate to all four of these figures (for example, 85% TI = HRR × (.85 + RHR).

Example. The 40, 50, 60, and 85 percent training intensities for a 20-year-old with a resting heart rate of 68 beats per minute (bpm) would be as follows:

MHR: 220 – 20 = 200 bpm

RHR: = 68 bpm

HRR: 200 – 68 = 132 beats

40% TI = (132 × .40) + 68 = 121 bpm

50% TI = (132 × .50) + 68 = 134 bpm

60% TI = (132 × .60) + 68 = 147 bpm

85% TI = (132 × .85) + 68 = 180 bpm

Low-intensity cardiorespiratory training zone: 121 to 134 bpm

Moderate-intensity cardiorespiratory training zone: 134 to 147 bpm

Optimal cardiorespiratory training zone: 147 to 180 bpm

When you exercise to improve the cardiorespiratory system, maintain your heart rate between the 60 and 85 percent training intensities to obtain adequate development (see Figure 7.1). If you have been physically inactive, you should train around the 40 to 60 percent intensity during the first 6 to 8 weeks of the exercise program. After that, you should exercise between 60 and 85 percent training intensity.

Following a few weeks of training, you may have a considerably lower resting heart rate (10 to 20 beats fewer in 8 to 12 weeks). Therefore, you should recompute your target zone periodically. You can compute your own cardiorespiratory training zone

Vigorous exercise Cardiorespiratory exercise that requires an intensity level above 60 percent of maximal capacity.

Intensity In cardiorespiratory exercise, how hard a person has to exercise to improve or maintain fitness.

Heart rate reserve (HRR) The difference between the maximal heart rate and the resting heart rate.

Maximal heart rate (MHR) Highest heart rate for a person, related primarily to age.

Resting heart rate (RHR) Heart rate after a person has been sitting quietly for 15–20 minutes.

Figure
7.1

Recommended cardiorespiratory or aerobic training pattern.

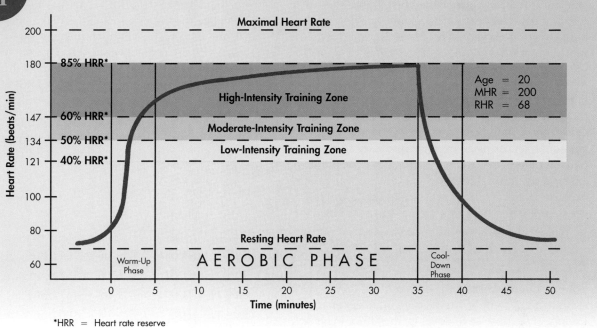

*HRR = Heart rate reserve

by using Lab 7B. You can also use the computer software available with this book and obtain a printout of your personalized cardiorespiratory exercise prescription (see Figure 7.2). You can also create and regularly update a computer file to keep a record of your activity program (see Figure 7.3). This file is based on the EXLOG computer program. Once you have reached an ideal level of cardiorespiratory endurance, continued training in the 60 to 85 percent range will allow you to maintain your fitness level.

During the first few weeks of an exercise program, you should monitor your exercise heart rate regularly to make sure you are training in the proper zone. Wait until you are about 5 minutes into your exercise session (aerobic phase) before taking your first reading. When you check your heart rate, count your pulse for 10 seconds and then multiply by 6 to get the per-minute pulse rate. The exercise heart rate will remain at the same level for about 15 seconds following exercise (aerobic phase). After 15 seconds, your heart rate will drop rapidly. Do not hesitate to stop during your exercise bout to check your pulse. If the rate is too low, increase the intensity of exercise. If the rate is too high, slow down.

To develop the cardiorespiratory system, you do not have to exercise above the 85 percent rate. From a fitness standpoint, training above this percentage

will not give extra benefits and actually may be unsafe for some individuals. Unconditioned people and older adults should train around the 50 percent rate to discourage potential problems associated with high-intensity exercise.

When determining the training intensity for your own program, you need to consider your personal fitness goals. Individuals who exercise at around the 50 percent training intensity will reap significant health benefits—in particular, improvements in the metabolic profile (see "Health Fitness Standards" in Chapter 1, page 12). Training at this lower percentage, however, may place you in only the "average" or "moderately fit" category (see Table 6.8 in Chapter 6). Exercising at this lower intensity does lower the risk for cardiovascular mortality (the health fitness standard), but will not allow you to achieve a "good" or "excellent" cardiorespiratory fitness rating (the physical fitness standard). The latter ratings are obtained by exercising closer to the 85 percent threshold.

Maintain your heart rate between the 50 and 85 percent training intensities to obtain adequate cardiorespiratory development.

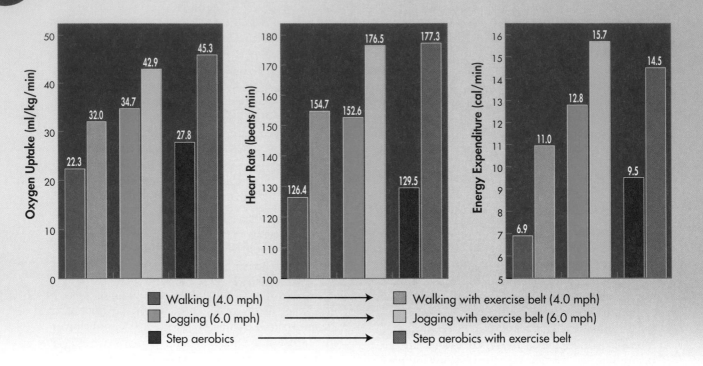

Figure 7.5 Oxygen uptake, heart rate, and energy expenditure response to walking, jogging, and step aerobics with and without an exercise belt with elastic cords (Aero-belt).

Legend:
- Walking (4.0 mph) → Walking with exercise belt (4.0 mph)
- Jogging (6.0 mph) → Jogging with exercise belt (6.0 mph)
- Step aerobics → Step aerobics with exercise belt

People who already exercise at high intensities need to realize that adding upper body activity may require them to decrease the rate of lower body work. For example, a runner who already trains at 85 percent intensity may have to decrease the pace when running with an exercise belt, because few people are able to sustain aerobic exercise for a prolonged time at an intensity above 85 percent.

Combined upper/lower body exercise is particularly useful for people who have functional limitations or injuries that keep them from doing a high-impact activity such as jogging. By adding upper body resistance, they can achieve high training intensities during a low-impact activity such as walking and low-impact aerobics. A word of caution: Combined upper/lower body activity may cause a slight increase in blood pressure during exercise. Although this increase in blood pressure usually does not pose a problem in people with normal blood pressure, individuals with elevated pressure should seek the advice of a physician before they participate in combined upper/lower body exercise.

Duration of Exercise

The general recommendation is that a person train between 20 and 60 minutes per session. The duration is based on how intensely a person trains.

If the training is done at around 85 percent, 20 minutes are sufficient. At 50 percent intensity, the person should train between 30 and 60 minutes. As mentioned under "Intensity of Exercise" above, unconditioned people and older adults should train at lower percentages; therefore, the activity should be carried out over a longer time.

Although most experts recommend 20 to 30 minutes of aerobic exercise per session, accumulating 30 minutes or more of moderate-intensity physical activity throughout the day can provide substantial health benefits.[8] Three 10-minute exercise sessions per day (separated by at least 4 hours), at approximately 70 percent of maximal heart rate, also produce training benefits.[9] Although the increases in maximal oxygen uptake with the latter program were not as large (57 percent) as those found in a group performing a continuous 30-minute bout of exercise per day, the researchers concluded that moderate-intensity exercise training, conducted for 10 minutes, three times per day, benefits the cardiorespiratory system significantly.

Results of this study are meaningful because people often mention lack of time as the reason for not taking part in an exercise program. Many think they have to exercise at least 20 continuous minutes

Mode Form of exercise.

to get any benefits at all. Even though 20 to 30 minutes are ideal, short, intermittent exercise bouts also are beneficial to the cardiorespiratory system.

Exercise sessions should always be preceded by a 5-minute **warm-up** and followed by a 5-minute **cool-down** period (see Figure 7.1). The warm-up should consist of general calisthenics, stretching exercises, or exercising at a lower intensity level than the actual target zone. In the cool-down, the intensity of exercise is decreased gradually. Stopping abruptly causes blood to pool in the exercised body parts, diminishing the return of blood to the heart. Less blood return can cause dizziness and faintness or even bring on cardiac abnormalities.

Frequency of Exercise

When you start an exercise program, a **frequency** of three to five 20- to 30-minute training sessions per week is recommended to improve maximal oxygen uptake. When training is conducted more than 5 days a week, further improvements are minimal.

For individuals on a weight-loss program, 45- to 60-minute exercise sessions of low to moderate intensity, conducted 5 to 6 days per week, are recommended. Longer exercise sessions increase caloric expenditure for faster weight reduction (see "Exercise: The Key to Weight Loss and Weight Maintenance," page 122). Three 20- to 30-minute training sessions per week, on nonconsecutive days, will maintain cardiorespiratory fitness as long as the heart rate is in the appropriate target zone. A summary of the cardiorespiratory exercise prescription guidelines according to the American College of Sports Medicine is provided in Figure 7.6.

Although three exercise sessions per week will maintain cardiorespiratory fitness, the importance of regular physical activity in preventing disease and enhancing quality of life was pointed out clearly in

1993 at a news briefing held at the National Press Club in Washington, DC. At this briefing, the American College of Sports Medicine and the U.S. Centers for Disease Control and Prevention, in conjunction with the President's Council on Physical Fitness and Sports, set forth recommendations on the types of physical activity needed to maintain and promote health.[10] This summary statement advocates at least 30 minutes of moderate-intensity physical activity almost daily. This routine has been promoted as an effective way to improve health.

These recommendations were subsequently upheld by the U.S. Surgeon General in its 1996 Report on Physical Activity and Health[11] and later in the 2000 Dietary Guidelines for Americans.[12] The Surgeon General's report states that people can improve their health and quality of life substantially by including moderate amounts of physical activity on most, preferably all, days of the week. Further, it states that no one, including older adults, is too old to enjoy the benefits of regular physical activity.

If you want to enjoy better health and fitness, physical activity must be pursued on a regular basis. According to Dr. William Haskell of Stanford University: "Most of the health-related benefits of exercise are relatively short-term, so people should think of exercise as medication and take it on a daily basis."[13] Many of the benefits of exercise and activity diminish within 2 weeks of substantially decreased physical activity. These benefits are completely lost within 2 to 8 months of inactivity.[14]

Ideally, a person should engage in physical activity six to seven times per week. Based on the above discussion, to reap both the high-fitness and health-fitness benefits of exercise, a person needs to exercise a minimum of three times per week in the appropriate target zone for high fitness maintenance and three to four additional times per week in moderate-intensity activities. All exercise/activity sessions should last about 30 minutes.

Fitness Benefits of Aerobic Activities

The contributions of different aerobic activities to the health-related components of fitness vary. Although an accurate assessment of the contributions to each fitness component is difficult to establish, a summary of likely benefits of several activities is provided in Table 7.1. Instead of a single rating or number, ranges are given for some of the categories. The benefits derived are based on the person's effort while participating in the activity.

The nature of the activity often dictates the potential aerobic development. For example, jogging is much more strenuous than walking. The effort during exercise also has an impact on the amount of

Figure 7.6 Cardiorespiratory exercise prescription guidelines.

Activity:	Aerobic (examples: walking, jogging, cycling, swimming, aerobics, racquetball, soccer, stair climbing)
Intensity:	40/50%–85% of heart rate reserve
Duration:	20–60 minutes of continuous aerobic activity
Frequency:	3 to 5 days per week

Based on American College of Sports Medicine, "Position Stand: The Recommended Quantity and Quality of Exercise for Developing and Maintaining Cardiorespiratory and Muscular Fitness, and Flexibility in Healthy Adults," *Medical Science Sports Exercise*, 30 (1998): 975–991.

Table 7.1 — Ratings for Selected Aerobic Activities

Activity	Recommended Starting Fitness Level[1]	Injury Risk[2]	Potential Cardiovascular Endurance Development (VO_{2max})[3,5]	Upper Body Strength Development[3]	Lower Body Strength Development[3]	Upper Body Flexibility Development[3]	Lower Body Flexibility Development[3]	Weight Control[3]	MET Level[4,5,6]	Caloric Expenditure (cal/hour)[5,6]
Walking	B	L	1–2	1	2	1	1	3	4–6	300–450
Walking/Water/Chest-Deep	I	L	2–4	2	3	1	1	3	6–10	450–750
Hiking	B	L	2–4	1	3	1	1	3	6–10	450–750
Jogging	I	M	3–5	1	3	1	1	5	6–15	450–1,125
Jogging/Deep Water	A	L	3–5	2	2	1	1	5	8–15	600–1,125
High-Impact Aerobics	A	H	3–4	2	4	3	2	4	6–12	450–900
Low-Impact Aerobics	B	L	2–4	2	3	3	2	3	5–10	375–750
Step Aerobics	I	M	2–4	2	3–4	3	2	3–4	5–12	375–900
Moderate-Impact Aerobics	I	M	2–4	2	3	3	2	3	6–12	450–900
Swimming (front crawl)	B	L	3–5	4	2	3	1	3	6–12	450–900
Water Aerobics	B	L	2–4	3	3	3	2	3	6–12	450–900
Stationary Cycling	B	L	2–4	1	4	1	1	3	6–10	450–750
Road Cycling	I	M	2–5	1	4	1	1	3	6–12	450–900
Cross-Training	I	M	3–5	2–3	3–4	2–3	1–2	3–5	6–15	450–1,125
Rope Skipping	I	H	3–5	2	4	1	2	3–5	8–15	600–1,125
Cross-Country Skiing	B	M	4–5	4	4	2	2	4–5	10–16	750–1,200
Aero-belt Exercise	B	M	4–5	4	4	3	2	4–5	10–16	750–1,200
In-Line Skating	I	M	2–4	2	4	2	2	3	6–10	450–750
Rowing	B	L	3–5	4	2	3	1	4	8–14	600–1,050
Stair Climbing	B	L	3–5	1	4	1	1	4–5	8–15	600–1,125
Racquet Sports	I	M	2–4	3	3	3	2	3	6–10	450–750

[1] B = Beginner, I = Intermediate, A = Advanced

[2] L = Low, M = Moderate, H = High

[3] 1 = Low, 2 = Fair, 3 = Average, 4 = Good, 5 = Excellent

[4] One MET represents the rate of energy expenditure at rest (3.5 ml/kg/min). Each additional MET is a multiple of the resting value. For example, 5 METs represents an energy expenditure equivalent to five times the resting value, or about 17.5 ml/kg/min.

[5] Varies according to the person's effort (intensity) during exercise.

[6] Varies according to body weight.

physiological development. The training benefits of just going through the motions of a low-impact aerobics routine, as compared with accentuating all motions, are of a different magnitude. Accentuating all motions increases training benefits by orders of magnitude.

Table 7.1 indicates a starting fitness level for each aerobic activity. Attempting to participate in high-intensity activities without proper conditioning often leads to injuries and discouragement. Beginners should start with low-intensity activities that carry a minimum risk for injuries.

In some cases, such as high-impact aerobics and rope skipping, the risk for injuries remains high even if the participants are adequately conditioned. These activities should be supplemental only and are not recommended as the sole mode of exercise.

Warm-up Starting a workout slowly.

Cool-down Tapering off an exercise session slowly.

Frequency How often a person engages in an exercise session.

Most exercise-related injuries occur as a result of high-impact activities, not high intensity of exercise.

Physicians who work with cardiac patients frequently use **METs** as an alternative method of prescribing exercise intensity. One MET represents the rate of energy expenditure at rest. The MET range for the various activities is included in Table 7.1. A 10-MET activity requires a tenfold increase in the resting energy requirement, or approximately 35 ml/kg/min. MET levels for a given activity vary according to the effort expended. The harder a person exercises, the higher is the MET level.

The effectiveness of various aerobic activities in weight management also is provided in Table 7.1. As a general rule, the greater the muscle mass involved in exercise, the better are the results. Rhythmic and continuous activities that involve large amounts of muscle mass are most effective in burning calories.

Higher-intensity activities increase caloric expenditure as well. Exercising longer, however, compensates for lower intensities. If carried out long enough (45 to 60 minutes five to six times per week), even walking can be an excellent exercise mode for weight loss. Additional information on a comprehensive weight management program is given in Chapter 5.

Specific Considerations

In addition to the exercise-related issues discussed previously, many concerns require clarification or are somewhat controversial. Let's examine some of these issues.

1. Does aerobic exercise make a person immune to heart and blood vessel disease?

Although aerobically fit individuals as a whole have a lower incidence of cardiovascular disease, a regular aerobic exercise program by itself does not offer an absolute guarantee against cardiovascular disease. Overall management of the risk factors is the best way to minimize the risk for cardiovascular disease. Many factors, including a genetic predisposition, can increase the person's risk. In any case, experts believe that a regular aerobic exercise program not only will delay the onset of cardiovascular problems but also will improve the chances of surviving a heart attack.

Even moderate increases in aerobic fitness significantly lower the incidence of premature cardiovascular deaths. Data from the research study illustrated in Chapter 1, Figure 1.7, indicate that the decrease in cardiovascular mortality is greatest between the unfit (group 1) and the moderately fit (2 and 3) groups. A further decrease in cardiovascular mortality is observed between the moderately fit and the highly fit groups (4 and 5),

although the difference is not as much as that between the unfit and moderately fit groups.

2. How much aerobic exercise is required to decrease the risk for cardiovascular disease?

Even though research has not yet indicated the exact amount of aerobic exercise required to lower the risk for cardiovascular disease, some general recommendations have been set forth. In their study, Dr. Ralph Paffenbarger and his co-researchers showed that expending 2,000 calories per week as a result of physical activity yielded the lowest risk for cardiovascular disease among a group of almost 17,000 Harvard alumni.[15] Two thousand calories per week represents about 300 calories per daily exercise session.

3. Do people get a "physical high" during aerobic exercise?

During vigorous exercise, **endorphins** are released from the pituitary gland in the brain. They can create feelings of euphoria and natural well-being. Higher levels of endorphins often are seen as a result of aerobic endurance activities and may remain elevated for as long as 30 to 60 minutes following exercise. Many experts believe these higher levels explain the physical high some people get during and after prolonged exercise.

Endorphin levels have also been shown to increase during pregnancy and childbirth. Endorphins act as pain killers. The higher levels could explain a woman's greater tolerance for the pain and discomfort of natural childbirth and her pleasant feelings shortly after the baby's birth. Several reports have indicated that well-conditioned women have shorter and easier labor. These women may attain higher endorphin levels during delivery, making childbirth less traumatic than it is for untrained women.

4. Can people with asthma exercise?

Asthma, a condition that causes difficulty breathing, is characterized by coughing, wheezing, and shortness of breath induced by narrowing of the airway passages because of contraction (bronchospasm) of the airway muscles, swelling of the mucous membrane, and excessive secretion of mucus. In a few people, asthma can be triggered by exercise itself, in particular exercise in cool and dry environments. This type of condition is referred to as exercise-induced asthma (EIA).

People with asthma need to obtain proper medication from a physician prior to initiating an exercise program. A regular program is best, because random exercise bouts are more likely to trigger asthma attacks. In the initial stages of exercise, an intermittent program (frequent rest periods during the exercise session) is recommended. Gradual

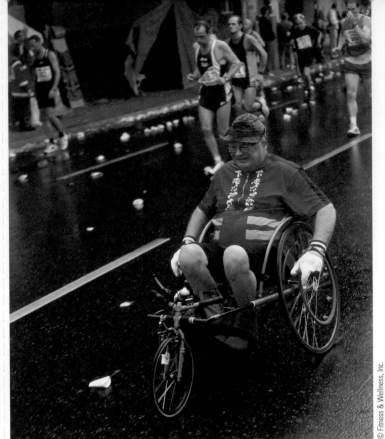

Physically challenged people can participate and derive health and fitness benefits through a high-intensity exercise program.

warm-up and cool-down are also essential to reduce the risk of an acute attack. Furthermore, exercise in warm and humid conditions (swimming) is better because it helps to moisten the airways and minimizes the asthmatic response. For land-based activities (walking, aerobics), drinking water before, during, and after exercise helps to keep the airways moist, thus decreasing the risk of an attack. During the winter months, wearing an exercise mask is recommended to increase warmth and humidity of inhaled air. People with asthma should not exercise alone and should always carry their medication with them during workouts.

5. What types of activities are recommended for people with arthritis?

Individuals who suffer from arthritis should participate in a combined stretching, aerobic, and strength-training program. Mild stretching should be performed prior to aerobic exercise to relax tight muscles. A regular flexibility program following aerobic exercise is encouraged to help maintain good joint mobility. For the aerobic portion of the exercise program, avoid high-impact activities, because they may cause greater trauma to arthritic joints. Low-impact activities like swimming, water aerobics, or cycling are recommended. A complete

strength-training program is recommended, with special emphasis on exercises that will help support the affected joint(s). As with any other program, start with low intensity or resistance and build up gradually to a higher fitness level.

6. What precautions should diabetics take with respect to exercise?

According to the Centers for Disease Control and Prevention, there are 10.3 million reported diabetics in the U.S. and an additional 5.4 million undiagnosed cases. There are two types of diabetes: Type I, or insulin-dependent diabetes (IDDM), and Type II, or non-insulin–dependent diabetes (NIDDM). In Type I, found primarily in young people, the pancreas produces little or no insulin. With Type II, the pancreas may not produce enough insulin or the cells become insulin-resistant, thereby keeping glucose from entering the cell. Type II accounts for over 90 percent of all diabetes cases, and it occurs mainly in adults over 40 who are also overweight. (A more thorough discussion of the types of diabetes is given in Chapter 12.)

If you are a diabetic, consult your physician before you start exercising. You may not be able to start until your diabetes is under control. Never exercise alone and always wear a bracelet that identifies your condition. If you take insulin, the amount and timing of each dose may need to be regulated with your physician. If you inject insulin, inject it over a muscle that won't be exercised and then wait one hour before exercising. For Type I diabetics, it is recommended that you ingest 15 to 30 grams of carbohydrate during each 30 minutes of intense exercise and follow it with a carbohydrate snack after exercise.

Both types of diabetes improve with exercise, although the results are more notable in patients with Type II diabetes. Exercise usually lowers blood sugar and helps the body use food more effectively. The degree to which blood glucose level can be controlled in overweight Type II diabetics appears to be directly related to how long and how hard a person exercises. Normal or near-normal blood glucose levels can be achieved through a proper exercise program.

As with any fitness program, the exercise must be done on a regular basis to be effective against

MET Represents the rate of resting energy expenditure at rest; MET is the equivalent of 3.5 ml/kg/min.

Endorphins Morphine-like substances released from the pituitary gland in the brain during prolonged aerobic exercise; thought to induce feelings of euphoria and natural well-being.

diabetes. The benefits of a single exercise bout on blood glucose are highest between 12 and 24 hours following exercise. These benefits are completely lost within 72 hours after exercise. Thus, regular participation is crucial to derive ongoing benefits. In terms of fitness, all diabetic patients can achieve higher fitness levels, including reductions in weight, blood pressure, and total cholesterol and triglycerides.

According to the ACSM, the following guidelines should be followed by diabetic patients to make their exercise program safe and derive the best benefits:[16]

- Burn a minimum of 1,000 calories per week through your exercise program.
- Exercise at a low to moderate intensity (40 to 70 percent of HRR). Start your program with 10 to 15 minutes per session, on at least three non-consecutive days, but preferably exercise five days per week. Gradually increase the time you exercise to 30 minutes until you achieve your goal of at least 1,000 weekly calories. Diabetic individuals with a weight problem should build up daily physical activity to 60 minutes per session.
- Choose an activity that you enjoy doing and stay with it. As you select your activity, be aware of your condition. For example, if you have lost sensation in your feet, swimming or stationary cycling is better than walking or jogging to minimize injury risk.
- Check blood glucose levels before and after exercise. If you are on insulin or diabetes medication, monitor blood glucose regularly and check it at least twice within 30 minutes of starting exercise.
- Schedule your exercise 1 to 3 hours after a meal and avoid exercise when your insulin is peaking.
- Be ready to treat low blood sugar with a fast-acting source of sugar, such as juice or raisins.
- Discontinue exercise immediately if you feel that a reaction is about to occur. Check your blood glucose level and treat the condition as needed.
- When you exercise outdoors, always do so with someone who knows what to do in a diabetes-related emergency.
- Strength training twice per week, using 8 to 10 exercises with a minimum of one set of 10 to 15 repetitions to near-fatigue is also recommended for individuals with diabetes. A complete description of strength-training programs is provided in Chapter 8.

7. Is exercise safe during pregnancy?

Women should not abandon exercise during pregnancy. If anything, they should exercise to strengthen the body and prepare for delivery. Moderate exercise during pregnancy helps to prevent excessive weight gain and speed up recovery following birth.

Pregnant women in Native American tribes used to do all of their difficult work chores up to the very day of delivery. A few hours after the baby's birth, they resumed many of their normal activities. Several women athletes have competed in sports during the early stages of pregnancy. Nevertheless, the woman and her personal physician should make the final decision regarding her exercise program.

Stretching exercises are to be performed gently because hormonal changes during pregnancy increase the laxity of muscles and connective tissue. Although these changes facilitate delivery, they also make women more susceptible to injuries during exercise.

In 1994 the American College of Obstetricians and Gynecologists set forth Guidelines for Exercise During Pregnancy. Among the recommendations for pregnant women with no additional risk factors are the following:

- Continue to exercise at a mild-to-moderate pace throughout the pregnancy, but decrease the exercise intensity by about 25 percent from the pre-pregnancy program.
- Exercise regularly a minimum of three times a week instead of doing occasional exercise.
- Pay attention to the body's signals of discomfort and distress. Stop exercising when tired. Never exercise to exhaustion. Stop if unusual symptoms arise, such as pain of any kind, cramping, nausea, bleeding, leaking of amniotic fluid, faintness, dizziness, palpitations, numbness in any part of the body, or less fetal activity.
- After the first trimester, avoid exercises that require lying on the back. This position can block blood flow to the uterus and the baby.
- Do non–weight-bearing activities such as cycling, swimming, or water aerobics, which minimize the risk of injury and may allow continuation of exercise throughout pregnancy.
- Avoid activities that could precipitate a loss of balance or cause even mild trauma to the abdomen.
- Get proper nourishment (pregnancy requires approximately 300 extra calories per day).
- During the first 3 months in particular, avoid exercising in the heat. Wear clothing that allows for proper dissipation of heat and drink plenty of water.

8. Does exercise help relieve dysmenorrhea?

Although exercise has not been shown to either cure or aggravate **dysmenorrhea**, it has been shown to relieve menstrual cramps because it improves circulation to the uterus. Less severe menstrual cramps also could be related to higher levels of endorphins produced during prolonged physical activity, which may counteract pain. Particularly, stretching exercises of the muscles in the pelvic

region seem to reduce and prevent painful menstruation that is not the result of disease.[17]

9. Does participation in exercise hinder menstruation?

In some instances, highly trained athletes develop **amenorrhea** during training and competition. This condition is seen most often in extremely lean women who also engage in sports that require strenuous physical effort over a sustained time. It is by no means irreversible. At present, we do not know whether the condition is caused by physical or emotional stress related to high-intensity training, excessively low body fat, or other factors.

Although, on the average, women have a lower physical capacity during menstruation, medical surveys at the Olympic games have shown that women have broken Olympic and world records at all stages of the menstrual cycle. Menstruation should not keep a woman from participating in athletics, and it will not necessarily have a negative impact on performance.

10. Does exercise offset the detrimental effects of cigarette smoking?

Physical exercise often motivates smoking cessation, but it does not offset any ill effects of smoking. If anything, smoking greatly decreases the ability of the blood to transport oxygen to working muscles.

Oxygen is carried in the circulatory system by hemoglobin, the iron-containing pigment of the red blood cells. Carbon monoxide, a byproduct of cigarette smoke, has 210 to 250 times greater affinity for hemoglobin over oxygen. Consequently, carbon monoxide combines much faster with hemoglobin, decreasing the oxygen-carrying capacity of the blood.

Chronic smoking also increases airway resistance, requiring the respiratory muscles to work much harder and consume more oxygen just to ventilate a given amount of air. If a person quits smoking, exercise does help increase the functional capacity of the pulmonary system.

A regular exercise program seems to be a powerful incentive to quit smoking. A random survey of 1,250 runners conducted at the 6.2-mile Peachtree Road Race in Atlanta provided impressive results. The survey indicated that 81 percent and 75 percent of the men and women, respectively, who smoked cigarettes when they started running had quit before the race date.

11. What type of clothing should I wear when I exercise?

The type of clothing you wear during exercise is important. In general, clothing should fit comfortably and allow free movement of the various body parts. Select clothing according to air temperature,

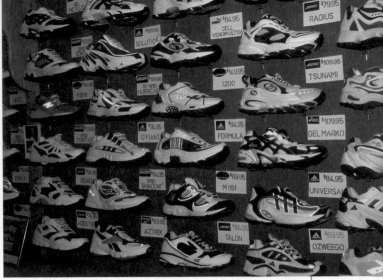
© Fitness & Wellness, Inc.

Activity-specific shoes are recommended to prevent lower-extremity injuries.

humidity, and exercise intensity. Avoid nylon and rubberized materials and tight clothes that interfere with the cooling mechanism of the human body or obstruct normal blood flow. Choose fabrics made from polypropylene, Capilene, or Thermax, or any synthetics that draw moisture away from the skin, enhancing evaporation and cooling of the body. It's also important to consider your exercise intensity, because the harder you exercise, the more heat your body produces.

When exercising in the heat, avoid the hottest time of the day—between 11:00 A.M. and 5:00 P.M. Surfaces such as asphalt, concrete, and artificial turf absorb heat, which then radiates to the body. Therefore, these surfaces are not recommended. (Also see the discussion about heat and humidity, below.)

Only a minimal amount of clothing is necessary during exercise in the heat, to allow for maximal evaporation. Clothing should be lightweight, light-colored, loose-fitting, airy, and absorbent. Examples of commercially available products that can be used during exercise in the heat are Asci's Perma Plus, Cool-max, and Nike's Dri-F.I.T. Double-layer acrylic socks are more absorbent than cotton and help to prevent blistering and chafing of the feet. A straw-type hat can be worn to protect the eyes and head from the sun. (Clothing for exercise in the cold is discussed below.)

A good pair of shoes is vital to prevent injuries to lower limbs. Shoes manufactured specifically for your choice of activity are a must (see Figure 7.7). When selecting proper footwear, you should

Dysmenorrhea Painful menstruation.

Amenorrhea Cessation of regular menstrual flow.

Figure
7.7

What to look for in a good pair of shoes.

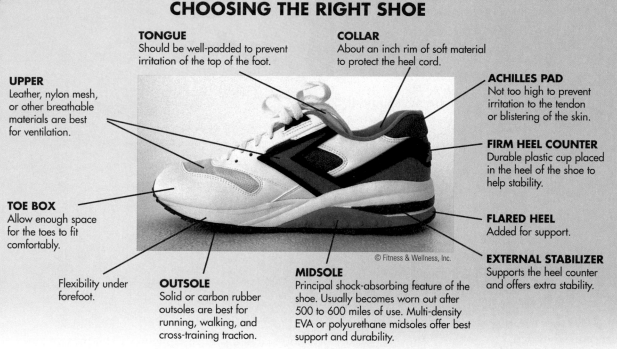

CHOOSING THE RIGHT SHOE

TONGUE
Should be well-padded to prevent irritation of the top of the foot.

COLLAR
About an inch rim of soft material to protect the heel cord.

UPPER
Leather, nylon mesh, or other breathable materials are best for ventilation.

ACHILLES PAD
Not too high to prevent irritation to the tendon or blistering of the skin.

FIRM HEEL COUNTER
Durable plastic cup placed in the heel of the shoe to help stability.

TOE BOX
Allow enough space for the toes to fit comfortably.

FLARED HEEL
Added for support.

Flexibility under forefoot.

OUTSOLE
Solid or carbon rubber outsoles are best for running, walking, and cross-training traction.

MIDSOLE
Principal shock-absorbing feature of the shoe. Usually becomes worn out after 500 to 600 miles of use. Multi-density EVA or polyurethane midsoles offer best support and durability.

EXTERNAL STABILIZER
Supports the heel counter and offers extra stability.

© Fitness & Wellness, Inc.

---

consider body type, tendency toward pronation (rotating foot outward) or supination (rotating foot inward), and exercise surfaces. Shoes should have good stability, motion control, and comfortable fit. Purchase shoes in the middle of the day when the feet have expanded and might be one-half size larger. For increased breathability, choose shoes with nylon or mesh uppers. Generally, salespeople at reputable athletic shoe stores are knowledgeable and can help you select a good shoe that fits your needs. After 300 to 500 miles or 6 months, examine your shoes and obtain a new pair if they are worn out. Old shoes frequently are responsible for lower-limb injuries.

12. How long should a person wait after a meal before exercising strenuously?

The length of time to wait before exercising after a meal depends on the amount of food eaten. On the average, after a regular meal, you should wait about 2 hours before participating in strenuous physical activity. A walk or some other light physical activity is fine following a meal, though. If anything, it helps burn extra calories and may help the body metabolize fats more efficiently.

13. What time of the day is best for exercise?

You can do intense exercise almost any time of the day, with the exception of about 2 hours following a heavy meal, or the noon and early afternoon hours

on hot, humid days. Moderate exercise seems to be beneficial shortly after a meal, because exercise enhances the **thermogenic response**. A walk shortly after a meal burns more calories than a walk several hours after a meal.

Many people enjoy exercising early in the morning because it gives them a boost to start the day. People who exercise in the morning also seem to stick with it more than others. Some prefer the lunch hour for weight-control reasons. By exercising at noon, they do not eat as big a lunch, which helps keep down the daily caloric intake. Highly stressed people seem to like the evening hours because of the relaxing effects of exercise.

14. Why is exercising in hot and humid conditions unsafe?

When a person exercises, only 30 to 40 percent of the energy the body produces is used for mechanical work or movement. The rest of the energy (60 to 70 percent) is converted into heat. If this heat cannot be dissipated properly because either the weather is too hot or the relative humidity is too high, body temperature increases and, in extreme cases, can result in death.

The specific heat of body tissue (the heat required to raise the temperature of the body by 1 degree C) is .38 calories per pound of body weight (.38 cal/lb). This indicates that if no body heat is

dissipated, a 150-pound person has to burn only 57 calories (150 × .38) to increase total body temperature by 1 degree C. If this person were to conduct an exercise session requiring 300 calories (e.g., running about 3 miles) without any heat dissipation, the inner body temperature would increase by 5.3 degrees C, which is the equivalent of going from 98.6 degrees F to 108.1 degrees F.

This example illustrates clearly the need for caution when exercising in hot or humid weather. If the relative humidity is too high, body heat cannot be lost through evaporation because the atmosphere already is saturated with water vapor. In one instance, a football casualty occurred when the temperature was only 64 degrees F—but the relative humidity was 100 percent. People must be cautious when air temperature is above 90 degrees F and the relative humidity is above 60 percent.

The American College of Sports Medicine recommends avoiding strenuous physical activity when the readings of a wet-bulb globe thermometer exceed 82.4 degrees F. With this type of thermometer, the wet bulb is cooled by evaporation, and on dry days it shows a lower temperature than the regular (dry) thermometer. On humid days, the cooling effect is less because of less evaporation; hence, the difference between the wet and dry readings is not as great.

Following are descriptions of and first-aid measures for the three major signs of trouble when exercising in the heat:

■ **Heat cramps**. Symptoms include cramps, spasms, and muscle twitching in the legs, arms, and abdomen. To relieve heat cramps, stop exercising, get out of the heat, massage the painful area, stretch slowly, and drink plenty of fluids (water, fruit drinks, or electrolyte beverages).
■ **Heat exhaustion**. Symptoms include fainting; dizziness; profuse sweating; cold, clammy skin; weakness; headache; and a rapid, weak pulse. If you incur any of these symptoms, stop and find a cool place to rest. If conscious, drink cool water. Do not give water to an unconscious person. Loosen or remove clothing, and rub your body with a cool/wet towel or ice packs. Place yourself in a supine position with the legs elevated 8 to 12 inches. If you are not fully recovered in 30 minutes, seek immediate medical attention.
■ **Heat stroke**. Symptoms include serious disorientation; warm, dry skin; no sweating; rapid, full pulse; vomiting; diarrhea; unconsciousness; and high body temperature. As the body temperature climbs, unexplained anxiety sets in. When the body temperature reaches 104 to 105 degrees F, the individual may feel a cold sensation in the

trunk of the body, goose bumps, nausea, throbbing in the temples, and numbness in the extremities. Most people become incoherent after this stage. When body temperature reaches 105 to 107 degrees F, disorientation, loss of fine-motor control, and muscular weakness set in. If the temperature exceeds 106 degrees F, serious neurologic injury and death may be imminent.

Heat stroke requires immediate emergency medical attention. Request help and get out of the sun and into a cool, humidity-controlled environment. While you are waiting to be taken to the hospital emergency room, you should be placed in a semi-seated position, and your body should be sprayed with cool water and rubbed with cool towels. If possible, cold packs should be placed in areas with abundant blood supply, such as the head, neck, armpits, and groin. Fluids should not be given if you are unconscious. In any case of heat-related illness, if the person refuses water, vomits, or starts to lose consciousness, call for an ambulance immediately. Proper initial treatment of heat stroke is critical.

15. What should a person do to replace fluids lost during prolonged aerobic exercise?

The main objective of fluid replacement during prolonged aerobic exercise is to maintain the blood volume so circulation and sweating can continue at normal levels. Adequate water replacement is the most important factor in preventing heat disorders. Drinking about 6 to 8 ounces of cool water every 15 to 20 minutes during exercise seems to be ideal to prevent dehydration. Cold fluids seem to be absorbed more rapidly from the stomach.

Other relevant points are the following:

■ Commercial fluid-replacement solutions (such as Exceed® and Gatorade®) contain about 6 to 8 percent glucose,

The main objective of fluid replacement during prolonged aerobic exercise is to maintain the blood volume so circulation and sweating can continue at normal levels.

Thermogenic response Amount of energy required to digest food.

Heat cramps Muscle spasms caused by heat-induced changes in electrolyte balance in muscle cells.

Heat exhaustion Heat-related fatigue.

Heat stroke Emergency situation resulting from the body being subjected to high atmospheric temperatures.

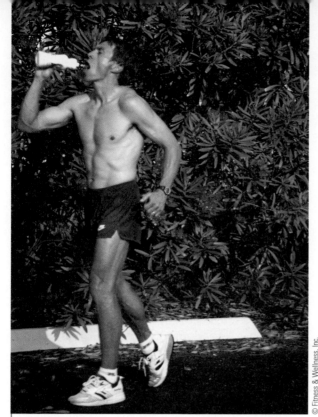

Fluid and carbohydrate replacement are essential when exercising in the heat or for a prolonged period.

which seems to be optimal for fluid absorption and performance. Sugar does not become available to the muscles until about 30 minutes after drinking a glucose solution.

Commercially prepared sports drinks are recommended when exercise will be strenuous and carried out for more than an hour. For exercise lasting less than an hour, water is just as effective in replacing lost fluid. The sports drinks you select should be based on your personal preference. Try different drinks at 6 to 8 percent glucose concentration to see which drink you tolerate best and suits your tastes as well.

■ Drinks high in fructose or with a glucose concentration above 8 percent are not recommended because they slow down water absorption when exercising in the heat.

■ Most soft drinks (cola, non-cola) contain between 10 and 12 percent glucose, an amount that is too high for proper rehydration during exercise in the heat.

16. What precautions must a person take when exercising in the cold?

When exercising in the cold, the two factors to consider are frostbite and **hypothermia**. In contrast to hot and humid conditions, exercising in the cold usually does not threaten health because clothing can be selected for heat conservation, and exercise itself increases the production of body heat.

Most people actually overdress for exercise in the cold. Because exercise increases body temperature, a moderate workout on a cold day makes a person feel that the temperature is 20 degrees to 30 degrees warmer than it actually is. Overdressing for exercise can make the clothes damp from excessive perspiration. The risk for hypothermia increases when a person is wet or not moving around sufficiently to increase body heat.

Initial warning signs of hypothermia include shivering, loss of coordination, and difficulty speaking. With a continued drop in body temperature, shivering stops, the muscles weaken and stiffen, and the person has feelings of elation or intoxication and eventually loses consciousness. To prevent hypothermia, use common sense, dress properly, and be aware of environmental conditions.

The popular belief that exercising in cold temperatures (32 degrees F and lower) freezes the lungs is false, because the air is warmed properly in the air passages before it reaches the lungs. Cold is not what poses a threat. Rather, wind velocity is what affects the chill factor greatly.

For example, exercising at a temperature of 25 degrees F with adequate clothing is not too cold, but if the wind is blowing at 25 miles per hour, the chill factor lowers the actual temperature to 15 degrees F. This effect is even worse if a person is wet and exhausted. When the weather is windy, exercise (jog or cycle) against the wind on the way out and with the wind when you return.

Even though the lungs are under no risk when exercising in the cold, the face, head, hands, and feet should be protected, because they are subject to frostbite. Watch for signs of frostbite—numbness and discoloration. In cold temperatures, as much as half of the body's heat can be lost through an unprotected head and neck. A wool or synthetic cap, hood, or hat will help to hold in body heat. Mittens are better than gloves, because they keep the fingers together so the surface area from which to lose heat is less. Inner linings of synthetic material to wick (draw) moisture away from the skin are recommended. Avoid cotton next to the skin because once cotton gets wet—whether from perspiration, rain, or snow—it loses its insulating properties.

Wearing several layers of lightweight clothing is preferable to wearing one single, thick layer because warm air is trapped between layers of clothes, enabling greater heat conservation. As body temperature increases, you can remove layers as necessary. For lengthy or long-distance workouts (cross-country skiing or long runs), take a small backpack to carry the clothing that is removed. You also can

carry extra warm and dry clothes in case you stop exercising away from shelter. If you remain outdoors following exercise, added clothing and continuous body movement are essential.

The first layer of clothes should wick moisture away from the skin. Polypropylene, Capilene, and Thermax are recommended materials. Next, a layer of wool, dacron, or polyester fleece insulates well even when wet. Lycra tights or sweatpants help protect the legs. The outer layer should be waterproof, wind-resistant, and breathable. A synthetic material such as Gortex is best, so moisture can still escape from the body. A ski mask or face mask helps protect the face. In extremely cold conditions, exposed skin, such as the nose, cheeks, or around the eyes, can be insulated with petroleum jelly.

17. Can I exercise when I have a cold or the flu?
The most important consideration is to use common sense and pay attention to your symptoms. Typically, you may continue to exercise if your symptoms include a runny nose, sneezing, or a scratchy throat. However, if you are running a fever or your muscles ache or if you are vomiting, have diarrhea, or have a hacking cough, you should avoid exercise. Following an illness, be sure to ease back gradually into your program. Do not attempt to return at the same intensity and duration that you were used to prior to your illness.

Exercise-Related Injuries

To enjoy and maintain physical fitness, preventing injury during a conditioning program is essential. Exercise-related injuries, nonetheless, are common in individuals who participate in exercise programs. Surveys indicate that more than half of all new participants incur injuries during the first 6 months of the conditioning program.

The four most common causes of injuries are

1. High-impact activities,
2. Rapid conditioning programs—doing too much too quickly,
3. Improper shoes or training surfaces, and
4. Anatomical predisposition (body propensity).

High-impact activities and a significant increase in quantity, intensity, and duration of activities are by far the most common causes of injuries. The body requires time to adapt to more intense activities. Most of these injuries can be prevented through a more gradual and correct conditioning (low-impact) program.

Proper shoes for specific activities are essential. Shoes should be replaced when they show a lot of wear and tear. Softer training surfaces, such as grass and dirt, produce less trauma than asphalt and concrete.

Because few people have perfect body alignment, injuries associated with overtraining may occur eventually. In case of injury, proper treatment can avert a lengthy recovery process. A summary of common exercise-related injuries and how to manage them follows.

Acute Sports Injuries

The best treatment always has been prevention itself. If an activity causes unusual discomfort or chronic irritation, you need to treat the cause by decreasing the intensity, switching activities, substituting equipment, or upgrading clothing (such as buying proper-fitting shoes).

In cases of acute injury, the standard treatment is rest, cold application, compression or splinting (or both), and elevation of the affected body part. This commonly is referred to as RICE:

R = rest
I = ice application
C = compression
E = elevation

Cold should be applied three to five times a day for 15 to 20 minutes at a time during the first 24 to 36 hours, by submerging the injured area in cold water, using an icebag, or applying ice massage to the affected part. An elastic bandage or wrap can be used for compression. Elevating the body part decreases blood flow (and therefore swelling) in that body part.

The purpose of these treatment modalities is to minimize swelling in the area, which hastens recovery time. After the first 36 to 48 hours, heat can be used if the injury shows no further swelling or inflammation. If you have doubts regarding the nature or seriousness of the injury (such as suspected fracture), you should seek a medical evaluation.

Obvious deformities (such as exhibited by fractures, dislocations, or partial dislocations) call for splinting, cold application with an icebag, and medical attention. Do not try to reset any of these conditions by yourself, because you could further damage muscles, ligaments, and nerves. Treatment of these injuries always should be in the hands of specialized medical personnel. A quick reference guide for the signs or symptoms and treatment of exercise-related problems is provided in Table 7.2.

Hypothermia A breakdown in the body's ability to generate heat; a drop in temperature below 95 degrees F.

Table 7.2 Reference Guide for Exercise-Related Problems

Injury	Signs/Symptoms	Treatment*
Bruise (contusion)	Pain, swelling, discoloration	Cold application, compression, rest
Dislocation / Fracture	Pain, swelling, deformity	Splinting, cold application, seek medical attention
Heat cramp	Cramps, spasms, and muscle twitching in the legs, arms, and abdomen	Stop activity, get out of the heat, stretch, massage the painful area, drink plenty of fluids
Heat exhaustion	Fainting, profuse sweating, cold/clammy skin, weak/rapid pulse, weakness, headache	Stop activity, rest in a cool place, loosen clothing, rub body with cool/wet towel, drink plenty of fluids, stay out of heat for 2–3 days
Heat stroke	Hot/dry skin, no sweating, serious disorientation, rapid/full pulse, vomiting, diarrhea, unconsciousness, high body temperature	**Seek immediate medical attention**, request help and get out of the sun, bathe in cold water/spray with cold water/rub body with cold towels, drink plenty of cold fluids
Joint sprain	Pain, tenderness, swelling, loss of use, discoloration	Cold application, compression, elevation, rest, heat after 36 to 48 hours (if no further swelling)
Muscle cramp	Pain, spasm	Stretch muscle(s), use mild exercises for involved area
Muscle soreness and stiffness	Tenderness, pain	Mild stretching, low-intensity exercise, warm bath
Muscle strain	Pain, tenderness, swelling, loss of use	Cold application, compression, elevation, rest, heat after 36 to 48 hours (if no further swelling)
Shin splints	Pain, tenderness	Cold application prior to and following any physical activity, rest, heat (if no activity is carried out)
Side stitch	Pain on the side of the abdomen below the rib cage	Decrease level of physical activity or stop altogether, gradually increase level of fitness
Tendonitis	Pain, tenderness, loss of use	Rest, cold application, heat after 48 hours

* Cold should be applied three to four times a day for 15 minutes. Heat can be applied three times a day for 15 to 20 minutes.

Muscle Soreness and Stiffness

Individuals who begin an exercise program or participate after a long layoff from exercise often develop muscle soreness and stiffness. The acute soreness that sets in the first few hours after exercise is thought to be related to a lack of blood (oxygen) flow and general fatigue of the exercised muscles.

Delayed muscle soreness that appears several hours after exercise (usually about 12 hours later) and lasts 2 to 4 days may be related to actual tiny tears in muscle tissue, muscle spasms that increase fluid retention (stimulating the pain nerve endings), and overstretching or tearing of connective tissue in and around muscles and joints.

Mild stretching before and adequately stretching after exercise help to prevent soreness and stiffness. Gradually progressing into an exercise program is important, too. A person should not attempt to do too much too quickly. To relieve pain, mild stretching, low-intensity exercise to stimulate blood flow, and a warm bath might help.

Exercise Intolerance

When starting an exercise program, participants should stay within the safe limits. The best method to determine whether you are exercising too strenuously—**exercise intolerance**—is to check your heart rate and make sure it does not exceed the limits of your target zone. Exercising above this target zone may not be safe for unconditioned or high-risk individuals. You do not have to exercise beyond your target zone to gain the desired cardiorespiratory benefits.

Several physical signs will tell you when you are exceeding your functional limitations. Signs of intolerance include rapid or irregular heart rate, difficult breathing, nausea, vomiting, lightheadedness, headache, dizziness, unusually flushed or pale skin, extreme weakness, lack of energy, shakiness, sore muscles, cramps, and tightness in the chest. Learn to listen to your body. If you notice any of these symptoms, seek medical attention before continuing your exercise program.

Recovery heart rate is another indicator of overexertion. To a certain extent, recovery heart rate is related to fitness level. The higher your cardiorespiratory fitness level, the faster your heart rate will decrease following exercise. As a rule of thumb, heart rate should be below 120 beats per minute 5 minutes into recovery. If your heart rate is above 120, you most likely have overexerted yourself or possibly could have some other cardiac abnormality. If you lower the intensity or duration of exercise, or both, and you still have a fast heart rate 5 minutes into recovery, you should consult your physician.

Side Stitch

Side stitch happens primarily in the early stages of participation in exercise. The exact cause is unknown. Some experts suggest that it could relate to a lack of blood flow to the respiratory muscles during strenuous physical exertion. Side stitch occurs primarily in unconditioned beginners and in trained individuals when they exercise at higher intensities than usual. As one's physical condition improves, this condition tends to disappear unless training is intensified. Some people encounter side stitch during downhill running. If side stitch is a problem for you, slow down, and if it persists, stop altogether. Lying down on your back and gently bringing both knees to the chest and holding that position for 30 to 60 seconds also helps.

Some people get side stitch if they eat or drink juice shortly before exercise. Drinking only water an hour to two prior to exercise sometimes prevents side stitch. Other individuals have problems with commercially available carbohydrate solutions during high-intensity exercise. Unless carbohydrate replacement is crucial to complete an event (such as a marathon or a triathlon), drink cool water for fluid replacement or try a different carbohydrate solution.

Shin Splints

Shin splints, one of the most common injuries to the lower limbs, usually results from one or more of the following: (a) lack of proper and gradual conditioning, (b) doing physical activities on hard surfaces (wooden floors, hard tracks, cement, or asphalt), (c) fallen arches, (d) chronic overuse, (e) muscle fatigue, (f) faulty posture, (g) improper shoes, and (h) participating in weight-bearing activities when excessively overweight.

To manage shin splints,

1. Remove or reduce the cause (exercise on softer surfaces, wear better shoes or arch supports, or completely stop exercise until the shin splints heal);

2. Do stretching exercises before and after physical activity;
3. Use ice massage for 10 to 20 minutes before and after exercise;
4. Apply active heat (whirlpool and hot baths) for 15 minutes, two to three times a day; or
5. Use supportive taping during physical activity (a qualified athletic trainer can teach you the proper taping technique).

Muscle Cramps

Muscle cramps are caused by the body's depletion of essential electrolytes or a breakdown in the coordination between opposing muscle groups. If you have a muscle cramp, you should first attempt to stretch the muscles involved. In the case of the calf muscle, for example, pull your toes up toward the knees. After stretching the muscle, rub it down gently, and finally, do some mild exercises requiring the use of that muscle.

In pregnant and lactating women, muscle cramps often are related to a lack of calcium. If women get cramps during these times, calcium supplements usually relieve the problem. Tight clothing also can cause cramps by decreasing blood flow to active muscle tissue.

Leisure-Time Physical Activity

Although individuals have notable differences, the average person in developed countries has about 3.5 hours of "free" or leisure time daily. In our current automated society, most of this time is spent in sedentary living. People would be better off doing some physical activities, based on personal interests. Motivational factors include health, aesthetics, weight control, competition and challenge, fun, social interaction, mental arousal, relaxation, and stress management.

Frequently, leisure-time physical activity does not include exercise performed during a regular exercise program. It consists of activities such as walking, hiking, gardening, yard work, occupational work and chores, and moderate sports such as tennis, table tennis, badminton, golf, or croquet.

Exercise intolerance Inability to function during exercise because of excessive fatigue or extreme feelings of discomfort.

Side stitch A sharp pain in the side of the abdomen.

Shin splints Injury to the lower leg characterized by pain and irritation in the shin region or front of the leg.

Every small increase in daily physical activity contributes to better health and wellness. Small increases in physical activity have a large impact in decreasing early risks for disease and premature death. Therefore, a new, concerted effort must be made to spend leisure-time in activities that will promote the expenditure of energy, provide a break from daily tasks, and contribute to health-related fitness.

Getting Started and Adhering to a Lifetime Exercise Program

Following the guidelines provided in Lab 7B, you may proceed to initiate your cardiorespiratory endurance program. If you have not been exercising regularly, you might begin by attempting to train five or six times a week for 30 minutes at a time. You may find this discouraging, however, and may drop out before getting too far because you will probably develop some muscle soreness and stiffness and possibly incur minor injuries.

Muscle soreness and stiffness and the risk for injuries can be lessened or eliminated by increasing the intensity, duration, and frequency of exercise progressively, as outlined in Lab 7B. Once you have determined your exercise prescription, the difficult part begins: starting and sticking to a lifetime exercise program. Although you may be motivated after reading the benefits to be gained from physical activity, lifelong dedication and perseverance are necessary to reap and maintain good fitness.

The first few weeks probably will be the most difficult, but where there's a will, there's a way. Once you begin to see positive changes, it won't be as hard. Soon you will develop a habit for exercise that will be deeply satisfying and will bring about a sense of self-accomplishment. The following suggestions have been used successfully to help change behavior and adhere to a lifetime exercise program.

1. Set aside a regular time for exercise. If you don't plan ahead, it is a lot easier to skip. On a weekly basis, using red ink, schedule your exercise time into your day planner. Next, hold your exercise hour "sacred." Give exercise priority equal to the most important school or business activity of the day.

    If you are too busy, attempt to accumulate 30 minutes of activity by doing three separate 10-minute sessions throughout the day. Try reading the mail while you walk, take stairs instead of elevators, walk the dog, or ride the stationary bike as you watch the evening news.

2. Exercise early in the day, when you will be less tired and the chances of something interfering

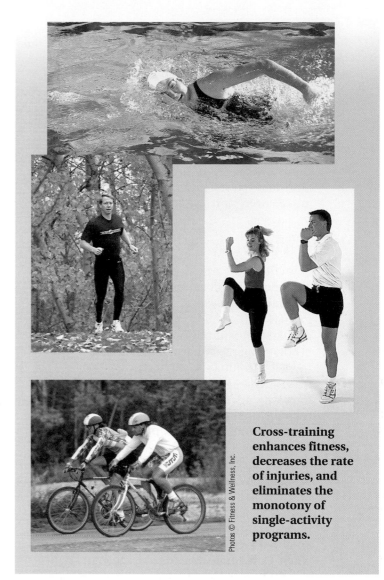

Cross-training enhances fitness, decreases the rate of injuries, and eliminates the monotony of single-activity programs.

Photos © Fitness & Wellness, Inc.

with your workout are minimal; thus you will be less likely to skip your exercise session.

3. Select aerobic activities you enjoy. Exercise should be as much fun as your favorite hobby. If you pick an activity you don't enjoy, you will be unmotivated and less likely to keep exercising. Don't be afraid to try out a new activity, even if that means learning new skills.

4. Combine different activities. You can train by doing two or three different activities the same week. This cross-training may deter the monotony of repeating the same activity every day. Try lifetime sports. Many endurance sports, such as racquetball, basketball, soccer, badminton, roller skating, cross-country skiing, and body surfing (paddling the board), provide a nice break from regular workouts.

5. Use the proper clothing and equipment for exercise. A poor pair of shoes, for example, can make you more prone to injury, discouraging you from the beginning.

6. Find a friend or group of friends to exercise with. Social interaction will make exercise more fulfilling. Besides, it's harder to skip if someone is waiting to go with you.

7. Set goals and share them with others. Quitting is tougher when someone else knows what you are trying to accomplish. When you reach a targeted goal, reward yourself with a new pair of shoes or a jogging suit.

8. Don't become a chronic exerciser. Learn to listen to your body. Overexercising can lead to chronic fatigue and injuries. Exercise should be enjoyable, and in the process you should stop and smell the roses.

9. Exercise in different places and facilities. This will add variety to your workouts.

10. Exercise to music. People who listen to fast-tempo music tend to exercise more vigorously and longer. Using headphones when exercising outdoors, however, can be dangerous. Even indoors, it is preferable not to use headphones, so that you can still be aware of your surroundings.

11. Keep a regular record of your activities. Keeping a record allows you to monitor your progress and compare it against previous months and years (see Figures 7.3 and 7.8, pp. 168 and 191).

12. Conduct periodic assessments. Improving to a higher fitness category is a reward in itself.

13. Listen to your body. Stop exercise if you experience pain or unusual discomfort. Pain and aches are an indication of potential injury. If you do suffer an injury, do not return to your regular workouts until you are fully recovered. You may cross-train using activities that do not aggravate your injury (for instance, swimming instead of jogging).

14. If a health problem arises, see a physician. When in doubt, it's better to be safe than sorry.

Exercise and Aging

Unlike any prior time in U.S. history, the elderly population constitutes the fastest growing segment. In 1880, less than 3 percent of the total population, or fewer than 2 million people, was older than 65. By 1980 the elderly population had reached approximately 25 million, more than 11.3 percent of the population. By the year 2030, more than 70 million people in the United States are expected to be older than age 65.

Historically, older adults have been neglected when developing fitness programs. Nevertheless, fitness is just as important for older people as it is for young people. Although much research remains to be done in this area, studies indicate that older individuals who are physically fit also enjoy better health and a higher quality of life.

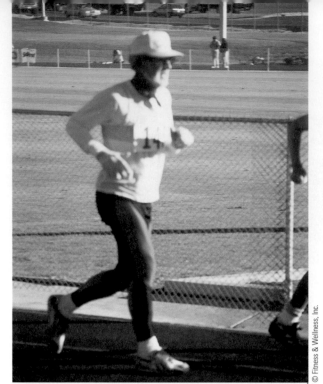

Older adults who exercise enjoy better health, increase their quality of life, and live longer than physically inactive adults.

The main objective of fitness programs for older adults should be to help them improve their functional status and contribute to healthy aging. This implies the ability to maintain independent living status and to avoid disability. The American Alliance of Health, Physical Education, Recreation and Dance (AAHPERD) has defined functional fitness for older adults as the physical capacity of the individual to meet ordinary and unexpected demands of daily life safely and effectively.[18] This definition clearly indicates the need for fitness programs that closely relate to activities this population normally encounters. Older adults are encouraged to participate in programs that will help develop cardiorespiratory endurance, muscular strength and endurance, muscular flexibility, agility and balance, and motor coordination.

Physical Training in the Older Adult

Regular participation in physical activity provides both physiological and physical benefits to older adults.[19] Cardiorespiratory endurance training helps to increase functional capacity, decrease the risk for disease, improve health status, and increase life expectancy. Strength training decreases the rate at which strength and muscle mass are lost. Among the psychological benefits are preserved cognitive function, reduced symptoms and behaviors related

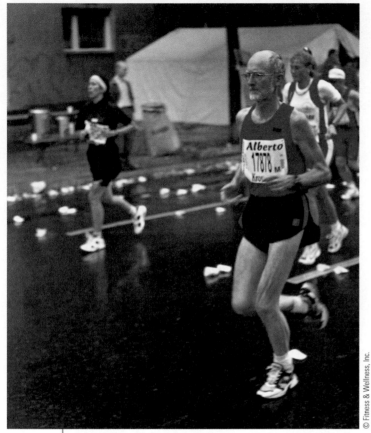

A high level of physical fitness can be maintained throughout the life span.

Table 7.3 Effects of Physical Activity and Inactivity on Older Men

	Exercisers	Non-exercisers
Age (yrs)	68.0	69.8
Weight (lbs)	160.3	186.3
Resting heart rate (bpm)	55.8	66.0
Maximal heart rate (bpm)	157.0	146.0
Heart rate reserve* (bpm)	101.2	80.0
Blood pressure (mm Hg)	120/78	150/90
Maximal oxygen uptake (ml/kg/min)	38.6	20.3

*Heart rate reserve = maximal heart rate − resting heart rate.

Data from F. W. Kash, J. L. Boyer, S. P. Van Camp, L. S. Verity, and J. P. Wallace, "The Effect of Physical Activity on Aerobic Power in Older Men (A Longitudinal Study)," *The Physician and Sports Medicine* 18, no. 4 (1990): 73–83.

to depression, and improved self-confidence and self-esteem.

The trainability of older men and women alike and the effectiveness of physical activity in enhancing health have been demonstrated in prior research. Older adults who increase their physical activity experience significant changes in cardiorespiratory endurance, strength, and flexibility. The extent of the changes depends on their initial fitness level and the types of activities they select for their training (walking, cycling, strength training, and so on).

Improvements in maximal oxygen uptake in older adults are similar to those of younger people, although older people seem to require a longer training period to achieve these changes. Declines in maximal oxygen uptake average about 1 percent per year between age 25 and 75.[20] A slower rate of decline is seen in people who maintain a lifetime aerobic exercise program.

Results of research on the effects of aging on the cardiorespiratory system of male exercisers versus nonexercisers showed that the maximal oxygen uptake of regular exercisers was almost twice that of the nonexercisers (see Table 7.3).[21] The study revealed a decline in maximal oxygen uptake

between ages 50 and 68, of only 13 percent in the active group, compared with 41 percent in the inactive group. These changes indicate that about one-third of the loss in maximal oxygen uptake results from aging and two-thirds of the loss comes from inactivity. Blood pressure, heart rate, and body weight also were remarkably better in the exercising group. Furthermore, aerobic training seems to decrease high blood pressure in the older patients at the same rate as in young hypertensive people.[22]

In terms of aging, muscle strength declines by 10 to 20 percent between the ages of 20 and 50, but between ages 50 and 70, it drops by another 25 to 30 percent. Through strength training, frail adults in their 80s or 90s can double or triple their strength in just a few months. The amount of muscle hypertrophy achieved, however, decreases with age. Strength gains close to 200 percent have been found in previously inactive adults over age 90.[23] In fact, research has shown that regular strength training improves balance, gait, speed, **functional independence**, morale, depression symptoms, and energy intake.[24] (The health-related components of strength and flexibility fitness are addressed in Chapters 8 and 9 respectively.)

Although muscle flexibility drops by about 5 percent per decade of life, 10 minutes of stretching every other day can prevent most of this loss as a person ages.[25] Improved flexibility enhances mobility skills.[26] The latter promotes independence because it helps older adults successfully perform activities of daily living.

In terms of body composition, inactive adults continue to gain body fat after age 60 despite the tendency toward lower body weight. The increase in

body fatness is most likely related to a decrease in basal metabolic rate and physical activity along with increased caloric intake above that required to maintain daily energy requirements.[27]

Older adults who wish to initiate or continue an exercise program are strongly encouraged to have a complete medical exam, including a stress electrocardiogram test (see Chapter 12). Recommended activities for older adults include calisthenics, walking, jogging, swimming, cycling, and water aerobics.

Older people should avoid isometric and very high intensity weight-training exercises (see Chapter 8). Activities that require all-out effort or require participants to hold their breath (e.g., the valsalva maneuver) tend to lessen blood flow to the heart and cause a significant increase in blood pressure and increases the load placed on the heart. Older adults should participate in activities that require continuous and rhythmic muscular activity (about 40 to 60 percent of HHR). These activities do not cause large increases in blood pressure or place an intense overload on the heart.

Predicting Oxygen Uptake and Caloric Expenditure

As indicated in Chapter 6, oxygen uptake can be expressed in liters per minute (l/min) or milliliters per kilogram per minute (ml/kg/min). The latter is used to classify individuals into the various cardio-respiratory fitness categories (see Table 6.8, page 156).

Oxygen uptake expressed in l/min is valuable in determining the caloric expenditure of physical activity. The human body burns about 5 calories for each liter of oxygen consumed. During aerobic exercise the average person trains between 60 and 75 percent of maximal oxygen uptake.[28]

A person with a maximal oxygen uptake of 3.5 l/min who trains at 60 percent of maximum uses 2.1 (3.5 × .60) liters of oxygen per minute of physical activity. This indicates that 10.5 calories are burned each minute of exercise (2.1 × 5). If the activity is carried out for 30 minutes, 315 calories (10.5 × 30) have been burned.

Applying the principle of 5 calories burned per liter of oxygen consumed, you can determine with reasonable accuracy your own caloric output for walking and jogging. Table 7.4 contains the oxygen requirement (uptake) for walking speeds between 50 and 100 meters per minute and for jogging speeds in excess of 80 meters per minute.

There is a transition period from walking to jogging for speeds in the range of 80 to 134 meters

Table 7.4 Oxygen Requirement Estimates for Selected Walking and Jogging Speeds

Walking		Jogging			
Speed (m/min)	VO₂ (ml/kg/min)	Speed (m/min)	VO₂ (ml/kg/min)	Speed (m/min)	VO₂ (ml/kg/min)
50	8.5	80	19.5	210	45.5
52	8.7	85	20.5	215	46.5
54	8.9	90	21.5	220	47.5
56	9.1	95	22.5	225	48.5
58	9.3	100	23.5	230	49.5
60	9.5	105	24.5	235	50.5
62	9.7	110	25.5	240	51.5
64	9.9	115	26.5	245	52.5
66	10.1	120	27.5	250	53.5
68	10.3	125	28.5	255	54.5
70	10.5	130	29.5	260	55.5
72	10.7	135	30.5	265	56.5
74	10.9	140	31.5	270	57.5
76	11.1	145	32.5	275	58.5
78	11.3	150	33.5	280	59.5
80	11.5	155	34.5		
82	11.7	160	35.5		
84	11.9	165	36.5		
86	12.1	170	37.5		
88	12.3	175	38.5		
90	12.5	180	39.5		
92	12.7	185	40.5		
94	12.9	190	41.5		
96	13.1	195	42.5		
98	13.3	200	43.5		
100	13.5	205	44.5		

m/min = meters per minute

ml/kg/min = milliliters per kilogram per minute

* Table developed using the metabolic calculations contained in *Guidelines for Exercise Testing and Exercise Prescription*, by the American College of Sports Medicine (Philadelphia: Lea & Febiger, 1995).

per minute. Consequently, the person must be truly jogging at these lower speeds to use the estimated oxygen uptakes for jogging in Table 7.4. Because these uptakes are expressed in ml/kg/min, you will need to convert this figure to l/min to predict caloric output. This is done by multiplying the oxygen uptake in ml/kg/min by your body weight in kilograms (kg) and then dividing by 1,000.

For example, let's estimate the caloric cost for an individual who weighs 145.5 pounds and runs 3 miles in 21 minutes. Each mile is about 1,600 meters, or four laps around a 400-meter (440-yard) track. Three miles then would be 4,800 meters

Functional independence Ability to carry out activities of daily living without assistance from other individuals.

(1,600 × 3). Therefore, 3 miles (4,800 meters) in 21 minutes represents a pace of 228.6 meters per minute (4,800 ÷ 21).

Table 7.4 indicates an oxygen requirement (uptake) of about 49.5 ml/kg/min for a speed of 228.6 meters per minute. A weight of 145.5 pounds equals 66 kilograms (145.5 ÷ 2.2046). The oxygen uptake in l/min now can be calculated by multiplying the value in ml/kg/min by body weight in kg and dividing by 1,000. In our example, it is (49.5 × 66) ÷ 1,000 = 3.3 l/min. This oxygen uptake in 21 minutes represents a total of 347 calories (3.3 × 5 × 21).

In Lab 7C you have an opportunity to determine your own oxygen uptake and caloric expenditure for walking and jogging. Using your oxygen uptake information in conjunction with exercise heart rates allows you to estimate your caloric expenditure for almost any activity, as long as the heart rate ranges from 110 to 180 beats per minute. To make an accurate estimate, you have to be skilled in assessing exercise heart rate. Also, as your level of fitness improves, you will need to reassess your exercise heart rate because it will drop (given the same workload) with improved physical condition.

A Lifetime Commitment to Fitness

The benefits of fitness can be maintained only through a regular lifetime program. Exercise is not like putting money in the bank. It does not help much to exercise 4 or 5 hours on Saturday and not do anything else the rest of the week. If anything, exercising only once a week is unsafe for unconditioned adults.

Even the greatest athletes on earth, if they were to stop exercising, would be, after just a few years, at a risk for disease similar to someone who never has done any physical activity. Staying with a physical fitness program long enough brings about positive physiological and psychological changes. Once you are there, you will not want to have it any other way.

The time involved in losing the benefits of exercise varies among the different components of physical fitness and also depends on the person's condition before the interruption. In regard to cardiorespiratory endurance, it has been estimated that 4 weeks of aerobic training are completely reversed in 2 consecutive weeks of physical inactivity. On the other hand, if you have been exercising regularly for months or years, 2 weeks of inactivity will not hurt you as much as it will someone who has exercised only a few weeks. As a rule of thumb, after 48 to 72 hours of aerobic inactivity, the cardiorespiratory system starts to lose some of its capacity.

To maintain fitness, you should keep up a regular exercise program, even during vacations. If you have to interrupt your program for reasons beyond your control, you should not attempt to resume training at the same level you left off, but rather build up gradually again.

Web Interactive

- American Council of Exercise Cardiovascular Fitness Facts. This site features information about a variety of cardiovascular forms of exercise, including walking, running, jumping rope, swimming, spinning, cross-training, interval training, and others.

  http://www.acefitness.org/fitfacts/fitfacts_list.cfm#1

- Improving Cardiovascular Health In African Americans. This document written by the National Heart, Lung, and Blood Institute provides information on the value of cardiovascular exercise to improving health.

  http://www.nhlbi.nih.gov/health/public/heart/other/chdblack/energize.htm

- Worldguide Online. This site provides information about various types of cardiorespiratory endurance exercises and how to treat exercise injuries.

  http://www.worldguide.com/Fitness/hf.html

Interactive Sites:

- Aerobics and Fitness Association of America. This interactive site features "Exercise Gets Personal™" where you can create a customized exercise program that includes activities you select, geared to your current level of fitness activity. Exercises include aerobics, muscular conditioning, and flexibility with descriptions and precautions for each activity.

  http://www.afaa.com

- Let's Get Physical Challenge. This site will describe an eight-week, interactive program designed to help individuals participate in regular, moderate physical activity. This is a fun, non-competitive program designed to educate people of all ages and abilities. You can do it!

  http://www.physicalfitness.org/lgpstart.html

Notes

1. W. M. Bortz II, "Disuse and Aging," *Journal of the American Medical Association* 248 (1982): 1203–1208.

2. R. K. Dishman, "Compliance/Adherence in Health-Related Exercise," *Health Psychology* 1 (1982): 237–267.

3. U.S. Department of Health and Human Services, *Physical Activity and Health: A Report of the Surgeon General* (Atlanta: U.S. Department of Health and Human Services, Centers for Disease Control and Prevention, National Center for Chronic Disease Prevention and Health Promotion, 1996).

4. American College of Sports Medicine, "Position Stand: The Recommended Quantity and Quality of Exercise for Developing and Maintaining Cardiorespiratory and Muscular Fitness, and Flexibility in Healthy Adults," *Medicine and Science in Sports and Exercise* 30 (1998): 975–991.

5. American College of Sports Medicine, *Guidelines for Exercise Testing and Prescription* (Baltimore: Williams & Wilkins, 2000).

6. See note 4.

7. W. W. K. Hoeger, C. Harris, W. L. Nurge, and M. L. Jensen, "Physiologic Responses to Step Aerobics Combined with Upper Work in Trained Subjects," *Journal for the International Council for Health Physical Education, Recreation, Sport, and Dance*, (In Press).

   D. R. Hopkins, W. W. K. Hoeger, D. E. Van Zee, and W. J. Nurge, "Physiologic Responses to Aero-belt Walking," *Medicine and Science in Sports and Exercise* 26 (1994): 243–245.

   W. J. Nurge, D. E. Van Zee, and W. W. K. Hoeger. "Physiologic Responses to Aero-belt Walking and Jogging," *Medicine and Science in Sports and Exercise* 26 (1994): 243–247.

8. S. Blair, "Surgeon General's Report on Physical Fitness: The Inside Story," *ACSM's Health & Fitness Journal* 1 (1997): 14–18.

9. R. F. DeBusk, U. Stenestrand, M. Sheehan, and W. L. Haskell, "Training Effects of Long Versus Short Bouts of Exercise in Healthy Subjects," *American Journal of Cardiology* 65 (1990): 1010–1013.

10. "Summary Statement: Workshop on Physical Activity and Public Health," *Sports Medicine Bulletin* 28 (1993): 7.

11. See note 3.

12. U.S. Department of Agriculture and U.S. Department of Health and Human Services, "Nutrition and Your Health: Dietary Guidelines for Americans," *Home and Garden Bulletin* 232 (2000).

13. "Scanning Sports," *Physician and Sportsmedicine* 21, no. 11 (1993): 34.

14. See note 4.

15. R. S. Paffenbarger, Jr., R. T. Hyde, A. L. Wing, and C. H. Steinmetz, "A Natural History of Athleticism and Cardiovascular Health," *Journal of the American Medical Association* 252 (1984): 491–495.

16. American College of Sports Medicine, "Position Stand: Exercise and Type 2 Diabetes," *Medicine and Science in Sports and Exercise* 32 (2000): 1345–1360.

17. University of California at Berkeley, *The Wellness Guide to Lifelong Fitness* (New York: Random House, 1993): 198.

18. W. Osness, M. Adrian, B. Clark, W. W. K. Hoeger, D. Raab, and R. Wiswell, "The AAHPERD Fitness Task Force, History and Philosophy," *Journal of Physical Education, Recreation and Dance* 60, no. 3 (1989): 64–65.

19. American College of Sports Medicine, "Position Stand: Exercise and Physical Activity for Older Adults," *Medicine and Science in Sports and Exercise* 30 (1998): 992–1008.

20. R. J. Shephard, "Exercise and Aging: Extending Independence in Older Adult," *Geriatrics* 48 (1993): 61–64.

21. F. W. Kash, J. L. Boyer, S. P. Van Camp, L. S. Verity, and J. P. Wallace, "The Effect of Physical Activity on Aerobic Power in Older Men (A Longitudinal Study)," *Physician and Sports Medicine* 18, no. 4 (1990): 73–83.

22. J. Hagberg, S. Blair, A. Ehsani, N. Gordon, N. Kaplan, C. Tipton, and E. Zambraski, "Position Stand: Physical Activity, Physical Fitness, and Hypertension," *Medicine and Science in Sports and Exercise* 25 (1993): i–x.

23. W. S. Evans, "Exercise, Nutrition and Aging," *Journal of Nutrition* 122 (1992): 796–801.

24. See note 19.

25. "Exercise for the Ages," *Consumer Reports on Health* (Yonkers, NY: The Editors, July, 1996).

26. J. M. Walker, D. Sue, N. Miles-Elkousy, G. Ford, and H. Trevelyan, "Active Mobility of the Extremities in Older Subjects," *Physical Therapy* 64 (1994): 919–923.

27. S. B. Roberts, et al., "What are the Dietary Needs of Adults?" *International Journal of Obesity* 16 (1992): 969–976.

28. R. K. Dishman, "Prescribing Exercise Intensity for Healthy Adults Using Perceived Exertion," *Medicine and Science in Sports and Exercise* 26 (1994): 1087–1094.

Suggested Readings

ACSM's Resource Manual for Guidelines for Exercise Testing and Prescription. Baltimore: Williams & Wilkins, 1998.

American College of Sports Medicine. *Guidelines for Exercise Testing and Prescription.* Baltimore: Williams & Wilkins, 2000.

Arnheim, D. D., and W. Prentice. *Principles of Athletic Training.* Dubuque, IA: Brown & Benchmark, 1996.

Borg, G. "Perceived Exertion: A Note on History and Methods." *Medicine and Science in Sports and Exercise* 5 (1993): 90–93.

Clark, B., W. Osness, W. W. K. Hoeger, M. Adrian, D. Raab, and R. Wiswell. "Tests for Fitness in Older Adults: AAHPERD Fitness Task Force." *Journal of Physical Education, Recreation and Dance* 60, no. 3 (1989): 66–71.

Coleman, E. *Eating for Endurance.* Palo Alto, CA: Bull Publishing, 1997.

Fox, E. L., R. W. Bowers, and M. L. Foss. *The Physiological Basis for Exercise and Sport.* Madison, WI: Brown & Benchmark, 1993.

Heyward, V. H. *Advanced Fitness Assessment & Exercise Prescription.* Champaign, IL: Human Kinetics, 1998.

Karvonen, M. J., E. Kentala, and O. Mustala. "The Effects of Training on the Heart Rate, a Longitudinal Study." *Annales Medicinae Experimetalis et Biologiae Fenniae* 35 (1957): 307–315.

Kushi, L. H. "Physical Activity and Mortality in Postmenopausal Women." *Journal of the American Medical Association* 277 (1997): 1287–1292.

McArdle, W. D., F. I. Katch, and V. L. Katch. *Exercise Physiology.* Baltimore: Williams & Wilkins, 1996.

Metcalf, J. A. "Exercising During Pregnancy." *Certified News* 5, no. 2 (1995): 10–11.

Pfeiffer, R. P., and B. C. Mangus. *Concepts of Athletic Training.* Boston: Jones and Bartlett Publishers, 1998.

Teitz, C. C. "Overuse Injuries." In *Scientific Foundations of Sports Medicine,* edited by C. C. Teitz, 299–328. Philadelphia: B. C. Decker, 1989.

Figure
7.8
Cardiorespiratory exercise record form.

Month _____

Date	Body Weight	Exercise Heart Rate	Type of Exercise	Distance In Miles	Time Hrs/Min	RPE*
1						
2						
3						
4						
5						
6						
7						
8						
9						
10						
11						
12						
13						
14						
15						
16						
17						
18						
19						
20						
21						
22						
23						
24						
25						
26						
27						
28						
29						
30						
31						
			Total			

*Rate of perceived exertion.

Month _____

Date	Body Weight	Exercise Heart Rate	Type of Exercise	Distance In Miles	Time Hrs/Min	RPE*
1						
2						
3						
4						
5						
6						
7						
8						
9						
10						
11						
12						
13						
14						
15						
16						
17						
18						
19						
20						
21						
22						
23						
24						
25						
26						
27						
28						
29						
30						
31						
			Total			

*Rate of perceived exertion.

Figure 7.8 Cardiorespiratory exercise record form.

Month _____

Date	Body Weight	Exercise Heart Rate	Type of Exercise	Distance In Miles	Time Hrs/Min	RPE*
1						
2						
3						
4						
5						
6						
7						
8						
9						
10						
11						
12						
13						
14						
15						
16						
17						
18						
19						
20						
21						
22						
23						
24						
25						
26						
27						
28						
29						
30						
31						
			Total			

*Rate of perceived exertion.

Month _____

Date	Body Weight	Exercise Heart Rate	Type of Exercise	Distance In Miles	Time Hrs/Min	RPE*
1						
2						
3						
4						
5						
6						
7						
8						
9						
10						
11						
12						
13						
14						
15						
16						
17						
18						
19						
20						
21						
22						
23						
24						
25						
26						
27						
28						
29						
30						
31						
			Total			

*Rate of perceived exertion.

Name:	Date:	Grade:
Instructor:	Course:	Section:

Necessary Lab Equipment
None required.

Objective
To determine your preparedness to start an exercise program.

Instructions
Read each statement carefully and circle the number that best describes your feelings in each statement. Please be completely honest with your answers. Interpret the results of this questionnaire using the guidelines provided on the next page.

	Strongly Agree	Mildly Agree	Mildly Disagree	Strongly Disagree
1. I can walk, ride a bike (or a wheelchair), swim, or walk in a shallow pool.	4	3	2	1
2. I enjoy exercise.	4	3	2	1
3. I believe exercise can help decrease the risk for disease and premature mortality.	4	3	2	1
4. I believe exercise contributes to better health.	4	3	2	1
5. I have previously participated in an exercise program.	4	3	2	1
6. I have experienced the feeling of being physically fit.	4	3	2	1
7. I can envision myself exercising.	4	3	2	1
8. I am contemplating an exercise program.	4	3	2	1
9. I am willing to stop contemplating and give exercise a try for a few weeks.	4	3	2	1
10. I am willing to set aside time at least three times a week for exercise.	4	3	2	1
11. I can find a place to exercise (the streets, a park, a YMCA, a health club).	4	3	2	1
12. I can find other people who would like to exercise with me.	4	3	2	1
13. I will exercise when I am moody, fatigued, and even when the weather is bad.	4	3	2	1
14. I am willing to spend a small amount of money for adequate exercise clothing (shoes, shorts, leotards, swimsuit).	4	3	2	1
15. If I have any doubts about my present state of health, I will see a physician before beginning an exercise program.	4	3	2	1
16. Exercise will make me feel better and improve my quality of life.	4	3	2	1

Scoring Your Test:

This questionnaire allows you to examine your readiness for exercise. You have been evaluated in four categories: mastery (self-control), attitude, health, and commitment. Mastery indicates that you can be in control of your exercise program. Attitude examines your mental disposition toward exercise. Health provides evidence of the wellness benefits of exercise. Commitment shows dedication and resolution to carry out the exercise program. Write the number you circled after each statement in the corresponding spaces below. Add the scores on each line to get your totals. Scores can vary from 4 to 16. A score of 12 and above is a strong indicator that that factor is important to you, and 8 and below is low. If you score 12 or more points in each category, your chances of initiating and adhering to an exercise program are good. If you fail to score at least 12 points in three categories, your chances of succeeding at exercise may be slim. You need to be better informed about the benefits of exercise, and a retraining process may be required.

Mastery:	1.		+	5.		+	6.		+	9.	=
Attitude:	2.		+	7.		+	8.		+	13.	=
Health:	3.		+	4.		+	15.		+	16.	=
Commitment:	10.		+	11.		+	12.		+	14.	=

II. Stage of Change for Cardiorespiratory Endurance Exercise

Using Figure 2.3 (page 40) and Table 2.3 (page 41), identify your current stage of change in regard to participation in a cardiorespiratory endurance exercise program:

III. Advantages and Disadvantages for Adding Aerobic Exercise to Your Lifestyle

Advantages: _____

_____

_____

_____

_____

_____

_____

_____

Disadvantages: _____

_____

_____

_____

_____

_____

_____

_____

Lab 7B

CARDIORESPIRATORY EXERCISE PRESCRIPTION

Name: _____   Date: _____   Grade: _____

Instructor: _____   Course: _____   Section: _____

Necessary Lab Equipment
None required.

Objective
To write your own cardiorespiratory exercise prescription.

I. Intensity of Exercise

1. Estimate your own maximal heart rate (MHR)

   MHR = 220 minus age (220 − age)

   MHR = 220 − _____ = _____ bpm

2. Resting Heart Rate (RHR) = _____ bpm

3. Heart Rate Reserve (HRR) = MHR − RHR

   HRR = _____ − _____ = _____ beats

4. Training Intensities (TI) = HRR × TI + RHR

   40 Percent TI = _____ × .40 + _____ = _____ bpm

   50 Percent TI = _____ × .50 + _____ = _____ bpm

   60 percent TI = _____ × .60 + _____ = _____ bpm

   85 Percent TI = _____ × .85 + _____ = _____ bpm

5. Cardiorespiratory Training Zone. The optimum cardiorespiratory training zone is found between the 60% and 85% training intensities. Older adults, individuals who have been physically inactive or are in the poor or fair cardiorespiratory fitness categories, however, should follow a 40% to 50% training intensity during the first few weeks of the exercise program.

   Cardiorespiratory Training Zone: _____ (60% TI) to _____ (85% TI)

   Rate of Perceived Exertion (see Figure 7.4, page 169): _____ to _____

II. Mode of Exercise

Select any activity or combination of activities that you enjoy doing. The activity has to be continuous in nature and must get your heart rate up to the cardiorespiratory training zone and keep it there for as long as you exercise. Indicate your preferred mode(s) of exercise:

1. _____   2. _____   3. _____

4. _____   5. _____   6. _____

III. Cardiorespiratory Exercise Program

The following is your weekly program for development of cardiorespiratory endurance. If you are in the average, good, or excellent fitness category, you may start at week 5. After completing this 12-week program, for you to maintain your fitness level, you should exercise in the 60% to 85% training zone for about 20 to 30 minutes, a minimum of three times per week, on nonconsecutive days. You should also recompute your target zone periodically because you will experience a significant reduction in resting heart rate with aerobic training (approximately 10 to 20 beats in about 8 to 12 weeks).

Week	Duration (min)	Frequency	Training Intensity	10-Sec Pulse Count*
1	15	3	Between 40% and 50%	
2	15	4	Between 40% and 50%	
3	20	4	Between 40% and 50%	____ beats
4	20	5	Between 40% and 50%	
5	20	4	Between 50% and 60%	
6	20	5	Between 50% and 60%	
7	30	4	Between 50% and 60%	____ beats
8	30	5	Between 50% and 60%	
9	30	4	Between 60% and 85%	
10	30	5	Between 60% and 85%	
11	30–40	5	Between 60% and 85%	____ to ____ beats
12	30–40	5	Between 60% and 85%	

*Fill out your own 10-second pulse count under this column.

Briefly State Your Experiences and Feelings Regarding Aerobic Exercise:

_____

_____

_____

_____

_____

_____

_____

_____

_____

_____

_____

_____

_____

_____

_____

_____

_____

_____

Name: **Date:**   **Grade:**

Instructor: **Course:**   **Section:**

Necessary Lab Equipment

A school track (or premeasured course) and a stopwatch. Each student also should bring a watch with a second hand.

Objective

To monitor exercise heart rate and determine the caloric cost of physical activity based on exercise heart rate.

Lab Preparation

Wear exercise clothing, including jogging shoes. Do not engage in vigorous physical activity prior to this lab. Read the information on predicting oxygen uptake and caloric expenditure in Chapter 7, pages 187–188.

Procedure

1. **Cardiorespiratory Training Zone.** Look up your cardiovascular training zone at 70 percent and 85 percent of heart rate reserve in Lab 7B. Record this information in beats per minute (bpm) and in 10-second pulse counts in the blank spaces provided below.

                         Beats/minute   **10-sec count**

   70% intensity   =

   85% intensity   =

2. **Resting Heart Rate (HR) and Body Weight (BW).** Determine your resting HR prior to exercise and your body weight in kilograms (divide pounds by 2.2046).

   Resting HR: bpm

   BW: lbs ÷ 2.2046 =   kg

3. **Walking HR, Oxygen Uptake (VO$_2$), and Caloric Expenditure.** Walk two laps around a 400-meter (440-yard) track at an average speed of 75 to 100 meters per minute. Try to maintain a constant speed around the track. You can monitor your speed by starting the walk at the beginning of the 100-meter straightway and making sure you have walked at least 75 meters and no more than 100 meters in one minute. As soon as you complete the two laps (800 meters), notice the time required to walk this distance and immediately check your exercise HR by taking a 10-second pulse count. Record this information in the spaces provided below. Do not record the time until after you have checked your pulse. Exercise HR will remain at the same rate for about 15 seconds following cessation of exercise. Therefore, you need to check your pulse as soon as you finish the walk, after noticing the 800-meter walk time.

   10-sec. pulse count: beats (from question 1 above)

   800-meter time: min   sec

   HR in bpm = 10-sec pulse count × 6

   HR in bpm =   × 6 =   bpm

   800-meter time in minutes = min + (sec ÷ 60)

   800-meter time in minutes =   + (÷ 60) =   min

   Speed in meters per minute (mts/min) = 800 ÷ 800-meter time in min

   Speed in mts/min = 800 ÷   =   mts/min

VO_2 in ml/kg/min at this walking speed (Use Table 7.4, page 187) = [____] ml/kg/min

VO_2 in l/min = VO_2 in ml/kg/min × BW in kg ÷ 1,000

VO_2 in l/min = [____] × [____] ÷ 1000 = [____] l/min

Caloric expenditure for 800-meter walk = VO_2 in l/min × 5 × 800-meter time in min

Caloric expenditure for 800-meter walk = [____] × 5 × [____] = [____] calories

4. **Slow-Jogging HR, VO_2, and Caloric Expenditure.** Slowly jog 800 meters (two laps) around the track. Try to maintain the same slow-jogging pace throughout the two laps. Do NOT jog fast or sprint. This is not a speed test and is intended to be a slow jog only. As soon as you complete the 800 meters, notice the time required to complete the distance and check your exercise HR immediately by taking another 10-second pulse count. Record this information below.

10-sec pulse count: [____] beats

800-meter time: [____] min [____] sec.

HR in bpm = 10-sec pulse count × 6

HR in bpm = [____] × 6 = [____] bpm

800-meter time in minutes = min + (sec ÷ 60)

800-meter time in minutes = [____] + ([____] ÷ 60) = [____] min

Speed in mts/min = 800 ÷ 800-meter time in min

Speed in mts/min = 800 ÷ [____] = [____] mts/min.

VO_2 in ml/kg/min at this slow-jogging speed (Use Table 7.4, page 187) = [____] ml/kg/min

VO_2 in l/min = VO_2 in ml/kg/min × BW in kg ÷ 1,000

VO_2 in l/min = [____] × [____] ÷ 1000 = [____] l/min

Caloric expenditure for 800-meter slow jog = VO_2 in l/min × 5 × 800-meter time in min

Caloric expenditure for 800-meter slow jog = [____] × 5 × [____] = [____] calories

5. **Fast-Jogging HR, VO_2, Caloric Expenditure, and Recovery HR.** Jog another 800 meters at a faster speed around the track. Again try to maintain the same jogging pace throughout the two laps. Do NOT sprint. Your HR should not exceed 180 bpm on this test. As soon as you complete the 800 meters, notice your time for the two laps and check your 10-second pulse count. Record this information below. You also should check your 2- and 5-minute recovery HRs after the run and record these rates below.

10-sec pulse count: [____] beats

800-meter time: [____] min [____] sec

HR in bpm = 10-sec pulse count × 6

HR in bpm = [____] × 6 = [____] bpm

800-meter time in minutes = min + (sec ÷ 60)

800-meter time in minutes = [____] + ([____] ÷ 60) = [____] min

Speed in mts/min = 800 ÷ 800-meter time in min

Speed in mts/min = 800 ÷ [____] = [____] mts/min

VO_2 in ml/kg/min at this fast-jogging speed (Use Table 7.4, page 187) = [____] ml/kg/min

$\text{VO}_2 \text{ in l/min } = \text{ VO}_2 \text{ in ml/kg/min } \times \text{ BW in kg } \div \text{ 1,000}$

$\text{VO}_2 \text{ in l/min } = \underline{\hspace{2cm}} \times \underline{\hspace{2cm}} \div \text{ 1,000 } = \underline{\hspace{2cm}} \text{ l/min}$

Caloric expenditure for 800-meter fast jog $= \text{ VO}_2 \text{ in l/min } \times \text{ 5 } \times \text{ 800-meter time in min}$

Caloric expenditure for 800-meter fast jog $= \underline{\hspace{2cm}} \times \text{ 5 } \times \underline{\hspace{2cm}} = \underline{\hspace{2cm}} \text{ calories}$

Recovery HRs

	10-sec count	bpm
2 minutes		
5 minutes*		

6. **Resting, Exercise, and Recovery HRs.** Plot your resting, exercise, and recovery HRs on the graph provided below.

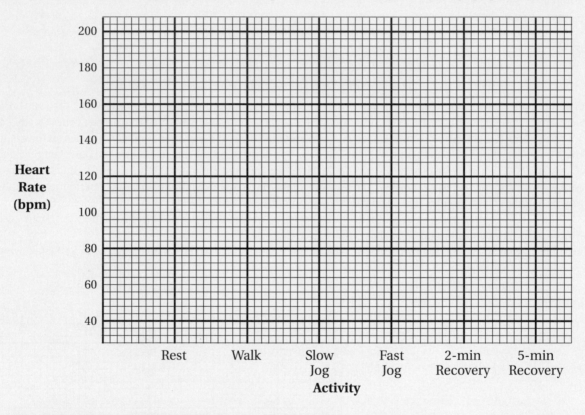

7. **Training Exercise HR and Equivalent Caloric Expenditure.** This part of the lab should be completed outside your regular lab time, during the next 2 or 3 days prior to turning in the assignment. According to the previous exercise HRs (items 3, 4, and 5), try to select a walking or jogging speed that will allow you to maintain your exercise HR in the appropriate cardiovascular training zone. Using a 400-meter track, walk or jog for 20 minutes at the selected speed and again try to maintain a constant speed throughout the exercise time. At the end of the 20 minutes, check your 10-second pulse count and estimate the distance covered in meters. Record this information below and estimate the VO$_2$ and caloric expenditure.

10-sec pulse count: $\underline{\hspace{2cm}}$ beats

HR in bpm $= \text{ 10-sec pulse count } \times \text{ 6}$

HR in bpm $= \underline{\hspace{2cm}} \times \text{ 6 } = \underline{\hspace{2cm}} \text{ bpm}$

Approximate distance covered in twenty minutes: $\underline{\hspace{2cm}}$ meters

---

* Your 5-minute recovery HR should be below 120 bpm. If it is above 120, you most likely have overexerted yourself and, therefore, need to decrease the intensity of exercise (and/or duration when exercising for long periods of time). If your 5-minute recovery HR is still above 120 after decreasing the intensity of exercise, you should consult a physician regarding this condition.

Speed in mts/min = distance in meters ÷ 20 minutes

Speed in mts/min = ⬚ ÷ 20 = ⬚ mts/min

VO_2 at this speed (see Table 7.4, page 187) = ⬚ ml/kg/min

VO_2 in l/min = VO_2 in ml/kg/min × BW in kg = 1,000

VO_2 in l/min = ⬚ × ⬚ ÷ 1,000 = ⬚ l/min

Caloric expenditure for 20-min walk/jog = VO_2 in l/min × 5 × 20 min

Caloric expenditure for 20-min walk/jog = ⬚ × 5 × 20 = ⬚ calories

Using the previous information, how many calories would you have burned if you had maintained this pace for:

10 minutes (VO_2 in l/min × 5 × 10) = ⬚ × 5 × 10 = ⬚ calories

30 minutes (VO_2 in l/min × 5 × 30) = ⬚ × 5 × 30 = ⬚ calories

60 minutes (VO_2 in l/min × 5 × 60) = ⬚ × 5 × 60 = ⬚ calories

PREDICTING CALORIC EXPENDITURE ACCORDING TO EXERCISE HR

Research indicates that there is a linear relationship between HR and VO_2, as long as the HR ranges from about 110 to 180 bpm. If you obtain two exercise HRs in this range and the equivalent oxygen uptakes (in l/min), you can easily predict your VO_2 and caloric expenditure for any given HR in the specified range. Plot your two exercise HRs and the corresponding VO_2 values on the graph provided below. Next, draw a line between these two points on the graph and extend the line to 110 and 180 bpm. You now may look up the VO_2 for any HR by finding the desired HR on the Y axis, then going across to the reference line and straight down to the X axis, where you will find the corresponding VO_2 in l/min. To obtain the caloric expenditure in calories per minute, simply multiply the VO_2 by 5. You also may predict your maximal VO_2 (in l/min) by extending the line up to your maximal HR. The maximal HR is estimated by subtracting your age from 220. To convert the maximal VO_2 to ml/kg/min, multiply the l/min value by 1,000 and divide by body weight in kilograms.

Using the results from your lab and the graph below, indicate the VO_2 in l/min and the caloric expenditure at the following HRs:

	VO_2 (l/min)	Caloric Expenditure (calories per minute)
120 bpm		
150 bpm		
170 bpm		

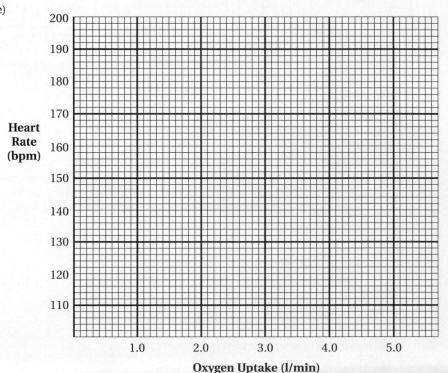

Chapter 8

Principles of Muscular Strength Assessment and Prescription

Objectives

- Understand the importance of adequate strength levels in maintaining good health and well-being.

- Clarify misconceptions about women who engage in strength-training programs.

- Define muscular strength and muscular endurance.

- Be able to assess muscular strength and endurance through two different strength-testing protocols.

- Learn to interpret strength-testing results according to health fitness and physical fitness standards.

- Identify the factors that affect strength.

- Name the different types of muscle fibers.

- Understand the overload principle for strength development.

- Recognize the principles that govern the development of muscular strength and muscular endurance (mode, resistance, sets, and frequency).

- Become acquainted with two distinct strength-training programs.

The evidence of the benefits of strength training in enhancing health and well-being is well documented. Many people, nonetheless, still have the impression that strength is necessary only for highly trained athletes, fitness enthusiasts, and individuals who hold jobs that require heavy muscular work. In fact, a well-planned strength training program leads to increased muscle strength and endurance, muscle tone, tendon and ligament strength, and bone density—all of which help to improve functional physical capacity.

Strength is a basic component of fitness and wellness and is crucial for optimal performance in daily activities such as sitting, walking, running, lifting and carrying objects, doing housework, and enjoying recreational activities. Strength also is of great value in improving posture, personal appearance, and self-image; in developing sports skills; promoting joint stability; and in meeting certain emergencies in life. From a health standpoint, increasing strength helps to increase or maintain muscle and a higher resting metabolic rate, lessens the risk for injury, helps to reduce chronic low-back pain, reduces arthritic pain, aids in childbearing, improves cholesterol levels, and may also help lower blood pressure and control blood sugar.

An important adaptation to strength training is that, with time, the heart rate and blood pressure response to lifting a heavy resistance (that is, a weight) decreases. This adaptation reduces the demands on the cardiovascular system when performing activities such as carrying a child, the groceries, or a suitcase.

Muscular strength may be the most important health-related component of physical fitness in the older adult population. Though proper cardio-respiratory endurance is necessary to help maintain a healthy heart, good strength contributes more to independent living than any other fitness component. Older adults with good strength levels can successfully perform most **activities of daily living**. Strength training helps to slow the age-related loss of muscle function.

More than anything else, older adults want to enjoy good health and function independently. Many of them, however, are confined to nursing homes because they lack sufficient strength to move about. They cannot walk very far, and many have to be helped in and out of beds, chairs, and tubs. Only people with advanced heart disease are advised to refrain from strength training.

A strength-training program can enhance quality of life tremendously. Inactive adults between the ages of 56 and 86 who participated in a 12-week strength-training program increased lean body mass by about 3 pounds, lost about 4 pounds of fat, and increased their resting metabolic rate by almost 7 percent.[1] In other research, leg strength improved by as much as 200 percent in previously inactive adults over age 90.[2] As strength improves, so does the ability to move about, the capacity for independent living, and enjoyment of life during the "golden years." More specifically, good strength enhances quality of life in the following ways:

- It improves balance and restores mobility.
- It makes lifting and reaching easier.
- It decreases the risk for injuries and falls.
- It stresses the bones and preserves bone mineral density, thus decreasing the risk for osteoporosis.

Relationship Between Strength and Metabolism

Perhaps one of the most significant benefits of maintaining a good strength level is its relationship to human **metabolism**. A primary outcome of a strength-training program is an increase in muscle mass or size (lean body mass), known as muscle **hypertrophy**.

Muscle tissue uses energy even at rest. In contrast, fatty tissue uses little energy and may be considered metabolically inert from the standpoint of caloric use (that is, unlike muscle, your body expends very few calories to maintain fat). As muscle size increases, so does **resting metabolism**. Even small increases in muscle mass may improve resting metabolism.

Each additional pound of muscle tissue increases resting metabolism by 35 calories per day.[3] All other factors being equal, if two individuals both weigh 150 pounds but have different amounts of muscle mass—let's say 5 pounds—the one with more muscle mass will have a higher resting metabolic rate, allowing this person to ingest more calories (which will be used to maintain the muscle tissue, not to create fat). Briefly, the higher your metabolic rate, the more you can eat without gaining fat.

Loss of lean tissue is also thought to be the main reason for the decrease in metabolism as people grow older. Contrary to some beliefs, metabolism does not have to slow down significantly with aging. It is not so much that metabolism slows down. It's that we slow down.

Lean body mass decreases with sedentary living, which, in turn, slows down the resting metabolic rate. If people continue eating at the same rate, body fat increases. The average decrease in resting metabolism from age 26 to age 60 is about 360 calories per day.[4] Hence, participating in a strength-training program is important in preventing and reducing excess body fat.

Gender Differences

One of the most common misconceptions about physical fitness is related to women and strength training. Because of the increase in muscle mass typically seen in men, some women think that a strength training program will be counterproductive because they, too, will develop large musculature. Even though the quality of muscle in men and women is the same, endocrinological differences do not allow women to achieve the same amount of muscle hypertrophy (size) as men. Men also have more muscle fibers and, because of the male sex-specific hormones, each individual fiber has more potential for hypertrophy.

The idea that strength training allows women to develop muscle hypertrophy to the same extent as men do is as false as the notion that playing basketball will turn women into giants. Masculinity and femininity are established by genetic inheritance, not by the amount of physical activity. Variations in the extent of masculinity and femininity are determined by individual differences in hormonal secretions of androgen, testosterone, estrogen, and progesterone. Women with a bigger-than-average build often are inclined to participate in sports because of their natural physical advantage. As a result, many women have associated participation in sports and strength training with large muscle size.

As the number of females who participate in sports has increased steadily during the last few years, the myth that strength training in women leads to large increases in muscle size has abated somewhat. For example, per pound of body weight, female gymnasts are considered among the strongest athletes in the world. These athletes engage regularly in serious strength-training programs. Yet, female gymnasts have some of the most well-toned and graceful figures of all women.

Improved body appearance is the rule rather than the exception for women who participate in strength-training programs.

In recent years improved body appearance has become the rule rather than the exception for women who participate in strength-training programs. Some of the most attractive female movie stars also train with weights to further improve their personal image.

Nonetheless, you may ask, "If weight training does not masculinize women, why do so many women body builders develop such heavy musculature?" In the sport of body building, the athletes follow intense training routines consisting of two or more hours of constant weight lifting with short rest intervals between sets. Many body-building training routines call for back-to-back exercises using the same muscle groups. The objective of this type of training is to pump extra blood into the muscles. This additional fluid makes the muscles appear much bigger than they do in a resting condition. Based on the intensity and the length of the training session, the muscles can remain filled with blood, appearing measurably larger for several hours after completing the training session. Therefore, in real life, these women are not as muscular as they seem when they are participating in a contest.

In the sport of body building, a big point of controversy is the use of **anabolic steroids** and human growth hormones, even among women participants. These hormones, however, produce detrimental and undesirable side effects (such as hypertension, fluid retention, decreased breast size, deepening of the voice, facial whiskers, and atypical body hair growth), which some women deem tolerable. Anabolic steroid use in general—except for medical reasons and when carefully monitored by a physician—can lead to serious health consequences.

Anabolic steroid use among female body builders is widespread. According to several sports medicine physicians and female body builders, about 80 percent of female body builders have used steroids. Furthermore, according to several female track-and-field coaches, as many as 95 percent of female athletes around the world in this sport have used anabolic steroids to remain competitive at the international level.

Women who take steroids undoubtedly will build heavy musculature and, if they take the steroids long enough, the steroids will produce masculinizing effects. As a result, the International Federation of Body Building instituted a mandatory steroid-testing program for females participating in the Miss Olympia contest. When drugs are not used to promote development, improved body image is

Activities of daily living Everyday behaviors that people normally do to function in life (cross the street, carry groceries, lift objects, do laundry, sweep floors).

Metabolism All energy and material transformations that occur within living cells; necessary to sustain life.

Hypertrophy An increase in the size of the cell (for example, muscle hypertrophy).

Resting metabolism Amount of energy (expressed in milliliters of oxygen per minute or total calories per day) an individual requires during resting conditions to sustain proper body function.

Anabolic steroids Synthetic versions of the male sex hormone testosterone, which promotes muscle development and hypertrophy.

SELECTED DETRIMENTAL EFFECTS OF ANABOLIC STEROID USE

- Liver tumors
- Hepatitis
- Hypertension
- Reduction of high-density lipoprotein (HDL) cholesterol
- Elevation of low-density lipoprotein (LDL) cholesterol
- Hyperinsulinism
- Impaired pituitary function
- Impaired thyroid function
- Mood swings
- Aggressive behavior
- Increased irritability
- Acne
- Fluid retention
- Decreased libido
- HIV infection (via injectable steroids)
- Prostate problems (men)
- Testicular atrophy (men)
- Reduced sperm count (men)
- Clitoral enlargement (women)
- Decreased breast size (women)
- Increased body and facial hair (nonreversible in women)
- Deepening of the voice (nonreversible in women)

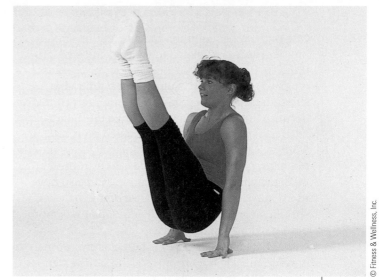

Female gymnast performs a strength skill.

the rule rather than the exception among females who participate in body building, strength training, or sports in general.

Changes in Body Composition

Another benefit of strength training, accentuated even more when combined with aerobic exercise, is a decrease in adipose or fatty tissue around muscle fibers themselves. The decrease in fatty tissue often is greater than the amount of muscle hypertrophy (see Figure 8.1). Therefore, losing inches but not body weight is common.

Because muscle tissue is more dense than fatty tissue (and despite the fact that inches are lost during a combined strength-training and aerobic program), people, especially women, often become discouraged because they cannot see the results readily on the scale. They can offset this discouragement by determining body composition regularly to monitor changes in percent body fat rather than simply measuring changes in total body weight (see Chapter 4).

Assessment of Muscular Strength and Endurance

Although muscular strength and endurance are interrelated, they do differ. **Muscular strength** is the ability to exert maximum force against resistance. **Muscular endurance** is the ability of a muscle to exert submaximal force repeatedly over time.

Muscular endurance (also referred to as "localized muscular endurance") depends to a large extent on muscular strength. Weak muscles cannot repeat an action several times or sustain it. Based upon these principles, strength tests and training programs have been designed to measure and develop absolute muscular strength, muscular endurance, or a combination of the two.

Muscular strength is usually determined by the maximal amount of resistance (weight)—**one repetition maximum**, or 1 RM—an individual is able to lift in a single effort. Although this assessment yields a good measure of absolute strength, it does require a considerable amount of time, because the 1 RM is determined through trial and error. For example, strength of the chest muscles is frequently measured through the bench press exercise. If an individual has not trained with weights, he may try 100 pounds and lift this resistance quite easily. After adding 50 pounds, he fails to lift the resistance. The resistance then is decreased by 10 or 20 pounds. Finally, after several trials, the 1 RM is established.

A true 1 RM might be difficult to obtain the first time an individual is tested, because fatigue becomes a factor. By the time the 1 RM is established, the person has already made several maximal or near-maximal attempts.

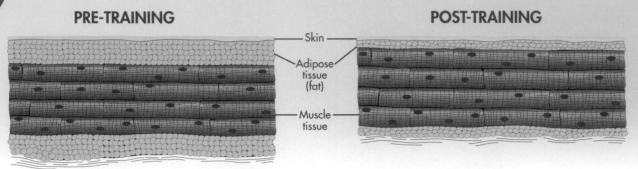

Figure 8.1

Changes in body composition as a result of a combined aerobic and strength-training program.

PRE-TRAINING   POST-TRAINING

Skin
Adipose tissue (fat)
Muscle tissue

Muscular endurance is typically established by the number of repetitions an individual can perform against a submaximal resistance or by the length of time a given contraction can be sustained. For example: How many push-ups can an individual do? Or how many times can she lift 30 pounds? Or how long can a person hold a chin-up?

In strength testing, several body sites should be assessed. Because different body parts have different strength levels, no single strength test provides a good assessment of overall body strength. As a minimum, a strength profile should include the upper body, the lower body, and the abdominal muscles.

If time is a factor and only one test item can be done, the Hand Grip Test, described in Figure 8.2, is commonly used to assess strength. This test, though, provides only a weak correlation with overall body strength.

For the most accurate assessment, use procedures in Figures 8.2, 8.3, and 8.4. Lab 8A also provides the opportunity to assess your own level of muscular strength or endurance with the three tests. You may take one or more of these tests according to your time and the facilities available.

Muscular strength and endurance are both highly specific. A high degree of strength or endurance in one body part does not necessarily indicate this is the case in other parts. Accordingly, exercises for the strength tests were selected to obtain a profile including the upper body, lower body, and abdominal regions.

Before taking the strength test, you should become familiar with the procedures for the respective tests. For safety reasons, always take a friend or group of friends with you whenever you train with weights or conduct any type of strength assessment. Also, these are different tests, so to make valid comparisons, the same test should be used for pre- and post-assessments. The following are your options.

Hand Grip Test

As indicated earlier, when time is a factor, the Hand Grip Test can be used to provide a rough estimate of strength. Unlike the next two tests, this is an isometric (static contraction) test. If the proper grip is used, no finger or body movement is visible during the test. The test procedure is given in Figure 8.2, and percentile ranks based on your results are provided in Table 8.1. The results of this test can be recorded in Lab 8A.

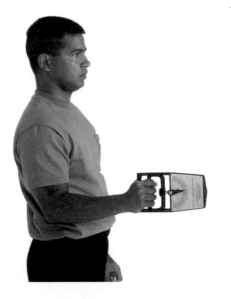

The hand grip tests strength.

© Fitness & Wellness, Inc.

Muscular strength The ability of a muscle to exert maximum force against resistance (for example, 1 repetition maximum [or 1 RM] of the bench press exercise).

Muscular endurance The ability of a muscle to exert submaximal force repeatedly over time.

One repetition maximum (1 RM) The maximum amount of resistance an individual is able to lift in a single effort.

Figure
8.2
Procedure for the Hand Grip Strength Test.

1. Adjust the width of the dynamometer* so the middle bones of your fingers rest on the distant end of the dynamometer grip.

2. Use your dominant hand for this test. Place your elbow at a 90° angle and about 2 inches away from the body.

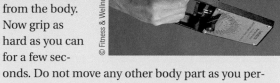

3. Now grip as hard as you can for a few seconds. Do not move any other body part as you perform the test (do not flex or extend the elbow, do not move the elbow away or toward the body, and do not lean forward or backward during the test).

4. Record the dynamometer reading in pounds (if reading is in kilograms, multiply by 2.2046).

5. Three trials are allowed for this test. Use the highest reading for your final test score. Look up your percentile rank for this test in Table 8.1.

6. Based on your percentile rank, obtain the hand grip strength fitness category according to the following guidelines:

Percentile Rank	Fitness Classification
≥81	Excellent
61–80	Good
41–60	Average
21–40	Fair
≤20	Poor

* A Lafayette model 78010 dynamometer is recommended for this test (Lafayette Instruments Co., Sagamore and North 9th Street, Lafayette, IN 47903).

Table
8.1

Scoring Table for Hand Grip Strength Test

Percentile Rank	MEN	WOMEN
99	153	101
95	145	94
90	141	91
80	139	86
70	132	80
60	124	78
50	122	74
40	114	71
30	110	66
20	100	64
10	91	60
5	76	58

 High physical fitness standard

Health fitness standard

Changes in strength may be more difficult to evaluate with this test. Most strength-training programs are dynamic in nature (body segments are moved through a range of motion), whereas this test provides an isometric assessment. Further, grip strength exercises are seldom used in strength training, and increases in strength are specific to the body parts exercised. This test also can be used to supplement the following strength tests.

Muscular Endurance Test

Three exercises were selected to assess the endurance of the upper body, lower body, and mid-body muscle groups (see Figure 8.3). The advantage of this test is that it does not require strength-training equipment—only a stopwatch, a metronome, a bench or gymnasium bleacher 16¼" high, a cardboard strip 3½" wide by 30" long, and a partner. A percentile rank is given for each exercise according to the number of repetitions performed (see Table 8.2). An overall endurance rating can be obtained by totaling the number of points obtained on each exercise. Record the results of this test in Lab 8A.

Figure 8.3 Muscular Endurance Test.

Three exercises are conducted on this test: bench-jumps, modified dips (men) or modified push-ups (women), and bent-leg curl-ups or abdominal crunches. All exercises should be conducted with the aid of a partner. The correct procedure for performing each exercise is as follows:

Bench-jump. Using a bench or gymnasium bleacher 16¼" high, attempt to jump up and down the bench as many times as possible in 1 minute. If you cannot jump the full minute, you may step up and down. A repetition is counted each time both feet return to the floor.

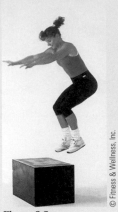

Figure 8.3a Bench jump

Modified dip. Men only: Using a bench or gymnasium bleacher, place the hands on the bench with the fingers pointing forward. Have a partner hold your feet in front of you. Bend the hips at approximately 90° (you also may use three sturdy chairs, put your hands on two chairs placed by the sides of your body, and place your feet on the third chair in front of you). Lower your body by flexing the elbows until they reach a 90° angle, then return to the starting position (also see Exercise 6, page 224). Perform the repetitions to a two-step cadence (down-up) regulated with a metronome set at 56 beats per minute. Perform as many continuous repetitions as possible. Do not count any more repetitions if you fail to follow the metronome cadence.

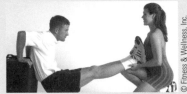

Figure 8.3b Modified dip

Modified push-up. Women: Lie down on the floor (face down), bend the knees (feet up in the air), and place the hands on the floor by the shoulders with the fingers pointing forward. The lower body will be supported at the knees (as opposed to the feet) throughout the test (see Figure 8.3c). The chest must touch the floor on each repetition. As with the modified-dip exercise (above), perform the repetitions to a two-step cadence (up-down) regulated with a metronome set at 56 beats per minute. Perform as many continuous repetitions as possible. Do not count any more repetitions if you fail to follow the metronome cadence.

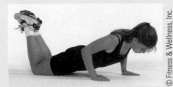

Figure 8.3c Modified push-up

Bent-leg curl-up. Lie down on the floor (face up) and bend both legs at the knees at approximately 100°. The feet should be on the floor, and you must hold them in place yourself throughout the test. Cross the arms in front of the chest, each hand on the opposite shoulder. Now raise the head off the floor, placing the chin against the chest. This is the starting and finishing position for each curl-up (see Figure 8.3d). **The back of the head may not come in contact**

with the floor, the hands cannot be removed from the shoulders, nor may the feet or hips be raised off the floor at any time during the test. The test is terminated if any of these four conditions occur. When you curl up, the upper body must come to an upright position before going back down (see Figure 8.3e). The repetitions are performed to a two-step cadence (up-down) regulated with the metronome set at 40 beats per minute. For this exercise, you should allow a brief practice period of 5 to 10 seconds to familiarize yourself with the cadence (the *up* movement is initiated with the

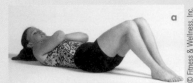

Figure 8.3d Bent-leg curl-up

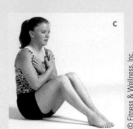

Figure 8.3e Bent-leg curl-up

first beat, then you must wait for the next beat to initiate the *down* movement; one repetition is accomplished every two beats of the metronome). Count as many repetitions as you are able to perform following the proper cadence. The test is also terminated if you fail to maintain the appropriate cadence or if you accomplish 100 repetitions. Have your partner check the angle at the knees throughout the test to make sure to maintain the 100° angle as close as possible.

Abdominal crunch. This test is recommended only for individuals who are unable to perform the bent-leg curl-up test because susceptibility to low-back injury. Exercise form must be carefully monitored during the test. Several authors and researchers have indicated that proper form during this test is extremely difficult to control. Subjects often slide their bodies, bend their elbows, or shrug their shoulders during the test. Such actions facilitate the performance of the test and misrepresent the actual test results. Biomechanical factors also limit the ability to perform this test. Further, lack of spinal flexibility keeps some individuals from being able to move the full 3½" range of motion. Others are unable to keep their heels on the floor during the test. The validity of this test as an effective measure of abdominal strength or abdominal endurance has also been questioned in recent research.

Tape a 3½" × 30" strip of cardboard onto the floor. Lie down on the floor in a supine position (face up) with the knees bent at approximately 100° and the legs slightly apart. The feet should be on the floor, and you must hold them in place yourself throughout the test. Straighten out your arms and place them on the floor alongside the trunk with the palms down and the fingers fully extended. The fingertips of both hands should barely touch the closest edge of the cardboard (see Figure 8.3f). Bring the head off the floor until the chin is 1" to 2" away from your chest. Keep the

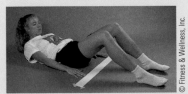

Figure 8.3f Abdominal crunch test

(Continued)

Figure 8.3 (Continued)

head in this position during the entire test (do not move the head by flexing or extending the neck). You are now ready to begin the test.

Perform the repetitions to a two-step cadence (up–down) regulated with a metronome set at 60 beats per minute. As you curl up, slide the fingers over the cardboard until the fingertips reach the far edge (3½") of the board (see Figure 8.3g), then return to the starting position.

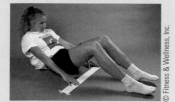

Allow a brief practice period of 5 to 10 seconds to familiarize yourself with the cadence. Initiate the *up* movement with the first beat and the *down* movement with the next beat. Accomplish one repetition every two beats of the metronome. Count as many repetitions as you are able to perform following the proper cadence. You may not count a repetition if the fingertips fail to reach the distant edge of the cardboard.

Figure 8.3g Abdominal crunch test

Terminate the test if you (a) fail to maintain the appropriate cadence, (b) bend the elbows, (c) shrug the shoulders, (d) slide the body, (e) lift heels off the floor, (f) raise the chin off the chest, (g) accomplish 100 repetitions, or (h) no longer can perform the test. Have your partner check the angle at the knees throughout the test to make sure that the 100° angle is maintained as close as possible.

For this test you may also use a Crunch-Ster Curl-Up Tester, available from Novel Products.* An illustration of the test performed with this equipment is provided in Figures 8.3h and 8.3i.

According to the results, look up your percentile rank for each exercise in the far left column of Table 8.2 and determine your

* Novel Products, Inc. Figure Finder Collection. P.O. Box 408, Rockton, IL 61072-0408. 1-800-323-5143, Fax 815-624-4866.

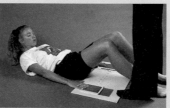
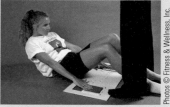

Figure 8.3h   **Figure 8.3i**
Abdominal crunch test performed with a Crunch-ster curl-up tester.

muscular endurance fitness category according to the following classification:

Average Score	Fitness Category	Points
≥90	Excellent	5
70–80	Good	4
50–60	Average	3
30–40	Fair	2
≤20	Poor	1

Look up the number of points assigned for each fitness category above. Total the number of points and determine your overall strength endurance fitness category according to the following ratings:

Total Points	Strength Endurance Category
≥13	Excellent
10–12	Good
7–9	Average
4–6	Fair
≤3	Poor

Table 8.2 Muscular Endurance Scoring Table

Percentile Rank	MEN Bench Jumps	MEN Modified Dips	MEN Bent-Leg Curl-Ups	MEN Abdominal Crunches	WOMEN Bench Jumps	WOMEN Modified Push-ups	WOMEN Bent-Leg Curl-Ups	WOMEN Abdominal Crunches
99	66	54	100	100	58	95	100	100
95	63	50	81	100	54	70	100	100
90	62	38	65	100	52	50	97	69
80	58	32	51	66	48	41	77	49
70	57	30	44	45	44	38	57	37
60	56	27	31	38	42	33	45	34
50	54	26	28	33	39	30	37	31
40	51	23	25	29	38	28	28	27
30	48	20	22	26	36	25	22	24
20	47	17	17	22	32	21	17	21
10	40	11	10	18	28	18	9	15
5	34	7	3	16	26	15	4	0

▨ High physical fitness standard   ▢ Health fitness standard

Muscular Strength and Endurance Test

In this test you will lift a submaximal resistance as many times as possible during six different strength-training exercises. The resistance for each lift is determined according to selected percentages of body weight (see Figure 8.4 and Lab 8A).

With this test, if an individual does only a few repetitions, the test will primarily measure absolute strength. For those who are able to do a lot of repetitions, the test will be an indicator of muscular endurance. If you are not familiar with the different lifts, review the illustrations on pages 227–234.

Strength/endurance ratings for this test can only be established if the same equipment is used at all times. Unfortunately, a certain resistance (for example, 50 pounds) is seldom the same on two different weight machines (for example, Universal Gym versus Nautilus). Thus no fitness ratings can be established. The industry has no standard calibration procedure for strength equipment. Consequently, if you lift a certain resistance on one machine, you may or may not be able to lift the same amount on a different machine.

Even though no fitness ratings are given, test results can be used to evaluate changes in fitness. For example, you may be able to do 7 repetitions at first attempt, but if you can perform 14 repetitions after 12 weeks of training, that's a measure of improvement. The results for the Muscular Strength and Endurance Test can also be recorded in Lab 8A.

Strength Training Prescription

The capacity of muscle cells to exert force increases and decreases according to the demands placed upon the muscular system. If muscle cells are overloaded beyond their normal use, such as in strength-training programs, the cells increase in size (a condition known as hypertrophy) and strength. If the demands placed on the muscle cells decrease, such as in sedentary living or required rest because of illness or injury, the cells **atrophy** and lose strength. A good level of muscular strength is important to develop and maintain fitness, health, and total well-being.

Factors that Affect Strength

Several physiological factors combine to create muscle contraction and subsequent strength gains: neural stimulation, type of muscle fiber, the overload principle, and specificity of training. Basic knowledge of these concepts is important to understand the principles involved in strength training.

Neural Stimulation

Within the neuromuscular system, single **motor neurons** branch and attach to multiple muscle

Atrophy Decrease in the size of a cell.

Motor neurons Nerves connecting the central nervous system to the muscle.

Figure 8.4 Muscular Strength and Endurance Test.

1. Familiarize yourself with the six lifts used for this test: lat pull-down, leg extension, bench press, bent-leg curl-up or abdominal crunch,* leg curl, and arm curl. Graphic illustrations for each lift are given on pages 230, 231, 227, 224, 229, and 228, respectively. For the leg curl exercise, the knees should be flexed to 90°. A description and illustration of the bent-leg curl-up and the abdominal crunch exercises is provided in Figure 8.3. For the lateral pull-down exercise, use a sitting position and have your partner hold you down by the waist or shoulders. On the leg extension lift, maintain the trunk in an upright position.
2. Determine your body weight in pounds.
3. Determine the amount of resistance to be used on each lift. To obtain this number, multiply your body weight by the percent given below for each lift.

Lift	Percent of Body Weight	
	MEN	WOMEN
Lat Pull-Down	.70	.45
Leg Extension	.65	.50
Bench Press	.75	.45
Bent-Leg Curl-Up or Abdominal Crunch*	NA**	NA**
Leg Curl	.32	.25
Arm Curl	.35	.18

 * The abdominal crunch exercise should be used only by individuals who suffer or are susceptible to low-back pain.
 ** NA = not applicable — see Figure 8.3

4. Perform the maximum continuous number of repetitions possible. Record these results in Lab 8A.

fibers. The motor neuron and the fibers it innervates (supplies with nerves) form a **motor unit**. The number of fibers a motor neuron can innervate varies from just a few in muscles that require precise control (eye muscles, for example) to as many as 1,000 or more in large muscles that do not perform refined or precise movements.

Stimulation of a motor neuron causes the muscle fibers to contract maximally or not at all. Variations in the number of fibers innervated and the frequency of their stimulation determine the strength of the muscle contraction. As the number of fibers innervated and frequency of stimulation increases, so does the strength of the muscular contraction.

> *Muscular strength seems to be the most important health-related component of physical fitness in the older adult population.*

Types of Muscle Fiber

The human body has two basic types of muscle fibers: (a) **slow-twitch** or red fibers and (b) **fast-twitch** or white fibers. Slow-twitch fibers have a greater capacity for aerobic work. Fast-twitch fibers have a greater capacity for anaerobic work and produce more overall force. The latter are important for quick and powerful movements commonly used in strength training activities.

The proportion of slow- and fast-twitch fibers is determined genetically, and consequently varies from one person to another. Nevertheless, training increases the functional capacity of both types of fiber and, more specifically, strength training increases their ability to exert force.

During muscular contraction, slow-twitch fibers always are recruited first. As the force and speed of muscle contraction increase, the relative importance of the fast-twitch fibers increases. To activate the fast-twitch fibers, an activity must be intense and powerful.

Overload Principle

Strength gains are achieved in two ways:

1. Through increased ability of individual muscle fibers to generate a stronger contraction.
2. By recruiting a greater proportion of the total available fibers for each contraction.

These two factors combine in the **overload principle**. The demands placed on the muscle must be increased systematically and progressively over time, and the resistance must be of a magnitude significant enough to cause physiological adaptation. In simpler terms, just like all other organs and systems of the human body, to increase in physical capacity, muscles have to be taxed repeatedly beyond their accustomed loads. Because of this principle, strength training also is called "progressive resistance training."

Specificity of Training

The principle of **specificity of training** states that, for a muscle to increase in strength or endurance, the training program must be specific to obtain the desired effects (also see discussion on Resistance on page 213).

Principles Involved in Strength Training

Because muscular strength and endurance are important in developing and maintaining overall fitness and well-being, the principles necessary to develop a strength-training program have to be followed, as in the prescription for cardiorespiratory exercise. These principles are mode of training, resistance, sets, and frequency of training.

Mode of Training

Two types of training methods are used to improve strength: isometric (static) and dynamic (previously called "isotonic"). In isometric training, muscle contractions produce little or no movement, such as pushing or pulling against an immovable object. In dynamic training, the muscle contractions produce movement, such as extending the knees with resistance on the ankles (leg extension exercise). The

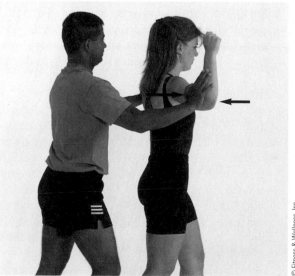

In isometric training, muscle contraction produces little or no movement.

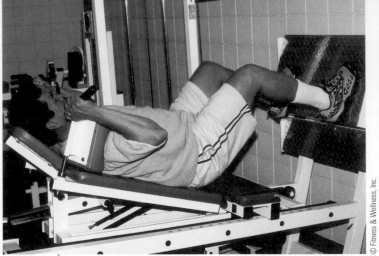

In dynamic training, muscle contraction produces movement in the respective joint.

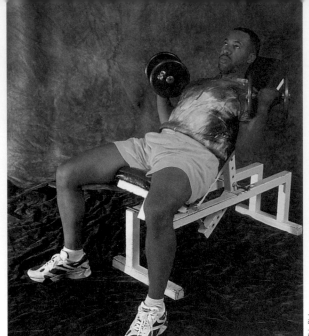

Strength-training can be done using free weights.

specificity of training principle applies here, too. To increase isometric versus dynamic strength, an individual must use static instead of dynamic training to achieve the desired results.

Isometric Training

Isometric training does not require much equipment, but its popularity of several years ago has waned. Because strength gains with isometric training are specific to the angle of muscle contraction, this type of training is beneficial in a sport such as gymnastics, which requires regular static contractions during routines.

Dynamic Training

With **dynamic training** there are two action phases when an exercise is performed: **concentric** or **positive resistance** and **eccentric** or **negative resistance**. In the concentric phase, the muscle shortens as it contracts to overcome the resistance. For example, during the bench press exercise, when the person lifts the resistance from the chest to full-arm extension, the triceps muscle on the back of the upper arm contracts and shortens to extend the elbow. During the eccentric phase, the muscle lengthens as it contracts. In the case of the bench press exercise, the same triceps muscle contracts to lower the resistance during elbow flexion, but the muscle lengthens slowly to avoid dropping the resistance. Both motions work the same muscle against the same resistance.

Eccentric muscle contractions allow us to lower weights in a smooth, gradual, and controlled manner. Without eccentric contractions, weights would be dropped on the way down. Because the same muscles work when you lift and lower a resistance, always be sure to execute both actions in a controlled manner. Failure to do so diminishes the benefits of the training program and increases the risk for injuries.

Dynamic training programs can be conducted without weights, or with exercise bands, **free weights**, **fixed-resistance** machines, variable-resistance machines, and isokinetic equipment. When you perform dynamic exercises without

Motor unit The combination of a motor neuron and the muscle fibers that neuron innervates.

Slow-twitch fibers Muscle fibers with greater aerobic potential and slow speed of contraction.

Fast-twitch fibers Muscle fibers with greater anaerobic potential and fast speed of contraction.

Overload principle Training concept that the demands placed on a system (cardiorespiratory or muscular) must be increased systematically and progressively over time to cause physiological adaptation (development or improvement).

Specificity of training Principle that training must be done with the specific muscle the person is attempting to improve.

Isometric training Strength-training method referring to a muscle contraction that produces little or no movement, such as pushing or pulling against an immovable object.

Dynamic training Strength-training method referring to a muscle contraction with movement.

Concentric Shortening of a muscle during muscle contraction.

Positive resistance The lifting, pushing, or concentric phase of a repetition during the performance of a strength-training exercise.

Eccentric Lengthening of a muscle during muscle contraction.

Negative resistance The lowering or eccentric phase of a repetition during the performance of a strength training exercise.

Free weights Barbells and dumbbells.

Fixed resistance Type of exercise in which a constant resistance is moved through a joint's full range of motion.

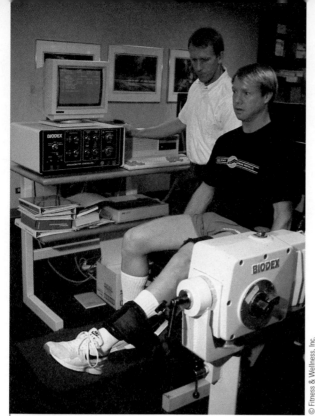

In isokinetic training, the speed of muscle contraction is constant.

© Fitness & Wellness, Inc.

weights (for example, pull-ups and push-ups), with free weights, or with fixed-resistance machines, you move a constant resistance through a joint's full **range of motion**. The greatest resistance that can be lifted equals the maximum weight that can be moved at the weakest angle of the joint. This is because of changes in muscle length and angle of pull as the joint moves through its range of motion.

As strength training became more popular, new strength-training machines were developed. This technology brought about **isokinetic training** and **variable-resistance training** programs, which require special machines equipped with mechanical devices that provide differing amounts of resistance, with the intent of overloading the muscle group maximally through the entire range of motion. A distinction of isokinetic training is that the speed of the muscle contraction is kept constant because the machine provides resistance to match the user's force through the range of motion. The mode of training an individual selects depends mainly on the type of equipment available and the specific objective the training program is attempting to accomplish.

Dynamic training is the most popular mode for strength training. The primary advantage is that strength is gained through the full range of motion. Most daily activities are dynamic in nature. We are constantly lifting, pushing, and pulling objects, and strength is needed through a complete range of motion. Another advantage is that improvements are measured easily by the amount lifted.

The benefits of isokinetic and variable-resistance training are similar to the other dynamic training methods. Theoretically, strength gains should be better because maximum resistance is applied at all angles. Research, however, has not shown this type of training to be more effective than other modes of dynamic training. A possible advantage, though, is that specific speeds used in various sport skills can be duplicated more closely with isokinetic strength training, which may enhance performance (specificity of training). A disadvantage is that the equipment is not readily available to many people.

Free Weights Versus Machines in Dynamic Training

Plate-loaded barbells (free weights) were the most popular weight training equipment available during the first half of the twentieth century. Strength-training machines were developed in the middle of the century, but did not become popular until the 1970s. With subsequent technological improvements on these machines, a stirring debate surfaced over which of the two training modalities was better.

Free weights require that the individual balance the resistance through the entire lifting motion. Thus, a logical assumption could be made that free weights are a better training modality because of the involvement of additional stabilizing muscles needed to balance the resistance as it is moved through its range of motion. Research studies, however, have not shown any differences in strength development between the two exercise modalities.[5] Although there are pros and cons to each modality, muscles do not know whether the source of a resistance is a barbell, a dumbbell, a Universal Gym machine, a Nautilus machine, or a simple cinder block. What determines the degree of a person's strength development is the quality of the program and the individual's effort during the training program itself—not the type of equipment used.

Advantages of Free Weights Following are the advantages of using free weights over machines in a strength-training program.

1. Cost: Free weights are much less expensive than most exercise machines. On a limited budget, free weights are a better option.
2. Variety: A bar and a few plates can be used to perform many exercises to strengthen most muscles in the body.
3. Portability: Free weights are portable and can be easily moved from one area or station to another.
4. Balance: Free weights require that a person balance the weight through the entire range of

motion. This feature requires the involvement of additional (stabilizing) muscles to keep the weight moving properly.

5. One size fits all: Free weights can be used by people of almost all ages. A drawback of machines is that individuals who are at the extremes in terms of height or limb length often do not fit into the machines. In particular, small women and adolescents are at a disadvantage.

Advantages of Machines Strength training machines have the following advantages over free weights.

1. Safety: Machines are safer because spotters are rarely needed to monitor exercises.
2. Selection: A few exercises—such as hip flexion, hip abduction, leg curls, lat pulldowns, and neck exercises—can be performed only with machines.
3. Variable resistance: Most machines provide variable resistance. Free weights provide only fixed resistance.
4. Isolation: Individual muscles are better isolated with machines because stabilizing muscles are not used to balance the weight during the exercise.
5. Time: Exercising with machines requires less time because the resistance is quickly set using a selector pin instead of having to manually change dumbbells or weight plates on both sides of a barbell.
6. Flexibility: Most machines can provide resistance over a greater range of movement during the exercise, thus contributing to greater flexibility in the joints. For example, a barbell pull-over exercise provides resistance over a range of 100 degrees, whereas a weight machine may allow for as much as 260 degrees.
7. Rehabilitation: Machines are more useful during injury rehabilitation. A knee injury, for instance is practically impossible to rehab using free weights, whereas small loads can be easily selected through a limited range of motion with a weight machine.
8. Skill acquisition: Learning a new exercise movement is faster because the machine controls the direction of the movement.

Resistance

Resistance in strength training is the equivalent of intensity in cardiorespiratory exercise prescription. The amount of resistance, load, or weight lifted, depends on whether the individual is trying to develop muscular strength or muscular endurance.

To stimulate strength development, a resistance of approximately 80 percent of the maximum

capacity (1 RM) is recommended.[6] For example, a person who can press 150 pounds should work with at least 120 pounds (150 × .80). Less than 80 percent will help increase muscular endurance rather than strength.

Because of the time factor involved in constantly determining the 1 RM on each lift to ensure that the person is indeed working above 80 percent, a rule of thumb accepted by many authors and coaches is that individuals should be able to perform more than 3 but no more than 12 repetitions (3 to 12 RM) for adequate strength gains. For example, if a person is training with a resistance of 120 pounds and cannot lift it more than 12 times, the training stimulus (weight) is adequate for development of strength.

Once the person can lift the resistance more than 12 times, the resistance should be increased by 5 to 10 pounds and the person again should build up to 12 repetitions. This is referred to as **progressive resistance training**.

Research on strength indicates that the closer a person trains to the 1 RM, the greater are the strength gains. A disadvantage of working constantly at or near the 1 RM is that it increases the risk for injury.

Highly trained athletes seeking maximum strength development often use 1 to 6 repetitions maximum. Working around 10 repetitions maximum seems to produce the best results in terms of muscular hypertrophy. If training is conducted with more than 12 repetitions, primarily muscular endurance will be developed.

Body builders tend to work with moderate resistance levels (60 to 85 percent of the 1 RM) and perform 8 to 20 repetitions to near-fatigue. A foremost objective of body building is to increase muscle size. Moderate resistance promotes blood flow to the muscles, "pumping up the muscles" (also known as "the pump") and making them look much larger than they do in a rested state.

From a health-fitness point of view, 8 to 12 repetitions maximum are recommended for

Range of motion Entire arc of movement of a given joint.

Isokinetic training Strength-training method in which the speed of the muscle contraction is kept constant because the equipment (machine) provides an accommodating resistance to match the user's force (maximal) through the range of motion.

Variable resistance Training using special machines equipped with mechanical devices that provide differing amounts of resistance through the range of motion.

Resistance Amount of weight that is lifted.

Progressive resistance training A gradual increase of resistance over a period of time.

adequate development. We live in a dynamic world in which muscular strength and endurance are both required to lead an enjoyable life. Therefore, working near a 10-repetition threshold seems to improve overall performance most effectively.

Sets

In strength training, a **set** is the number of repetitions performed for a given exercise. For example, a person lifting 120 pounds eight times has performed one set of 8 repetitions (1 × 8 × 120).

When working with 8 to 12 repetitions maximum, three sets per exercise are recommended. Because of the characteristics of muscle fiber, the number of sets that can be done is limited. As the number of sets increases, so does the amount of muscle fatigue and subsequent recovery time. Therefore, strength gains may be lessened by performing too many sets.

A recommended program for beginners in their first year of training is three heavy sets, up to the maximum number of repetitions, preceded by one or two light warm-up sets using about 50 percent of the 1 RM (no warm-up sets are necessary for subsequent exercises that use the same muscle group). Because of the lower resistances used in body building, four to eight sets can be done for each exercise.

To avoid muscle soreness and stiffness, new participants ought to build up gradually to the three sets of maximal repetitions. This can be done by performing only one set of each exercise with a lighter resistance on the first day, two sets of each exercise on the second day—one light and the second with the regular resistance—and three sets on the third day—one light and two heavy. After that, a person should be able to do all three heavy sets.

The time necessary to recover between sets depends mainly on the resistance used during each set. In strength training, the energy to lift heavy weights is derived primarily from the ATP-CP or phosphagen system (see Chapter 3, "Energy (ATP) Production"). Ten seconds of maximal exercise nearly depletes the CP stores in the exercised muscle(s). These stores are replenished in about 3 minutes of recovery.

Based on this principle, a rest period of about 3 minutes between sets is necessary for people who are trying to maximize their strength gains. Individuals training for health-fitness purposes might allow 2 minutes of rest between sets. Body builders should rest no more than 1 minute to maximize the "pumping" effect. The exercise program will be more time-effective by alternating two or three exercises that require different muscle groups (called "**circuit training**"). In this way, an individual will not have to wait 2 to 3 minutes before proceeding to a new set on a different exercise. For example, the bench

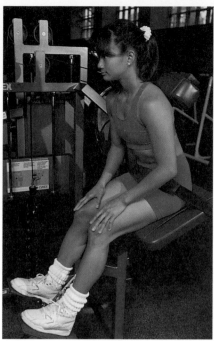

From a health-fitness standpoint, one strength-training session per week is sufficient to maintain strength.

Eric Risberg

press, leg extension, and abdominal curl-up exercises may be combined so the person can go almost directly from one set to the next.

Frequency of Training

Strength training should be done either through a total body workout two to three times a week, or more frequently if using a split-body routine (upper body one day, lower body the next). After a maximum strength workout, the muscles should be rested for about 2 to 3 days to allow adequate recovery. If not completely recovered in 2 to 3 days, the person most likely is overtraining and therefore not reaping the full benefits of the program. In that case, the person should do fewer sets of exercises than in the previous workout. A summary of strength training guidelines for health-fitness purposes is provided in Figure 8.5.

To achieve significant strength gains, a minimum of 8 weeks of consecutive training is necessary. After achieving a recommended strength level, from a health-fitness standpoint, one training session per week will be sufficient to maintain the new strength level. Highly trained athletes will need to train two times per week to maintain their strength level.

Frequency of strength training for body builders varies from person to person. Because they use moderate resistance, daily or even two-a-day workouts are common. The frequency depends on the amount of resistance, number of sets performed per session, and the person's ability to recover from the previous exercise bout (see Table 8.3). The latter often is dictated by level of conditioning.

Figure 8.5 Strength-training guidelines.

Mode:	8 to 10 dynamic strength-training exercises involving the body's major muscle groups
Resistance:	Enough resistance to perform 8 to 12 repetitions to near-fatigue (10 to 15 repetitions for older and more frail individuals)
Sets:	A minimum of 1 set
Frequency:	At least two times per week

Based on "The Recommended Quantity and Quality of Exercise for Developing and Maintaining Cardiorespiratory and Muscular Fitness, and Flexibility in Healthy Adults," *Medicine and Science in Sports and Exercise* 30 (1998): 975–991.

Table 8.3 Guidelines for Various Strength-Training Programs

Strength-Training Program	Resistance	Sets	Rest Between Sets*	Frequency (workouts per week)**
Health fitness	8–12 reps max	3	2 min	2–3
Maximal strength	1–6 reps max	3–6	3 min	2–3
Muscular endurance	10–30 reps	3–6	2 min	3–6
Body building	8–20 reps near max	3–8	0–1 min	4–12

* Recovery between sets can be decreased by alternating exercises that use different muscle groups.

** Weekly training sessions can be increased by using a split-body routine.

Plyometrics

Strength, speed, and explosiveness are all crucial for success in athletics. All three of these factors are enhanced with a progressive resistance training program, but greater increases in speed and explosiveness are thought possible with plyometric exercise. The objective is to generate the greatest amount of force in the shortest time. A sound strength base is necessary before attempting **plyometric exercises**.

Plyometric training is popular in sports that require powerful movements, such as basketball, volleyball, sprinting, jumping, and gymnastics. A typical plyometric exercise involves jumping off and back onto a box, attempting to rebound as quickly as possible on each jump. Box heights are increased progressively from about 12 to 22 inches.

The bounding action attempts to take advantage of the stretch-recoil and stretch reflex characteristics of muscle. The rapid stretch applied to the muscle during contact with the ground is thought to augment muscle contraction, leading to more explosiveness. Plyometrics can be used, too, for strengthening upper body muscles. An example is push-ups with a forceful extension of the arms to drive the hands (and body) completely off the floor during each repetition.

A drawback of plyometric training is its higher risk for injuries compared with conventional modes of progressive resistance training. For instance, the rebound exercise's potential for injury escalates as the box height or the number of repetitions, increases.

Strength-Training Exercises

The two strength-training programs introduced below provide a complete body workout. The major muscles of the human body referred to in the exercises are pointed out in Figure 8.6 (pages 219–220).

Only a minimum of equipment is required for the first program, Strength Training Exercises Without Weights (Exercises 1 through 12). This program can be conducted within your own home. Your body weight is used as the primary resistance for most exercises. A few exercises call for a friend's help or some basic implements from around your house to provide greater resistance.

Strength Training Exercises with Weights (Exercises 13 through 32), require machines such as those shown in the accompanying photographs on pages 227–234. These exercises can be conducted on either fixed-resistance or variable-resistance equipment. Many of these exercises can also be performed with free weights. The first twelve exercises (13 to 24) are recommended to get a complete workout. You can do these exercises as circuit training. If time is a factor, as a minimum, perform the first eight (13 through 20) exercises. Exercises 25 to 32 are supplemental or can be used to replace some of the basic twelve (for instance, substitute Exercise 25 or 26 for 13; 27 for 14; 28 for 17; 29 for 18; 30 for 21; 31 or 32 for 23).

Set A fixed number of repetitions. One set of bench presses might be 10 repetitions.

Circuit training Alternating exercises by performing them in a sequence of three to six or more.

Plyometric exercise Explosive jump training, incorporating speed and strength training to enhance explosiveness.

Exercise Guidelines

As you prepare to design your strength training program, keep the following guidelines in mind:

1. Select exercises that will involve all major muscle groups: chest, shoulders, back, legs, arms, hip, and trunk.
2. Never lift weights alone. Always have someone work out with you in case you need a spotter or help with an injury. When using free weights, one to two spotters are recommended for certain exercises (bench press, squats, overhead press).
3. Warm up properly prior to lifting weights by performing a light- to moderate-intensity aerobic activity (5 to 7 minutes) and some gentle stretches for a few minutes.
4. Exercise larger muscle groups (such as those in the chest, back, and legs) before exercising smaller muscle groups (arms, abdominals, ankles, neck). For example, the bench press exercise works the chest, shoulders, and back of the upper arms (triceps), whereas the triceps extension works the back of the upper arms only.
5. Exercise opposing muscle groups for a balanced workout. When you work the chest (bench press), also work the back (rowing torso). If you work the biceps (arm curl), also work the triceps (triceps extension).
6. Perform all exercises in a controlled manner. Avoid fast and jerky movements and do not throw the entire body into the lifting motion. Failure to do so increases the risk of injury and decreases the effectiveness of the exercise. Do not arch the back when lifting a weight.
7. Perform each exercise through the entire possible range of motion.
8. Breathe naturally. Inhale during the eccentric phase (bringing the weight down) and exhale during the concentric phase (lifting or pushing the weight up). Practice proper breathing with lighter weights when you are learning a new exercise.
9. Avoid holding your breath while straining to lift a weight. Holding your breath greatly increases the pressure inside the chest and abdominal cavity, making it practically impossible for the blood in the veins to return to the heart. Although rare, a sudden high intrathoracic pressure may lead to dizziness, a blackout, a stroke, a heart attack, or a hernia.
10. Based on the program selected, allow adequate recovery time between sets of exercises (see Table 8.3).
11. Discontinue training if you experience unusual discomfort or pain. High tension loads used in strength training can exacerbate potential injuries. Discomfort and pain are signals to stop and determine what's wrong. Be sure to properly evaluate your condition before you continue training.
12. Stretch out for a few minutes at the end of each strength-training workout to help muscles return to their normal resting length and to minimize muscle soreness and risk of injury.

Setting Up Your Own Strength-Training Program

The same pre-exercise guidelines outlined for cardiorespiratory endurance training apply to strength training (see Lab 1B, page 237). If you have any concerns about your present health status or ability to safely participate in strength training, consult a physician before you start. Strength training is not advised for people with advanced heart disease.

Before you proceed to write your strength-training program, you should determine your stage of change for this fitness component in Lab 8B. Next, if you are prepared to do so and depending on the facilities available, you can choose one of the training programs outlined in this chapter. Once you begin your strength-training program, you may use the form provided in Figure 8.7 (page 221) to keep a record of your training sessions.

The resistance and the number of repetitions you use with your program should be based on whether you want to increase muscular strength or muscular endurance. For strength gains, do up to 12 repetitions maximum, and, for muscular endurance, more than 12. For most people, three training sessions per week on nonconsecutive days is an ideal arrangement for proper development.

Because both strength and endurance are required in daily activities, three sets of about 12 repetitions maximum for each exercise are recommended. In doing this, you will obtain good strength gains and yet be close to the endurance threshold. If you are training for reasons other than health fitness, review Table 8.3 for a summary of the guidelines.

Perhaps the only exercise that calls for more than 12 repetitions is the abdominal group of exercises. The abdominal muscles are considered primarily antigravity or postural muscles. Hence, a little more endurance may be required. When doing abdominal work, most people perform about 20 repetitions.

If time is a concern in completing a strength training exercise program, the American College of Sports Medicine[7] recommends as a minimum

(a) one set of 8 to 12 repetitions performed to near-fatigue, and (b) 8 to 10 exercises involving the major muscle groups of the body, conducted twice a week. The recommendation is based on research showing that this training generates 70 to 80 percent of the improvements reported in other programs using three sets of about 10 RM.

Web Interactive

- Strength Training: This site features several types of exercises designed to increase your power and speed, complete with step-by-step instructions and photographs.

  http://www.worldguide.com/Fitness/stex.html

- Muscle Building: Do Andro and Creatine Really Work? A brief description written by the Mayo Clinic, of the benefits, risks, and mostly unknowns about two popular dietary supplements which claim to enhance muscle mass and strength.

  http://mayohealth.org./mayo/9811/htm/muscle.htm

- Health and Fitness Worldguide. This site features exercises that develop muscular strength and endurance, featuring photographs and step-by-step instructions.

  http://www.worldguide.com/Fitness/stex.html

- Ten Tips To Maximize Your Weight Training. This site gives simple tips to have a healthy workout that will best enable to reach your muscle strength and endurance training goals.

  http://www.vitality.com/vfm/weight_train.html

- Comprehensive information about muscle strength exercises, provided by the American Medical Association. This site includes three simple exercises using light weights and six others that do not require weights.

  http://www.ama-assn.org/insight/gen_hlth/trainer/strength.htm

Interactive Sites:

- Strength Training Muscle Map & Explanation. This site provides an anatomical map of the body's muscles. Click on the muscle for exercises designed to specifically strengthen that particular muscle, complete with a video and safety information.

  http://www.global-fitness.com/strength/s_map.html

Notes

1. W. Campbell, M. Crim, V. Young, and W. J. Evans, "Increased Energy Requirements and Changes in Body Composition with Resistance Training in Older Adults," *Journal of Clinical Nutrition* 60 (1994): 167–175.

2. W. J. Evans, "Exercise, Nutrition and Aging," *Journal of Nutrition* 122 (1992): 796–801.

3. W. W. Campbell, M. C. Crim, V. R. Young, and W. J. Evans, "Increased Energy Requirements and Changes in Body Composition with Resistance Training in Older Adults," *American Journal of Clinical Nutrition* 60 (1994): 167–175.

4. P. E. Allsen, *Strength Training* (Dubuque, IA: Kendall/Hunt, 1996).

5. S. P. Messier, and M. Dill, "Alterations in Strength and Maximal Oxygen Uptake Consequent to Nautilus Circuit Weight Training," *Research Quarterly for Exercise and Sport* 56 (1985): 345–351.

T. V. Pipes, "Variable Resistance Versus Constant Resistance Strength Training in Adult Males," *European Journal of Applied Physiology* 39 (1978): 27–35.

6. W. W. K. Hoeger, D. R. Hopkins, S. L. Barette, and D. F. Hale, "Relationship Between Repetitions and Selected Percentages of One Repetition Maximum: A Comparison Between Untrained and Trained Males and Females," *Journal of Applied Sport Science Research* 4, no. 2 (1990): 47–51.

7. "The Recommended Quantity and Quality of Exercise for Developing and Maintaining Cardiorespiratory and Muscular Fitness and Flexibility in Healthy Adults," *Medicine and Science in Sports and Exercise* 30 (1998): 975–991.

Suggested Readings

Allsen, P. E. *Strength Training*. Dubuque, IA: Kendall/Hunt, 1996.

Brzycki, M. "Free Weights and Machines." *Fitness Management* 15 (1999): 36–37, 40.

Foss, M. L., and S. J. Keteyian. *Fox's Physiological Basis for Exercise and Sport*. Boston: WCB McGraw-Hill, 1998.

Hesson, J. L. *Weight Training for Life*. Belmont, CA: Wadsworth/Thomson Learning, 2000.

Heyward, V. H. *Advanced Fitness Assessment & Exercise Prescription*. Champaign, IL: Human Kinetic Press, 1998.

Hoeger, W. W. K., and S. A. Hoeger. *Lifetime Physical Fitness and Wellness*. Belmont, CA: Wadsworth/Thomson Learning, 2000.

Mannie, K. "Barbells Versus Machines: Balancing a Weighty Issue." *Coach and Athletic Director* 67 (1998): 6–7.

McArdle, W. D., F. I. Katch, and V. L. Katch. *Essentials of Exercise Physiology*. Philadelphia: Lippincott Williams & Wilkins, 2000.

Munnings, F. "Strength Training: Not Only for the Young." *Physician and Sportsmedicine* 21 (1993): 133–140.

Wescott, W. L., and T. R. Baechle. *Strength Training for Seniors*. Champaign, IL: Human Kinetic Press, 1999.

Wilmore, J. H., and D. L. Costill. *Physiology of Sport and Exercise*. Champaign, IL: Human Kinetic Press, 1999.

Figure 8.6 Major muscles of the human body.

THE MUSCULAR SYSTEM

Temporalis (closes jaw)

Masseter (flexes and closes jaw)

Sterno-cleido-mastoid (rotates head)

Intercostals (breathing)

Pectoralis minor (abducts ribs)

Biceps brachii (flexes elbow)

Serratus (adducts shoulder)

Rectus abdominus

Deep flexors (flex fingers)

Internal oblique (flattens abdomen)

Tendons from forearm flexors to fingers

Sartorius (rotates thigh)

Rectus femoris (extends knee)

Gastrocnemius (points toe, flexes knee)

Soleus (points toe)

Tendons of toes

Frontalis (raises eyebrow)

Orbicularis oculi (closes eye)

Orbicularis oris (purses lips)

Throat muscles (aid swallowing)

Pectoralis major (adducts arm)

Deltoid (abducts arm)

Brachialis (flexes arm)

External oblique (flattens abdomen)

Superficial flexors (flex fingers)

Vastus lateralis (extends knee)

Vastus medialis (extends knee)

Tibialis anterior (raises feet)

From E. Chaffee and F. Lytle, *Basic Physiology and Anatomy* (Philadelphia: Lippincott Co., 1980). Reproduced by permission.

Figure 8.6   Major muscles of the human body *(continued).*

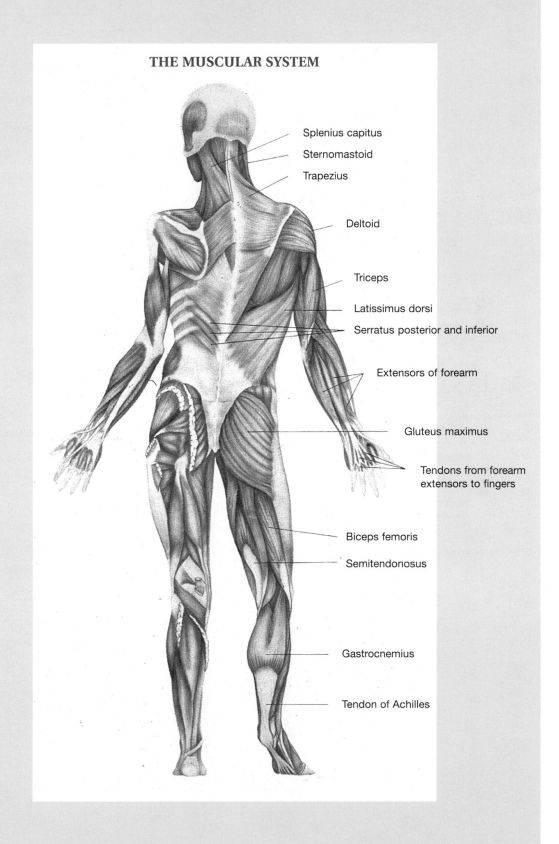

THE MUSCULAR SYSTEM

Splenius capitus

Sternomastoid

Trapezius

Deltoid

Triceps

Latissimus dorsi

Serratus posterior and inferior

Extensors of forearm

Gluteus maximus

Tendons from forearm
extensors to fingers

Biceps femoris

Semitendonosus

Gastrocnemius

Tendon of Achilles

Figure
8.7

Strength training record form.

Name

Date										
Exercise	St/Reps/Res*	St/Reps/Res*	St/Reps/Res*	St/Reps/Res*	St/Reps/Res*	St/Reps/Res*	St/Reps/Res*	St/Reps/Res*	St/Reps/Res*	St/Reps/Res*

*Sets, Repetitions, and Resistance (e.g., 1/6/125 = 1 set of 6 repetitions with 125 pounds)

Figure 8.7

Strength training record form.

Name

Date	Exercise	St/Reps/Res*	St/Reps/Res*	St/Reps/Res*	St/Reps/Res*	St/Reps/Res*	St/Reps/Res*	St/Reps/Res*	St/Reps/Res*	St/Reps/Res*	St/Reps/Res*

*Sets, Repetitions, and Resistance (e.g., 1/6/125 = 1 set of 6 repetitions with 125 pounds)

Strength-Training Exercises without Weights

Exercise 1
Step-Up

Action Step up and down using a box or chair approximately 12 to 15 inches high (a). Conduct one set using the same leg each time you go up, and then conduct a second set using the other leg. You also could alternate legs on each step-up cycle. You may increase the resistance by holding an object in your arms (b). Hold the object close to the body to avoid increased strain in the lower back.

Muscles Developed Gluteal muscles, quadriceps, gastrocnemius, and soleus

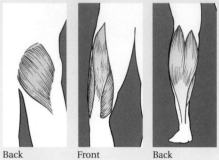

Back   Front   Back

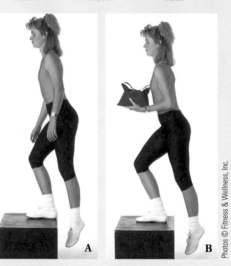

A   B

Photos © Fitness & Wellness, Inc.

Exercise 2
Rowing Torso

Action Raise your arms laterally (abduction) to a horizontal position and bend your elbows to 90°. Have a partner apply enough pressure on your elbows to gradually force your arms forward (horizontal flexion) while you try to resist the pressure. Next, reverse the action, horizontally forcing the arms backward as your partner applies sufficient forward pressure to create resistance.

Muscles Developed Posterior deltoid, rhomboids, and trapezius

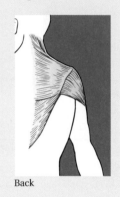

Back

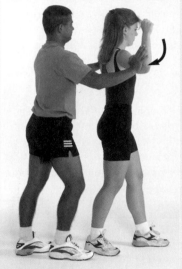

© Fitness & Wellness, Inc.

Exercise 3
Push-Up

Action Maintaining your body as straight as possible (a), flex the elbows, lowering the body until you almost touch the floor (b), then raise yourself back up to the starting position. If you are unable to perform the push-up as indicated, decrease the resistance by supporting the lower body with the knees rather than the feet (c) or using an incline plane and supporting your hands at a higher point than the floor (d). If you wish to increase the resistance, have someone else add resistance to your shoulders as you are coming back up (e).

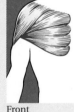 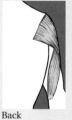 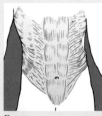

Back   Front   Front

Muscles Developed Triceps, deltoid, pectoralis major, abdominals, and erector spinae

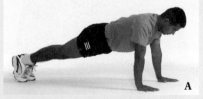

A

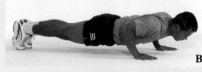

B

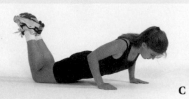

C

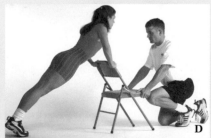

D

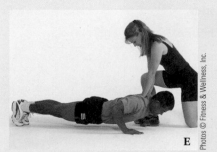

E

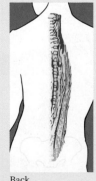

Back

Photos © Fitness & Wellness, Inc.

Exercise 4
Abdominal Crunch and Bent-leg Curl-Up

Action   Start with your head and shoulders off the floor, arms crossed on your chest, and knees slightly bent (a). The greater the flexion of the knee, the more difficult the curl-up. Now curl up to about 30° (abdominal crunch — illustration b) or curl up all the way (abdominal curl-up — illustration c), then return to the starting position without letting the head or shoulders touch the floor or allowing the hips to come off the floor. If you allow the hips to raise off the floor and the head and shoulders to touch the floor, you most likely will "swing up" on the next crunch or curl-up, which minimizes the work of the abdominal muscles. If you cannot curl up with the arms on the chest, place the hands by the side of the hips or even help yourself up by holding on to your thighs (illustrations d and e). Do not perform the sit-up exercise with your legs completely extended, because this will strain the lower back. For additional resistance during the abdominal crunch, have a partner add slight resistance to your shoulders as you "crunch up."

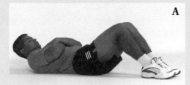
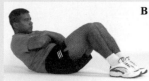
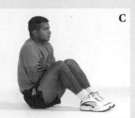
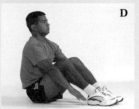

Muscles Developed   Abdominal muscles and hip flexors

Note: The abdominal curl-up exercise should be used only by individuals of at least average fitness without a history of lower back problems. New participants and those with a history of lower back problems should use the abdominal crunch exercise in its place.

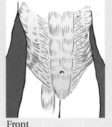
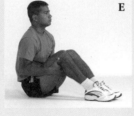

Front

Exercise 5
Leg Curl

Action   Lie on the floor face down. Cross the right ankle over the left heel (a). Apply resistance with your right foot while you bring the left foot up to 90° at the knee joint (b). Apply enough resistance so the left foot can only be brought up slowly. Repeat the exercise, crossing the left ankle over the right heel.

Muscles Developed Hamstrings (and quadriceps)

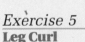
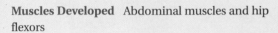

Front   Back

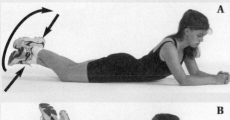
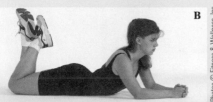

Exercise 6
Modified Dip

Action   Place your hands on two opposite chairs; feet on a third chair with knees slightly bent (make sure that the chairs are well stabilized). Dip down at least to a 90° angle at the elbow joint, then return to the initial position. To increase the resistance, have someone else hold you down by the shoulders on the way up (see illustration c). You may also perform this exercise using a gymnasium bleacher or box and with the help of a partner, as illustrated in photo d.

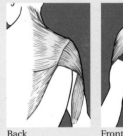
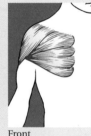

Back   Front

Muscles Developed   Triceps, deltoid, and pectoralis major

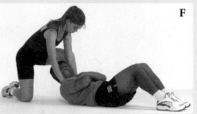
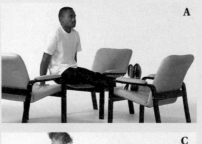
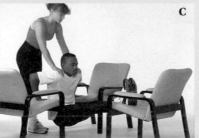
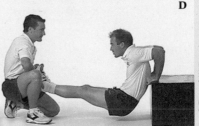
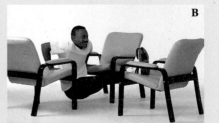
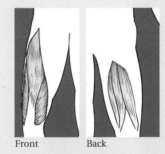
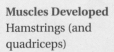

Photos © Fitness & Wellness, Inc.

Exercise 7
Pull-Up

Action   Suspend yourself from a bar with a pronated (thumbs-in) grip (a). Pull your body up until your chin is above the bar (b), then lower the body slowly to the starting position. If you are unable to perform the pull-up as described, either have a partner hold your feet to push off and facilitate the movement upward (illustrations c and d) or use a lower bar and support your feet on the floor (e).

Muscles Developed   Biceps, brachioradialis, brachialis, trapezius, and latissimus dorsi

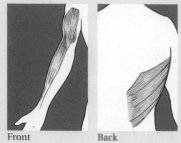

Front   Back

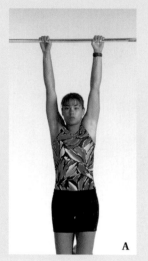
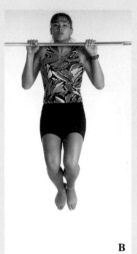
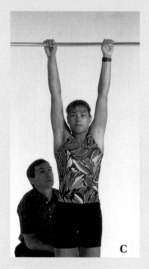
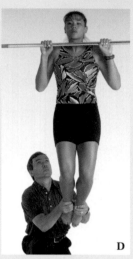
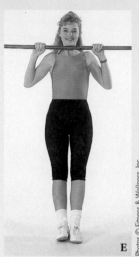

A   B   C   D   E

Photos © Fitness & Wellness, Inc.

Exercise 8
Arm Curl

Action   Using a palms-up grip, start with the arm completely extended and, with the aid of a sandbag or bucket filled (as needed) with sand or rocks (a), curl up as far as possible, (b) then return to the initial position. Repeat the exercise with the other arm.

Muscles Developed   Biceps, brachioradialis, and brachialis

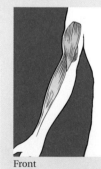

Front

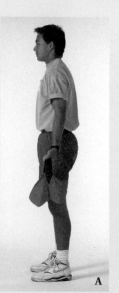
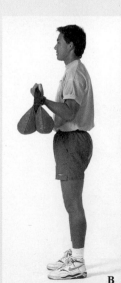

A   B

Photos © Fitness & Wellness, Inc.

Exercise 9
Heel Raise

Action   From a standing position with feet flat on the floor (a), raise and lower your body weight by moving at the ankle joint only (b). For added resistance, have someone else hold your shoulders down as you perform the exercise.

Muscles Developed   Gastrocnemius and soleus

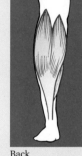

Back

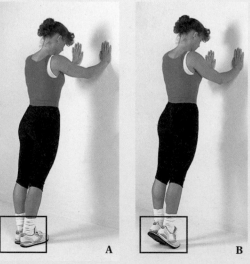

A   B

Photos © Fitness & Wellness, Inc.

Exercise 10
Leg Abduction and Adduction

Action   Both participants sit on the floor. The person on the left places the feet on the inside of the other person's feet. Simultaneously, the person on the left presses the legs laterally (to the outside—abduction), while the person on the right presses the legs medially (adduction). Hold the contraction for 5 to 10 seconds. Repeat the exercise at all three angles, and then reverse the pressing sequence. The person on the left places the feet on the outside and presses inward, while the person on the right presses outward.

Muscles Developed   Hip abductors (rectus femoris, sartori, gluteus medius and minimus) and adductors (pectineus, gracilis, adductor magnus, adductor longus, and adductor brevis)

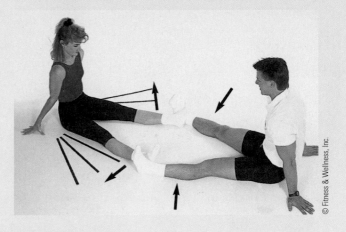

Exercise 11
Reverse Crunch

Action   Lie on your back with arms crossed on your chest and knees and hips flexed at 90° (a). Now attempt to raise the pelvis off the floor by lifting vertically from the knees and lower legs (b). This is a challenging exercise that may be difficult for beginners to perform.

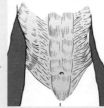

Muscles Developed
Abdominals

Front

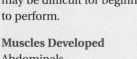

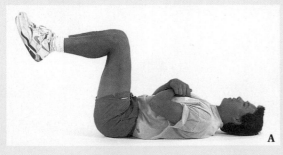

A

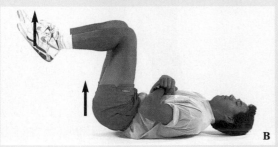

B

Exercise 12
Pelvic Tilt

Action   Lie flat on the floor with the knees bent at about a 90° angle (a). Tilt the pelvis by tightening the abdominal muscles, flattening your back against the floor, and raising the lower gluteal area ever so slightly off the floor (b). Hold the final position for several seconds. The exercise can also be performed against a wall (c).

Front   Back

Areas Stretched   Low back muscles and ligaments

Areas Strengthened   Abdominal and gluteal muscles

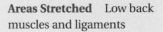

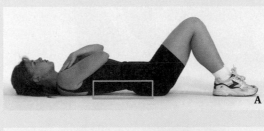

A

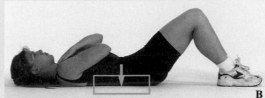

B

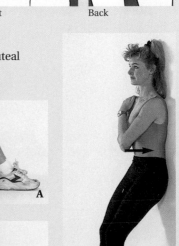

C

Strength-Training Exercises with Weights

Exercise 13
Bench Press

Machine Lie down on the bench with the head by the weight stack, the bench press bar above the chest, and the knees bent so the feet rest on the far end of the bench (a). Grasp the bar handles and press upward until the arms are completely extended (b), then return to the original position. Do not arch the back during this exercise.

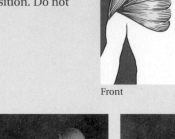

Front   Back

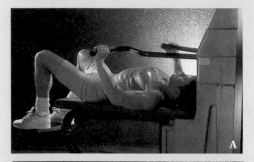

Photos © Nautilus Sports/Medical Industries, Inc.

Muscles Developed Pectoralis major, triceps, and deltoid

Free Weights Lie on the bench with arms extended and have one or two spotters help you place the barbell directly over your shoulders (a). Lower the weight to your chest (b) and then push it back up until you achieve full extension of the arms. Do not arch the back during this exercise.

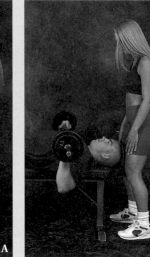

Eric Risberg

Exercise 14
Leg Press

Action From a sitting position with the knees flexed at about 90° and both feet on the footrest (a), extend the legs fully (b), then return slowly to the starting position.

Muscles Developed Quadriceps and gluteal muscles

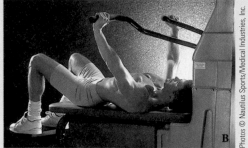

Front   Back

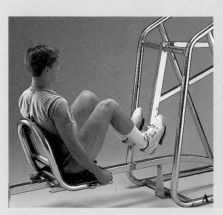

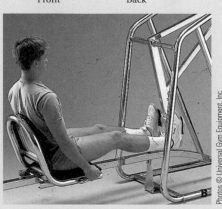

Photos © Universal Gym Equipment, Inc.

Exercise 15
Abdominal Crunch

Action Sit in an upright position. Grasp the handles over your shoulders and crunch forward. Return slowly to the original position.

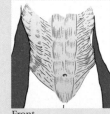

Front

Muscles Developed Abdominals

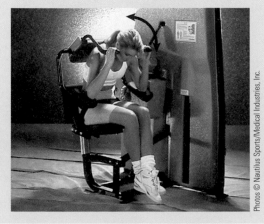

Photos © Nautilus Sports/Medical Industries, Inc.

Exercise 16
Rowing Torso

Action Sit in the machine with your arms in front of you, elbows bent and resting against the padded bars (a). Press back as far as possible, drawing the shoulder blades together (b). Return to the original position.

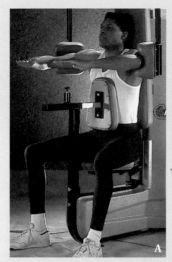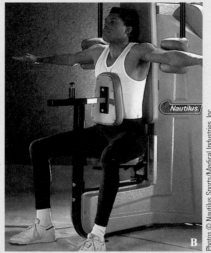

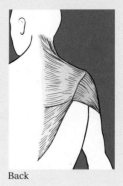

Back

Muscles Developed
Posterior deltoid, rhomboids, and trapezius

Bent-Over Lateral Raise

Action Bend over with your back straight and knees bent at about 5 to 10° (a). Hold one dumbbell in each hand. Raise the dumbbells laterally to about shoulder level (b) and then slowly return them to the starting position.

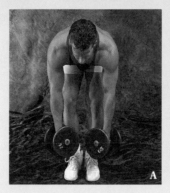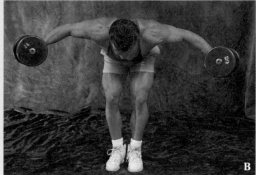

Exercise 17
Arm Curl

Machine Using a supinated or palms-up grip, start with the arms almost completely extended (a). Curl up as far as possible (b), then return to the starting position.

Free Weights Standing upright, hold a barbell in front of you at about shoulder width with arms extended and the hands in a thumbs-out position (supinated grip) (a). Raise the barbell to your shoulders (b) and slowly return it to the starting position.

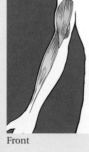

Front

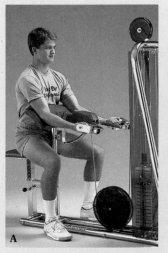

Muscles Developed Biceps, brachioradialis, and brachialis

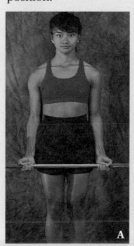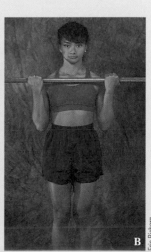

Exercise 18
Leg Curl

Action Lie with the face down on the bench, legs straight, and place the back of the feet under the padded bar (a). Curl up to at least 90° (b), and return to the original position.

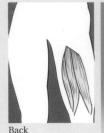

Back

Muscles Developed Hamstrings

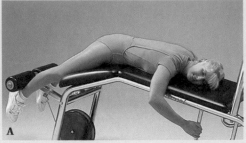

A

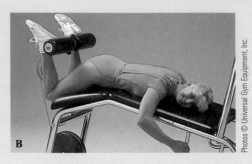

B

Photos © Universal Gym Equipment, Inc.

Exercise 19
Seated Back

Action Sit in the machine with your trunk flexed and the upper back against the shoulder pad. Place the feet under the padded bar and hold on with your hands to the bars on the sides (a). Start the exercise by pressing backward, simultaneously extending the trunk and hip joints (b). Slowly return to the original position.

Muscles Developed Erector spinae and gluteus maximus

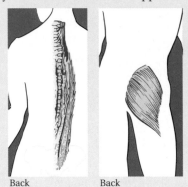

Back   Back

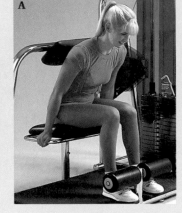

A

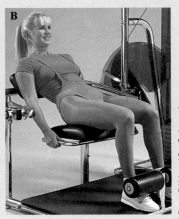

B

Photos © Universal Gym Equipment, Inc.

Exercise 20
Heel Raise

Machine Start with your feet either flat on the floor or the front of the feet on an elevated block (a), then raise and lower yourself by moving at the ankle joint only (b). If additional resistance is needed, you can use a squat strength-training machine.

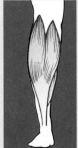

Back

Muscles Developed Gastrocnemius, soleus

Free Weights In a standing position, place a barbell across the shoulders and upper back. Grip the bar away from the shoulders as far out as needed (a). Place the ball of your feet over a weight plate or a small board so that your heels are lower than the front of your feet. Raise your heels off the floor as far as possible (b) and then slowly return them to the starting position.

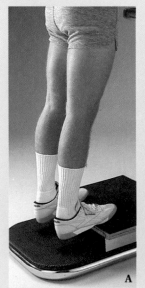

A

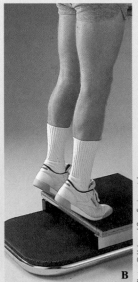

B

Photos © Universal Gym Equipment, Inc.

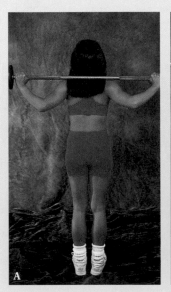

A   B

Eric Risberg

Exercise 21
Lat Pull-Down

Action Starting from a sitting position, hold the exercise bar with a wide grip (a). Pull the bar down in front of you until it reaches the base of the neck (b), then return to the starting position. (If heavy resistance is used, stabilization of the body may be required either by using equipment as shown or by having someone else hold you down by the waist or shoulders.

Muscles Developed Latissimus dorsi, pectoralis major, and biceps

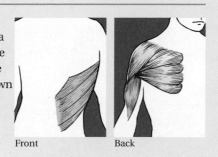

Front   Back

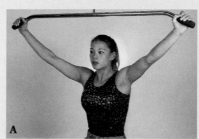

A

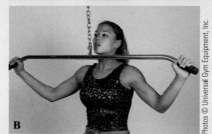

B

Photos © Universal Gym Equipment, Inc.

Exercise 22
Rotary Torso

Machine Sit upright in the machine and place the elbows behind the padded bars. Rotate the torso as far as possible to one side and then return slowly to the starting position. Repeat the exercise to the opposite side.

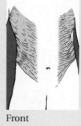

Front

Free Weights Stand with your feet slightly apart. Place a barbell across your shoulders and upper back, holding on to the sides of the barbell. Now gently, and in a controlled manner, twist your torso to one side as far as possible and then do so in the opposite direction.

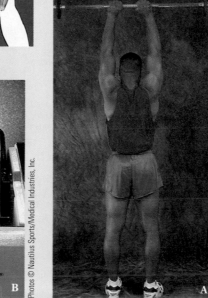

© Fitness & Wellness, Inc.

Photos © Nautilus Sports/Medical Industries, Inc.

Muscles Developed Internal and external obliques (abdominal muscles)

Exercise 23
Triceps Extension

Machine Sit in an upright position, arms up, elbows bent, and place the little finger side of the hands and wrists against the pads, palms of the hands facing each other (a). Fully extend one arm at a time (b), and then return to the original position. Repeat with the other arm.

Muscles Developed Triceps

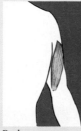

Back

Free Weights In a standing position, hold a barbell with both hands overhead and with the arms in full extension (a). Slowly lower the barbell behind your head (b) and then return it to the starting position.

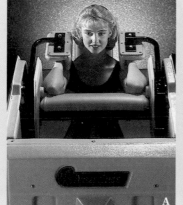

A

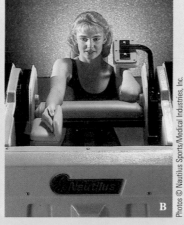

B

Photos © Nautilus Sports/Medical Industries, Inc.

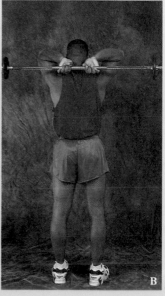

A   B

Eric Risberg

Exercise 24
Leg Extension

Action Sit in an upright position with the feet under the padded bar and grasp the handles at the sides (a). Extend the legs until they are completely straight (b), then return to the starting position.

Muscles Developed
Quadriceps

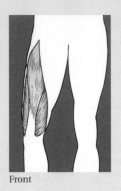

Front

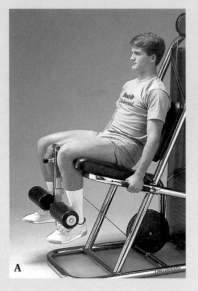

A

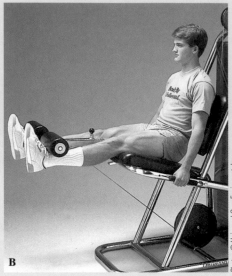

B

Exercise 25
Shoulder Press

Machine Sit in an upright position and grasp the bar wider than shoulder width (a). Press the bar all the way up until the arms are fully extended (b), then return to the initial position.

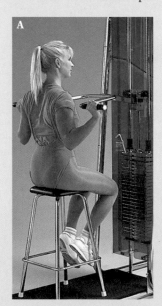

A

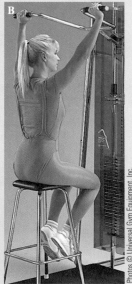

B

Muscles Developed
Triceps, deltoid, and pectoralis major

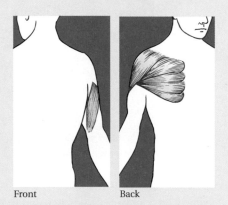

Front   Back

Free Weights Place a barbell on your shoulders in front of the body (a) and press the weight overhead until complete extension of the arms is achieved (b). Then return the weight to the original position. Be sure not to arch the back or lean back during this exercise.

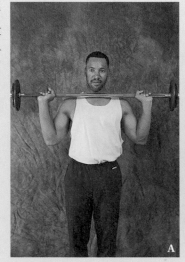

A

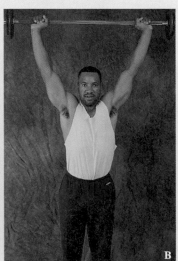

B

Exercise 26
Chest Press

Action Start with the arms up to the side, hands resting against the handle bars, and elbows bent at 90° (a). Press the movement arms forward as far as possible, leading with the elbows (b). Slowly return to the starting position.

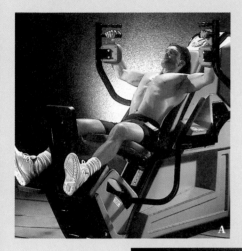

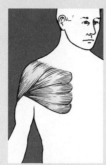

Front

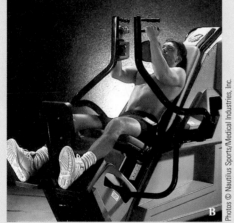

Muscles Developed
Pectoralis major and deltoid

Bent-arm Flyes

Action Lie down on your back on a bench and hold a dumbbell in each hand directly overhead (a). Keeping your elbows slightly bent, lower the weights laterally to a horizontal position (b) and then bring them back up to the starting position.

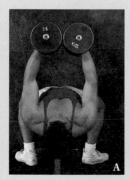

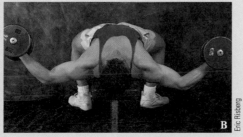

Photos © Nautilus Sports/Medical Industries, Inc.

Eric Risberg

Exercise 27
Squat

Machine Sit in an upright position with the feet under the padded bar and grasp the handles at the sides (a). Extend the legs until they are completely straight (b), then return to the starting position.

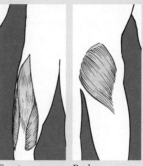

Front   Back

Back

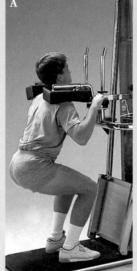 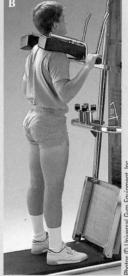

Muscles Developed
Quadriceps, gluteus maximus, erector spinae

Photos © Universal Gym Equipment, Inc.

Free Weights From a standing position, and with a spotter to each side, support a barbell over your shoulders and upper back (a). Keeping your head up and back straight, bend at the knees and the hips until you achieve an approximate 120° angle at the knees (b). Then return to the starting position. *Do not perform this exercise alone.* If no spotters are available, use a squat rack to ensure that you will not get trapped under a heavy weight.

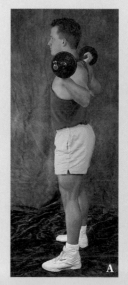

Eric Risberg

Exercise 28
Upright Rowing

Machine Start with the arms extended and grip the handles with the palms down (a). Pull all the way up to the chin (b), then return to the starting position.

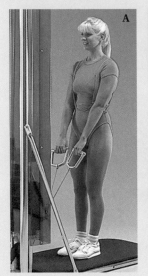
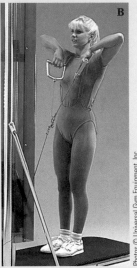

Muscles Developed Biceps, brachioradialis, brachialis, deltoid, and trapezius

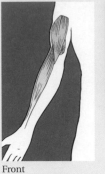
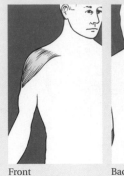
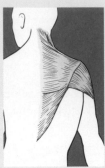

Front   Front   Back

Free Weights Hold a barbell in front of you, with the arms fully extended and hands in a thumbs-in grip (pronated) less than shoulder-width apart (a). Pull the barbell up until it reaches shoulder level (b) and then slowly return it to the starting position.

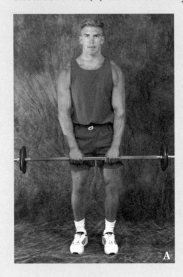
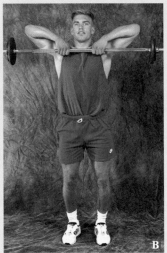

Exercise 29
Seated Leg Curl

Action Sit in the unit and place the strap over the upper thighs. With legs extended, place the back of the feet over the padded rollers (a). Flex the knees until you reach a 90° to 100° angle (b). Slowly return to the starting position.

Muscles Developed
Hamstrings

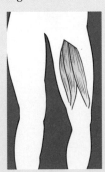

Back

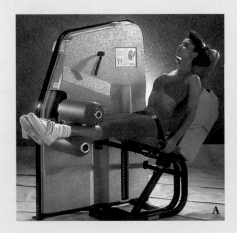
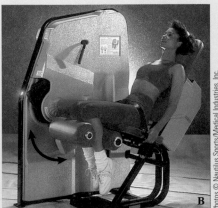

Exercise 30
Bent-arm Pullover

Machine   Sit back into the chair and grasp the bar behind your head (a). Pull the bar over your head all the way down to your abdomen (b) and slowly return to the original position.

Muscles Developed   Latissimus dorsi, pectoral muscles, deltoid, and serratus anterior

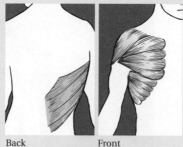

Back   Front

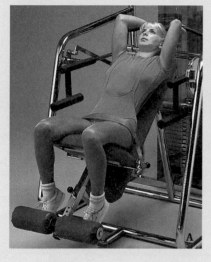

Free Weights   Lie on your back on an exercise bench with the head over the edge of the bench. Hold a barbell over your chest with the hands less than shoulder-width apart (a). Keeping the elbows shoulder-width apart, lower the weight over your head until your shoulders are completely extended (b). Slowly return the weight to the starting position.

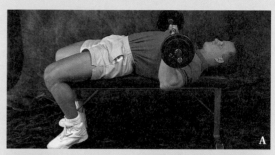

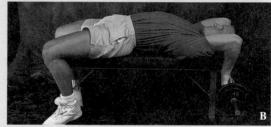

Exercise 31
Triceps Extension

Action   Using a palms-down grip, grasp the bar slightly closer than shoulder width and start with the elbows almost completely bent (a). Extend the arms fully (b), then return to starting position.

Muscles Developed   Triceps

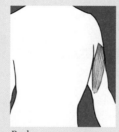

Back

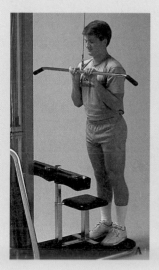
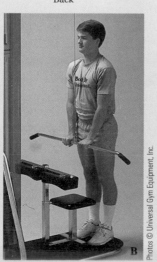

Exercise 32
Dip

Action   Start with the elbows flexed (a), then extend the arms fully and return slowly to the initial position.

Muscles Developed Triceps, deltoid, and pectoralis major

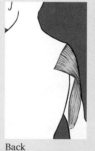
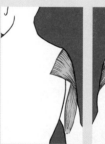

Back   Front

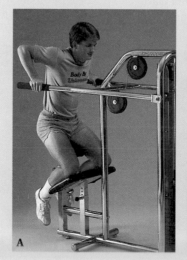

MUSCULAR STRENGTH AND ENDURANCE ASSESSMENT

Name: _____   Date: _____   Grade: _____

Instructor: _____   Course: _____   Section: _____

Necessary Lab Equipment

A Lafayette hand grip dynamometer model 78010 is recommended for the Hand Grip Test. A metronome, gymnasium bleachers, and a stopwatch are needed for the Muscular Endurance Test. A metronome is also needed for the Muscular-Strength and Endurance Test.

Objective

To determine muscular strength and/or endurance and the respective fitness classification.

Lab Preparation

Wear exercise clothing and avoid strenuous strength training 48 hours prior to this lab.

I. Hand Grip Strength Test

The instructions for the Hand Grip Strength Test are provided in Figure 8.2, page 206. Perform the test according to the instructions and look up your results in Table 8.1, page 206.

Hand used: ☐ Right   ☐ Left

Reading: _____ lbs.

Fitness category (see Figure 8.2, page 206): _____

II. Muscular Endurance Test

Conduct this test using the guidelines provided in Figure 8.3 and Table 8.2, pages 207–208. Record your repetitions, fitness category, and points in the spaces provided below.

Exercise	Metronome Cadence	Repetitions	Fitness Category	Points
Bench jumps	none			
Modified dips — men only	56 bpm			
Modified push-ups — women only	56 bpm			
Bent-leg curl-ups	40 bpm			
Abdominal crunches	60 bpm			

Total Points: _____

Overall muscular endurance fitness category (see Figure 8.3, page 208): _____

III. Muscular Strength and Endurance Test

Perform the Muscular Strength and Endurance Test according to the procedure outlined in Figure 8.4, page 209. Record the results, fitness category, and points in the appropriate blanks provided below.

Body weight: [   ] lbs.

Lift	Body Weight	Percent of (pounds)	Resistance	Repetitions
	Men	Women		
Lat pull-down	.70	.45		
Leg extension	.65	.50		
Bench press	.75	.45		
Bent-leg curl-up or abdominal crunch	NA*	NA		
Leg curl	.32	.25		
Arm curl	.35	.18		

*Not applicable—no resistance required. Use test described in Figure 8.3, page 207–208.

IV. Muscular Strength and Endurance Goals

Indicate the muscular strength/endurance classification that you would like to achieve by the end of the term:

Briefly state your feelings about your current strength level and indicate how you are planning to achieve your strength objective: _____

Name:		Date:		Grade:	
Instructor:		Course:		Section:	

Necessary Lab Equipment

Free weights, strength-training machines, or no equipment if the "Strength-Training Exercises Without Weights" program is selected.

Objective

To develop your personal strength-training exercise program.

Lab Preparation

Wear exercise clothing and prepare to participate in a sample strength-training exercise session. All of the strength-training exercises are illustrated on pages 223–234.

I. Stage of Change for Muscular Strength or Endurance

Using Figure 2.3 (page 40) and Table 2.3 (page 41), identify your current stage of change for participation in a muscular strength or muscular endurance program:

II. Instructions

Select one of the two strength-training exercise programs. Perform all of the recommended exercises and, with the exception of the abdominal curl-up exercises, determine the resistance required to do approximately 10 repetitions maximum. For "Strength-Training Exercises Without Weights," simply indicate the total number of repetitions performed. For the abdominal crunches or curl-up exercises, perform or build up to about 20 repetitions.

1. **Strength-Training Exercises Without Weights**

Exercise	Repetitions
Rowing torso	
Push-up	
Abdominal curl-up or abdominal crunch	
Leg curl	
Modified dip	
Pull-up or arm curl	
Heel raise	
Leg abduction and adduction	
Reverse crunch	
Pelvic tilt	

2. Strength-Training Exercises with Weights

Exercise	Repetitions	Resistance
Bench press, shoulder press, or chest press (select and circle one)		
Leg press or squat (select one)		
Abdominal curl-up or abdominal crunch		N/A
Rowing torso		
Arm curl or upright rowing (select one)		
Leg curl or seated leg curl (select one)		
Seated back		
Heel raise		
Lat pull-down or bent-arm pullover (select one)		
Rotary torso		
Triceps extension or dip (select one)		
Leg extension		

III. Your Personalized Strength-Training Program

Once you have performed activity 1 or 2 above (or both), and depending on your personal preference (strength versus endurance), design your strength-training program selecting a minimum of eight exercises. Indicate the number of sets, repetitions, and approximate resistance that you will use. Also state the days of the week, time, and facility that will be used for this program.

Strength-training days: M ☐ T ☐ W ☐ Th ☐ F ☐ Sa ☐ Su ☐   Time of day: ☐   Facility: ☐

	Exercise	Sets / Reps / Resistance		Exercise	Sets / Reps / Resistance
1.			9.		
2.			10.		
3.			11.		
4.			12.		
5.			13.		
6.			14.		
7.			15.		
8.			16.		

Chapter 9

Principles of Muscular Flexibility Assessment and Prescription

Objectives

- Understand the importance of muscular flexibility to adequate fitness and preventive health care.

- Identify the factors that affect muscular flexibility.

- Become familiar with a battery of tests to assess overall body flexibility (Modified Sit-and-Reach Test, Total Body Rotation Test, Shoulder Rotation Test).

- Learn to interpret flexibility test results according to health-fitness and physical-fitness standards.

- Define ballistic stretching, slow-sustained stretching, and proprioceptive neuromuscular facilitation stretching.

- Understand the factors that contribute to the development of muscular flexibility.

- Be introduced to a program for the prevention and rehabilitation of low back pain.

Health-care professionals and practitioners generally have underestimated and overlooked the contribution of good muscular flexibility to overall fitness and preventive health care. **Flexibility** is defined as the ability of a joint to move freely through its full range of motion. Most people who exercise don't take the time to stretch. And a large number of those who do stretch don't stretch properly.

Sports medicine specialists believe that many muscular/skeletal problems and injuries are related to a lack of flexibility. In daily life, we often have to make rapid or strenuous movements we are not accustomed to making. A tight muscle that is abruptly forced beyond its normal range of motion often leads to injuries.

A decline in flexibility can cause poor posture and subsequent aches and pains that lead to limited and painful joint movement. Inordinate tightness is uncomfortable and debilitating. Approximately 80 percent of all low back problems in the United States stem from improper alignment of the vertebral column and pelvic girdle, a direct result of inflexible and weak muscles. This backache syndrome costs U.S. industry billions of dollars each year in lost productivity, health services, and worker compensation.[1]

Improving and maintaining good range of motion in the joints enhances the quality of life. Good flexibility promotes healthy muscles and joints. Improving elasticity of muscles and connective tissue around joints enhances freedom of movement and the individual's ability to participate in all types of activities.

Taking part in a regular stretching program also increases resistance to muscle injury and soreness, prevents low back and other spinal column problems, improves and maintains good postural alignment, promotes proper and graceful body movement, improves personal appearance and self-image, and helps to develop and maintain motor skills throughout life. In addition, flexibility exercises have been prescribed successfully to treat **dysmenorrhea**[2] (painful menstruation) and general neuromuscular tension (stress). Regular **stretching** helps decrease the aches and pains caused by psychological stress and contributes to a decrease in anxiety, blood pressure, and breathing rate.[3]

Further, stretching exercises, in conjunction with calisthenics, are helpful in warm-up routines to prepare the human body for more vigorous aerobic or strength-training exercises, as well as in cooldown routines following exercise to help the person return to a normal resting state. Fatigued muscles tend to contract to a shorter-than-average resting length, and stretching exercises help fatigued muscles reestablish their normal resting length.

Similar to muscular strength, good range of motion is critical in older life. Because of decreased flexibility, older adults lose mobility and are unable to perform simple daily tasks such as bending forward or turning. Many older adults do not turn their head or rotate their trunk to look over their shoulder but, rather, step around 90° to 180° to see behind them.

Physical activity and exercise can also be hampered severely by lack of good range of motion. Because of the pain during activity, older people who have tight hip flexors (muscles) cannot jog or walk very far. A vicious circle ensues, because the condition usually worsens with further inactivity. A simple stretching program can alleviate or prevent this problem and help people return to an exercise program.

Lack of physical activity and excessive sitting lead to chronic back pain.

© Fitness & Wellness, Inc.

Factors Affecting Flexibility

Total range of motion around a joint is highly specific and varies from one joint to another (hip, trunk, shoulder), as well as from one individual to the next. Muscular flexibility relates primarily to genetic factors and to physical activity. Beyond that, factors such as joint structure, ligaments, tendons, muscles, skin, tissue injury, adipose tissue (fat), body temperature, age, and sex influence range of motion about a joint. Because of the specificity of flexibility, indicating an "ideal" level of flexibility is difficult. Nevertheless, flexibility is important to health and independent living.

The range of motion about a given joint depends mostly on the structure of that joint. Greater range of motion, however, can be attained through plastic and elastic elongation. **Plastic elongation** is the permanent lengthening of soft

tissue. Even though joint capsules, ligaments, and tendons are basically nonelastic, they can undergo plastic elongation. This permanent lengthening, accompanied by increases in range of motion, is best attained through slow-sustained stretching exercises.

Elastic elongation is the temporary lengthening of soft tissue. Muscle tissue has elastic properties and responds to stretching exercises by undergoing elastic or temporary lengthening. This elastic elongation increases the extensibility of the muscles.

> *Plastic elongation is permanent lengthening of soft tissue. Elastic elongation is the temporary lengthening of soft tissue.*

Changes in muscle temperature can increase or decrease flexibility by as much as 20 percent. Properly warmed-up individuals have better flexibility than non–warmed-up people. Cool temperatures have the opposite effect, impeding range of motion. Because of the effects of temperature on muscular flexibility, many people prefer to do their stretching exercises after the aerobic phase of their workout. Aerobic activities raise body temperature, facilitating plastic elongation.

Another factor that influences flexibility is the amount of adipose (fat) tissue in and around joints and muscle tissue. Excess adipose tissue will increase resistance to movement, and the added bulk also hampers joint mobility because of the contact between body surfaces.

On the average, women have more flexibility than men do, and they seem to retain this advantage throughout life. Aging does decrease the extensibility of soft tissue, though, resulting in less flexibility in both sexes.

The two most significant contributors to lower flexibility levels are sedentary living and lack of exercise. With less physical activity, muscles lose their elasticity and tendons and ligaments tighten and shorten. Inactivity also tends to be accompanied by an increase in adipose tissue, which further decreases joint range of motion. Finally, injury to muscle tissue and tight skin from excessive scar tissue have negative effects on joint range of motion.

Assessment of Flexibility

Most of the flexibility tests developed over the years are specific to certain sports and are not practical for the general population. Their application in health and fitness programs is limited. For example, the front-to-rear splits test and the bridge-up test have applications in sports such as gymnastics and several track-and-field events, but they do not

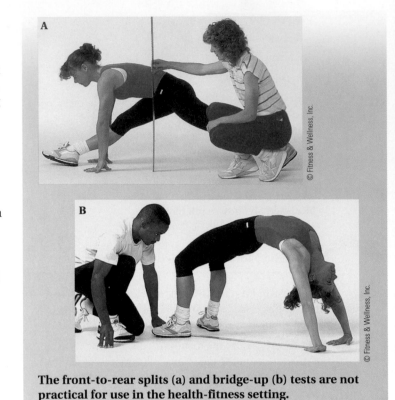

The front-to-rear splits (a) and bridge-up (b) tests are not practical for use in the health-fitness setting.

represent actions most people encounter in daily life.

Because of the lack of practical flexibility tests, most health and fitness centers rely strictly on the sit-and-reach test as an indicator of overall flexibility. This test measures flexibility of the hamstring muscles (back of the thigh) and, to a lesser extent, the lower back muscles.

Flexibility is joint-specific. This means that a lot of flexibility in one joint does not necessarily indicate that other joints are just as flexible. Therefore, the total body rotation test and the shoulder rotation test—indicators of everyday movements such as reaching, bending, and turning—are included to determine your flexibility profile.

The sit-and-reach test has been modified from the traditional test so that arm and leg lengths are taken into consideration to determine the score (see Figure 9.1). In the original sit-and-reach test, the 15-inch mark of the yardstick used to measure

Flexibility The ability of a joint to move freely through its full range of motion.

Dysmenorrhea Painful menstruation.

Stretching Moving the joints beyond the accustomed range of motion.

Plastic elongation Permanent lengthening of soft tissue.

Elastic elongation Temporary lengthening of soft tissue.

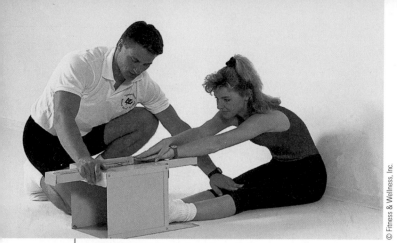

Modified sit-and-reach test.

Figure 9.1 Procedure for the modified sit-and-reach test.

To perform this test, you will need the Acuflex I* Sit-and-Reach Flexibility Tester, or you may simply place a yardstick on top of a box approximately 12" high.

1. Warm up properly before the first trial.
2. Remove your shoes for the test. Sit on the floor with the hips, back, and head against a wall, the legs fully extended, and the bottom of the feet against the Acuflex I or sit-and-reach box.
3. Place the hands one on top of the other and reach forward as far as possible without letting the head and back come off the wall (the shoulders may be rounded as much as possible, but neither the head nor the back should come off the wall at this time). The technician then can slide the reach indicator on the Acuflex I (or yardstick) along the top of the box until the end of the indicator touches the participant's fingers. The indicator then must be held firmly in place throughout the rest of the test.
4. Now your head and back can come off the wall. Gradually reach forward three times, the third time stretching forward as far as possible on the indicator (or yardstick) and holding the final position for at least 2 seconds. Be sure that during the test you keep the backs of the knees flat against the floor.
5. Record the final number of inches reached to the nearest one-half inch.

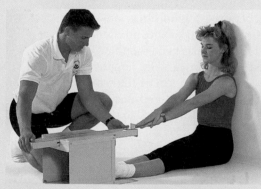

Determining the starting position for the modified sit-and-reach test.

You are allowed two trials, and an average of the two scores is used as the final test score. The respective percentile ranks and fitness categories for this test are given in Tables 9.1 and 9.4.

* The Acuflex I Flexibility Tester for the Modified Sit-and-Reach Test can be obtained from Figure Finder Collection, Novel Products, P. O. Box 408, Rockton, IL 61072-0480. Phone: 800-323-5143, Fax 815-624-4866.

flexibility was always set at the edge of the box where the feet are placed. This does not take into consideration an individual with long arms and/or short legs or one with short arms and/or long legs.[4] All other factors being equal, an individual with longer arms or shorter legs, or both, receives a better rating because of the structural advantage.

The procedures and norms for the flexibility tests are described in Figures 9.1 through 9.3 and Tables 9.1 through 9.3. The flexibility test results in these three tables are provided both in inches and centimeters (cm). Be sure to use the proper column to read your percentile score based on your test results. For the flexibility profile, you should take all three tests. You will be able to assess your flexibility profile in Lab 9A.

Table 9.1 Percentile Ranks for the Modified Sit-and-Reach Test

Age Category—Men

Percentile Rank	≤18 in.	≤18 cm	19–35 in.	19–35 cm	36–49 in.	36–49 cm	≥50 in.	≥50 cm
99	20.8	52.8	20.1	51.1	18.9	48.0	16.2	41.1
95	19.6	49.8	18.9	48.0	18.2	46.2	15.8	40.1
90	18.2	46.2	17.2	43.7	16.1	40.9	15.0	38.1
80	17.8	45.2	17.0	43.2	14.6	37.1	13.3	33.8
70	16.0	40.6	15.8	40.1	13.9	35.3	12.3	31.2
60	15.2	38.6	15.0	38.1	13.4	34.0	11.5	29.2
50	14.5	36.8	14.4	36.6	12.6	32.0	10.2	25.9
40	14.0	35.6	13.5	34.3	11.6	29.5	9.7	24.6
30	13.4	34.0	13.0	33.0	10.8	27.4	9.3	23.6
20	11.8	30.0	11.6	29.5	9.9	25.1	8.8	22.4
10	9.5	24.1	9.2	23.4	8.3	21.1	7.8	19.8
05	8.4	21.3	7.9	20.1	7.0	17.8	7.2	18.3
01	7.2	18.3	7.0	17.8	5.1	13.0	4.0	10.2

Age Category—Women

Percentile Rank	≤18 in.	≤18 cm	19–35 in.	19–35 cm	36–49 in.	36–49 cm	≥50 in.	≥50 cm
99	22.6	57.4	21.0	53.3	19.8	50.3	17.2	43.7
95	19.5	49.5	19.3	49.0	19.2	48.8	15.7	39.9
90	18.7	47.5	17.9	45.5	17.4	44.2	15.0	38.1
80	17.8	45.2	16.7	42.4	16.2	41.1	14.2	36.1
70	16.5	41.9	16.2	41.1	15.2	38.6	13.6	34.5
60	16.0	40.6	15.8	40.1	14.5	36.8	12.3	31.2
50	15.2	38.6	14.8	37.6	13.5	34.3	11.1	28.2
40	14.5	36.8	14.5	36.8	12.8	32.5	10.1	25.7
30	13.7	34.8	13.7	34.8	12.2	31.0	9.2	23.4
20	12.6	32.0	12.6	32.0	11.0	27.9	8.3	21.1
10	11.4	29.0	10.1	25.7	9.7	24.6	7.5	19.0
05	9.4	23.9	8.1	20.6	8.5	21.6	3.7	9.4
01	6.5	16.5	2.6	6.6	2.0	5.1	1.5	3.8

▮ High physical fitness standard
▯ Health fitness standard

Figure 9.2

Procedure for the total body rotation test.

An Acuflex II* Total Body Rotation Flexibility Tester or a measuring scale with a sliding panel is needed to administer this test. The Acuflex II or scale is placed on the wall at shoulder height and should be adjustable to accommodate individual differences in height. If you need to build your own scale, use two measuring tapes and glue them above and below the sliding panel centered at the 15" mark. Each tape should be at least 30" long. If no sliding panel is available, simply tape the measuring tapes onto a wall oriented in opposite directions as shown below. A line also must be drawn on the floor and centered with the 15" mark.

1. Warm up properly before beginning this test.
2. Stand with one side toward the wall, an arm's length away from the wall, with the feet straight ahead, slightly separated, and the toes touching the center line drawn on the floor. Hold out the arm away from the wall horizontally from the body, making a fist with the hand. The Acuflex II measuring scale, or tapes should be shoulder height at this time.
3. Rotate the trunk, the extended arm going backward (always maintaining a horizontal plane) and making contact with the panel, gradually sliding it forward as far as possible. If no panel

is available, slide the fist alongside the tapes as far as possible. Hold the final position at least 2 seconds. Position the hand with the little finger side forward during the entire sliding movement. **Proper hand position is crucial. Many people attempt to open the hand, or push with extended fingers, or slide the panel with the knuckles — none of which is acceptable.** During the test the knees can be bent slightly, but **the feet cannot be moved or rotated** — they must point forward. The body must be kept as straight (vertical) as possible.

4. Conduct the test on either the right or the left side of the body. Perform two trials on the selected side. Record the farthest point reached, measured to the nearest half inch and held for at least 2 seconds. Use the average of the two trials as the final test score. Refer to Tables 9.2 and 9.4 to determine the percentile rank and flexibility fitness classification for this test.

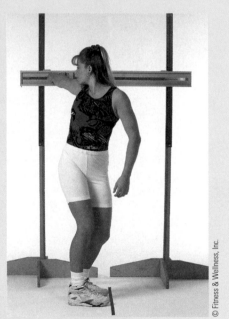

Total body rotation test.

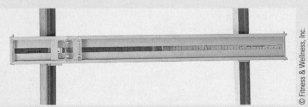

Acuflex II measuring device for the total body rotation test.

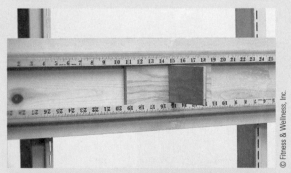

Homemade measuring device for the total body rotation test.

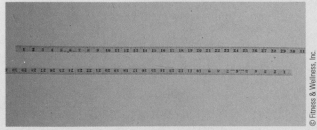

Measuring tapes for the total body rotation test.

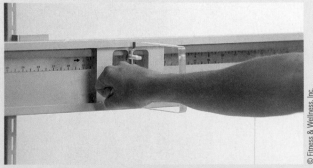

Proper hand position for the total body rotation test.

* The Acuflex II Flexibility Tester for the Total Body Rotation Test can be obtained from Figure Finder Collection, Novel Products, P.O. Box 408, Rockton, IL 61072-0408. Phone: 800-323-5143, Fax 815-624-4866.

Table 9.2

Percentile Ranks for the Total Body Rotation Test

Percentile Rank	Left Rotation								Right Rotation							
	≤18		19–35		36–49		≥50		≤18		19–35		36–49		≥50	
	in.	cm	in.	cm	in.	cm	in.	cm	in.	cm	in.	cm	in.	cm	in.	cm
Men																
99	29.1	73.9	28.0	71.1	26.6	67.6	21.0	53.3	28.2	71.6	27.8	70.6	25.2	64.0	22.2	56.4
95	26.6	67.6	24.8	63.0	24.5	62.2	20.0	50.8	25.5	64.8	25.6	65.0	23.8	60.5	20.7	52.6
90	25.0	63.5	23.6	59.9	23.0	58.4	17.7	45.0	24.3	61.7	24.1	61.2	22.5	57.1	19.3	49.0
80	22.0	55.9	22.0	55.9	21.2	53.8	15.5	39.4	22.7	57.7	22.3	56.6	21.0	53.3	16.3	41.4
70	20.9	53.1	20.3	51.6	20.4	51.8	14.7	37.3	21.3	54.1	20.7	52.6	18.7	47.5	15.7	39.9
60	19.9	50.5	19.3	49.0	18.7	47.5	13.9	35.3	19.8	50.3	19.0	48.3	17.3	43.9	14.7	37.3
50	18.6	47.2	18.0	45.7	16.7	42.4	12.7	32.3	19.0	48.3	17.2	43.7	16.3	41.4	12.3	31.2
40	17.0	43.2	16.8	42.7	15.3	38.9	11.7	29.7	17.3	43.9	16.3	41.4	14.7	37.3	11.5	29.2
30	14.9	37.8	15.0	38.1	14.8	37.6	10.3	26.2	15.1	38.4	15.0	38.1	13.3	33.8	10.7	27.2
20	13.8	35.1	13.3	33.8	13.7	34.8	9.5	24.1	12.9	32.8	13.3	33.8	11.2	28.4	8.7	22.1
10	10.8	27.4	10.5	26.7	10.8	27.4	4.3	10.9	10.8	27.4	11.3	28.7	8.0	20.3	2.7	6.9
05	8.5	21.6	8.9	22.6	8.8	22.4	0.3	0.8	8.1	20.6	8.3	21.1	5.5	14.0	0.3	0.8
01	3.4	8.6	1.7	4.3	5.1	13.0	0.0	0.0	6.6	16.8	2.9	7.4	2.0	5.1	0.0	0.0
Women																
99	29.3	74.4	28.6	72.6	27.1	68.8	23.0	58.4	29.6	75.2	29.4	74.7	27.1	68.8	21.7	55.1
95	26.8	68.1	24.8	63.0	25.3	64.3	21.4	54.4	27.6	70.1	25.3	64.3	25.9	65.8	19.7	50.0
90	25.5	64.8	23.0	58.4	23.4	59.4	20.5	52.1	25.8	65.5	23.0	58.4	21.3	54.1	19.0	48.3
80	23.8	60.5	21.5	54.6	20.2	51.3	19.1	48.5	23.7	60.2	20.8	52.8	19.6	49.8	17.9	45.5
70	21.8	55.4	20.5	52.1	18.6	47.2	17.3	43.9	22.0	55.9	19.3	49.0	17.3	43.9	16.8	42.7
60	20.5	52.1	19.3	49.0	17.7	45.0	16.0	40.6	20.8	52.8	18.0	45.7	16.5	41.9	15.6	39.6
50	19.5	49.5	18.0	45.7	16.4	41.7	14.8	37.6	19.5	49.5	17.3	43.9	14.6	37.1	14.0	35.6
40	18.5	47.0	17.2	43.7	14.8	37.6	13.7	34.8	18.3	46.5	16.0	40.6	13.1	33.3	12.8	32.5
30	17.1	43.4	15.7	39.9	13.6	34.5	10.0	25.4	16.3	41.4	15.2	38.6	11.7	29.7	8.5	21.6
20	16.0	40.6	15.2	38.6	11.6	29.5	6.3	16.0	14.5	36.8	14.0	35.6	9.8	24.9	3.9	9.9
10	12.8	32.5	13.6	34.5	8.5	21.6	3.0	7.6	12.4	31.5	11.1	28.2	6.1	15.5	2.2	5.6
05	11.1	28.2	7.3	18.5	6.8	17.3	0.7	1.8	10.2	25.9	8.8	22.4	4.0	10.2	1.1	2.8
01	8.9	22.6	5.3	13.5	4.3	10.9	0.0	0.0	8.9	22.6	3.2	8.1	2.8	7.1	0.0	0.0

■ High physical fitness standard   □ Health fitness standard

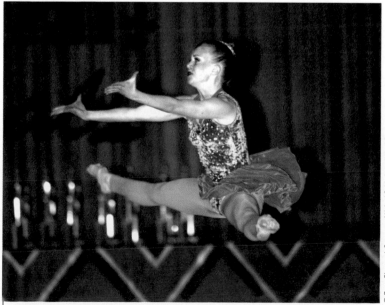

Adequate flexibility helps to develop and maintain sports skill throughout life.

© Doug Olmstead. Courtesy of United Spirit Association, Sunnyvale, CA.

Figure
9.3

Procedure for the shoulder rotation test.

This test can be done using the Acuflex III* Flexibility Tester, which consists of a shoulder caliper and a measuring device for shoulder rotation. If this equipment is unavailable, you can construct your own device quite easily. The caliper can be built with three regular yardsticks. Nail and glue two of the yardsticks at one end at a 90° angle, and use the third one as the sliding end of the caliper. Construct the rotation device by placing a 60" measuring tape on an aluminum or wood stick, starting at about 6" or 7" from the end of the stick.

1. Warm up before the test.
2. Using the shoulder caliper, measure the biacromial width to the nearest one-fourth inch (use the top scale on the Acuflex III). Measure biacromial width between the lateral edges of the acromion processes of the shoulders.
3. Place the Acuflex III or homemade device behind the back and use a reverse grip (thumbs out) to hold on to the device. Place the index finger of the right hand next to the zero point of the scale or tape (lower scale on the Acuflex III) and hold it firmly in place throughout the test. Place the left hand on the other end of the measuring device wherever comfortable.

4. Standing straight up and extending both arms to full length, with elbows locked, slowly bring the measuring device over the head until it reaches about forehead level. For subsequent trials, depending on the resistance encountered when rotating the shoulders, move the left grip in ½" to 1" at a time, and repeat the task until you no longer can rotate the shoulders without undue strain or starting to bend the elbows. Always keep the right-hand grip against the zero point of the scale. Measure the last successful trial to the nearest one-half inch. Take this measurement at the inner edge of the left hand on the side of the little finger.
6. Determine the final score for this test by subtracting the biacromial width from the best score (shortest distance) between both hands on the rotation test. For example, if the best score is 35" and the biacromial width is 15", the final score is 20" (35 − 15 = 20). Using Tables 9.3 and 9.4, determine the percentile rank and flexibility fitness classification for this test.

* The Acuflex III Flexibility Tester for the Shoulder Rotation Test can be obtained from Figure Finder Collection, Novel Products, Inc., P. O. Box 408, Rockton, IL 61072-0408. Phone: (800) 323-5143, Fax 815-624-4866.

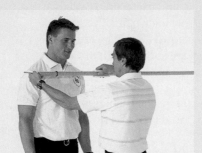

Measuring biacromial width.

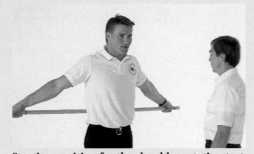

Starting position for the shoulder rotation test (note the reverse grip used for this test).

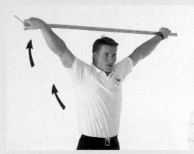

Shoulder rotation test.

Photos © Fitness & Wellness, Inc.

Table
9.3

Percentile Ranks for the Shoulder Rotation Test

Percentile Rank	Age Category—Men								Percentile Rank	Age Category—Women							
	≤18		19–35		36–49		≥50			≤18		19–35		36–49		≥50	
	in.	cm	in.	cm	in.	cm	in.	cm		in.	cm	in.	cm	in.	cm	in.	cm
99	2.2	5.6	−1.0	−2.5	18.1	46.0	21.5	54.6	99	2.6	6.6	−2.4	−6.1	11.5	29.2	13.1	33.3
95	15.2	38.6	10.4	26.4	20.4	51.8	27.0	68.6	95	8.0	20.3	6.2	15.7	15.4	39.1	16.5	41.9
90	18.5	47.0	15.5	39.4	20.8	52.8	27.9	70.9	90	10.7	27.2	9.7	24.6	16.8	42.7	20.9	53.1
80	20.7	52.6	18.4	46.7	23.3	59.2	28.5	72.4	80	14.5	36.8	14.5	36.8	19.2	48.8	22.5	57.1
70	23.0	58.4	20.5	52.1	24.7	62.7	29.4	74.7	70	16.1	40.9	17.2	43.7	21.5	54.6	24.3	61.7
60	24.2	61.5	22.9	58.2	26.6	67.6	29.9	75.9	60	19.2	48.8	18.7	47.5	23.1	58.7	25.1	63.8
50	25.4	64.5	24.4	62.0	28.0	71.1	30.5	77.5	50	21.0	53.3	20.0	50.8	23.5	59.7	26.2	66.5
40	26.3	66.8	25.7	65.3	30.0	76.2	31.0	78.7	40	22.2	56.4	21.4	54.4	24.4	62.0	28.1	71.4
30	28.2	71.6	27.3	69.3	31.9	81.0	31.7	80.5	30	23.2	58.9	24.0	61.0	25.9	65.8	29.9	75.9
20	30.0	76.2	30.1	76.5	33.3	84.6	33.1	84.1	20	25.0	63.5	25.9	65.8	29.8	75.7	31.5	80.0
10	33.5	85.1	31.8	80.8	36.1	91.7	37.2	94.5	10	27.2	69.1	29.1	73.9	31.1	79.0	33.1	84.1
05	34.7	88.1	33.5	85.1	37.8	96.0	38.7	98.3	05	28.0	71.1	31.3	79.5	33.4	84.8	34.1	86.6
01	40.8	103.6	42.6	108.2	43.0	109.2	44.1	112.0	01	32.5	82.5	37.1	94.2	34.9	88.6	35.4	89.9

High physical fitness standard   Health fitness standard

Interpreting Flexibility Test Results

After obtaining your scores and fitness ratings for each test, you can determine the fitness category for each flexibility test using the guidelines given in Table 9.4. You also should look up the number of points assigned for each fitness category in this table. The overall flexibility fitness classification is obtained by totaling the number of points from all three tests and using the ratings given in Table 9.5.

Evaluating Body Posture

Posture tests are used to detect deviations from normal body alignment and prescribe corrective exercises or procedures to improve alignment. These analyses are best conducted early in life, because certain postural deviations are more difficult to correct in older people. If deviations are allowed to go uncorrected, they usually become more serious as the person grows older. Consequently, corrective exercises or other medical procedures should be used to stop or slow down postural degeneration.

Faulty posture and weak and inelastic muscles are a leading cause of chronic low back problems. Evaluating these areas is crucial to prevent and rehabilitate low back pain. The results of these tests can be used to prescribe corrective exercises.

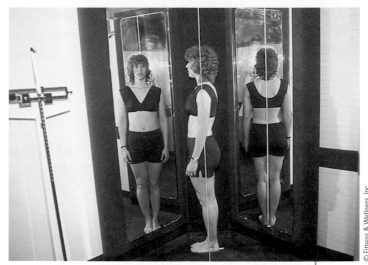

Photographic technique used for posture evaluation.

© Fitness & Wellness, Inc.

Adequate body mechanics also aid in reducing chronic low-back pain. Proper body mechanics means using correct positions in all the activities of daily life, including sleeping, sitting, standing, walking, driving, working, and exercising. Because of the high incidence of low back pain, illustrations of proper body mechanics and a series of corrective and preventive exercises are shown in Figure 9.6 on pages 253–254.

Most people are unaware of how faulty their posture is until they see themselves in a photograph. This can be quite a shock and is often enough to motivate them to change.

Besides engaging in the recommended exercises to elicit changes in postural alignment, people need to be continually aware of the corrections they are trying to make. As their posture improves, people frequently become motivated to change other aspects, such as improving muscular strength and flexibility and decreasing body fat.

Proper body alignment has been difficult to evaluate because most experts still don't know exactly what constitutes good posture. To objectively analyze a person's posture, an observer either must be adequately trained or must have some guidelines to identify abnormalities and assign ratings according to the amount of deviation from "normal" posture.

A posture rating chart, such as that in Lab 9B, provides simple guidelines for evaluating posture. Assuming the drawings in the left column to be proper alignment and the drawings in the right column to be extreme deviations from normal, an observer is able to rate each body segment on a scale from 1 to 5.

Postural analysis can be done with more precision with the aid of a plumb line, two mirrors, and a Polaroid camera. The mirrors are placed at an 80 to 85° angle, and the plumb line is centered in front

Table 9.4 — Flexibility Fitness Categories According to Percentile Ranks

Percentile Rank	Fitness Category	Points
≥ 90	Excellent	5
70–80	Good	4
50–60	Average	3
30–40	Fair	2
≤ 20	Poor	1

Table 9.5 — Overall Flexibility Fitness Category

Total Points	Flexibility Category
≥ 13	Excellent
10–12	Good
7–9	Average
4–6	Fair
≤ 3	Poor

of the mirrors. Another line is drawn down the center of the mirror on the right. The person should stand with the left side to the plumb line. The plumb line is used as a reference to divide the body into front and back halves (try to center the line with the hip joint and the shoulder). The line on the back (right) mirror should divide the body into right and left halves. A picture then is taken (like the photo on page 246) that can be compared to the rating chart given in Lab 9B.

The photographic procedure allows for a better comparison of the different body segment alignments and a more objective analysis. If no mirrors and camera are available, the participant should stand with his or her side to the line, and then repeat with the back to the line, while the evaluator does the assessment.

A final posture score is determined according to the sum of the ratings obtained for each body segment. Table 9.6 contains the various categories as determined by the final posture score.

Principles of Muscular Flexibility Prescription

Even though heredity, or genetics, plays a crucial role in body flexibility, the range of joint mobility can be increased and maintained through a regular flexibility exercise program. Because range of motion is highly specific to each body part (ankle, trunk, shoulder), a comprehensive stretching program should include all body parts and follow the basic guidelines for flexibility development.

The overload and specificity of training principles (discussed in conjunction with strength development in Chapter 8) apply as well to the development of muscular flexibility. To increase the total range of motion of a joint, the specific muscles surrounding that joint have to be stretched progressively beyond their accustomed length. The principles of mode, intensity, repetitions, and frequency of exercise also can be applied to flexibility programs.

Mode of Training

Three modes of stretching exercises can increase flexibility:

1. Ballistic stretching.
2. Slow-sustained stretching.
3. Proprioceptive neuromuscular facilitation (PNF) stretching.

Although research has indicated that all three types of stretching are effective in improving flexibility, each technique has certain advantages.

Ballistic Stretching

Ballistic (or **dynamic**) **stretching** exercises are done with jerky, rapid, and bouncy movements that provide the necessary force to lengthen the muscles. This type of stretching helps to develop flexibility, but the ballistic actions may cause muscle soreness and injury from small tears to the soft tissue.

Precautions must be taken not to overstretch ligaments, because they undergo plastic or permanent elongation. If the stretching force cannot be controlled, as in fast, jerky movements, ligaments easily can be overstretched. This, in turn, leads to excessively loose joints, increasing the risk for injuries, including joint dislocation and **subluxation**. Slow, gentle, and **controlled-ballistic stretching** (instead of jerky, rapid, and bouncy movements), however, is quite effective in developing flexibility and can be performed safely by most individuals.

Slow-Sustained Stretching

With the **slow-sustained stretching** technique, muscles are lengthened gradually through a joint's complete range of motion, and the final position is held for a few seconds. A slow-sustained stretch causes the muscles to relax and thereby achieve greater length. This type of stretch causes little pain and has a low risk for injury. Slow-sustained stretching exercises are the most frequently used and recommended in flexibility-development programs.

Table 9.6 Posture Evaluation Standards	
Total Points	**Classification**
≥ 45	Excellent
40–44	Good
30–39	Average
20–29	Fair
≤ 19	Poor

Source: W. W. K. Hoeger, *The Complete Guide for the Development and Implementation of Health Promotion Programs,* (Englewood, CO: Morton Publishing, 1987). Reproduced by permission.

Ballistic stretching Exercises done with jerky, rapid, bouncy movements.

Subluxation Partial dislocation of a joint.

Controlled ballistic stretching Exercises done with slow, short, and sustained movements.

Slow-sustained stretching Exercises in which the muscles are lengthened gradually through a joint's complete range of motion.

Proprioceptive Neuromuscular Facilitation (PNF)

Proprioceptive neuromuscular facilitation (PNF) stretching has become more popular in the last few years. This technique, based on a "contract-and-relax" method, requires the assistance of another person. The procedure is as follows:

1. The person assisting with the exercise provides initial force by pushing slowly in the direction of the desired stretch. This first stretch does not cover the entire range of motion.
2. The person being stretched then applies force in the opposite direction of the stretch, against the assistant, who tries to hold the initial degree of stretch as close as possible. This results in an isometric contraction at the angle of the stretch.
3. After 4 or 5 seconds of isometric contraction, the muscle being stretched is relaxed completely. The assistant then increases the degree of stretch slowly to a greater angle.
4. The isometric contraction is repeated for another 4 or 5 seconds, following which the muscle is relaxed again. The assistant then can increase the degree of stretch, slowly, one more

time. Steps 1 through 4 are repeated two to five times, until the exerciser feels mild discomfort. On the last trial, the final stretched position should be held for several seconds.

Theoretically, with the PNF technique, the isometric contraction helps relax the muscle being stretched, which results in greater muscle length. Some fitness leaders believe PNF is more effective than slow-sustained stretching. Another benefit of PNF is an increase in strength of the muscle(s) being stretched. Research has shown approximately 17 and 35 percent increases in absolute strength and muscular endurance, respectively, in the hamstring muscle group after 12 weeks of PNF stretching.[5] The results were consistent in both men and women. These increases are attributed to the isometric contractions performed during PNF. The disadvantages of PNF are (1) more pain, (2) need for a second person to assist, and (3) need for more time to conduct each session.

Intensity

The **intensity**, or degree of stretch, when doing flexibility exercises should be only to a point of mild discomfort. Pain does not have to be part of the stretching routine. Excessive pain is an indication that the load is too high and may cause injury.

All stretching should be done to slightly below the pain threshold. As participants reach this point, they should try to relax the muscle being stretched as much as possible. After completing the stretch, the body part is brought back gradually to the starting point.

> *Pain does not have to be part of the stretching routine. Excessive pain is an indication that the load is too high and may cause injury.*

Repetitions

The time required for an exercise session for flexibility development is based on the number of repetitions and the length of time each **repetition** (final stretched position) is held. The general recommendation is that each exercise be done four or five times, holding the final position each time for about 10 to 30 seconds.

As flexibility increases, a person can gradually increase the time each repetition is held, to a maximum of 1 minute. Individuals who are susceptible to flexibility injuries, however, should limit each stretch to 20 seconds.

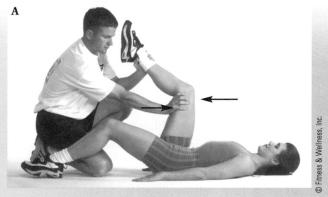

A

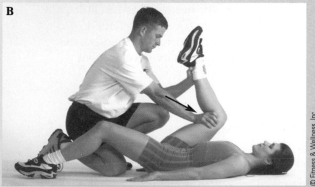

B

© Fitness & Wellness, Inc.

Proprioceptive neuromuscular facilitation (PNF) stretching technique (a) isometric phase (b) stretching phase.

Frequency of Exercise

Flexibility exercises should be conducted five to six times a week in the early stages of the program. After a minimum of 6 to 8 weeks of almost daily stretching, flexibility levels can be maintained with only two or three sessions per week, doing about three repetitions of 10 to 15 seconds each. Figure 9.4 summarizes the flexibility development guidelines.

When to Stretch?

Many people do not differentiate a warm-up from stretching. Warming up means starting a workout slowly with walking, cycling, or slow jogging, followed by gentle stretching (not through the entire range of motion). Stretching implies movement of joints through their full range of motion and holding the final degree of stretch according to recommended guidelines.

Gentle stretching is recommended in conjunction with warm-up routines. Two to three minutes are recommended before steady activities (walking, jogging, cycling) and up to ten minutes before stop-and-go activities (racquet sports, basketball, soccer) and athletic participation in general (football, gymnastics). Activities that require abrupt changes in direction are more likely to cause muscle strains if performed without proper warm-up that includes mild stretching.

A good time to do flexibility exercises is after aerobic workouts. Surveys have shown that individuals who stretch intensely before workouts without an adequate warm-up actually have a higher rate of injuries than those who do not stretch at all. Higher body temperature in itself helps to increase the joint range of motion. Muscles also are fatigued following exercise. A fatigued muscle tends to shorten, which can lead to soreness and spasms. Stretching exercises help fatigued muscles re-establish their normal resting length and prevent unnecessary pain.

Flexibility Exercises

To improve body flexibility, each major muscle group should be subjected to at least one stretching exercise. A complete set of exercises for developing muscular flexibility is presented on pages 255–257.

You may not be able to hold a final stretched position with some of these exercises (such as lateral head tilts and arm circles), but you still should perform the exercise through the joint's full range of motion. Depending on the number and length of repetitions, a complete workout will last between 15 and 30 minutes.

Preventing and Rehabilitating Low Back Pain

Few people make it through life without having low back pain at some point. An estimated 75 million Americans have chronic low back pain each year. Back pain is considered chronic if it persists longer than three months. About 80 percent of the time, backache syndrome is preventable and is caused by (a) physical inactivity, (b) poor postural habits and body mechanics, or (c) excessive body weight.

People tend to think of back pain as a skeleton problem. In fact, the spine's curvature, alignment, and movement are controlled by surrounding muscles. Lack of physical activity is the most common reason for chronic low back pain. In particular, a major contributor to back pain is excessive sitting, which causes back muscles to shorten, stiffen, and become weaker.

Faulty posture and weak and inelastic muscles are the leading causes of chronic low back problems in the United States.

Figure 9.4 Guidelines for flexibility development.

Mode:	Static or dynamic (slow ballistic or proprioceptive neuromuscular facilitation) stretching to include every major joint of the body
Intensity:	Stretch to the point of mild discomfort
Repetitions:	Repeat each exercise at least 4 times and hold the final stretched position for 10 to 30 seconds
Frequency:	2–3 days per week

Based on American College of Sports Medicine, "Position Stand: The Recommended Quantity and Quality of Exercise for Developing and Maintaining Cardiorespiratory and Muscular Fitness, and Flexibility in Healthy Adults," *Medical Science Sports Exercise* 30 (1998): 975–991.

Proprioceptive neuromuscular facilitation (PNF) Stretching technique in which muscles are stretched out sequentially with intermittent isometric contractions.

Intensity (for flexibility exercises) Degree of stretch when doing flexibility exercises.

Repetitions Number of times a given stretch is performed.

Deterioration or weakening of the abdominal and gluteal muscles, along with tightening of the lower back (erector spinae) muscles, brings about an unnatural forward tilt of the pelvis (Figure 9.5). This tilt puts extra pressure on the spinal vertebrae, causing pain in the lower back. Accumulation of fat around the midsection of the body contributes to the forward tilt of the pelvis, which further aggravates the condition.

Low back pain frequently is associated with faulty posture and improper body mechanics (body positions in all of life's daily activities, including sleeping, sitting, standing, walking, driving, working, and exercising). Incorrect posture and poor mechanics, as explained in Figure 9.6, increase strain not only on the lower back, but on many other bones, joints, muscles, and ligaments as well.

Back pain can be reduced greatly by including some specific stretching and strengthening exercises in the regular fitness program. In most cases back pain is present only with movement and physical activity.

If the pain is severe and persists even at rest, the first step is to consult a physician, who can rule out any disc damage and may prescribe proper bed rest using several pillows under the knees for leg support (see Figure 9.6). This position helps release muscle spasms by stretching the muscles involved. In addition, a physician may prescribe a muscle relaxant or anti-inflammatory medication (or both) and some type of physical therapy.

In most cases of low back pain, even with severe pain, people feel better within days or weeks without treatment from health care professionals.[6] To relieve symptoms, you may use over-the-counter pain relievers and hot or cold packs. You should also stay active to avoid further weakening of the back muscles. Low-impact activities like walking, swimming, water aerobics, and cycling are recommended. Once you are pain-free in the resting state, you need to start correcting the muscular imbalance by stretching the tight muscles and strengthening the weak ones. Stretching exercises always are performed first.

If there is no indication of disease or injury (such as leg numbness or pain), a herniated disk, or fractures, spinal manipulation by a chiropractor or other health care professional can provide pain relief. Spinal manipulation as a treatment modality for low back pain has been endorsed by the federal Agency for Health Care Policy and Research. The

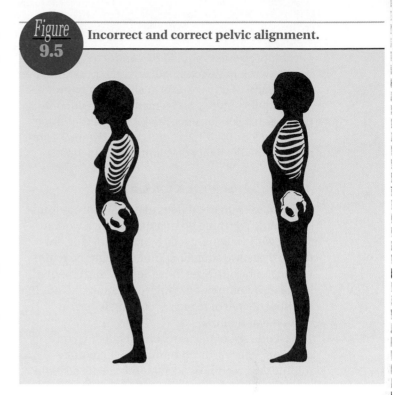

Figure 9.5 Incorrect and correct pelvic alignment.

guidelines suggest that spinal manipulation may help to alleviate discomfort and pain during the first few weeks of an acute low back pain episode. Generally, benefits are seen within ten treatments. People who have had chronic pain for over 6 months should avoid spinal manipulation until they have been thoroughly examined by a physician.

Several exercises for preventing and rehabilitating the backache syndrome are given on pages 257–258. These exercises can be done twice or more daily when a person has back pain. Under normal circumstances, doing these exercises three to four times a week is enough to prevent the syndrome. Lab 9C allows you to develop your own flexibility and low back conditioning programs.

Psychological stress may also lead to back pain.[7] Excessive stress causes muscles to contract. In the case of the lower back, frequent tightening of the muscles can throw the back out of alignment and constrict blood vessels that supply oxygen and nutrients to the back. If you suffer from excessive stress and back pain at the same time, proper stress management (see Chapter 11) should be a part of your comprehensive back-care program.

Web Interactive

- Stretching and Flexibility: Everything You Never Wanted to Know. This is a very comprehensive and academic site describing the physiology of muscles, types of flexibility, types of stretching, factors limiting flexibility, how to stretch, specific exercises, as well as references.

  http://www.enteract.com/~bradapp/docs/rec/stretching

- Ten Basic Stretches. This site features ten exercises to improve flexibility, complete with photographs.

  http://www.drkoop.com/wellness/fitness/exercise/stretch.asp

Interactive Sites:

- Warm-up and stretching exercises to enhance your performance. Learn several techniques on proper warm-ups and stretches to help you reduce your risk of injury and enhance your performance. This site lists specific types of warm-ups for basketball, baseball, running, walking, racquet sports, and golf.

  http://www.vitality.com/vfm/performance.html

Notes

1. S. A. Plowman, "Physical Fitness and Healthy Low Back Function," President's Council on Physical Fitness and Sports: *Physical Activity and Fitness Research Digest*, Series 1 (3):3, 1993.

2. American College of Obstetricians and Gynecologists, *Guidelines for Exercise During Pregnancy*, 1994.

3. "Stretch Yourself Younger," *Consumer Reports on Health* 11 (August 1999): 6–7.

4. W. W. K. Hoeger and D. R. Hopkins, "A Comparison Between the Sit and Reach and the Modified Sit and Reach in the Measurement of Flexibility in Women," *Research Quarterly for Exercise and Sport* 63 (1992): 191–195.

   W. W. K. Hoeger, D. R. Hopkins, S. Button, and T. A. Palmer, "Comparing the Sit and Reach with the Modified Sit and Reach in Measuring Flexibility in Adolescents," *Pediatric Exercise Science* 2 (1990): 156–162.

   D. R. Hopkins and W. W. K. Hoeger, "A Comparison of the Sit and Reach and the Modified Sit and Reach in the Measurement of Flexibility for Males," *Journal of Applied Sports Science Research* 6 (1992): 7–10.

5. J. Kokkonen and S. Lauritzen, "Isotonic Strength and Endurance Gains Through PNF Stretching," *Medicine and Science in Sports and Exercise* 27 (1995): S22, 127.

6. R. Deyo, "Chiropractic Care for Back Pain: The Physician's Perspective," *HealthNews* 4 (September 10, 1998).

7. A. Brownstein, "Chronic Back Pain Can Be Beaten," *Bottom Line Health* 13 (October 1999): 3–4.

Suggested Readings

Alter, M. J. *The Science of Stretching*. Champaign, IL: Human Kinetic Press, 1996.

Alter, M. J. *Sports Stretch*. Champaign, IL: Human Kinetic Press, 1997.

Anderson, B. *Stretching*. Bolinas, CA: Shelter Publications, 1999.

Heyward, V. H. *Advanced Fitness Assessment and Exercise Prescription*. Champaign, IL: Human Kinetic Press, 1998.

Hoeger, W. W. K., and D. R. Hopkins. "Assessing Muscular Flexibility." *Fitness Management* 6, no. 2 (1990): 34–36, 42.

Kurz, T. *Stretching Scientifically: A Guide to Flexibility Training*. Island Pond, VT: Stadion Publishers, 1994.

McAtee, R. E. *Facilitated Stretching*. Champaign, IL: Human Kinetic Press, 1993.

Figure 9.6 Your back and how to care for it.

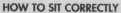

Your back and how to care for it

Whatever the cause of low back pain, part of its treatment is the correction of faulty posture. But good posture is not simply a matter of "standing tall." It refers to correct use of the body at all times. In fact, for the body to function in the best of health it must be so used that no strain is put upon the muscles, joints, bones, and ligaments. To prevent low back pain, avoiding strain must become a way of life, practiced while lying, sitting, standing, walking, working, and exercising. When body position is correct, internal organs have enough room to function normally and blood circulates more freely.

With the help of this guide, you can begin to correct the positions and movements that bring on or aggravate backache. Particular attention should be paid to the positions recommended for resting, since it is possible to strain the muscles of the back and neck even while lying in bed. By learning to live with good posture, under all circumstances, you will gradually develop the proper carriage and stronger muscles needed to protect and support your hard-working back.

HOW TO STAY ON YOUR FEET WITHOUT TIRING YOUR BACK

To prevent strain and pain in everyday activities, it is restful to change from one task to another before fatigue sets in. Housewives can lie down between chores; others should check body position frequently, drawing in the abdomen, flattening the back, bending the knees slightly.

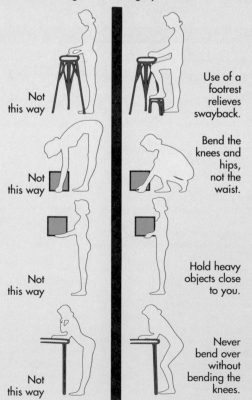

Not this way

Use of a footrest relieves swayback.

Not this way

Bend the knees and hips, not the waist.

Not this way

Hold heavy objects close to you.

Not this way

Never bend over without bending the knees.

CHECK YOUR CARRIAGE HERE

In correct, fully erect posture, a line dropped from the ear will go through the tip of the shoulder, middle of hip, back of kneecap, and front of anklebone.

Incorrect
Lower back is arched or hollow.

Incorrect
Upper back is stooped, lower back is arched, abdomen sags.

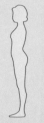

Incorrect
Note how, in strained position, pelvis tilts forward, chin is out, and ribs are down, crowding internal organs.

Correct
In correct position, chin is in, head up back flattened, pelvis held straight.

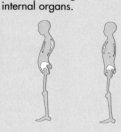

To find the correct standing position: Stand one foot away from wall. Now sit against wall, bending knees slightly. Tighten abdominal and buttock muscles. This will tilt the pelvis back and flatten the lower spine. Holding this position, inch up the wall to standing position, by straightening the legs. Now walk around the room, maintaining the same posture. Place back against wall again to see if you have held it.

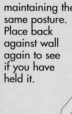

HOW TO SIT CORRECTLY

A back's best friend is a straight, hard chair. If you can't get the chair you prefer, learn to sit properly on whatever chair you get. To correct sitting position from forward slump: Throw head well back, then bend it forward to pull in the chin. This will straighten the back. Now tighten abdominal muscles to raise the chest. Check position frequently.

Relieve strain by sitting well forward, flatten back by tightening abdominal muscles, and cross knees.

Use of footrest relieves swayback. Aim is to have knees higher than hips.

Correct way to sit while driving, close to pedals. Use seat belt or hard backrest, available commercially.

TV slump leads to "dowager's hump," strains neck and shoulders.

If chair is too high, swayback is increased.

Keep neck and back in as straight a line as possible with the spine. Bend forward from hips.

Driver's seat too far from pedals emphasizes curve in lower back.

Strained reading position. Forward thrusting strains muscles of neck and head.

Figure 9.6 Your back and how to care for it (continued).

HOW TO PUT YOUR BACK TO BED

For proper bed posture, a firm mattress is essential. Bedboards, sold commercially, or devised at home, may be used with soft mattresses. Bedboards, preferably, should be made of 3/4-inch plywood. Faulty sleeping positions intensify swayback and result not only in backache but in numbness, tingling, and pain in arms and legs.

Incorrect:

Lying flat on back makes swayback worse.

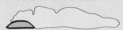

Use of high pillow strains neck, arms, shoulders.

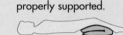

Sleeping face down exaggerates swayback, strains neck and shoulders.

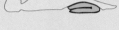

Bending one hip and knee does not relieve swayback.

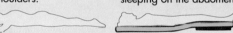

Correct:

Lying on side with knees bent effectively flattens the back. Flat pillow may be used to support neck, especially when shoulders are broad.

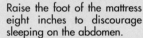

Sleeping on back is restful and correct when knees are properly supported.

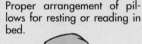

Raise the foot of the mattress eight inches to discourage sleeping on the abdomen.

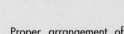

Proper arrangement of pillows for resting or reading in bed.

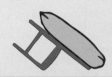

A straight-back chair used behind a pillow makes a serviceable backrest.

WHEN DOING NOTHING, DO IT RIGHT

Rest is the first rule for the tired, painful back. The following positions relieve pain by taking all pressure and weight off the back and legs.

Note pillows under knees to relieve strain on spine.

For complete relief and relaxing effect, these positions should be maintained from 5 to 25 minutes.

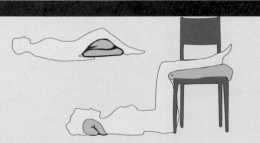

EXERCISE — WITHOUT GETTING OUT OF BED

Exercises to be performed while lying in bed are aimed not so much at strengthening muscles as at teaching correct positioning. But muscles used correctly become stronger and in time are able to support the body with the least amount of effort.

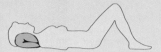

Do all exercises in this position. Legs should not be straightened.

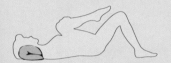

Bring knee up to chest. Lower slowly but do not straighten leg. Relax. Repeat with each leg 10 times.

Bring both knees slowly up to chest. Tighten muscles of abdomen, press back flat against bed. Hold knees to chest 20 seconds, then lower slowly. Relax. Repeat 5 times. This exercise gently stretches the shortened muscles of the lower back, while strengthening abdominal muscles. Clasp knees, bring them up to chest, at the same time coming to a sitting position. Rock back and forth.

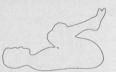

EXERCISE — WITHOUT ATTRACTING ATTENTION

Use these inconspicuous exercises whenever you have a spare moment during the day, both to relax tension and improve the tone of important muscle groups.

1. Rotate shoulders, forward and backward.
2. Turn head slowly side to side.
3. Watch an imaginary plane take off, just below the right shoulder. Stretch neck, follow it slowly as it moves up, around and down, disappearing below the other shoulder. Repeat, starting on left side.
4. Slowly, slowly, touch left ear to left shoulder, right ear to right shoulder. Raise both shoulders to touch ears, drop them as far down as possible.
5. At any pause in the day — waiting for an elevator to arrive, for a specific traffic light to change — pull in abdominal muscles, tighten, hold it for the count of eight without breathing. Relax slowly. Increase the count gradually after the first week, practice breathing normally with the abdomen flat and contracted. Do this sitting, standing, and walking.

RULES TO LIVE BY — FROM NOW ON

1. Never bend from the waist only; bend the hips and knees.
2. Never lift a heavy object higher than your waist.
3. Always turn and face the object you wish to lift.
4. Avoid carrying unbalanced loads; hold heavy objects close to your body.
5. Never carry anything heavier than you can manage with ease.
6. Never lift or move heavy furniture. Wait for someone to do it who knows the principles of leverage.
7. Avoid sudden movements, sudden "overloading" of muscles. Learn to move deliberately, swinging the legs from the hips.
8. Learn to keep the head in line with the spine, when standing, sitting, lying in bed.
9. Put soft chairs and deep couches on your "don't sit" list. During prolonged sitting, cross your legs to rest your back.
10. Your doctor is the only one who can determine when low back pain is due to faulty posture and he is the best judge of when you may do general exercises for physical fitness. When you do, omit any exercise that arches or overstrains the lower back: backward bends, or forward bends, touch-ing the toes with the knees straight.
11. Wear shoes with moderate heels, all about the same height. Avoid changing from high to low heels.
12. Put a footrail under the desk and a footrest under the crib.
13. Diaper the baby sitting next to him or her on the bed.
14. Don't stoop and stretch to hang the wash; raise the clothesbasket and lower the washline.
15. Beg or buy a rocking chair. Rocking rests the back by changing the muscle groups used.
16. Train yourself vigorously to use your abdominal muscles to flatten your lower abdomen. In time, this muscle contraction will become habitual, making you the envied possessor of a youthful body-profile!
17. Don't strain to open windows or doors.
18. For good posture, concentrate on strengthening "nature's corset" — the abdominal and buttock muscles. The pelvic roll exercise is especially recommended to correct the postural relation between the pelvis and the spine.

Flexibility Exercises

Exercise 1
Lateral Head Tilt

Action Slowly and gently tilt the head laterally. Repeat several times to each side.

Areas Stretched Neck flexors and extensors and ligaments of the cervical spine

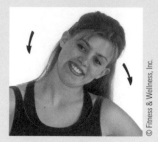

© Fitness & Wellness, Inc.

Exercise 2
Arm Circles

Action Gently circle your arms all the way around. Conduct the exercise in both directions.

Areas Stretched Shoulder muscles and ligaments

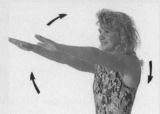

© Fitness & Wellness, Inc.

Exercise 3
Side Stretch

Action Stand straight up, feet separated to shoulder width, and place your hands on your waist. Now move the upper body to one side and hold the final stretch for a few seconds. Repeat on the other side.

Areas Stretched Muscles and ligaments in the pelvic region

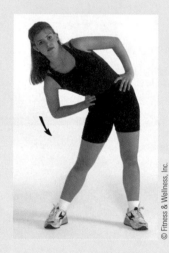

© Fitness & Wellness, Inc.

Exercise 4
Body Rotation

Action Place your arms slightly away from your body and rotate the trunk as far as possible, holding the final position for several seconds. Conduct the exercise for both the right and left sides of the body. You also can perform this exercise by standing about 2 feet away from the wall (back toward the wall) and then rotating the trunk, placing the hands against the wall.

Areas Stretched Hip, abdominal, chest, back, neck, and shoulder muscles; hip and spinal ligaments

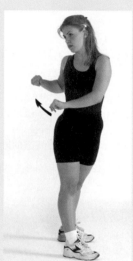

© Fitness & Wellness, Inc.

Exercise 5
Chest Stretch

Action Place your hand on the shoulder of your partner, who will in turn push you down by your shoulders. Hold the final position for a few seconds.

Areas Stretched Chest (pectoral) muscles and shoulder ligaments

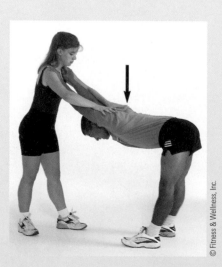

© Fitness & Wellness, Inc.

Exercise 6
Shoulder Hyperextension Stretch

Action Have a partner grasp your arms from behind by the wrists and slowly push them upward. Hold the final position for a few seconds.

Areas Stretched Deltoid and pectoral muscles; ligaments of the shoulder joint

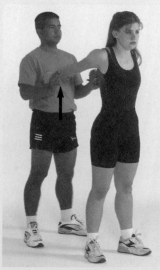

© Fitness & Wellness, Inc.

Exercise 7
Shoulder Rotation Stretch

Action   With the aid of surgical tubing or an aluminum or wood stick, place the tubing or stick behind your back and grasp the two ends using a reverse (thumbs-out) grip. Slowly bring the tubing or stick over your head, keeping the elbows straight. Repeat several times (bring the hands closer together for additional stretch).

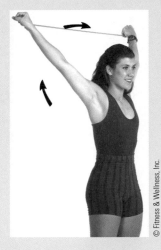

Areas Stretched   Deltoid, latissimus dorsi, and pectoral muscles; shoulder ligaments

Exercise 8
Quad Stretch

Action   Lie on your side and move one foot back by flexing the knee. Grasp the front of the ankle and pull the ankle toward the gluteal region. Hold for several seconds. Repeat with the other leg.

Areas Stretched   Quadriceps muscle, hip flexors; knee and ankle ligaments

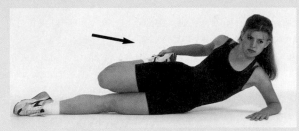

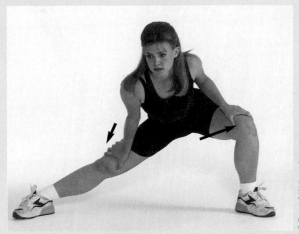

Exercise 10
Adductor Stretch

Action   Stand with your feet about twice shoulder width apart and place your hands slightly above the knees. Flex one knee and slowly go down as far as possible, holding the final position for a few seconds. Repeat with the other leg.

Areas Stretched   Hip adductor muscles

Exercise 9
Heel Cord Stretch

Action   Stand against the wall or at the edge of a step and stretch the heel downward, alternating legs. Hold the stretched position for a few seconds.

Areas Stretched   Heel cord (Achilles tendon), gastrocnemius and soleus muscles

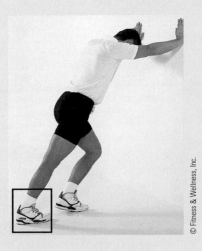

Exercise 11
Sitting Adductor Stretch

Action   Sit on the floor and bring your feet in close to you, allowing the soles of the feet to touch each other. Now place your forearms (or elbows) on the inner part of the thighs and push the legs downward, holding the final stretch for several seconds.

Areas Stretched   Hip adductor muscles

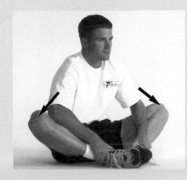

Exercise 12
Sit-and-Reach Stretch

Action   Sit on the floor with legs together and gradually reach forward as far as possible. Hold the final position for a few seconds. This exercise also may be performed with the legs separated, reaching to each side as well as to the middle.

Areas Stretched
Hamstrings and lower back muscles; lumbar spine ligaments

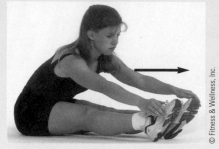

Exercise 13
Triceps Stretch

Action   Place the right hand behind your neck. Grasp the right arm above the elbow with the left hand. Gently pull the elbow backward. Repeat the exercise with the opposite arm.

Areas Stretched   Back of upper arm (triceps muscle); shoulder joint

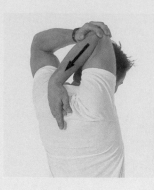

Exercises for the Prevention and Rehabilitation of Low-Back Pain

Exercise 14
Hip Flexors Stretch

Action   Kneel down on an exercise mat, a soft surface, or place a towel under your knees. Raise the left knee off the floor and place the left foot about three feet in front of you. Place your left hand over your left knee and the right hand over the back of the right hip. Keeping the lower back flat, slowly move forward and downward as you apply gentle pressure over the right hip. Repeat the exercise with the opposite leg forward

Areas Stretched   Flexor muscles in front of the hip joint

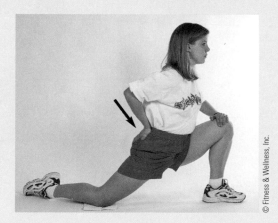

Exercise 15
Single-Knee to Chest Stretch

Action   Lie down flat on the floor. Bend one leg at approximately 100° and gradually pull the opposite leg toward your chest. Hold the final stretch for a few seconds. Switch legs and repeat the exercise.

Areas Stretched   Lower back and hamstring muscles; lumbar spine ligaments

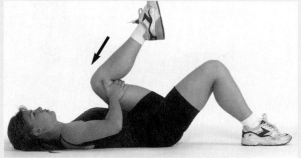

Exercise 16
Double-Knee to Chest Stretch

Action   Lie flat on the floor and then curl up slowly into a fetal position. Hold for a few seconds.

Areas Stretched   Upper and lower back and hamstring muscles; spinal ligaments

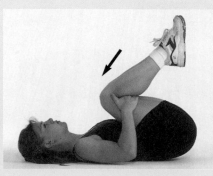

Exercise 17
Upper and Lower Back Stretch

Action   Sit on the floor and bring your feet in close to you, allowing the soles of the feet to touch each other. Holding on to your feet, bring your head and upper chest gently toward your feet.

Areas Stretched Upper and lower back muscles and ligaments

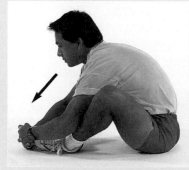

Exercise 18
Sit-and-Reach Stretch

(see Exercise 12 on page 257)

Exercise 19
Gluteal Stretch

Action　Sit on the floor, bend your right leg and place your right ankle slightly above the left knee. Grasp the left thigh with both hands and gently pull the leg toward your chest. Repeat the exercise with the opposite leg.

Areas Stretched　Buttock area (gluteal muscles)

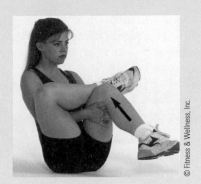

Exercise 20
Back Extension Stretch

Action　Lie face down on the floor with the elbows by the chest, forearms on the floor, and the hands beneath the chin. Gently raise the trunk by extending the elbows until you reach an approximate 90° angle at the elbow joint. Be sure the forearms remain in contact with the floor at all times. DO NOT extend the back beyond this point. Hyperextension of the lower back may lead to or aggravate an existing back problem. Hold the stretched position for about 10 seconds.

Areas Stretched　Abdominal region

Additional Benefits　Restore lower back curvature

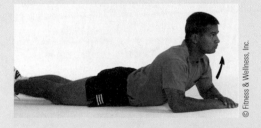

Exercise 21
Trunk Rotation and Lower Back Stretch

Action　Sit on the floor and bend the right leg, placing the right foot on the outside of the left knee. Place the left elbow on the right knee and push against it. At the same time, try to rotate the trunk to the right (clockwise). Hold the final position for a few seconds. Repeat the exercise with the other side.

Areas Stretched　Lateral side of the hip and thigh; trunk and lower back

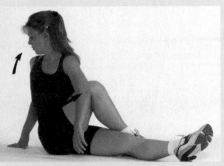

Exercise 22
Pelvic Tilt

(see Exercise 12 in Chapter 8, page 226)

Note:

This is perhaps the most important exercise for the care of the lower back. It should be included as a part of the your daily exercise routine and should be performed several times throughout the day when pain in the lower back is present as a result of muscle imbalance.

Exercise 23
Cat Stretch

Action　Kneel on the floor and place your hands in front of you (on the floor) about shoulder width apart. Relax your trunk and lower back (a). Now arch the spine and pull in your abdomen as far as you can and hold this position for a few seconds (b). Repeat the exercise 4–5 times.

Areas Stretched　Low back muscles and ligaments

Areas Strengthened Abdominal and gluteal muscles

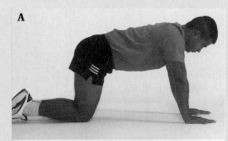

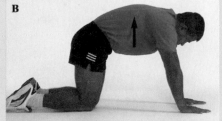

Exercise 24
Abdominal Crunch or Abdominal Curl-Up

(see Exercise 4 in Chapter 8, page 224)

It is important that you do not stabilize your feet when performing either of these exercises, because doing so decreases the work of the abdominal muscles. Also, remember not to "swing up" but, rather, to curl up as you perform these exercises.

Lab 9A

MUSCULAR FLEXIBILITY ASSESSMENT

Name: _____ Date: _____ Grade: _____

Instructor: _____ Course: _____ Section: _____

Necessary Lab Equipment

Acuflex I, Acuflex II, and Acuflex III Flexibility Testers* or homemade flexibility testing equipment as described in Figures 9.1, 9.2, and 9.3.

Objective

To assess muscular flexibility and the respective fitness categories.

Lab Preparation

The procedures for the flexibility tests* administered in this lab are explained in Chapter 9 (Figures 9.1, 9.2, and 9.3, pages 242, 243, and 245. It is important that you warm up properly before you perform any of these tests. Do gentle stretching exercises specific to the tests that will be administered. Wear loose exercise clothing for this lab. Be sure to circle either inches or cm, depending on which system you use.

I. Modified Sit-and-Reach Test

Trials: 1. _____ inches _____ cm 2. _____ inches _____ cm (circle either inches or cm)

Average score: _____ inches _____ cm Percentile rank: _____ Points: _____

Fitness classification: _____

II. Total Body Rotation Test

Right Side   Left Side   (circle one)

Trials: 1. _____ inches _____ cm 2. _____ inches _____ cm (circle either inches or cm)

Average score: _____ inches _____ cm Percentile rank: _____ Points: _____

Fitness classification: _____

III. Shoulder Rotation Test

Biacromial width: _____ inches _____ cm   Rotation score: _____ inches _____ cm

Final score = Rotation score − biacromial width

Final score = _____ − _____ = _____ inches / cm (circle one)   Percentile rank: _____

Fitness classification: _____   Points: _____

IV. Overall Flexibility Rating

Test	Points
Modified sit-and-reach:	
Total body rotation (right, left — circle one):	
Shoulder rotation:	
Total Points:	

Overall flexibility classification (see Table 9.5, page 246): _____

---

* The Acuflex I, II, and III Flexibility Testers can be obtained from Figure Finder Collection, Novel Products, Inc., P. O. Box 408, Rockton, IL 61072-0408, Phone (800) 623-5143, Fax 815-624-4866.

V. Flexibility Goals

1. Indicate the flexibility classification that you would like to achieve by the end of the term:

2. Describe your feelings about your current body flexibility and any potential implications that your current flexibility levels may have on your health and wellness. Also, briefly state how you plan to achieve your flexibility objective by the end of the term.

Name: _____   Date: _____   Grade: _____

Instructor: _____   Course: _____   Section: _____

Necessary Lab Equipment

A plumb line, two large mirrors set at about an 85° angle, and a Polaroid camera (the mirrors and the camera are optional — see "Evaluating Body Posture" (page 246).

Objective

To determine current body alignment.

Lab Preparation

To conduct the posture analysis, men should wear shorts only and women, shorts and a tank top. Shoes should also be removed for this test.

Lab Assignment

The class should be divided in groups of four students each. The group should carefully study the posture form given in this lab, then proceed to fill out the form for each member according to the instructions given under "Evaluating Body Posture." If no mirrors and camera are available, three members of the group are to rate the fourth person's posture while he/she first stands with the side of the body and then with the back to the plumb line. A final score is obtained by totaling the points given for each body segment and looking up the posture rating according to the total score found in the table provided below.

Results

Total points: _____

Classification: _____

Posture Evaluation Standards	
Total Points	Classification
≥45	Excellent
40–44	Good
30–39	Average
20–29	Fair
≤19	Poor

Posture Improvement

Indicate how you feel about your posture, identify areas to correct, and specify the steps you can take to make those improvements.

_____

_____

_____

_____

_____

_____

_____

_____

		Good — 5	Fair — 3	Poor — 1	Score
HEAD Left Right		head erect, gravity passes directly through center	head twisted or turned to one side slightly	head twisted or turned to one side markedly	
SHOULDERS Left Right		shoulders level horizontally	one shoulder slightly higher	one shoulder markedly higher	
SPINE Left Right		spine straight	spine slightly curved	spine markedly curved laterally	
HIPS Left Right		hips level horizontally	one hip slightly higher	one hip markedly higher	
KNEES and ANKLES		feet pointed straight ahead, legs vertical	feet pointed out, legs deviating outward at the knee	feet pointed out markedly, legs deviate markedly	
NECK and UPPER BACK		neck erect, head in line with shoulders, rounded upper back	neck slightly forward, chin out, slightly more rounded upper back	neck markedly forward, chin markedly out, markedly rounded upper back	
TRUNK		trunk erect	trunk inclined to rear slightly	trunk inclined to rear markedly	
ABDOMEN		abdomen flat	abdomen protruding	abdomen protruding and sagging	
LOWER BACK		lower back normally curved	lower back slightly hollow	lower back markedly hollow	
LEGS		legs straight	knees slightly hyper-extended	knees markedly hyperextended	
				Total Score	

Adapted with permission from *The New York Physical Fitness Test: A Manual for Teachers of Physical Education*, New York State Education Department (Division of HPER), 1958.

Name: _____ Date: _____ Grade: _____

Instructor: _____ Course: _____ Section: _____

Necessary Lab Equipment

Minor implements such as a chair, a table, an elastic band (surgical tubing or a wood or aluminum stick), and a stool or steps.

Objective

To develop a flexibility exercise program and a conditioning program for the prevention and rehabilitation of low-back pain.

Lab Preparation

Wear exercise clothing and prepare to participate in a sample stretching exercise session. All of the flexibility and low-back conditioning exercises are illustrated on pages 255–258.

I. Stage of Change for Flexibility Training

Using Figure 2.3 (page 40) and Table 2.3 (page 41), identify your current stage of change for participation in a muscular stretching program: _____

II. Instruction

Perform all of the recommended flexibility exercises given on pages 255–257. Use a combination of slow-sustained and proprioceptive neuromuscular facilitation stretching techniques. Indicate the technique(s) used for each exercise and, where applicable, the number of repetitions performed and the length of time that the final degree of stretch was held.

Stretching Exercises

Exercise	Stretching Technique	Repetitions	Length of Final Stretch
Lateral head tilt			NA*
Arm circles			NA
Side stretch			
Body rotation			
Chest stretch			
Shoulder hyperextension stretch			
Shoulder rotation stretch			NA
Quad stretch			
Heel cord stretch			
Adductor stretch			
Sitting adductor stretch			
Sit-and-reach stretch			
Triceps stretch			

*Not Applicable

Stretching Schedule (Indicate days, time, and place where you will stretch:

Strength-training days: M ☐ T ☐ W ☐ Th ☐ F ☐ Sa ☐ Su ☐   Time of day: ☐   Place: ☐

Low-Back Conditioning Program

Perform all of the recommended exercises for the prevention and rehabilitation of low back pain given on pages 257–258. Indicate the number of repetitions performed for each exercise.

Exercise	Repetitions
Hip flexors stretch	
Single knee-to-chest stretch	
Double knee-to-chest stretch	
Upper and lower back stretch	
Sit-and-reach stretch	
Gluteal stretch	
Back extension stretch	
Trunk rotation and lower back stretch	
Pelvic tilt	
Cat stretch	
Abdominal crunch or abdominal curl-ip	

Proper Body Mechanics

Perform the following tasks using the proper body mechanics given in Figure 9.6 (pages 253–254). Check off each item as you perform the task:

☐ Standing (carriage) position   ☐ Resting position for tired and painful back

☐ Sitting position   ☐ Lifting an object

☐ Bed posture

"Rules To Live By — From Now On"

Read the 18 "Rules To Live By—From Now On" given in Figure 9.6 (pages 253–254) and indicate below those rules what you need to work on to improve posture and body mechanics and prevent low back pain.

_____

_____

_____

_____

_____

_____

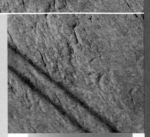

Chapter 10

Skill-Related Components of Physical Fitness

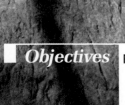

Objectives

- Learn the benefits of good skill-related fitness.

- Identify and define the six components of skill-related fitness.

- Become familiar with performance tests to assess skill-related fitness.

265

Skill-related fitness is important for successful motor performance in athletic events and in lifetime sports and activities such as basketball, racquetball, golf, hiking, soccer, and water skiing. Good skill-related fitness also enhances overall quality of life by helping people cope more effectively in emergency situations.

Outstanding gymnasts, for example, must achieve good skill-related fitness in all components. A significant amount of agility is necessary to perform a double back somersault with a full twist — a skill during which the athlete must simultaneously rotate around one axis and twist around a different one. Static balance is essential for maintaining a handstand or a scale. Dynamic balance is needed to perform many of the gymnastics routines (such as balance beam, parallel bars, and pommel horse). Coordination is important to successfully integrate various skills requiring varying degrees of difficulty into one routine. Power and speed are needed to propel the body into the air, such as when tumbling or vaulting. Reaction time is necessary to determine when to end rotation upon a visual clue, such as spotting the floor on a dismount.

As with the health-related fitness components, the principle of specificity of training applies to skill-related components. In the case of agility, balance, coordination, and reaction time, development of these components is highly task-specific. To develop a certain task or skill, the individual must practice that same task many times. There seems to be very little crossover learning effect.

For instance, properly practicing a handstand (balance) will lead eventually to successfully performing the skill, but complete mastery of this skill does not ensure that the person will have immediate success when attempting to perform other static-balance positions in gymnastics. Power and speed may improve with a specific strength-training program or frequent repetition of the specific task to be improved, or both.

The rate of learning in skill-related fitness varies from person to person, mainly because these components seem to be determined to a large extent by genetics. Individuals with good skill-related fitness tend to do better and learn faster when performing a wide variety of skills. Nevertheless, few individuals enjoy complete success in all skill-related components. Furthermore, though skill-related fitness can be enhanced with practice, improvements in reaction time and speed are limited and seem to be related primarily to genetic endowment.

Although we do not know how much skill-related fitness is desirable, everyone should attempt to develop and maintain a better-than-average level. As pointed out earlier, this type of fitness is crucial for athletes, and it also enables one to lead a better and happier life. Improving skill-related fitness not only affords an individual more enjoyment and success in lifetime sports (for example, tennis, racquetball, basketball), but it also can help a person cope more effectively in emergency situations. Some of the benefits are as follows:

1. Good reaction time, balance, coordination, and agility can help you avoid a fall or break a fall and thereby minimize injury.
2. The ability to generate maximum force in a short time (power) may be crucial to ameliorate injury or even preserve life in a situation in which you may be called upon to lift a heavy object that has fallen on another person or even on yourself.
3. In our society, where the average lifespan continues to expand, maintaining speed can be especially important for elderly people. Many of these individuals and, for that matter, many unfit/overweight young people no longer have the speed they need to cross an intersection safely before the light changes for oncoming traffic.

Regular participation in a health-related fitness program can heighten performance of skill-related components. For example, significantly overweight people do not have good agility or speed. Because participating in aerobic and strength-training programs helps take off body fat, an overweight individual who loses weight through such an exercise program can improve agility and speed. A sound flexibility program decreases resistance to motion about body joints, which may increase agility, balance, and overall coordination. Improvements in strength definitely help develop power. People who have good skill-related fitness usually participate in lifetime sports and games, which in turn helps develop health-related fitness.

Performance Tests for Skill-Related Fitness

Several performance tests have been developed over the years to assess the various components of skill-related fitness. Results of the performance tests, expressed in percentile ranks, are given in Table 10.1 (men) and Table 10.2 (women), at the end of the chapter. Fitness categories for skill-fitness components are established according to percentile

> *To develop a given component, the training program must be specific to the type of development the individual is trying to achieve.*

rankings only. The categories are similar to those given for muscular strength and endurance and for flexibility (see Table 10.3).

Agility

Agility is the ability to quickly and efficiently change body position and direction. Agility is important in sports such as basketball, soccer, and racquetball, in which the participant must change direction rapidly and also maintain proper body control.

Agility Test

SEMO Agility Test[1]

Objective
To measure general body agility

Procedure
The free-throw area of a basketball court or any other smooth area 12 by 19 feet with adequate running space around it can be used for this test. Four plastic cones or similar objects are placed on each corner of the free-throw lane, as shown in Figure 10.1.

Start on the outside of the free-throw lane at point A, with your back to the free-throw line. When given the "go" command, sidestep from A to B (do not make crossover steps), backpedal from B to D, sprint forward from D to A, again backpedal from A

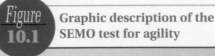

Figure 10.1 Graphic description of the SEMO test for agility

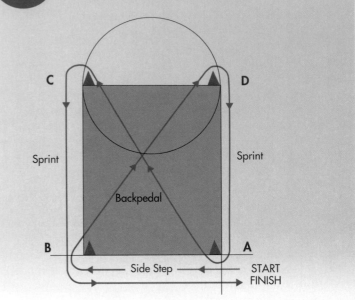

to C, sprint forward from C to B, and sidestep from B to the finish line at A.

During the test, always go around (outside) each corner cone. A stopwatch is started at the "go" command and stopped when the subject crosses the finish line. Use the best of two trials, preceded by a practice trial, as the final test score. Record the time to the nearest tenth of a second.

Balance

The ability to maintain the body in proper equilibrium, **balance,** is vital in activities such as gymnastics, diving, ice skating, skiing, and even football and wrestling, in which the athlete attempts to upset the opponent's equilibrium.

Balance Test

1-Foot Stand Test (preferred foot, without shoes)

Objective
To measure static balance

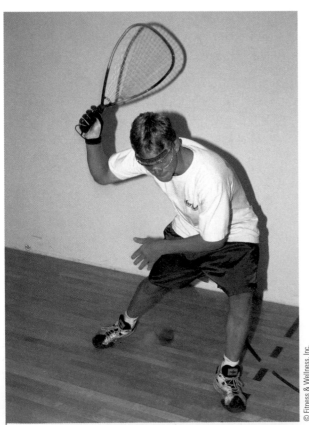

Successful racquetball players demonstrate high levels of skill-fitness.

© Fitness & Wellness, Inc.

Skill-related fitness Fitness components important for success in skillful activities and athletic events; encompasses agility, balance, coordination, power, reaction time, and speed.

Agility Ability to change body position and direction quickly and efficiently.

Balance Ability to maintain the body in proper equilibrium.

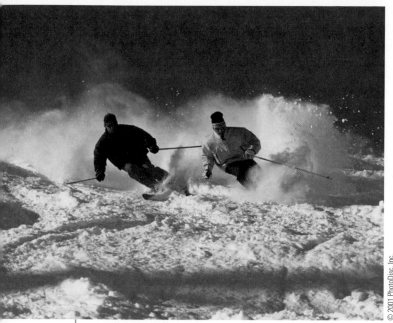

Nordic skiing requires good balance, a skill-related component of fitness.

maintains balance on the selected foot, starting with the "go" command. The best of two trials, preceded by a practice trial, is used as the final performance score. Record the time to the nearest tenth of a second.

Coordination

Coordination is the integration of the nervous and the muscular systems to produce correct, graceful, and harmonious body movements. This component is important in a wide variety of motor activities such as golf, baseball, karate, soccer, and racquetball, in which hand-eye or foot-eye movements, or both, must be integrated.

Coordination test

Soda Pop Test

Objective

To assess overall motor/muscular control and movement time

Procedure

Administrator: Homemade equipment is necessary to perform this test. Draw a straight line lengthwise through the center of a piece of cardboard approximately 32 inches long by 5 inches wide. Draw six marks exactly 5 inches away from each other on this line (draw the first mark about 2½ inches from the edge of the cardboard). Using a compass, draw six circles 3¼ inches in diameter (a radius of 1 centimeter larger than a can of soda pop), which must be centered on the six marks along the line. See Figure 10.2.

For purpose of this test, each circle is assigned a number starting with 1 for the first circle on the right of the testee, all the way to 6 for the last circle on the

Procedure

A flat, smooth floor, not carpeted, is used for this test. Remove your shoes and socks and stand on your preferred foot, placing the other foot on the inside of the supporting knee and the hands on the sides of the hips. When the "go" command is given, raise your heel off the floor and balance yourself as long as possible without moving the ball of the foot from its initial position.

The test is terminated when any of the following conditions occur:

1. The supporting foot moves (shuffles).
2. The raised heel touches the floor.
3. The hands are moved from the hip.
4. A minute has elapsed.

The test is scored by recording the number of seconds that the testee

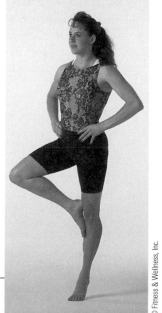

1-Foot Stand Test for balance.

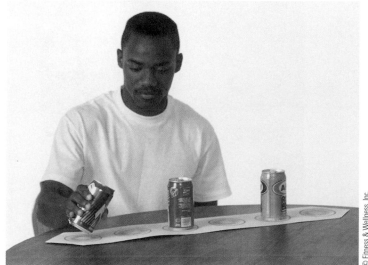

"Soda Pop" Test for coordination.

left. The cardboard, three unopened (full) cans of soda pop, a table, a chair, and a stopwatch are needed to perform the test.

Place the cardboard on a table and have the person sit in front of it with the center of the cardboard bisecting the body. Use the preferred hand for this test. If this is the right hand, place the three cans of soda pop on the cardboard in the following manner: can 1 centered in circle 1 (farthest to the right), can 2 in circle 3, and can 3 in circle 5.

Participant: To start the test, place the right hand, with the thumb up, on can 1 with the elbow joint bent at about 100°–120°. When the tester gives the signal and the stopwatch is started, turn the cans of soda pop upside down, placing can 1 inside circle 2, followed by can 2 inside circle 4, and then can 3 inside circle 6. Immediately return all three cans, starting with can 1, then can 2, and can 3, turning them right side up to their original placement. On this "return trip," grasp the cans with the hand in a thumb-down position.

The entire procedure is done twice, without stopping, and is counted as one trial. Two "trips" down and up are required to complete one trial. The watch is stopped when the last can of soda pop is returned to its original position, following the second trip back. The preferred hand (in this case, the right hand) is used throughout the entire task, and the objective of the test is to perform the task as fast as possible, making sure the cans are always placed within each circle. If the person misses a circle at any time during the test (a can placed on a line or outside a circle), the trial must be repeated from the start. A graphic illustration of this test is provided in Figure 10.2.

If using the left hand, the participant follows the same procedure, except the cans are placed starting from the left, with can 1 in circle 6, can 2 in circle 4, and can 3 in circle 2. The procedure is initiated by turning can 1 upside down onto circle 5, can 2 onto circle 3, and so on.

Prior to initiating the test, two practice trials are allowed. Two test trials then are administered, and the best time, recorded to the nearest tenth of a second, is used as the test score. If the person has a mistrial (misses a circle), the test is repeated until two successful trials are accomplished.

Power

Power is defined as the ability to produce maximum force in the shortest time. The two components of power are speed and force (strength). An effective combination of these two components allows a person to produce explosive movements such as in jumping, putting the shot, and spiking/throwing/hitting a ball.

Power Test

Standing Long Jump Test [2]

Objective
To measure leg power

Procedure
Administrator: Draw a takeoff line on the floor and place a 10-foot-long tape measure perpendicular to this line. Have the participant stand with feet several inches apart, centered with the tape measure and toes just behind the takeoff line (see Figure 10.3).

Participant: Prior to the jump, swing your arms backward and bend your knees. Perform the jump by extending your knees and swinging your arms forward at the same time.

The distance is recorded from the takeoff line to the heel or other body part that touches the floor nearest the takeoff line. Three trials are allowed, and the best trial, measured to the nearest inch, becomes the final test score.

Figure 10.2 Graphic illustration of "Soda Pop" Test

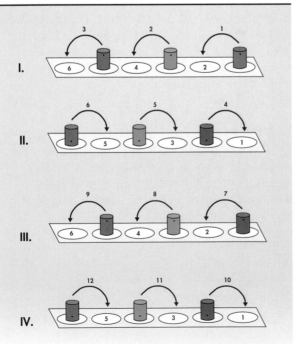

Coordination Integration of the nervous and the muscular systems to produce correct, graceful, and harmonious body movements.

Power The ability to produce maximum force in the shortest time.

Figure 10.3 Correct placement of feet for start of standing long jump.

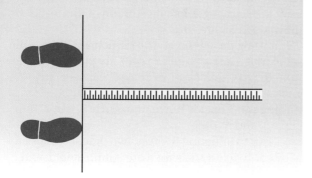

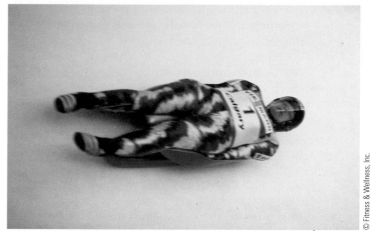

Luge athletes must exhibit excellent reaction time and coordination.

© Fitness & Wellness, Inc.

Reaction Time

Reaction time is defined as the time required to initiate a response to a given stimulus. Good reaction time is important for starts in track and swimming, when playing tennis at the net, and in sports such as ping pong, boxing, and karate.

Reaction Time Test

Yardstick Test (preferred hand)

Objective

To measure hand reaction time in response to a visual stimulus

Procedure

Administrator: For this test you will need a regular yardstick with a shaded "concentration zone" marked on the first 2 inches of the stick. Administer the test with the participant sitting in a chair adjacent to a table and the preferred forearm and hand resting on the table.

Participant: Hold the tips of the thumb and fingers in a "ready-to-pinch" position, about 1 inch apart and 3 inches beyond the edge of the table,

with the upper edges of the thumb and index finger parallel to the floor. With the person administering the test holding the yardstick near the upper end and the zero point of the stick even with the upper edge of your thumb and index finger (the administrator may steady the middle of the stick with the other hand), look at the "concentration zone" and react by catching the stick when it is dropped. Do not look at the administrator's hand or move your hand up or down while trying to catch the stick.

Twelve trials make up the test, each preceded by the preparatory command "ready." The administrator makes a random 1- to 3-second count between the "ready" command and each drop of the stick. Each trial is scored to the nearest half inch, read just above the upper edge of the thumb. Three practice trials are given before the actual test to be sure the person understands the procedure. The three lowest and the three highest scores are discarded, and the average of the middle six is used as the final test score. The testing area should be as free from distractions as possible.

Speed

Speed is the ability to rapidly propel the body or a part of the body from one point to another. Examples of activities that require good speed for success are soccer, basketball, sprints in track, and stealing a base in baseball.

Speed Test

50-Yard Dash[3]

Objective

To measure speed

Procedure

Two participants are preferable. Take your positions behind the starting line. The starter raises

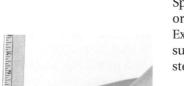
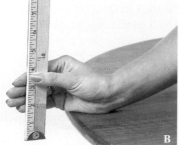

"Yardstick" Test for reaction time.

© Fitness & Wellness, Inc.

Chapter 11

Stress Assessment and Management Techniques

Objectives

- Define stress, eustress, and distress.

- Explain the role of stress in maintaining health and optimal performance.

- Identify the major sources of stress in life.

- Define the two major types of behavior patterns.

- Learn to lower your vulnerability to stress.

- Develop time-management skills.

- Define the role of physical exercise in reducing stress.

- Learn to use various stress-management techniques.

Learning to live and get ahead today is nearly impossible without stress. To succeed in an unpredictable world that changes with every new day, working under pressure has become the rule rather than the exception for most people. As a result, stress has become one of the most common problems we face. Current estimates indicate that the annual cost of stress and stress-related diseases in the United States exceeds $100 billion, a direct result of health-care costs, lost productivity, and absenteeism.

The good news is that stress can be self-controlled. Most people have accepted stress as a normal part of daily life and, even though everyone has to deal with it, few seem to understand it or know how to cope effectively. Stress should not be avoided entirely, because a certain amount is necessary for optimum health, performance, and well-being. It is difficult to succeed and have fun in life without "hits, runs, and errors."

Just what is **stress**? Dr. Hans Selye, one of the foremost authorities on stress, defined it as "the non-specific response of the human organism to any demand that is placed upon it."[1] "Nonspecific" indicates that the body reacts in a similar fashion regardless of the nature of the event that leads to the stress response. In simpler terms, stress is the body's mental, emotional, and physiological response to any situation that is new, threatening, frightening, or exciting.

The body's response to stress has been the same ever since humans were first put on the earth. Stress prepares the organism to react to the stress-causing event, also called the **stressor**. The problem, though, is the way in which we react to stress. Many people thrive under stress; others under similar circumstances are unable to handle it. An individual's reaction to a stress-causing agent determines whether stress is positive or negative.

Dr. Selye defined the ways in which we react to stress as either **eustress** or **distress**. In both cases, the nonspecific response is almost the same. In the case of eustress, health and performance continue to improve even as stress increases. On the other hand, distress refers to the unpleasant or harmful stress under which health and performance begin to deteriorate. The relationship between stress and performance is illustrated in Figure 11.1.

Stress is a fact of modern life, and every person does need an optimal level of stress that is most conducive to adequate health and performance. When stress levels reach mental, emotional, and physiological limits, however, stress becomes distress and the person no longer functions effectively.

Chronic distress raises the risk for many health disorders—including coronary heart disease, hypertension, eating disorders, ulcers, diabetes, asthma, depression, migraine headaches, sleep disorders, and chronic fatigue—and may even play a role in the development of certain types of cancers. Recognizing this and overcoming the problem quickly and efficiently are crucial in maintaining emotional and physiological stability.

Sources of Stress

Several instruments have been developed to assess sources of stress in life. The most practical instrument is the **Life Experiences Survey**, presented in Lab 11A. This survey identifies a person's life changes within the last 12 months that may have an impact on that person's physical and psychological well-being.

The Life Experiences Survey is divided into two sections. Section 1, to be completed by all respondents, contains a list of 47 life events plus three blank

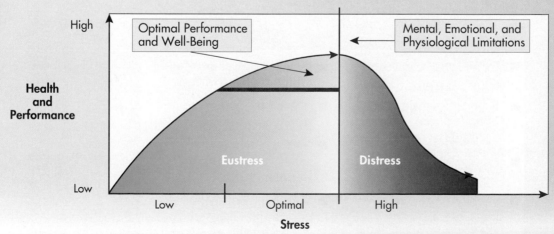

Figure 11.1 Relationship between stress and health and performance.

spaces for other events experienced but not listed in the survey. Section 2 contains an additional 10 questions designed for students only (students should fill out both sections).

The survey requires the person to rate the extent to which the life events he or she experienced had a positive or negative impact on his or her life at the time these events occurred. The ratings are on a 7-point scale. A rating of -3 indicates an extremely undesirable impact. A rating of zero (0) suggests neither a positive nor a negative impact. A rating of $+3$ indicates an extremely desirable impact.

After the subject determines the life events that have taken place, the negative and the positive points are totaled separately. Both scores are expressed as positive numbers (for example, positive ratings of 2, 1, 3, and 3 = 9 points positive score; negative ratings of -3, -2, -2, -1, and $-2 = 10$ points negative score). A final "total life change" score can be obtained by adding the positive score and the negative score together as positive numbers (total life change score: 9 + 10 = 19 points).

Because negative and positive changes alike can produce nonspecific responses, the total life change score is a good indicator of total life stress. Most research in this area, however, suggests that the negative change score is a better predictor of potential physical and psychological illness than the total change score. More research is necessary to establish the role of total change and the role of the ratio of positive to negative stress. Therefore, only the negative score is used as part of the stress profile.

Behavior Patterns

Common life events are not the only source of stress in life. All too often individuals bring on stress as a result of their behavior patterns. The two main types of behavior patterns are Type A and Type B. Each type is based on several observable characteristics.

Several attempts have been made to develop an objective scale to identify Type A individuals properly, but these questionnaires are not as valid and reliable as researchers would like them to be. Consequently, the main assessment tool to determine behavioral type is still the **structured interview,** during which a person is asked to reply to several questions that describe **Type A** and **Type B** behavior patterns. The interviewer notes not only the responses to the questions but also mental, emotional, and physical behaviors the individual

A Type A person is usually a hard-driving, overambitious, aggressive, at times hostile and overly competitive person.

exhibits as he or she replies to each question.

Based on the answers and the associated behaviors, the interviewer rates the person along a continuum, ranging from Type A to Type B. Along this continuum behavioral patterns are classified into five categories: A-1, A-2, X (a mix of Type A and Type B), B-3, and B-4. The Type A-1 exhibits all of the Type A characteristics, and the B-4 shows a relative absence of Type A behaviors. The Type A-2 does not exhibit a complete Type A pattern, and the Type B-3 exhibits only a few Type A characteristics.

Type A behavior characterizes a primarily hard-driving, overambitious, aggressive, at times hostile and overly competitive person. Type A individuals often set their own goals, are self-motivated, try to accomplish many tasks at the same time, are excessively achievement-oriented, and have a high degree of time urgency.

In contrast, Type B behavior is characteristic of calm, casual, relaxed, easy-going individuals. Type B people take one thing at a time, do not feel pressured or hurried, and seldom set their own deadlines.

Over the years, experts have indicated that individuals classified as Type A are under too much stress and have a significantly higher incidence of coronary heart disease. Based on these findings, Type A individuals have been counseled to lower their stress level by modifying many of their Type A behaviors.

A Type B person is usually calm, casual, relaxed, and easy-going.

Many of the Type A characteristics are learned behaviors. Consequently, if people can learn to identify the sources of stress and make changes in

Stress The mental, emotional, and physiological response of the body to any situation that is new, threatening, frightening, or exciting.

Stressor Stress-causing event.

Eustress Positive stress: Health and performance continue to improve, even as stress increases.

Distress Negative stress: Unpleasant or harmful stress under which health and performance begin to deteriorate.

Life Experiences Survey Questionnaire used to assess sources of stress in life.

Structured interview Assessment tool used to determine behavioral patterns that define Type A and B personalities.

Type A Behavior pattern characteristic of a hard-driving, overambitious, aggressive, at times hostile, and overly competitive person.

Type B Behavior pattern characteristic of a calm, casual, relaxed, and easy-going individual.

their behavioral responses, they can move along the continuum and respond more like Type B's. The debate, however, has centered on which Type A behaviors should be changed, because not all of them are undesirable.

Even though personality questionnaires are not as valid and reliable as the structured interview in identifying Type A individuals, Drs. Meyer Friedman and Ray Rosenman, two San Francisco scientists, constructed a Type A personality assessment form, adapted from the structured interview method, to give people a general idea of Type A behavioral patterns. This assessment form is found in Lab 11A. You can use it to understand your own behavioral patterns better. If you obtain a "high" rating, you probably are Type A.

We also know that many individuals perform well under pressure. They typically are classified as Type A but do not demonstrate any of the detrimental effects of stress. Drs. Robert and Marilyn Kriegel came up with the term **Type C** to characterize people with these behaviors.[2]

Type C individuals are just as highly stressed as Type A's but do not seem to be at higher risk for disease than Type B's. The keys to successful Type C performance seem to be commitment, confidence, and control. Type C people are highly committed to what they are doing, have a great deal of confidence in their ability to do their work, and are in constant control of their actions. In addition, they enjoy their work and maintain themselves in top physical condition to be able to meet the mental and physical demands of their work.

Type A behavior by itself is no longer viewed as a major risk factor for coronary heart disease. Type A individuals who commonly express anger and hostility are the ones at higher risk. Therefore, many behavioral modification counselors now work on changing the latter behaviors to prevent disease. The questionnaire provided at the end of Lab 11A can

CHANGING A TYPE A PERSONALITY

- Make a contract with yourself to slow down and take it easy. Put it in writing. Post it in a conspicuous spot, then stick to the terms you set up. Be specific. Abstracts ("I'm going to be less uptight") don't work.
- Work on only one or two things at a time. Wait until you change one habit before you tackle the next one.
- Eat more slowly and eat only when you are relaxed and sitting down.
- If you smoke, quit.
- Cut down on your caffeine intake, because it increases the tendency to become irritated and agitated.
- Take regular breaks throughout the day, even as brief as 5 or 10 minutes, when you totally change what you're doing. Get up, stretch, get a drink of cool water, walk around for a few minutes.
- Work on fighting your impatience. If you're standing in line at the grocery store, study the interesting things people have in their carts instead of getting upset.
- Work on controlling hostility. Keep a written log. When do you flare up? What causes it? How do you feel at the time? What preceded it? Look for patterns and figure out what sets you off. Then do something about it. Either avoid the situations that cause you hostility or practice reacting to them in different ways.
- Plan some activities just for the fun of it. Load a picnic basket in the car and drive to the country with a friend. After a stressful physics class, stop at a theater and see a good comedy.
- Choose a role model, someone you know and admire who does not have a Type A personality. Observe the person carefully, then try out some techniques the person demonstrates.

- Simplify your life so you can learn to relax a little bit. Figure out which activities or commitments you can eliminate right now, then get rid of them.
- If morning is a problem time for you and you get too hurried, set your alarm clock half an hour earlier.
- Take time out during even the most hectic day to do something truly relaxing. Because you won't be used to it, you may have to work at it at first. Begin by listing things you'd really enjoy that would calm you. Include some things that take only a few minutes: Watch a sunset, lie out on the lawn at night and look at the stars, call an old friend and catch up on news, take a nap, sauté a pan of mushrooms and savor them slowly.
- If you're under a deadline, take short breaks. Stop and talk to someone for 5 minutes, take a short walk, or lie down with a cool cloth over your eyes for 10 minutes.
- Pay attention to what your own body clock is saying. You've probably noticed that every 90 minutes or so, you lose the ability to concentrate, get a little sleepy, and have a tendency to daydream. Instead of fighting the urge, put down your work and let your mind wander for a few minutes. Use the time to imagine and let your creativity run wild.
- Learn to treasure unplanned surprises: a friend dropping by unannounced, a hummingbird outside your window, a child's tightly clutched bouquet of wildflowers.
- Savor your relationships. Think about the people in your life. Relax with them and give yourself to them. Give up trying to control others and resist the urge to end relationships that don't always go as you'd like them to.

From W. W. K. Hoeger, L. W. Turner, and B. Q. Hafen, *Wellness: Guidelines for a Healthy Lifestyle* (3d ed.) (Belmont, CA: Wadsworth/Thomson Learning, 2002).

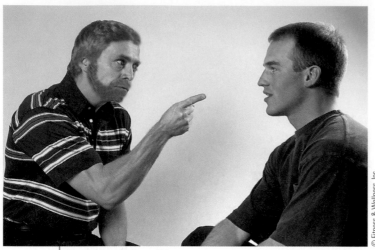

Anger and hostility can increase the risk for disease.

help you determine whether you have a hostile personality.

Many experts also believe that emotional stress is far more likely than physical stress to trigger a heart attack. People who are impatient and readily annoyed when they have to wait for someone or something—an employee, a traffic light, a table in a restaurant—are especially vulnerable.

Research also is focusing on individuals who have anxiety, depression, and feelings of helplessness when they encounter setbacks and failures in life. People who lose control of their lives or who give up on their dreams in life, knowing that they could and should be doing better, probably are more likely to have heart attacks than hard-driving people who enjoy their work.

Vulnerability to Stress

Researchers have identified a number of factors that can affect the way in which people handle stress. How people deal with these factors actually can increase or decrease vulnerability to stress. The questionnaire provided in Lab 11B lists these factors so you can determine your vulnerability rating. Many of the items on this questionnaire are related to health, social support, self-worth, and nurturance (sense of being needed). All of the factors are crucial to a person's physical, social, mental, and emotional well-being. The questionnaire will help you identify specific areas in which you can make improvements to help you cope more efficiently.

The health benefits of physical fitness have already been discussed extensively. Further, social support, self-worth, and nurturance are essential to cope effectively with stressful life events. All of these factors play a supportive and protective role in people's lives. The more integrated people are in society, the less vulnerable they are to stress and illness.

Positive correlations have been found between social support and health outcomes. People can draw upon social support to weather crises. Knowing that someone else cares, that people are there to lean on, that support is out there, is valuable for survival (or growth) in times of need.

As you take the test, you will notice that many of the items describe situations and behaviors that are within your own control. To make yourself less vulnerable to stress, you will want to improve the behaviors that make you more vulnerable to stress. You should start by modifying the behaviors that are easiest to change before undertaking some of the most difficult ones.

Time Management

According to Benjamin Franklin, "Time is the stuff life is made of." The present "hurry-up" style of life of the American people is not conducive to wellness. The hassles involved in getting through a routine day often lead to stress-related illnesses. People who do not manage their time properly will quickly experience chronic stress, fatigue, despair, discouragement, and illness.

Surveys indicate that almost 80 percent of Americans reported that time moves too fast for them, and 54 percent felt they had to get everything done. The younger the respondents, the more they struggled with lack of time. Almost half wished they had more time for exercise and recreation, hobbies, and family.

Healthy and successful people are good time managers, able to maintain a pace of life within their comfort zone. In a survey of 1954 Harvard graduates from the school of business, only 27 percent had reached the goals they established in college. Every one had rated himself a superior time manager, and

Type C Behavior pattern of individuals who are just as highly stressed as the Type A but do not seem to be at higher risk for disease than the Type B.

only 8 percent of the remaining graduates perceived themselves as superior time managers. The successful graduates attributed their success to "smart work," not necessarily "hard work."

Five Steps to Time Management

Trying to achieve one or more goals in a limited time can create a tremendous amount of stress. Many people just don't seem to have enough hours in the day to accomplish their tasks. The greatest demands on our time, nonetheless, frequently are self-imposed: trying to do too much, too fast, too soon.

Some time killers, such as eating, sleeping, and recreation, are necessary for health and wellness, but, in excess, they'll lead to stress in life. You can follow five basic steps to make better use of your time (also see Lab 11C):

1. Find the time killers. Many people do not know how they spend each part of the day. Keep a 4- to 7-day log and record at half-hour intervals the activities you do. Record the activities as you go through your typical day, so you will remember all of them. At the end of each day, decide when you wasted time. You may be shocked by the amount of time you spent on the phone, on the Internet, sleeping (more than 8 hours per night), or watching television.
2. Set long-range and short-range goals. Setting goals requires some in-depth thinking and helps put your life and daily tasks in perspective. What do I want out of life? Where do I want to

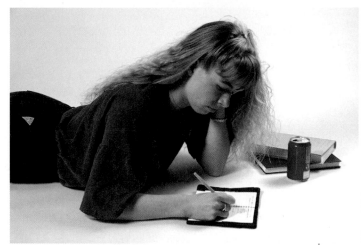

Planning and prioritizing activities simplifies your days.

be 10 years from now? Next year? Next week? Tomorrow? You can use Lab 11C to list these goals.

3. Identify your immediate goals and prioritize them for today and this week (Use Lab 11C—make as many copies as necessary). Each day sit down and determine what you need to accomplish that day and that week. Rank your "today" and "this week" tasks in four categories: (a) top-priority, (b) medium-priority, (c) low-priority, and (d) "trash."

Top-priority tasks are the most important ones. If you were to reap most of your productivity from 30 percent of your activities, which would they be? Medium-priority activities are those that must be done but can wait a day or two. Low-priority activities are those to be done only upon completing all top- and middle-priority activities. Trash activities are not worth your time (for example, cruising the hallways, channel-surfing).

4. Use a daily planner to help you organize and simplify your day. In this way you can access your priority list, appointments, notes, references, names, places, phone numbers, and addresses conveniently from your coat pocket or purse. Many individuals think that planning daily and weekly activities is a waste of time. A few minutes to schedule your time each day, however, may pay off in hours saved.

As you plan your day, be realistic and find your comfort zone. Determine what is the best way to organize your day. Which is the most productive time for work, study, errands? Are you a morning person, or are you getting most of your work done when people are quitting for the day? Pick your best hours for top-priority activities. Be sure to schedule enough time for

COMMON TIME KILLERS

- Watching television
- Listening to radio/music
- Sleeping
- Eating
- Daydreaming
- Shopping
- Socializing/parties
- Recreation
- Talking on the telephone
- Worrying
- Procrastinating
- Drop-in visitors
- Confusion (unclear goals)
- Indecision (what to do next)
- Interruptions
- Perfectionism (every detail must be done)

exercise and relaxation. Recreation is not necessarily wasted time. You need to take care of your physical and emotional well-being. Otherwise your life will be seriously imbalanced.

5. Conduct nightly audits. Take 10 minutes each night to figure out how well you accomplished your goals that day. Successful time managers evaluate themselves daily. This simple task will help you see the entire picture. Cross off the goals you accomplished and carry over to the next day those you did not get done. You also may realize that some goals can be moved down to low-priority or be trashed.

Time-Management Skills

In addition to the five major steps, the following can help you make better use of your time:

■ Delegate. If possible, delegate activities that someone else can do for you. Having another person type your paper while you prepare for an exam might be well worth the expense and your time.

■ Say "no." Learn to say no to activities that keep you from getting your top priorities done. You can do only so much in a single day. Nobody has enough time to do everything he or she would like to get done. Don't overload either. Many people are afraid to say no because they feel guilty if they do. Think ahead, and think of the consequences. Are you doing it to please others? What will it do to your well-being? Can you handle one more task? At some point you have to balance your activities and look at life and time realistically.

■ Protect against boredom. Doing nothing can be a source of stress. People need to feel that they are contributing and that they are productive members of society. It also is good for self-esteem and self-worth. Set realistic goals and work toward them each day.

■ Plan ahead for disruptions. Even a careful plan of action can be disrupted. An unexpected phone call or visitor can ruin your schedule. Planning your response ahead will help you deal with these saboteurs.

■ Get it done. Select only one task at a time, concentrate on it, and see it through. Many people do a little here, do a little there, then do something else. In the end, nothing gets done. An exception to working on just one task at a time is when you are doing a difficult task. Rather than "killing yourself," interchange with another activity that is not as hard.

■ Eliminate distractions. If you have trouble adhering to a set plan, remove distractions and trash activities from your eyesight. Television, radio, magazines, open doors, or studying in a park might distract you and become time killers.

■ Set aside "overtimes." Regularly schedule time you did not think you would need as overtime to complete unfinished projects. Most people underschedule rather than overschedule time. The result is usually late-night burnout! If you schedule overtimes and get your tasks done, enjoy some leisure time, get ahead on another project, or work on some of your trash activities.

■ Plan time for you. Set aside special time for yourself daily. Life is not meant to be all work. Use your time to walk, read, or listen to your favorite music.

■ Reward yourself. As with any other healthy behavior, positive change or a job well done deserves a reward. We often overlook the value of rewards, even if they are self-given. People practice behaviors that are rewarded and discontinue those that are not.

One more activity that you should perform weekly is to go through the list of strategies in Lab 11C to determine if you are becoming a good time manager. Provide a yes or no answer to each statement. If you are able to answer yes to most questions, congratulations. You are becoming a good time manager.

Coping with Stress

The ways in which people perceive and cope with stress seem to be more important in the development of disease than the amount and type of stress itself. If individuals perceive stress as a definite problem in their lives or when it interferes with optimal level of health and performance, several excellent stress management techniques can help them cope more effectively.

First, of course, the person must recognize that a problem exists. Many people either do not want to believe they are under too much stress or they fail to recognize some of the typical symptoms of distress. Noting some of the stress-related symptoms (see box on the following page) will help a person respond more objectively and initiate an adequate coping response.

When people have stress-related symptoms, they should first try to identify and remove the stressor or stress-causing agent. This is not as simple as it may seem, because in some situations

The ways in which people perceive and cope with stress seem to be more important in the development of disease than the amount and type of stress itself.

eliminating the stressor is not possible, or a person may not even know the exact causing agent. If the cause is unknown, keeping a log of the time and days when the symptoms occur, as well as the events preceding and following the onset of symptoms, may be helpful.

For instance, a couple noted that every afternoon around 6 o'clock, the wife became nauseated and had abdominal pain. After seeking professional help, both were instructed to keep a log of daily events. It soon became clear that the symptoms did not occur on weekends but always started just before the husband came home from work during the week. Following some personal interviews with the couple, it was determined that the wife felt a lack of attention from her husband and responded subconsciously by becoming ill to the point at which she required personal care and affection from her husband. Once the stressor was identified, appropriate behavior changes were initiated to correct the situation.

In many instances, however, the stressor cannot be removed. Examples of such situations are the death of a close family member, the first year on the job, an intolerable boss, or a change in work responsibility. Nevertheless, stress can be managed through relaxation techniques.

The body responds to stress by activating the **fight-or-flight** mechanism, which prepares a person to take action by stimulating the vital defense systems. This stimulation originates in the hypothalamus and the pituitary gland in the brain. The hypothalamus activates the sympathetic nervous system, and the pituitary activates the release of catecholamines (hormones) from the adrenal glands.

These hormonal changes increase heart rate, blood pressure, blood flow to active muscles and the brain, glucose levels, oxygen consumption, and strength—all necessary for the body to fight or flee. For the body to relax, one of these actions must take place. However, if the person is unable to take action, the muscles tense up and tighten (see Figure 11.2). This increased tension and tightening can be dissipated effectively through some coping techniques.

Physical Activity

Physical activity is one of the simplest tools to control stress. The value of exercise in reducing stress is related to several factors, the main one being a decrease in muscular tension. For example, a person can be distressed because he or she has had a miserable 8 hours of work in a smoke-filled room with an intolerable boss. To make matters worse, it is late and, on the way home, the car in front is going much slower than the speed limit. The fight-or-flight mechanism is activated, catecholamines rise, heart rate and blood pressure shoot up, breathing quickens and deepens, muscles tense up, and all systems say "go." No action can be initiated or stress dissipated, though, because the person cannot just hit the car in front.

A real remedy would be to take action by "hitting" the swimming pool, the tennis ball, the weights, or the jogging trail. By engaging in physical activity, a person is able to reduce the muscular tension and metabolize the increased catecholamines that brought about the physiological changes triggering the fight-or-flight mechanism. Although exercise does not solve problems at work or take care of slow drivers, it certainly can help a person cope with stress and can prevent stress from becoming a chronic problem.

The early evening hours are becoming the most popular time to exercise for a lot of highly stressed executives. On the way home from work, they stop at the health club or the fitness center. Exercising at this time helps them to dissipate the stress accumulated during the day. Not only does evening exercise help to get rid of the stress, but it also provides an opportunity to enjoy the evening more. At home, the family will appreciate Dad or Mom coming

COMMON SYMPTOMS OF STRESS

- Headaches
- Muscular aches (mainly in neck, shoulders, and back)
- Grinding teeth
- Nervous tick, finger tapping, toe tapping
- Increased sweating
- Increase in or loss of appetite
- Insomnia
- Nightmares
- Fatigue
- Dry mouth
- Stuttering
- High blood pressure
- Tightness or pain in the chest

- Impotence
- Hives
- Dizziness
- Depression
- Irritation
- Anger
- Hostility
- Fear, panic, anxiety
- Stomach pain, flutters
- Nausea
- Cold, clammy hands
- Poor concentration
- Pacing
- Restlessness
- Rapid heart rate
- Low-grade infection
- Loss of sex drive
- Rash or acne

You cannot hit your boss or the car in front of you, but you can certainly "hit" the swimming pool, the tennis ball, the weights, or the jogging trail.

Figure
11.2

**Physiological response to stress:
fight or flight mechanism.**

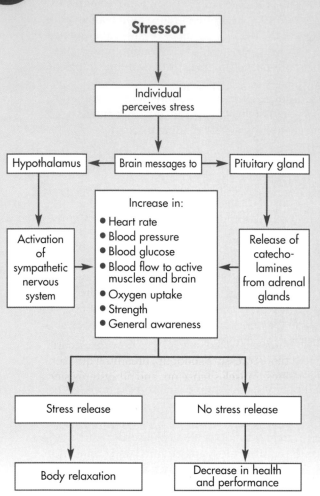

home more relaxed, leaving work problems behind, and being able to dedicate all energy to family activities.

Most people can relate to exercise as a means of managing stress by remembering how good they felt the last time they concluded a strenuous exercise session after a long, difficult day at the office. A fatigued muscle is a relaxed muscle. For this reason, many people have said that the best part of exercise is the shower afterward.

Research has also shown that physical exercise requiring continuous and rhythmic muscular activity, such as aerobic exercise, stimulates alpha-wave activity in the brain. These are the same wave patterns seen commonly during meditation and relaxation.

Further, during vigorous aerobic exercise lasting 30 minutes or longer, morphine-like substances referred to as **endorphins** are thought to be released from the pituitary gland in the brain. These

substances not only act as painkillers but also seem to induce the soothing, calming effect often associated with aerobic exercise.

Another way that exercise helps lower stress is by deliberately diverting stress to various body systems. Dr. Hans Selye explains in his book *Stress Without Distress* that, when one specific task becomes difficult, a change in activity can be as good or better than rest itself. For example, if a person is having trouble with a task and does not seem to be getting anywhere, jogging or swimming for a while is better than sitting around and getting frustrated. In this way the mental strain is diverted to the working muscles, and one system helps the other to relax.[3]

Other psychologists indicate that, when muscular tension is removed from the emotional strain, the emotional strain disappears. In many cases, the change of activity suddenly clears the mind and helps put the pieces together.

Researchers have found that physical exercise gives people a psychological boost because exercise does all the following:

- Lessens feelings of anxiety, depression, frustration, aggression, anger, and hostility.
- Alleviates insomnia.
- Provides an opportunity to meet social needs and develop new friendships.
- Allows the person to share common interests and problems.
- Develops discipline.
- Provides the opportunity to do something enjoyable and constructive that will lead to better health and total well-being.

Beyond the short-term benefits of exercise in lessening stress, another benefit of a regular aerobic exercise program is in actually strengthening the cardiovascular system itself. Because the cardiovascular system seems to be affected seriously by stress, a stronger system should be able to cope more effectively. For instance, good cardiovascular endurance has been shown to lower resting heart rate and blood pressure. Because both heart rate and blood pressure rise in stressful situations, initiating the stress response at a lower baseline will counteract the negative effects of stress. Cardiovascularly fit individuals can cope more effectively and are less affected by the stresses of daily living.

Fight or flight   Physiological response of the body to stress that prepares the individual to take action by stimulating the vital defense systems.

Endorphines   Morphine-like substances released from the pituitary gland in the brain during prolonged aerobic exercise. They are thought to induce feelings of euphoria and natural well-being.

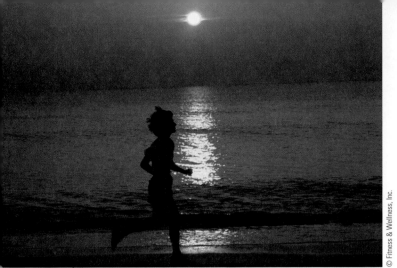

Physical activity: An excellent tool to control stress.

Relaxation Techniques

Although benefits are reaped immediately after engaging in any of the several relaxation techniques, several months of regular practice may be necessary for total mastery. The relaxation exercises that follow should not be considered cure-alls. If these exercises do not prove to be effective, more specialized textbooks and professional help are called for. In some instances a person's symptoms may not be caused by stress but rather may be related to a different medical disorder.

Biofeedback

Clinical application of **biofeedback** to treat various medical disorders has become popular in the last few years. Besides its successful application in managing stress, it is used commonly in treating medical disorders such as essential hypertension, asthma, heart rhythm and rate disturbances, cardiac neurosis, eczematous dermatitis, fecal incontinence, insomnia, and stuttering. Biofeedback as a treatment modality has been defined as

> A process in which a person learns to reliably influence physiological responses of two kinds: either responses which are not ordinarily under voluntary control or responses which ordinarily are easily regulated but for which regulation has broken down due to trauma or disease.[4]

In simpler terms, biofeedback is the interaction with the interior self. This interaction allows a person to learn the relationship between the mind and the biological response. The person actually can "feel" how thought processes influence biological responses (such as heart rate, blood pressure, body temperature, and muscle tension) and how biological responses influence the thought process.

As an illustration of this process, consider the association between a strange noise in the middle of a dark, quiet night and the heart rate response.

At first the heart rate shoots up because of the stress the unknown noise induces. The individual may even feel the heart palpitating in the chest and, while still uncertain about the noise, attempts not to panic to prevent an even faster heart rate. Upon realizing that all is well, the person can take control and influence the heart rate to come down. The mind now is able to exert almost complete control over the biological response.

Complex electronic instruments are required to conduct biofeedback. The process itself entails a three-stage, closed-loop feedback system:

1. A biological response to a stressor is detected and amplified.
2. The response is processed.
3. Results of the response are fed back to the individual immediately.

The person uses this new input and attempts to change the physiological response voluntarily—this attempt, in turn, is detected, amplified, and processed. The results then are fed back to the person. The process continues with the intent of teaching the person to reliably influence the physiological response for the better (see Figure 11.3). The most common methods used to measure physiological responses are heart rate, finger temperature, blood pressure equipment, electromyograms, and electroencephalograms.

Although biofeedback has significant applications in treating various medical disorders, including stress, it requires adequately trained personnel and, in many cases, costly equipment. Therefore, several alternative methods that yield similar results are

Figure 11.3 Biofeedback mechanism.

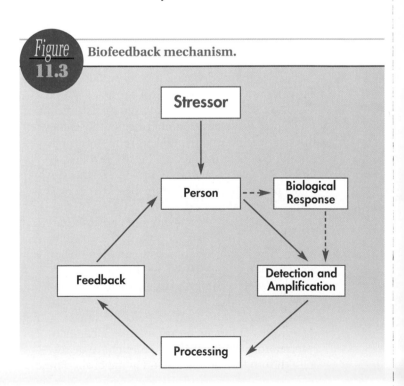

frequently substituted for biofeedback. For example, research has shown that physical exercise and progressive muscle relaxation, used successfully in stress management, seem to be just as effective as biofeedback in treating essential hypertension.

Progressive Muscle Relaxation

Progressive muscle relaxation was developed by Dr. Edmund Jacobsen in the 1930s. This technique enables individuals to relearn the sensation of deep relaxation. The technique involves progressively contracting and relaxing muscle groups throughout the body. Because chronic stress leads to high levels of muscular tension, acute awareness of how progressively tightening and relaxing the muscles feels can release the tension on the muscles and teach the body to relax at will.

Feeling the tension during the exercises also helps the person to be more alert to signs of distress, because this tension is similar to that experienced in stressful situations. In everyday life, these feelings then can cue the person to do relaxation exercises.

Relaxation exercises should be done in a quiet, warm, well-ventilated room. The recommended exercises and the duration of the routine vary from one person to the next. Most important is that the individual pay attention to the sensation he or she feels each time the muscles are tensed and relaxed.

The exercises should encompass all muscle groups of the body. Following is an example of a sequence of progressive muscle relaxation exercises. The instructions for these exercises can be read to the person, memorized, or tape-recorded. At least 20 minutes should be set aside to complete the entire sequence. Doing the exercises any faster will defeat their purpose. Ideally, the sequence should be done twice a day.

Example Relaxation Routine The individual performing the exercises stretches out comfortably on the floor, face up, with a pillow under the knees, and assumes a passive attitude, allowing the body to relax as much as possible. Each muscle group is to be contracted in sequence, taking care to avoid any strain. Muscles should be tightened to only about 70 percent of the total possible tension to avoid cramping or some type of injury to the muscle itself.

To produce the relaxation effects, the person must pay attention to the sensation of tensing up and relaxing. The person holds each contraction about 5 seconds and then allows the muscles to go totally limp. The person should take enough time to contract and relax each muscle group before going on to the next. An example of a complete progressive muscle relaxation sequence is as follows:

1. Point your feet, curling the toes downward. Study the tension in the arches and the top of the feet. Hold, continue to note the tension, then relax. Repeat once.
2. Flex the feet upward toward the face and note the tension in your feet and calves. Hold and relax. Repeat once.
3. Push your heels down against the floor as if burying them in the sand. Hold and note the tension at the back of the thigh. Relax. Repeat once.
4. Contract the right thigh by straightening the leg, gently raising the leg off the floor. Hold and study the tension. Relax. Repeat with the left leg. Hold and relax. Repeat each leg.
5. Tense the buttocks by raising your hips ever so slightly off the floor. Hold and note the tension. Relax. Repeat once.
6. Contract the abdominal muscles. Hold them tight and note the tension. Relax. Repeat once.
7. Suck in your stomach. Try to make it reach your spine. Flatten your lower back to the floor. Hold and feel the tension in the stomach and lower back. Relax. Repeat once.
8. Take a deep breath and hold it, then exhale. Repeat. Note your breathing becoming slower and more relaxed.
9. Place your arms at the sides of your body and clench both fists. Hold, study the tension, and relax. Repeat.
10. Flex the elbow by bringing both hands to the shoulders. Hold tight and study the tension in the biceps. Relax. Repeat.
11. Place your arms flat on the floor, palms up, and push the forearms hard against the floor. Note the tension on the triceps. Hold, and relax. Repeat.
12. Shrug your shoulders, raising them as high as possible. Hold and note the tension. Relax. Repeat.
13. Gently push your head backward. Note the tension in the back of the neck. Hold, relax. Repeat.
14. Gently bring the head against the chest, push forward, hold, and note the tension in the neck. Relax. Repeat.
15. Press your tongue toward the roof of your mouth. Hold, study the tension, and relax. Repeat.
16. Press your teeth together. Hold, and study the tension. Relax. Repeat.

Biofeedback A stress-management technique in which a person learns to reliably influence physiological responses of two kinds: either responses that are not ordinarily under voluntary control or responses that ordinarily are easily regulated but for which regulation has broken down because of trauma or disease.

Progressive muscle relaxation A stress management technique that involves progressive contraction and relaxation of muscle groups throughout the body.

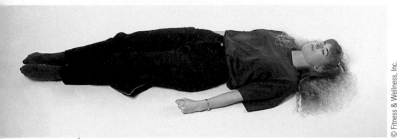

Practicing progressive muscle relaxation on a regular basis helps reduce stress.

17. Close your eyes tightly. Hold them closed and note the tension. Relax, leaving your eyes closed. Do this one more time.
18. Wrinkle your forehead and note the tension. Hold and relax. Repeat.

When time is a factor during the daily routine and an individual is not able to go through the entire sequence, he or she may do only the exercises specific to the area that feels most tense. Performing a partial sequence is better than not doing the exercises at all. Completing the entire sequence, of course, yields the best results.

Breathing Techniques For Relaxation

Breathing exercises also can be an antidote to stress. These exercises have been used for centuries in the Orient and India to improve mental, physical, and emotional stamina. In breathing exercises, the person concentrates on "breathing away" the tension and inhaling a large amount of air with each breath. Breathing exercises can be learned in only a few minutes and require considerably less time than the progressive muscle relaxation exercises.

As with any other relaxation technique, these exercises should be done in a quiet, pleasant, well-ventilated room. Any of the three examples of breathing exercises presented here will help relieve tension induced by stress.

1. Deep breathing. Lie with your back flat against the floor and place a pillow under your knees. Feet are slightly separated, with toes pointing outward. (The exercise also may be done while sitting up in a chair or standing straight up.) Place one hand on your abdomen and the other hand on your chest.

   Slowly breathe in and out so the hand on your abdomen rises when you inhale and falls as you exhale. The hand on the chest should not move much at all. Repeat the exercise about 10 times. Next, scan your body for tension and compare your present tension with the tension you felt at the beginning of the exercise. Repeat the entire process once or twice.

2. Sighing. Using the abdominal breathing technique, breathe in through your nose to a specific count (e.g., 4, 5, or 6). Now exhale through pursed lips to double the intake count (e.g., 8, 10, or 12). Repeat the exercise eight to ten times whenever you feel tense.

3. Complete natural breathing. Sit in an upright position or stand straight up. Breathing through your nose, gradually fill your lungs from the bottom up. Hold your breath for several seconds. Now exhale slowly by allowing your chest and abdomen to relax completely. Repeat the exercise eight to ten times.

> *In breathing exercises, concentrate on "breathing away" the tension and inhaling a large amount of air with each breath.*

Autogenic Training

Autogenic training is a form of self-suggestion in which people are able to place themselves in an autohypnotic state by repeating and concentrating on feelings of heaviness and warmth in the extremities. This technique was developed by Johannes Schultz, a German psychiatrist who noted that hypnotized individuals developed sensations of warmth and heaviness in the limbs and torso. The sensation of warmth is caused by dilation of blood vessels, which increases blood flow to the limbs. Muscular relaxation produces the feeling of heaviness.

In this technique the person lies down or sits in a comfortable position, eyes closed, and

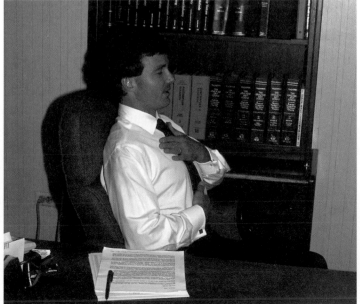

Breathing exercises help dissipate stress.

concentrates progressively on six fundamental stages and says (or thinks) the following:

1. Heaviness
   My right (left) arm is heavy.
   Both arms are heavy.
   My right (left) leg is heavy.
   Both legs are heavy.
   My arms and legs are heavy.
2. Warmth
   My right (left) arm is warm.
   Both arms are warm.
   My right (left) leg is warm.
   Both legs are warm.
   My arms and legs are warm.
3. Heart
   My heartbeat is calm and regular (repeat four or five times).
4. Respiration
   My body breathes itself (repeat four or five times).
5. Abdomen
   My abdomen is warm (repeat four or five times).
6. Forehead
   My forehead is cool (repeat four or five times).

The autogenic training technique is more difficult to master than any of those mentioned previously. The person should not move too fast through the entire exercise, because this actually may interfere with learning and relaxation. Each stage must be mastered before proceeding to the next.

Meditation

Meditation is a mental exercise that can bring about psychological and physical benefits. The objective of meditation is to gain control over one's attention by clearing the mind and blocking out the stressor(s) responsible for the higher tension. This technique can be learned rather quickly and can be used frequently during times of increased tension and stress.

Initially the person who is learning to meditate should choose a room that is comfortable, quiet, and free of all disturbances (including telephones). After learning the technique, the person will be able to meditate just about anywhere. A time block of approximately 15 minutes, twice a day, is needed to meditate.

1. Sit in a chair in an upright position with the hands resting either in your lap or on the arms of the chair. Close your eyes and focus on your breathing. Allow your body to relax as much as possible. Do not try to consciously relax, because trying means work. Rather, assume a passive attitude and concentrate on your breathing.
2. Allow the body to breathe regularly, at its own rhythm, and repeat in your mind the word "one" every time you inhale, and the word "two" every

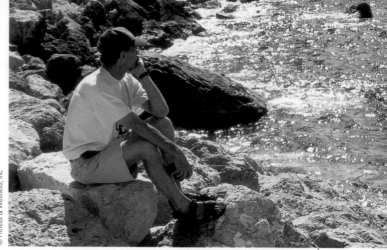

Meditation is an effective stress-reducing technique.

time you exhale. Paying attention to these two words keeps distressing thoughts from entering into your mind.

3. Continue to breathe in this way about 15 minutes. Because the objective of meditation is to bring about a hypometabolic state leading to body relaxation, do not use an alarm clock to remind you that the 15 minutes have expired. The alarm will only trigger your stress response again, defeating the purpose of the exercise. Opening your eyes once in a while to keep track of the time is fine, but do not rush or anticipate the end of the 15 minutes. This time has been set aside for meditation, and you need to relax, take your time, and enjoy the exercise.

Which Technique Is Best?

Each person reacts to stress differently. Therefore, the best coping strategy depends mostly on the individual. Which technique is used does not really matter as long as it works. An individual may want to experiment with all of them to find out which works best. A combination of two or more works best for many people.

All of the coping strategies discussed here help to block out stressors and promote mental and physical relaxation by diverting the attention to a different, nonthreatening action. Some of the

Breathing exercise   A stress management technique wherein the individual concentrates on "breathing away" the tension and inhaling fresh air to the entire body.

Autogenic training   Stress management technique using a form of self-suggestion, wherein an individual is able to place him/herself in an autohypnotic state by repeating and concentrating on feelings of heaviness and warmth in the extremities.

Meditation   A stress management technique used to gain control over one's attention by clearing the mind and blocking out the stressor(s) responsible for the increased tension.

15. Serious illness or injury of close family member:

a. father	-3	-2	-1	0	+1	+2	+3
b. mother	-3	-2	-1	0	+1	+2	+3
c. sister	-3	-2	-1	0	+1	+2	+3
d. brother	-3	-2	-1	0	+1	+2	+3
e. grandfather	-3	-2	-1	0	+1	+2	+3
f. grandmother	-3	-2	-1	0	+1	+2	+3
g. spouse	-3	-2	-1	0	+1	+2	+3
h. other (specify)	-3	-2	-1	0	+1	+2	+3
16. Sexual difficulties	-3	-2	-1	0	+1	+2	+3
17. Trouble with employer (in danger of losing job or of being suspended or demoted, etc.)	-3	-2	-1	0	+1	+2	+3
18. Trouble with in-laws	-3	-2	-1	0	+1	+2	+3
19. Major change in financial status (a lot better off or a lot worse off)	-3	-2	-1	0	+1	+2	+3
20. Major change in closeness of family members (increased or decreased closeness)	-3	-2	-1	0	+1	+2	+3
21. Gaining a new family member (through birth, adoption, family member moving in, etc.)	-3	-2	-1	0	+1	+2	+3
22. Change of residence	-3	-2	-1	0	+1	+2	+3
23. Marital separation from mate (due to conflict)	-3	-2	-1	0	+1	+2	+3
24. Major change in church activities (increased or decreased attendance)	-3	-2	-1	0	+1	+2	+3
25. Marital reconciliation with mate	-3	-2	-1	0	+1	+2	+3
26. Major change in number of arguments with spouse (a lot more or a lot less arguments)	-3	-2	-1	0	+1	+2	+3
27. Married male: Change in wife's work outside the home (beginning work, ceasing work, changing to a new job, etc.)	-3	-2	-1	0	+1	+2	+3
28. Married female: Change in husband's work (loss of job, beginning new job, retirement, etc.)	-3	-2	-1	0	+1	+2	+3
29. Major change in usual type and/or amount of recreation	-3	-2	-1	0	+1	+2	+3
30. Borrowing more than $10,000 (buying home, business etc.)	-3	-2	-1	0	+1	+2	+3
31. Borrowing less than $ 10,000 (buying car or TV, getting school loan, etc.)	-3	-2	-1	0	+1	+2	+3
32. Being fired from job	-3	-2	-1	0	+1	+2	+3
33. Male: Wife/girlfriend having abortion	-3	-2	-1	0	+1	+2	+3
34. Female: Having abortion	-3	-2	-1	0	+1	+2	+3
35. Major personal illness or injury	-3	-2	-1	0	+1	+2	+3
36. Major change in social activities (participation in parties, movies, visiting, etc.)	-3	-2	-1	0	+1	+2	+3
37. Major change in living conditions of family (building new home or remodeling, deterioration of home or neighborhood, etc.)	-3	-2	-1	0	+1	+2	+3
38. Divorce	-3	-2	-1	0	+1	+2	+3
39. Serious injury or illness of close friend	-3	-2	-1	0	+1	+2	+3
40. Retirement from work	-3	-2	-1	0	+1	+2	+3
41. Son or daughter leaving home (because of marriage, college, etc.)	-3	-2	-1	0	+1	+2	+3
42. End of formal schooling	-3	-2	-1	0	+1	+2	+3
43. Separation from spouse (because of work, travel, etc.)	-3	-2	-1	0	+1	+2	+3
44. Engagement	-3	-2	-1	0	+1	+2	+3

45. Breaking up with boyfriend/girlfriend | −3 | −2 | −1 | 0 | +1 | +2 | +3

46. Leaving home for the first time | −3 | −2 | −1 | 0 | +1 | +2 | +3

47. Reconciliation with boyfriend/girlfriend | −3 | −2 | −1 | 0 | +1 | +2 | +3

48. Others ______________________________ | −3 | −2 | −1 | 0 | +1 | +2 | +3

49. ______________________________ | −3 | −2 | −1 | 0 | +1 | +2 | +3

50. ______________________________ | −3 | −2 | −1 | 0 | +1 | +2 | +3

Section 2

51. Beginning a new school experience at a higher academic level (college, graduate school, professional school, etc.) | −3 | −2 | −1 | 0 | +1 | +2 | +3

52. Changing to a new school at the same academic level (undergraduate, graduate, etc.) | −3 | −2 | −1 | 0 | +1 | +2 | +3

53. Academic probation | −3 | −2 | −1 | 0 | +1 | +2 | +3

54. Being dismissed from dormitory or other residence | −3 | −2 | −1 | 0 | +1 | +2 | +3

55. Failing an important exam | −3 | −2 | −1 | 0 | +1 | +2 | +3

56. Changing a major | −3 | −2 | −1 | 0 | +1 | +2 | +3

57. Failing a course | −3 | −2 | −1 | 0 | +1 | +2 | +3

58. Dropping a course | −3 | −2 | −1 | 0 | +1 | +2 | +3

59. Joining a fraternity/sorority | −3 | −2 | −1 | 0 | +1 | +2 | +3

60. Financial problems concerning school (in danger of not having sufficient money to continue) | −3 | −2 | −1 | 0 | +1 | +2 | +3

How to Score

After determining the life events that have taken place, sum the negative and the positive points separately (e.g., positive ratings: 3, 2, 1, 2 = 11 points positive score; negative ratings: −1, −3, −1, −3, −2, −3 = 13 negative points score). A final "total life change" score is obtained by adding the positive and negative scores together as positive numbers (e.g., total life change score: 11 + 13 = 24 points). The various stress ratings for the Life Experiences Survey are given below. Your negative score is the best indicator of stress (distress or negative stress) in your life.

Score Interpretation*

	Negative Score		Total Score	
Category	**Men**	**Women**	**Men**	**Women**
Poor	≥13	≥15	≥27	≥27
Fair	7–12	8–14	17–26	18–26
Average	6	7	16	17
Good	1–5	1–6	5–15	6–16
Excellent	0	0	1–4	1–5

Life Experiences Survey Results

	Points	Stress Category
Negative score:		
Positive score:		
Total life change score:		

*Adapted from I. G. Sarason et al. "Assessing the Impact of Life Changes: Development of the Life Experiences Survey." *Journal of Consulting and Clinical Psychology* 46 (1978): 932–946.

II. Type A Behavior

Instructions

Please answer "yes" or "no" for each of the items listed below. For questions 7, 15, and 16, give yourself one point for each "yes" answer. For the rest of the questions, give yourself one point for each "no" answer.

Yes   No

1. Do you feel your job carries heavy responsibility?

2. Would you describe yourself as a hard-driving, ambitious type of person?

3. Do you usually try to get things done as quickly as possible?

4. Would family members and close friends describe you as hard-driving and ambitious?

5. Have people close to you ever asked you to slow down in your work?

6. Do you think you drive harder to accomplish things than most of your associates do?

7. When you play games with people your own age, do you play just for the fun of it?

8. If there's competition in your job, do you enjoy this?

9. When you are driving and there is a car in your lane going much too slowly for you, do you mutter and complain? Would anyone riding with you know you are annoyed?

10. If you make an appointment with someone, are you there on time in almost all cases?

11. If you are kept waiting, do you resent it?

12. If you see someone doing a job rather slowly and you know you could do it faster and better yourself, does it make you restless to watch him or her?

13. Would you be tempted to step in and do it yourself?

14. Do you eat rapidly? Walk rapidly?

15. After you've finished eating, do you like to sit around the table and chat?

16. When you go out to a restaurant and find eight or ten people waiting ahead of you for a table, will you wait?

17. Do you really resent having to wait in line at the bank or post office?

18. Do you always feel anxious to get going and finish whatever you have to do?

19. Do you have the feeling that time is passing too rapidly for you to accomplish all the things you'd like to get done in one day?

20. Do you often feel a sense of time urgency or time pressure?

21. Do you hurry in doing most things?

Form revised from *The Structured Interview from the Forum on Type A Behavior, National Heart/Lung/Blood Institute*, Ray M. Rosenman, MD, 1981. This form is reproduced with permission from R. W. Patton et. al, *Implementing Health/Fitness Programs* (Champaign, IL: Human Kinetics Publisher, 1986).

How to Score

Results   **Points**

Questions 7, 15, 16: _____ (1 point for each "yes" answer)

All other questions: _____ (1 point for each "no" answer)

Total score: _____

Your level of Type A: _____

Score Interpretation

Rating	Points
High	0–7
Medium	8–13
Low	14–21

III. Hostile Personality Assessment

Hostility could harm your heart. Experts now conclude that feelings of hostility increase your risk of heart disease. Dr. Redford Williams, of Duke University Medical Center, designed a questionnaire to help you determine whether you have a hostile personality. Circle the answer that most closely fits how you would respond to the given situation:

1. **A teenager drives by my yard blasting the car stereo:**
   A. I begin to understand why teenagers can't hear.
   B. I can feel my blood pressure starting to rise.

2. **A boyfriend/girlfriend calls at the last minute "too tired to go out tonight." I'm stuck with two $15 tickets:**
   A. I find someone else to go with.
   B. I tell my friend how inconsiderate he/she is.

3. **Waiting in the express checkout line at the supermarket where a sign says "No More Than 10 Items Please":**
   A. I pick up a magazine and pass the time.
   B. I glance to see if anyone has more than 10 items.

4. **Most homeless people in large cities:**
   A. Are down and out because they lack ambition.
   B. Are victims of illness or some other misfortune.

5. **At times when I've been very angry with someone:**
   A. I was able to stop short of hitting him/her.
   B. I have, on occasion, hit or shoved him/her.

6. **When I am stuck in a traffic jam:**
   A. I am usually not particularly upset.
   B. I quickly start to feel irritated and annoyed.

7. **When there's a really important job to be done:**
   A. I prefer to do it myself.
   B. I am apt to call on my friends to help.

8. **The cars ahead of me start to slow and stop as they approach a curve:**
   A. I assume there is a construction site ahead.
   B. I assume someone ahead had a fender-bender.

9. **An elevator stops too long above where I'm waiting:**
   A. I soon start to feel irritated and annoyed.
   B. I start planning the rest of my day.

10. **When a friend or co-worker disagrees with me:**
    A. I try to explain my position more clearly.
    B. I am apt to get into an argument with him or her.

11. **At times when I was really angry in the past:**
    A. I have never thrown things or slammed a door.
    B. I've sometimes thrown things or slammed a door.

12. **Someone bumps into me in a store:**
    A. I pass it off as an accident.
    B. I feel irritated at their clumsiness.

13. **When my spouse (significant other) is fixing a meal:**
    A. I keep an eye out to make sure nothing burns.
    B. I talk about my day or read the paper.

14. **Someone is hogging the conversation at a party:**
    A. I look for an opportunity to put him/her down.
    B. I soon move to another group.

15. **In most arguments:**
    A. I am the angrier one.
    B. The other person is angrier than I am.

How to Score

Score one point for each of these answers: 1. B, 2. B, 3. B, 4. A, 5. B, 6. B, 7. A, 8. B, 9. A, 10. B, 11. B, 12. B, 13. A, 14. A, 15. A. If you scored 4 or more points you may be hostile. Questions 1, 6, 9, 12 and 15 reflect anger. Questions 2, 5, 10, 11, 14, reflect aggression. Questions 3, 4, 7, 8, 13 reflect cynicism. If you scored 2 points in any category, you should work on that area of your personality.

Hostility Score		Anger Score		Aggression Score		Cynicism Score	

From Redford B. Williams, M.D., and Virginia Williams, Ph.D., *Anger Kills*. Copyright © 1993 by Redford B. Williams, M.D. and Virginia Williams, Ph.D. Reprinted by permission of Random House, Inc.

IV. In your own words, summarize the results of all three assessment tools and express your feelings about how stress and your personality affect you in daily life.

STRESS VULNERABILITY QUESTIONNAIRE

Name:	Date:	Grade:
Instructor:	Course:	Section:

Necessary Lab Equipment

None required.

Objective

To determine your stress vulnerability rating and identify areas where you can reduce your vulnerability to stress.

Instructions

Carefully read each statement and circle the number that best describes your feelings or behavior. Please be completely honest with your answers.

I. Stress Vulnerability Questionnaire

Item	Strongly Agree	Mildly Agree	Mildly Disagree	Strongly Disagree
1. I try to incorporate as much physical activity as possible in my daily schedule.	1	2	3	4
2. I exercise aerobically for 20 minutes or more at least three times per week.	1	2	3	4
3. I regularly sleep 7 to 8 hours per night.	1	2	3	4
4. I take my time eating at least one hot balanced meal a day.	1	2	3	4
5. I drink fewer than two cups of coffee (or equivalent) per day.	1	2	3	4
6. I am at recommended body weight.	1	2	3	4
7. I enjoy good health.	1	2	3	4
8. I do not use tobacco in any form.	1	2	3	4
9. I limit my alcohol intake to no more than one drink per day.	1	2	3	4
10. I do not use hard drugs (chemical dependency).	1	2	3	4
11. There is someone I love, trust, and can rely on for help if I have a problem or need to make an essential decision.	1	2	3	4
12. There is love in my family.	1	2	3	4
13. I routinely give and receive affection.	1	2	3	4
14. I have close personal relationships with other people that provide me with a sense of emotional security.	1	2	3	4
15. There are people close by whom I can turn to for guidance in time of stress.	1	2	3	4
16. I can speak openly about feelings, emotions, and problems with people I trust.	1	2	3	4
17. Other people rely on me for help.	1	2	3	4
18. I am able to keep my feelings of anger and hostility under control.	1	2	3	4
19. I have a network of friends who enjoy the same social activities that I do.	1	2	3	4
20. I take time to do something fun at least once a week.	1	2	3	4
21. My religious beliefs provide guidance and strength in my life.	1	2	3	4
22. I often provide service to others.	1	2	3	4
23. I enjoy my job (or major or school).	1	2	3	4
24. I am a competent worker.	1	2	3	4
25. I get along well with co-workers (or students).	1	2	3	4
26. My income is sufficient for my needs.	1	2	3	4
27. I manage time adequately.	1	2	3	4

Continued

Item	Strongly Agree	Mildly Agree	Mildly Disagree	Strongly Disagree
28. I have learned to say "no" to additional commitments when I already am pressed for time.	1	2	3	4
29. I take daily quiet time for myself.	1	2	3	4
30. I practice stress management as needed.	1	2	3	4

Total Points:

Test Interpretation

Rating	Points
Excellent (great stress resistance)	0–30 points
Good (little vulnerability to stress)	31–40 points
Average (somewhat vulnerable to stress)	41–50 points
Fair (vulnerable to stress)	51–60 points
Poor (very vulnerable to stress)	≥ 61 points

This questionnaire helps you identify areas where improvements can be made to help you cope with stress more effectively. As you take this test, you will notice that most of the items describe situations and behaviors that are within your control. To make yourself less vulnerable to stress, improve the behaviors that make you more vulnerable to stress. Start by modifying behaviors that are easiest to change before undertaking the most difficult ones.

II. In the space provided below, list, in order of priority, behaviors that you would like to change to help you decrease your vulnerability to stress. Also, briefly outline how you intend to accomplish these changes.

GOALS AND TIME MANAGEMENT SKILLS

Name: _____   Date: _____   Grade: _____

Instructor: _____   Course: _____   Section: _____

Necessary Lab Equipment
None required.

Objective
To help you develop time management skills.

Instructions
If you think you don't have enough hours during the day to get everything done, this lab is for you. Be sure to read the Time Management section and fill out all the forms provided with this lab.

I. Long- and Short-Term Goals

In the spaces provided below, list your goals as indicated. You may want to keep this form and review it in years to come.

1. List three goals you wish to accomplish in this life:

_____
_____
_____

2. List three goals you wish to see accomplished ten years from now:

_____
_____
_____

3. List three goals you wish to accomplish this year:

_____
_____
_____

4. List three goals you wish to accomplish this month:

_____
_____
_____

5. List three goals you wish to accomplish this week:

_____
_____
_____

Signature: _____   Date: _____

II. Finding Time Killers

Keep a 4- to 7-day log and record at half-hour intervals the activities you do (make additional copies of this form as needed). Record the activities as you go through your typical day, so you will remember them all. At the end of each day, decide when you wasted time. Using a highlighter, identify the time killers on this form and plan necessary changes for the next day.

6:00	
6:30	
7:00	
7:30	
8:00	
8:30	
9:00	
9:30	
10:00	
10:30	
11:00	
11:30	
12:00	
12:30	
1:00	
1:30	
2:00	
2:30	
3:00	
3:30	
4:00	
4:30	
5:00	
5:30	
6:00	
6:30	
7:00	
7:30	
8:00	
8:30	
9:00	
9:30	
10:00	
10:30	
11:00	
11:30	
12:00	

III. Daily and Weekly Goals and Priorities

Take 10 minutes each morning to write down the goals or tasks you wish to accomplish that day. Rank them as top, medium, low, or "trash" priorities. (Make as many copies of this form as needed.) At the end of the day, evaluate how well you accomplished your tasks for the day. Cross off the goals you accomplished and carry over to the next day those you did not get done.

Date: _____   Day of the Week: _____

Top-Priority Goals

1. _____
2. _____
3. _____
4. _____

Medium-Priority Goals

1. _____
2. _____
3. _____
4. _____

Low-Priority Goals

1. _____
2. _____
3. _____
4. _____

Trash (do only after all other goals have been accomplished)

1. _____
2. _____
3. _____
4. _____

Take a few minutes each Sunday night to write down the goals or tasks you wish to accomplish that week. As with your daily goals, rank them as top, medium, low, or "trash" priorities. (Make as many copies of this form as needed.) At the end of the week, evaluate how well you accomplished your goals. Cross off the goals you accomplished and carry over to the next week those you did not get done.

Week: _____ / _____ / _____ to _____ / _____ / _____

Top-Priority Goals

1. _____
2. _____
3. _____
4. _____

Medium-Priority Goals

1. _____
2. _____
3. _____
4. _____

Low-Priority Goals

1. _____
2. _____
3. _____
4. _____

Trash (do only after all other goals have been accomplished)

1. _____
2. _____
3. _____
4. _____

IV. Time Management Evaluation

On a weekly basis, go through the list of strategies below and provide a "yes" or "no" answer to each statement. If you are able to answer "yes" to most questions, congratulations, you are becoming a good time manager.

Strategy Date:															
1. I evaluate my time killers periodically.															
2. I have written down my long-range goals.															
3. I have written down my short-range goals.															
4. I use a daily planner.															
5. I conduct nightly audits.															
6. I conduct weekly audits.															
7. I delegate activities that others can do.															
8. I have learned to say "no" to additional tasks when I am already in "overload."															
9. I plan activities to avoid boredom.															
10. I plan ahead for distractions.															
11. I work on one task at a time, until it's done.															
12. I have removed distractions from my work.															
13. I set aside "overtimes."															
14. I set aside special time for myself daily.															
15. I reward myself for a job well done.															

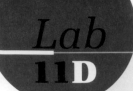

Lab 11D

STRESS MANAGEMENT

Name: _____   Date: _____   Grade: _____

Instructor: _____   Course: _____   Section: _____

Necessary Lab Equipment
None required.

Objective
To participate in a stress management session.

I. Stage of Change for Stress Management

Using Figure 2.3 (page 40) and Table 2.3 (page 41), identify your current stage of change for a stress management program:

_____

II. Stress Management

Instructions: The class should be divided into groups of about five students per group. Each group should select and go through a minimum of two of the following stress management techniques outlined in Chapter 11:

1. Progressive Muscle Relaxation
2. Breathing Techniques for Relaxation
3. Autogenic Training
4. Meditation

A group leader is chosen who will lead the exercise according to the instructions provided for each relaxation technique in Chapter 11. Be sure this experience is conducted in a comfortable room that is as free of noise as possible. If trained personnel or a tape-recording for progressive muscle relaxation exercises is available, the entire class may participate in this experience at once. Institutions that have biofeedback equipment may use it in this laboratory as well. After completing this lab, answer the four questions given below.

1. Indicate the two relaxation techniques used in your lab:

A. _____   B. _____

2. In your own words, relate your feelings as you were going through exercises A and B above:

Exercise A: _____
_____

Exercise B: _____
_____

3. Indicate how you felt mentally, emotionally, and physically after participating in this experience:

_____
_____

4. Are there situations in your daily life in which you think you would benefit from practicing the selected stress-management exercises?

_____
_____

III. Self-Assessment Stress Evaluation

1. Do you currently perceive stress to be a problem in your life?　☐ Yes　☐ No

2. Do you experience any of the typical stress symptoms listed in the box on page 282? If so, which ones?

3. Indicate any specific events in your life that trigger a stress response.

4. Write specific objectives to either avoid or help you manage the various stress-inducing events listed above, including one or more stress-management techniques.

5. Do you have any behavior patterns you would like to modify? List those you would like to change.

6. List specific techniques of change you will use to change undesirable behaviors (see Table 2.2, page 39).

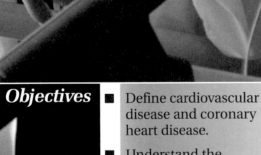
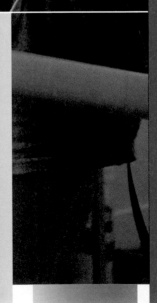

Chapter 12

Preventing Cardiovascular Disease

Objectives

- Define cardiovascular disease and coronary heart disease.

- Understand the importance of a healthy lifestyle in preventing cardiovascular disease.

- Understand the major risk factors that lead to the development of coronary heart disease, including physical inactivity, hypertension, smoking, and abnormal cholesterol profile.

- Assess your own risk for developing coronary heart disease.

- Become acquainted with a comprehensive program for reducing coronary heart disease risk and managing overall risk for cardiovascular disease.

The most prevalent degenerative conditions in the United States are **cardiovascular diseases**. About 20 percent of the population have some form of cardiovascular disease. One in three men and one in ten women will develop a major cardiovascular problem before age 60.[1] Based on 1998 statistics, 40 percent of all deaths in the United States were attributable to heart and blood vessel disease.[2]

Some examples of cardiovascular diseases are coronary heart disease, **peripheral vascular disease**, congenital heart disease, rheumatic heart disease, atherosclerosis, strokes, high blood pressure, and congestive heart failure. According to estimates, if all deaths from the major cardiovascular diseases were eliminated, life expectancy in the United States would increase by about 10 years.[3]

The estimated cost of heart and blood vessel disease in the United States exceeded $286 billion in 1998. About 1.1 million people have heart attacks each year, and more than 350,000 of them die as a result. More than half of these deaths occur within 1 hour of the onset of symptoms, before the person reaches the hospital.[4]

Although heart and blood vessel disease is still the number-one health problem in the United States, the incidence declined by 32 percent between 1960 and 2000 (see Figure 12.1), in large part because of health education. More people now are aware of the risk factors for cardiovascular disease and are changing their lifestyle to lower their potential risk for these diseases.

The heart and the coronary arteries are illustrated in Figure 12.2. The major form of cardiovascular disease is **coronary heart disease (CHD)**. In CHD the arteries that supply the heart muscle with oxygen and nutrients are narrowed by fatty deposits

SIGNS OF HEART ATTACK AND STROKE

These signs or symptoms may not all be present during a heart attack or a stroke. If any start to occur and last longer than a few minutes, do not delay, seek medical attention immediately. Call 911 or the emergency medical service (EMS) for an ambulance. If ambulance service is not available, immediately have someone drive you to the nearest hospital emergency room. Failure to do so may result in death.

Warning Signs of a Heart Attack

- Discomfort, pressure, fullness, squeezing, or pain in the middle of the chest that persists for several minutes. It may go away and return later.
- Pain that radiates to the shoulders, neck, or arms.
- Chest discomfort with lightheadedness, shortness of breath, nausea, sweating, or fainting.

Warning Signs of Stroke

- Sudden numbness or weakness of the face, arm, or leg—particularly on one side of the body.
- Sudden confusion, difficulty in speech or understanding.
- Sudden trouble seeing out of one or both eyes.
- Sudden trouble walking, dizziness, loss of balance or coordination.
- A sudden severe headache of unknown cause.

Adapted from American Heart Association, *Heart Stroke Facts*, Dallas: AHA, 1999.

such as cholesterol and triglycerides. Narrowing of the coronary arteries diminishes the blood supply to the heart muscle, which can precipitate a heart attack.

CHD is the single leading cause of death in the United States, accounting for approximately 20 percent of all deaths and about half of all cardiovascular deaths[5] (see Figure 12.3). More than half of the people who died suddenly from CHD had no previous symptoms of the disease. Further, approximately 80 percent of deaths from CHD in people under age 65 occur during the first heart attack. The risk of death is also greater in the least-educated segment of the population.[6] Almost all of the risk factors for CHD are preventable and reversible, therefore individuals can reduce their risk by adhering to a healthy lifestyle.

According to the American Heart Association, each year, more than 330,000 coronary bypass operations and 190,000 coronary **angioplasty** procedures are performed in the United States. Health-care costs for a coronary bypass average

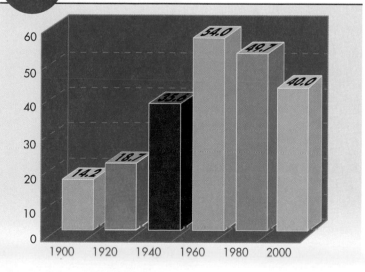

Figure 12.1

Incidence of cardiovascular disease in the United States for selected years: 1900–2000.

Figure 12.2

The heart and its blood vessels.

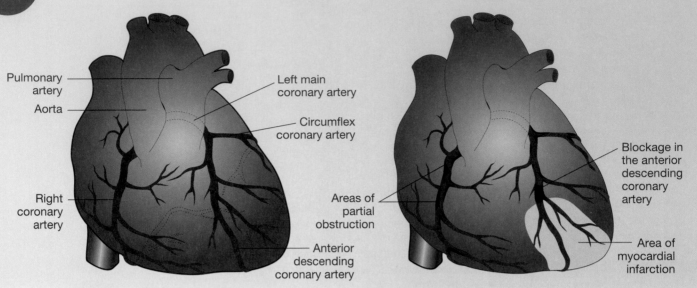

Normal Healthy Heart

Myocardial infarction (heart attack) as a result of acute reduction in blood flow through the anterior descending coronary artery

Figure 12.3

Death rates for cardiovascular disease in the United States, years 1940 and 2000.

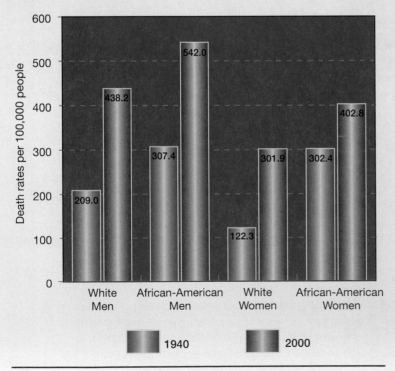

Source: American Heart Association, *Heart and Stroke Facts: 2000* (Statistical Supplement), Dallas: AHA, 1999.

more than $44,000 and for an angioplasty procedure over $21,000—or about $11 billion per year for coronary heart disease surgery.

Coronary Heart Disease Risk Profile

Although genetic inheritance plays a role in CHD, the most important determinant is personal lifestyle. CHD risk factor analyses are administered to evaluate the impact of a person's lifestyle and genetic endowment as potential factors contributing to the

Cardiovascular diseases The array of conditions that affect the heart and the blood vessels.

Peripheral vascular disease Narrowing of the peripheral blood vessels (excludes the cerebral and coronary arteries).

Coronary heart disease (CHD) Condition in which the arteries that supply the heart muscle with oxygen and nutrients are narrowed by fatty deposits, such as cholesterol and triglycerides.

Angioplasty A procedure in which a balloon-tipped catheter is inserted, then inflated, to widen the inner lumen of one or more arteries.

development of coronary disease. The specific objectives of a CHD risk factor analysis are the following:

- To screen individuals who may be at high risk for the disease.
- To educate people regarding the leading risk factors for developing CHD.
- To implement programs aimed at reducing the risks.
- To use the analysis as a starting point with which to compare changes induced by the intervention program.

The leading **risk factors** contributing to CHD are listed in Table 12.1. A self-assessment of risk factors for CHD is given in Lab 12A. This analysis can be done by people who have little or no medical information about their cardiovascular health, as well as those who have had a thorough medical examination. The guidelines for zero risk are outlined for each factor, making this self-analysis a valuable tool for managing CHD risk factors.

For example, a person who fills out the form will learn that the ideal blood pressure is around 120/80 or lower, that risk is reduced by smoking less or quitting altogether, that HDL-cholesterol should be 45 mg/dl (milligrams per deciliter) or higher for men and 55 mg/dl or higher for women, and that LDL-cholesterol should be less than 170 mg/dl (if unknown, basic nutritional guidelines also are given). (The role of HDL- and LDL-cholesterol in protecting and causing heart disease is discussed later in this chapter.)

To provide a meaningful score for CHD risk, a weighting system was developed to show the impact of each risk factor on developing the disease. This system is based on current research and on the work done at leading preventive medical facilities in the United States. The most significant risk factors are given the heaviest numerical weight.

For example, a poor cholesterol profile seems to be the largest predictor for developing CHD. Up to 12 risk points are assigned to individuals with "very high" LDL-cholesterol levels and "very low" HDL-cholesterol levels. On the other hand, the least heavily weighted risk factor is triglycerides. A maximum of only 2 risk points is assigned to this factor. Each risk factor also is assigned a zero risk level—the level at which it does not appear to increase the risk for disease at all.

> *Almost all of the risk factors for coronary heart disease are preventable and reversible, so the individual can reduce risks for acquiring CHD.*

Table 12.1	Coronary Heart Disease Risk Factors	
Risk Factors		**Maximal Risk Points**
Abnormal cholesterol profile		12
Low HDL-cholesterol		6
High LDL-cholesterol		6
Physical inactivity		8
Smoking		8
Hypertension		8
Systolic blood pressure		4
Diastolic blood pressure		4
Personal history of heart disease		8
Abnormal stress electrocardiogram		8
Diabetes		6
High blood glucose		3
Known diabetes		3
Family history of heart disease		6
Elevated homocysteine		4
Age		4
Excessive body fat		3
Tension and stress		3
Abnormal resting electrocardiogram		3
Elevated triglycerides		2

Based on actual test results, a person receives a score anywhere from zero to the maximum number of points for each factor. When the risk points from all of the risk factors are totaled, the final number is used to rate an individual in one of five overall risk categories for potential development of CHD (see Lab 12A).

A "very low" CHD risk category designates the group at lowest risk for developing heart disease based on age and gender. "Low" CHD suggests that, even though people in this category are taking good care of their cardiovascular health, they can improve it (unless all of the risk points come from age and family history). "Moderate" CHD risk means that the person can definitely improve his or her lifestyle to lower the risk for disease, or medical treatment may be required. A score in the "high" or "very high" CHD risk category points to a strong probability of developing heart disease within the next few years and calls for immediate implementation of a personal risk-reduction program, including professional medical, nutritional, and exercise intervention.

> *A risk factor analysis helps to determine the potential effect of lifestyle in the development of coronary heart disease.*

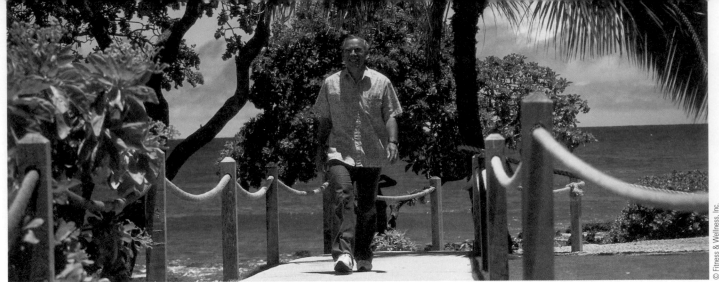

Regular physical activity helps to control most of the major risk factors that lead to heart disease.

With the exceptions of age, family history of heart disease, and certain electrocardiogram (ECG) abnormalities, the risk factors are preventable and reversible. The leading risk factors for CHD are discussed next, along with the general recommendations for risk reduction.

Physical Inactivity

Physical inactivity is responsible for low levels of cardiorespiratory endurance (the ability of the heart, lungs, and blood vessels to deliver enough oxygen to the cells to meet the demands of prolonged physical activity). The level of cardiorespiratory endurance (or fitness) is given most commonly by the maximal amount of oxygen (in milliliters) that every kilogram (2.2 pounds) of body weight is able to utilize per minute of physical activity (ml/kg/min). As maximal oxygen uptake increases, so does the efficiency of the cardiorespiratory system.

Even though physical inactivity has not been assigned the most risk points (8 points for a poor level of fitness, versus 12 for a poor cholesterol profile—see Table 12.1), improving cardiorespiratory endurance through daily physical activity and aerobic exercise has a great impact on reducing the overall risk for heart disease.

Although specific recommendations can be followed to improve each risk factor, daily physical activity and a regular aerobic exercise program help to control most of the major risk factors that lead to heart disease. Physical activity and aerobic exercise will

- Increase cardiorespiratory endurance.
- Decrease and control blood pressure.
- Reduce body fat.
- Lower blood lipids (cholesterol and triglycerides).
- Improve HDL-cholesterol.
- Help control diabetes.

- Increase and maintain good heart function, sometimes improving certain ECG abnormalities.
- Motivate toward smoking cessation.
- Alleviate tension and stress.
- Counteract a personal history of heart disease.

The significance of physical inactivity in contributing to cardiovascular risk was clearly shown in 1992, when the American Heart Association added physical inactivity to the major risk factors for cardiovascular disease. (The other five factors are smoking, a poor cholesterol profile, high blood pressure, diabetes, and obesity.) Based on the overwhelming amount of scientific data in this area, evidence of the benefits of aerobic exercise in reducing heart disease is far too impressive to be ignored.

Research at the Aerobics Research Institute in Dallas, Texas, clearly shows the tie between physical activity and mortality, regardless of age and other risk factors.[7] (See Figure 1.9, page 10 and Figures 12.8, page 312, and Figure 12.9, page 320.) A higher level of physical fitness benefits even those who have other risk factors, such as high blood pressure and serum cholesterol, cigarette smoking, and a family history of heart disease. In most cases, unfit people in the study (group 1) without these risk factors had higher death rates than fit people (groups 4 and 5) with these same risk factors.

Although the findings show that the higher the level of cardiorespiratory fitness, the longer the life, the largest drop in premature death is seen between the unfit and the moderately fit groups. Even small improvements in cardiorespiratory endurance greatly decrease the risk for cardiovascular mortality. Most adults who engage in a moderate exercise

Risk factors Lifestyle and genetic variables that may lead to disease.

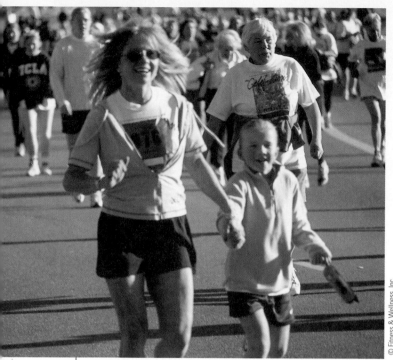

Lifetime participation in aerobic activities is one of the most important factors in the prevention of cardiovascular disease.

| Table 12.2 | Minimum Amount of Walking (Aerobic Activity) Required for Moderate Fitness in Adults |

Program 1	Days/Week	Distance (miles)	Time (min)
Women	≥3	2	≤30
Men	≥3	2	≤27
Program 2			
Women	5–6	2	30–40
Men	6–7	2	30–40

From S. N. Blair, *Fitness and Mortality* (Dallas: Aerobics Research Center, 1991).

program can attain these fitness levels easily. The minimum amount of exercise recommended for adults to achieve moderate fitness is presented in Table 12.2. Program 1 is of higher intensity than Program 2, thus only three exercise sessions per week are required for Program 1 (as compared to five to seven times per week for Program 2).

Subsequent research published in the *New England Journal of Medicine* substantiated the importance of exercise in preventing CHD.[8] Dr. Ralph Paffenbarger and his colleagues indicated that the benefits (to previously inactive adults) of starting a moderate-to-vigorous physical activity program were as important as quitting smoking, managing blood pressure, or controlling cholesterol. In relative risk for death from CHD, the increase in physical activity led to the same decrease as giving up cigarette smoking.

Even though aerobically fit individuals have a lower incidence of cardiovascular disease, regular physical activity and aerobic exercise by themselves do not guarantee a lifetime free of cardiovascular problems. Poor lifestyle habits—such as smoking, eating too many fatty/salty/sweet foods, being overweight, and having high stress levels—increase cardiovascular risk and will not be eliminated completely through an active lifestyle.

Overall management of risk factors is the best guideline to lower the risk for cardiovascular disease. Still, aerobic exercise is one of the most important

factors in preventing and reducing cardiovascular problems. The basic principles for cardiorespiratory exercise are given in Chapter 7.

As more research studies are conducted, the addition of strength training is increasingly recommended for good heart function. The American Heart Association recommends it even for individuals who have had a heart attack or have high blood pressure, as long as they do so under a physician's advice. Strength training helps control body weight and blood sugar and lowers cholesterol and blood pressure.

Abnormal Electrocardiograms

The **electrocardiogram** (**ECG** or **EKG**) is a valuable measure of the heart's function. The ECG provides a record of the electrical impulses that stimulate the heart to contract (see Figure 12.4). In reading an ECG, doctors interpret five general areas: heart rate, heart rhythm, axis of the heart, enlargement or hypertrophy of the heart, and myocardial infarction.

During a standard 12-lead ECG, 10 electrodes are placed on the person's chest. From these 10 electrodes, 12 "pictures" or leads of the electrical impulses as they travel through the heart muscle (**myocardium**) are studied from 12 different positions. By looking at ECG tracings, doctors can identify abnormalities in heart functioning (see Figure 12.5). Based on the findings, the ECG may be interpreted as normal, equivocal, or abnormal. An ECG will not always identify problems, so a normal tracing is not an absolute guarantee. Conversely, an abnormal tracing does not necessarily signal a serious condition.

ECGs are taken at rest, during the stress of exercise, and during recovery. A **stress**

Figure
12.4

Normal electrocardiogram.

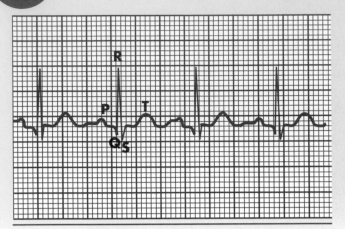

P wave = atrial depolarization
QRS complex = ventricular depolarization
T wave = ventricular repolarization

Figure
12.5

Abnormal electrocardiogram showing a depressed S-T segment.

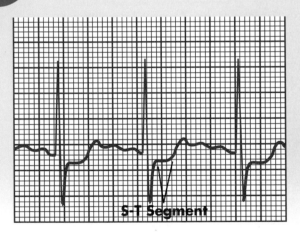

S-T Segment

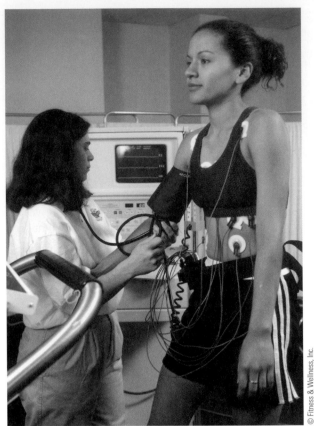

Exercise tolerance test with twelve-lead electrocardiographic monitoring (an exercise stress–ECG).

to monitor the return of the heart's activity to normal conditions.

Not every adult who wishes to start or continue an exercise program needs a stress ECG. This type of test, however, should be administered to all of the following:

1. Men over age 40 and women over age 50.
2. Anyone with total cholesterol level above 200 mg/dl or an HDL-cholesterol below 35 mg/dl.

A stress electrocardiogram reveals the tolerance of the heart to increases in physical activity.

electrocardiogram is also known as a "graded exercise stress test" or a "maximal exercise tolerance test." Similar to a high-speed test on a car, a stress ECG reveals the tolerance of the heart to increased physical activity. It is a much better test than a resting ECG to discover CHD.

Stress ECGs also are used to assess cardio-respiratory fitness levels, to screen individuals for preventive and cardiac rehabilitation programs, to detect abnormal blood pressure response during exercise, and to establish actual or functional maximal heart rate for exercise prescription. The recovery ECG is another important diagnostic tool

Electrocardiogram (ECG or EKG) A recording of the electrical activity of the heart.

Myocardium Heart muscle.

Stress electrocardiogram An exercise test during which the workload is gradually increased (until the subject reaches maximal fatigue) with blood pressure and 12-lead electrocardiographic monitoring throughout the test.

3. Hypertensive and diabetic patients.
4. Cigarette smokers.
5. Individuals with a family history of CHD, syncope, or sudden death before age 60.
6. People with an abnormal resting ECG.
7. All individuals with symptoms of chest discomfort, dysrhythmias (abnormal heartbeat), syncope, or chronotropic incompetence (heart rate that increases slowly during exercise and never reaches maximum).

At times the stress ECG has been questioned as a reliable predictor of CHD. Nevertheless, it remains the most practical, inexpensive, noninvasive procedure available to diagnose latent (undiagnosed/unknown) CHD. The test is accurate in diagnosing CHD about 65 percent of the time.

Part of the problem with reliability is that many times those who administer stress ECGs do so without clearly understanding the test's indications and limitations. In any event, sensitivity of the test increases along with the severity of the disease. The test also produces more accurate results in people who are at high risk for cardiovascular disease, in particular men over age 40 and women over age 50 with a poor cholesterol profile, high blood pressure, or a family history of heart disease.

Test protocols, number of leads, electrocardiographic criteria, and the skill of technicians administering the test also affect its sensitivity. In spite of its limitations, it is still a useful tool for identifying people who are at high risk for CHD and exercise-related sudden death.

Abnormal Cholesterol Profile

Blood lipids (fats) are carried in the bloodstream by molecules of protein known as **high-density lipoproteins (HDLs)**, **low-density lipoproteins (LDLs)**, **very low-density lipoproteins** (VLDLs), and **chylomicrons**. Although subcategories of these lipoproteins have been identified recently, the discussion here focuses primarily on the four major categories.

Cholesterol has received much attention because direct relationships have been established between high total cholesterol, high LDL-cholesterol, low HDL-cholesterol, and the rate of CHD in men and women. An abnormal cholesterol profile contributes to **atherosclerosis**, the build-up of fatty tissue in the walls of the arteries (see Figures 12.6 and 12.7). As the plaque builds up, it blocks the blood vessels that supply the myocardium with oxygen and nutrients (the coronary arteries), and these obstructions can trigger a **myocardial infarction**, or heart attack.

Figure 12.6 The atherosclerotic process.

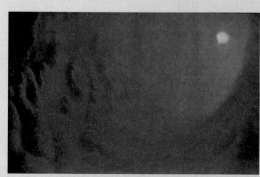

Early stage of atherosclerosis

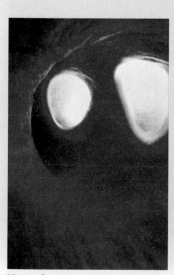

Normal artery

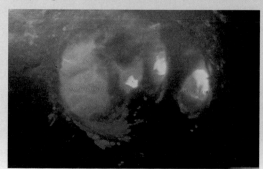

Progression of the atherosclerotic plaque

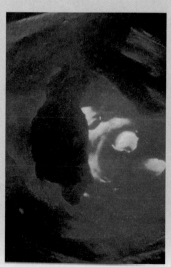

Advanced stage of atherosclerosis

Figure 12.7

Comparison of a normal healthy artery (a) and diseased arteries (b and c).

THE ATHEROSCLEROTIC PROCESS

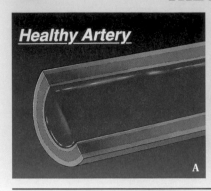
Healthy Artery — A

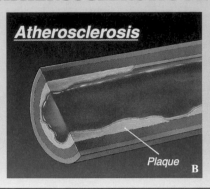
Atherosclerosis — Plaque — B

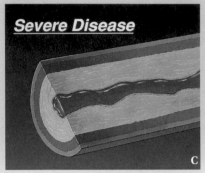
Severe Disease — C

From *Heart of a Healthy Life*. Courtesy of the American Heart Association, © 1992.

Unfortunately, the heart disguises its problems quite well, and typical symptoms of heart disease, such as **angina pectoris**, do not start until the arteries are about 75 percent blocked. In many cases, the first symptom is sudden death.

Based on research conducted at the Aerobics Research Institute in Dallas, Texas, the relative risk for all causes of mortality by physical fitness and total cholesterol levels is given in Figure 12.8. A closer look at this figure shows that a man with high cholesterol (greater than 260 mg/dl) but who is highly fit (groups 4 and 5) or moderately fit (groups 2 and 3) has a lower relative risk of early mortality than an unfit man (group 1) with low cholesterol (less than 200 mg/dl). The data indicate that, at least in men, it is better to be fit with high cholesterol than to be unfit with low cholesterol. The data aren't quite as strong for women, because fewer women have been included in the study. As the number of women studied increases, the data are expected to show a trend similar to men. The lowest mortality rate, of course, is seen in fit people with low total cholesterol levels.

The general recommendation by the National Cholesterol Education Program (NCEP) is to keep total cholesterol levels below 200 mg/dl. Other health professionals recommend that total cholesterol in individuals age 30 and younger should not be higher than 180 mg/dl, and for children the level should be below 170 mg/dl. Cholesterol levels between 200 and 239 mg/dl are borderline high, and levels of 240 mg/dl and above indicate high risk for disease (see Table 12.3). The risk for heart attack increases 2 percent for every 1 percent increase in total cholesterol.[9] Approximately 52 percent, or 98.1 million U.S. adults, have total cholesterol values of 200 mg/dl or higher, and 20 percent (37.7 million adults) have values at or above 240 mg/dl.[10]

Many preventive medicine practitioners recommend a range between 160 and 180 mg/dl as ideal for total cholesterol. In the Framingham Heart Study (a 50-year ongoing project in the community of Framingham, Massachusetts), not a single individual with a total cholesterol level of 150 mg/dl or lower has had a heart attack. Dr. William Castelli, director of the Framingham Study, recommends a total

Blood lipids (fat)   Cholesterol and triglycerides.

High density lipoproteins (HDLs)   Cholesterol-transporting molecules in the blood ("good" cholesterol) that help clear cholesterol from the blood.

Low-density lipoproteins (LDLs)   Cholesterol-transporting molecules in the blood ("bad" cholesterol) that tend to increase blood cholesterol.

Very low-density lipoproteins (VLDLs)   Triglyceride, cholesterol, and phospholipid-transporting molecules in the blood that tend to increase blood cholesterol.

Chylomicron   Triglyceride-transporting molecules.

Cholesterol   A waxy substance, technically a steroid alcohol, found only in animal fats and oil; used in making cell membranes, as a building block for some hormones, in the fatty sheath around nerve fibers, and in other necessary substances.

Atherosclerosis   Fatty/cholesterol deposits in the walls of the arteries leading to plaque formation.

Myocardial infarction   Heart attack; damage to or death of an area of the heart muscle as a result of an obstructed artery to that area.

Angina pectoris   Chest pain associated with coronary heart disease.

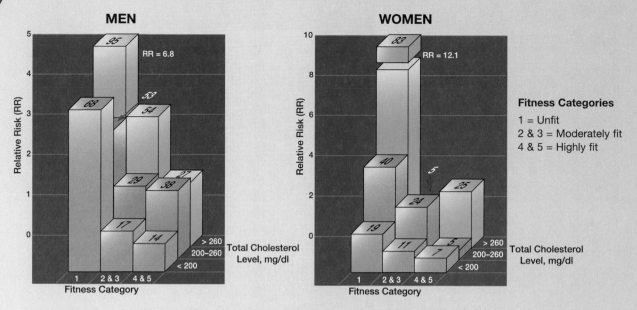

Figure 12.8

Relative risks of all-cause mortality by physical fitness and serum cholesterol level.

Numbers on top of the bars are all-cause death rates per 10,000 person-years of follow-up for each cell; 1 person-year indicates one person who was followed up one year later.

Source: S. N. Blair, H. W. Kohl III, R. S. Paffenbarger, Jr., D. G. Clark, K. H. Cooper, and L. W. Gibbons, "Physical Fitness and All-Cause Mortality: A Prospective Study of Healthy Men and Women," *Journal of the American Medical Association* 262 (1989): 2395–2401. © American Medical Association. Reproduced by permission.

Table 12.3

Cholesterol Guidelines

	Amount	Rating
Total Cholesterol	<200 mg/dl	Desirable
	200–239 mg/dl	Borderline high
	≥240 mg/dl	High risk
LDL-Cholesterol	<130 mg/dl	Desirable
	130–159 mg/dl	Borderline high
	≥160 mg/dl	High risk

	Men	Women	
HDL-Cholesterol	≥45 mg/dl	≥55 mg/dl	Desirable
	36–44 mg/dl	46–54 mg/dl	Moderate risk
	≤35 mg/dl	≤45 mg/dl	High risk

From National Cholesterol Education Program.

Cholesterol is transported primarily in the form of high-density lipoprotein (HDL) cholesterol and low-density lipoprotein (LDL) cholesterol.

In a process known as **reverse cholesterol transport**, HDLs act as "scavengers," removing cholesterol from the body and preventing plaque from forming in the arteries. The strength of HDL is in the protein molecules found in its coating. When HDL comes in contact with cholesterol-filled cells, these protein molecules attach to the cells and take their cholesterol.

LDL-cholesterol, on the other hand, tends to release cholesterol, which then may penetrate the lining of the arteries and speed up the process of atherosclerosis. The NCEP guidelines given in Table 12.3 state that an LDL-cholesterol value below 130 mg/dl is desirable, between 130 and 159 mg/dl is borderline-high, and 160 mg/dl and above presents high risk for cardiovascular disease. For people with atherosclerosis, Dr. Castelli recommends an LDL-cholesterol level of 100 mg/dl or lower.[11] A genetic variation of LDL-cholesterol, known as Lp(a), is noteworthy because a high level of these particles leads to an earlier development of atherosclerosis. It is thought that certain substances in the arterial wall interact with Lp(a) leading to premature formation of plaque.

cholesterol level of less than 150 mg/dl for possible plaque regression in people with atherosclerosis.

As important as it is, total cholesterol no longer is the best predictor for cardiovascular risk. Many heart attacks occur in people with only slightly elevated total cholesterol. More significant is the way in which cholesterol is carried in the bloodstream.

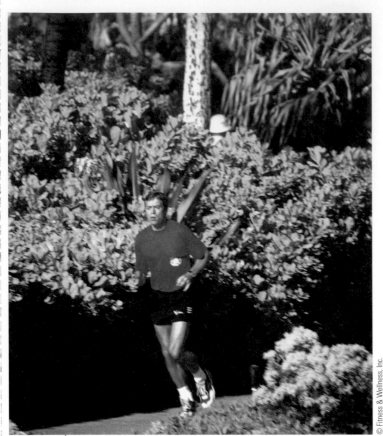

Habitual aerobic exercise helps to increase HDL-cholesterol ("good" cholesterol).

The more HDL-cholesterol (particularly the subcategory HDL$_2$), the better. HDL-cholesterol, the "good cholesterol," offers some protection against heart disease. Actually, low levels of HDL-cholesterol could be the best predictor of CHD and may be more significant than the total value. A low level of HDL-cholesterol has the strongest relationship to CHD at all levels of total cholesterol, including levels below 200 mg/dl.[12]

People with low total cholesterol (less than 200 mg/dl) and also low HDL-cholesterol (under 40 mg/dl) may have three times greater risk for heart disease than those with high cholesterol but with good HDL-cholesterol levels. Research, based on 797 patients whose total cholesterol was lower than 200 mg/dl, showed that 60 percent of the patients had heart disease, and almost 75 percent of this group had HDL-cholesterol levels below 40 mg/dl. Data also suggests that for every 1 mg/dl increase in HDL-cholesterol, the risk for CHD drops up to 3 percent in men and 5 percent in women.[13] The recommended HDL-cholesterol values to minimize the risk for CHD are a minimum of 45 mg/dl for men and 55 mg/dl for women. HDL-cholesterol levels above 60 mg/dl actually may reduce the risk for CHD.

For the most part, HDL-cholesterol is determined genetically. Generally, women have higher levels than men. The female sex hormone estrogen tends to raise HDL, so premenopausal women have a much lower incidence of heart disease. African-American children and adult men have higher HDL values than whites. HDL-cholesterol also decreases with age.

Increasing HDL-cholesterol improves the cholesterol profile and lessens the risk for CHD. Habitual aerobic exercise, weight loss, niacin, and quitting smoking help raise HDL-cholesterol.[14] Beta-carotene and drug therapy (see below) may also promote higher HDL-cholesterol levels.[15]

HDL-cholesterol and a regular aerobic exercise program (preferably high intensity, or above 6 METs, for at least 20 minutes three times per week—see Chapter 7) are clearly related. Individual responses to aerobic exercise differ, but, generally, the more the exercise, the higher the HDL-cholesterol level.

Even when more LDL-cholesterol is present than the cells can use, cholesterol seems not to cause a problem until it is oxidized by free radicals. After oxidization, white blood cells invade the arterial wall, take up the cholesterol, and clog the arteries.

As discussed in Chapter 3, the antioxidant effect of vitamins C and E and beta-carotene also can reduce the risk for CHD.[16] Data suggests that a single unstable free radical (an oxygen compound produced during metabolism) can damage LDL particles, accelerating the atherosclerotic process. Vitamin C seems to inactivate free radicals, and vitamin E protects LDL from oxidation. Beta-carotene not only absorbs free radicals, keeping them from causing damage, but it also may help increase HDL levels. One to two medium-size raw carrots per day provide the recommended daily amount of beta-carotene antioxidant nutrients.

Certain cholesterol-lowering drugs also may help raise HDL levels. These agents include colestipol, niacin, cholestyramine, and gemfibrozil.[17] Some experts believe that HDL levels below 35 mg/dl in combination with triglycerides above 160 mg/dl should be treated with medication (see discussion on triglycerides on page 316).

Many authorities also believe the ratio of LDL-cholesterol to HDL-cholesterol is a strong indicator of potential risk for cardiovascular disease. An LDL-cholesterol to HDL-cholesterol ratio of 3.5 or lower is excellent for men, and 3.0 or lower is best for

Reverse cholesterol transport A process in which HDL molecules attract cholesterol and carry it to the liver, where it is changed to bile and eventually excreted in the stool.

women. For instance, 50 mg/dl of HDL-cholesterol, as compared with 150 mg/dl of LDL-cholesterol, translates to a ratio of 3.0 (150 ÷ 50 = 3.0).

Although the average adult in the United States consumes between 400 and 600 mg of cholesterol daily, the body actually manufactures more than that. Saturated fats raise cholesterol levels more than anything else in the diet. Saturated fats produce approximately 1,000 mg of cholesterol per day.[18] Because of individual differences, some people can have a higher-than-normal intake of saturated fats and still maintain normal levels. Others who have a lower intake can have abnormally high levels.

Saturated fats are found mostly in meats and dairy products and seldom in foods of plant origin (see Table 12.4). Poultry and fish contain less saturated fat than beef does, but should be eaten in moderation (about 3 to 6 ounces per day—see Chapter 3). Unsaturated fats are mainly of plant origin and cannot be converted to cholesterol.

If one's LDL-cholesterol is higher than ideal, it can be lowered by losing body fat, manipulating the diet, taking medication, and participating in a regular aerobic exercise program. Cholesterol-lowering drugs, most notably the statins group, can lower cholesterol by 25 to 50 percent in two to three months. These medications decrease absorption in the intestines or block cholesterol formation by the cells. It is better to lower LDL-cholesterol without medication, because these drugs can cause muscle and joint pain and alter liver enzyme levels. People with heart disease must often take cholesterol-lowering medication, but it is best if medication is combined with lifestyle changes to augment the cholesterol-lowering effect.

BLOOD CHEMISTRY TEST GUIDELINES

People who have never had a blood chemistry test should do so, to establish a baseline for future reference. The blood test should include total cholesterol, LDL-cholesterol, HDL-cholesterol, triglycerides, and blood glucose.

Following an initial normal baseline test no later than age 20, for a person who adheres to the recommended dietary and exercise guidelines, a blood analysis at least every 5 years prior to age 40 should suffice. Thereafter, a blood lipid test is recommended every year, in conjunction with a regular preventive medicine physical examination.

A single baseline test is not necessarily a valid measure. Cholesterol levels vary from month to month and sometimes even from day to day. If the initial test reveals cholesterol abnormalities, the test should be repeated within a few weeks to confirm the results.

Table 12.4 Cholesterol and Saturated Fat Content of Selected Foods

Food	Serving Size	Cholesterol (mg)	Sat. Fat (gr)
Avocado	1/8 med.	—	3.2
Bacon	2 slices	30	2.7
Beans (all types)	any	—	—
Beef — lean, fat trimmed off	3 oz	75	6.0
Beef heart (cooked)	3 oz	150	1.6
Beef liver (cooked)	3 oz	255	1.3
Butter	1 tsp	12	0.4
Caviar	1 oz	85	—
Cheese			
American	2 oz	54	11.2
Cheddar	2 oz	60	12.0
Cottage (1% fat)	1 cup	10	0.4
Cottage (4% fat)	1 cup	31	6.0
Cream	2 oz	62	6.0
Muenster	2 oz	54	10.8
Parmesan	2 oz	38	9.3
Swiss	2 oz	52	10.0
Chicken (no skin)	3 oz	45	0.4
Chicken liver	3 oz	472	1.1
Chicken thigh, wing	3 oz	69	3.3
Egg (yolk)	1	250	1.8
Frankfurter	2	90	11.2
Fruits	any	—	—
Grains (all types)	any	—	—
Halibut, flounder	3 oz	43	0.7
Ice cream	1/2 cup	27	4.4
Lamb	3 oz	60	7.2
Lard	1 tsp	5	1.9
Lobster	3 oz	170	0.5
Margarine (all vegetable)	1 tsp	—	0.7
Mayonnaise	1 tbsp	10	2.1
Milk			
Skim	1 cup	5	0.3
Low fat (2%)	1 cup	18	2.9
Whole	1 cup	34	5.1
Nuts	1 oz	—	1.0
Oysters	3 oz	42	—
Salmon	3 oz	30	0.8
Scallops	3 oz	29	—
Sherbet	1/2 cup	7	1.2
Shrimp	3 oz	128	0.1
Trout	3 oz	45	2.1
Tuna (canned — drained)	3 oz	55	—
Turkey dark meat	3 oz	60	0.6
Turkey light meat	3 oz	50	0.4
Vegetables (except avocado)	any		

To decrease LDL-cholesterol, a diet low in fat, saturated fat, and cholesterol, and high in fiber is recommended. Saturated fat should be replaced with monounsaturated and polyunsaturated fats because the latter tend to decrease LDL-cholesterol (see the section titled "Simple Fats" in Chapter 3). Exercise is important, because dietary manipulation by itself is not as effective in lowering LDL-cholesterol as a combination of diet plus aerobic exercise.[19]

To lower LDL-cholesterol significantly, total daily fiber intake must be in the range of 25 to 30 grams per day (see "Fiber" in Chapter 3), total fat consumption must be significantly lower than the current 30 percent of total daily caloric intake guideline, saturated fat consumption has to be under 10 percent of the total daily caloric intake, and the average cholesterol consumption should be much lower than 300 mg per day.

Most people's fiber intake in the United States averages less than 12 grams per day. Fiber, in particular the soluble type, has been shown to lower cholesterol. Soluble fiber dissolves in water and forms a gel-like substance that encloses food particles. This property helps bind and excrete fats from the body. The incidence of heart disease is very low in populations where daily fiber intake exceeds 30 grams per day. Further, a 1996 Harvard University Medical School study of 43,000 middle-aged men who were followed for more than 6 years showed that increasing fiber intake to 30 daily grams resulted in a 41 percent reduction in heart attacks.[20]

Research on the effects of a 30 percent–fat diet have shown that it has little or no effect in lowering cholesterol, and that CHD actually continues to progress in people who have the disease. The good news came in a study published in the *Archives of Internal Medicine*.[21] Men and women in the study lowered their cholesterol by an average of 23 percent in only 3 weeks following a 10 percent or less fat-calorie diet combined with a regular aerobic exercise program, primarily walking. In this diet, cholesterol intake was less than 25 mg/day. The author of the study concluded that the exact percent-fat guideline (10 or 15 percent) is unknown (it also varies from individual to individual), but that 30 percent total fat calories is definitely too much when attempting to lower cholesterol.

A daily 10 percent total–fat diet requires the person to limit fat intake to an absolute minimum. Some health care professionals contend that a diet like this is difficult to follow indefinitely. People with high cholesterol levels, however, may not have to follow that diet indefinitely but should adopt the 10 percent–fat diet while attempting to lower cholesterol. Thereafter, eating a 20 to 30 percent–fat diet may be adequate to maintain recommended cholesterol levels (national data indicate that

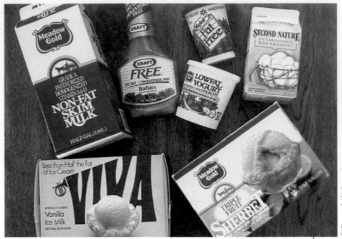

© Fitness & Wellness, Inc.

As long as the number of servings are not increased, substituting low-fat for high-fat products in the diet significantly decreases the risk for disease.

current fat consumption in the United States averages 34 percent of total calories—see Figure 3.7, page 56).

A drawback of very low-fat diets (less than 25 percent fat) is that they tend to lower HDL-cholesterol and increase triglycerides. If HDL-cholesterol is already low, monounsaturated and polyunsaturated fats should be added to the diet. Olive, canola, corn, and soybean oils and nuts are sample food items that are high in monounsaturated fats and polyunsaturated fats. A specialized nutrition book should be consulted to determine food items that are high in monounsaturated and polyunsaturated fats (also see Figure 3.11, page 62).

Soy protein is also recommended to lower total LDL-cholesterol. Over time, a diet low in saturated fat and cholesterol that includes 25 grams of soy protein a day will lower cholesterol by an additional 5 to 7 percent, compared with the same diet without the soy protein. This benefit is seen primarily in people with total cholesterol levels above 200 mg/dl. Some people may have to consume up to 60 grams a day to see an effect. Additional information on soy foods and their health benefits is given in Chapters 3 and 13.

Margarines and salad dressings that contain stanol ester, a plant-derived compound that lowers cholesterol, are now also on the market. Over the course of several weeks, about 3 grams of margarine or 6 tablespoons of salad dressing containing stanol ester lowers LDL-cholesterol by 14 percent.

To lower LDL-cholesterol levels, the following general dietary guidelines are recommended:

■ Consume between 25 and 30 grams of fiber daily, including a minimum of 10 grams of soluble fiber (good sources are oats, fruits, barley, and legumes).
■ Consume 25 grams of soy protein a day.

- Consume red meats (3 ounces per serving) fewer than three times per week and no organ meats (such as liver and kidneys).
- Do not eat commercially baked foods.
- Avoid foods that contain transfatty acids, hydrogenated fat, or partially hydrogenated vegetable oil.
- Drink low-fat milk (1 percent or less fat, preferably) and low-fat dairy products.
- Do not use coconut oil, palm oil, or cocoa butter.
- Limit egg consumption to less than three eggs per week (this is for people with high cholesterol only; others may consume eggs in moderation).
- Eat fish instead of red meat.
- Bake, broil, grill, poach, or steam food instead of frying.
- Refrigerate cooked meat before adding to other dishes. Remove fat hardened in the refrigerator before mixing the meat with other foods.
- Avoid fatty sauces made with butter, cream, or cheese.
- Maintain recommended body weight.

The combination of a healthy diet, a sound aerobic exercise program, and weight control is the best prescription for controlling blood lipids. If this does not work, a physician can administer a blood test to break down the lipoproteins into their various subcategories. Most U.S. laboratories do not conduct these tests. The American Heart Association, however, has established Lipid Disorder Training Centers that administer comprehensive blood tests. Your local American Heart Association can provide further information.

The NCEP guidelines recommend that people consider drug therapy if, after 6 months on a low-cholesterol, low-fat diet, cholesterol remains unacceptably high. An unacceptable level is an LDL-cholesterol above 190 mg/dl for people with fewer than two risk factors and no signs of heart disease. For people with more than two risk factors and with a history of heart disease, LDL-cholesterol above 160 mg/dl is unacceptable.

Elevated Triglycerides

Triglycerides are also known as free fatty acids. They make up most of the fat in our diet and most of the fat that circulates in the blood. In combination with cholesterol, triglycerides speed up formation of plaque in the arteries. Triglycerides are carried in the bloodstream primarily by very low-density lipoproteins (VLDLs) and chylomicrons.

Although they are found in poultry skin, lunch meats, and shellfish, these fatty acids are manufactured mainly in the liver from refined sugars, starches, and alcohol. High intake of alcohol and sugars (honey and fruit juices included) significantly raises triglyceride levels. Triglycerides can be lowered by cutting down on these foods and on overall fat consumption, quitting smoking, reducing weight (if overweight), and doing aerobic exercise. An optimal blood triglyceride level is less than 125 mg/dl (see Table 12.5). For people with cardiovascular problems, this level should be below 100 mg/dl.[22]

Some people consistently have slightly elevated triglyceride levels (above 140 mg/dl) and HDL-cholesterol levels below 35 mg/dl. About 80 percent of these people have a genetic condition called LDL phenotype B (approximately 40 percent of the U.S. population falls in this category). Although the blood lipids may not be notably high, these people are at higher risk for atherosclerosis and CHD.[23]

A single cholesterol test may not be a true indicator of a person's regular cholesterol values.

Elevated Homocysteine

Clinical data indicating that many heart attack and stroke victims have normal cholesterol levels has led researchers to look for other risk factors that may contribute to atherosclerosis. Although it is not a blood lipid, a high concentration of the amino acid **homocysteine** in the blood is thought to enhance plaque formation and subsequent blockage of the arteries.[24]

The body uses homocysteine to help build proteins and carry out cellular metabolism. It is an intermediate amino acid in the interconversion of two other amino acids—methionine and cysteine. This interconversion requires the B vitamin folate (folic acid) and vitamins B_6 and B_{12}. Typically, homocysteine is metabolized rapidly, so it does not accumulate in the blood or damage the arteries.

A large number of people, however, have high blood levels of homocysteine. This might result from either a genetic inability to metabolize homocysteine or a deficiency in the vitamins required for its conversion. Homocysteine is typically measured in micromoles per liter (μmol/l). In a 10-year follow-up study of people with high homocysteine levels,

Table 12.5	**Triglycerides Guidelines**	
	Amount	**Rating**
	≤125 mg/dl	Desirable
	126–499 mg/dl	Borderline high
	≥500 mg/dl	High risk

the data showed that those individuals with a level above 14.25 µmol/l had almost twice the risk of stroke compared with individuals whose level was below 9.25 µmol/l.[25] It is theorized that homocysteine accumulation is toxic because it may

1. cause damage to the inner lining of the arteries (the initial step in the process of atherosclerosis),
2. stimulate the proliferation of cells that contribute to plaque formation, and
3. encourage clotting, which may completely obstruct an artery and lead to a heart attack or stroke.

Keeping homocysteine from accumulating in the blood seems to be as simple as eating the recommended daily servings of vegetables, fruits, grains, and some meat and legumes. Increasing evidence that folate can prevent heart attacks has led to the recommendation that people consume 400 mcg per day. Unfortunately, estimates indicate that less than 88 percent of Americans get 400 daily mcg of folate.[26] Five servings of fruits and vegetables daily can provide sufficient levels of folate and vitamin B_6 to remove and clear homocysteine from the blood. People who consume five servings are unlikely to derive extra benefits from a vitamin B complex supplement (400 mcg of daily folate also are recommended for women of child-bearing age to prevent birth defects).

Vitamin B_{12} is found primarily in animal flesh and animal products. Vitamin B_{12} deficiency is rarely a problem, because 1 cup of milk or an egg provides the daily requirement. The body also recycles most of this vitamin; therefore, a deficiency takes years to develop.

For people who have elevated cholesterol, 500 mg of niacin (also a B vitamin) daily can help lower cholesterol. Niacin supplementation, nonetheless, may produce side effects such as flushing, tingling, and itching. These symptoms usually disappear in a few days but may return if the dose is altered or the supplement is not taken at the same time each day. Supplements, nonetheless, are not a replacement for a diet with ample amounts of fruits, vegetables, and whole grains daily.

Diabetes

Diabetes mellitus is a condition in which blood glucose is unable to enter the cells because the pancreas totally stops producing **insulin**, or it does not produce enough to meet the body's needs, or the cells develop **insulin resistance**. The role of insulin is to "unlock" the cells and escort glucose into the cell. Diabetes affects more than 16 million people in the United States, and the National Institutes of Health estimate the cost of diabetes to be $98 billion annually.

The incidence of cardiovascular disease and death in the diabetic population is quite high. More than 80 percent of people with diabetes mellitus die from cardiovascular disease. People with chronically elevated blood glucose levels may have problems metabolizing fats, which can make them more susceptible to atherosclerosis, coronary heart disease, heart attacks, high blood pressure, and strokes. Diabetics also have lower HDL-cholesterol and higher triglyceride levels.

Chronic high blood sugar can also lead to nerve damage, vision loss, kidney damage, and decreased immune function (making the individual more susceptible to infections). Diabetics are 4 times as likely to become blind and 20 times more likely to develop kidney failure. Nerve damage in the lower extremities decreases the person's awareness of injury and infection. A small, untreated sore can cause severe infection, gangrene, and even lead to an amputation.[27]

An 8-hour fasting blood glucose level above 126 mg/dl on two separate tests confirms a diagnosis of diabetes (see Table 12.6). A level of 126 or higher should be brought to the attention of a physician. (This guideline is a change from previous years. A level above 140 had been used to diagnose diabetes, but this guideline was revised to 126 in 1997.)

Diabetes is of two types: **Type I**, or insulin-dependent diabetes mellitus (IDDM), and **Type II**,

Adult-onset diabetes is related closely to overeating, obesity, and lack of physical activity.

Triglycerides   Fats formed by glycerol and three fatty acids.

Homocysteine   An amino acid that, when allowed to accumulate in the blood, may lead to plaque formation and blockage of arteries.

Diabetes mellitus   A disease in which the body doesn't produce or utilize insulin properly.

Insulin   Hormone secreted by the pancreas; essential for proper metabolism of blood glucose (sugar) and maintenance of blood glucose level.

Insulin resistance   The inability of the cells to respond appropriately to insulin.

Type I diabetes   Insulin-dependent diabetes mellitus (IDDM), a condition in which the pancreas produces little or no insulin. Also known as juvenile diabetes.

Type II diabetes   Non-insulin-dependent diabetes mellitus (NIDDM), a condition in which insulin is not processed properly. Also known as adult-onset diabetes.

Table
12.6

Blood Glucose Guidelines

Amount	Rating
≤126 mg/dl	Desirable
127–149 mg/dl	High
≥150 mg/dl	Very High

or non-insulin–dependent diabetes mellitus (NIDDM). Type I also is called "juvenile diabetes," because it is found mainly in young people. With Type I, the pancreas produces little or no insulin. With Type II, the pancreas either does not produce sufficient insulin or it produces adequate amounts but the cells become insulin-resistant, thereby keeping glucose from entering the cell. Type II accounts for 90 to 95 percent of all diabetes cases.

Although diabetes has a genetic predisposition, Type II, or adult-onset, diabetes is related closely to overeating, obesity, and lack of physical activity. Type II diabetes, once limited primarily to overweight adults, now accounts for almost one-half of the new cases diagnosed in children. More than 80 percent of all Type II diabetics are overweight or have a history of excessive weight. In most cases this condition can be corrected through a special diet, a weight-loss program, and a regular exercise program.

Aerobic exercise helps prevent diabetes in middle-aged men.[28] The protective effect is even greater in those with risk factors such as obesity, high blood pressure, and family propensity. The preventive effect is attributed to less body fat and better sugar and fat metabolism resulting from the regular exercise program. At 3,500 calories per week, the risk was cut in half versus sedentary men. This preventive effect, according to one of the authors of the study, should hold for women, too.

Both moderate-intensity and vigorous physical activity are associated with increased insulin sensitivity and decreased risk for diabetes.[29] The key to increase and maintain proper insulin sensitivity, however, is regularity of the exercise program. Failure to maintain habitual physical activity voids these benefits. A diet high in complex carbohydrates and water-soluble fibers (found in fruits, vegetables, oats, and beans), low in saturated fat, and low in sugar is helpful in treating diabetes. A simple aerobic exercise program (walking, cycling, or swimming four to five times per week) often is prescribed because it increases the body's sensitivity to insulin. Aggressive weight loss, especially if combined with exercise, often allows diabetic patients to normalize their blood sugar level without the use of medication. Individuals who have high blood

glucose levels should consult a physician to decide on the best treatment. Exercise guidelines for diabetic patients are discussed in detail in Chapter 7.

Although complex carbohydrates are recommended in the diet, diabetics need to pay careful attention to the glycemic index (explained in Chapter 5 and detailed in Table 5.1). Refined and starchy foods are of a high glycemic index (small-particle carbohydrates, which are quickly digested); whereas grains, fruits, and vegetables are low-glycemic foods. Foods with a high glycemic index cause a rapid increase in blood sugar. A diet that includes many high-glycemic foods increases the risk for cardiovascular disease in people with high insulin resistance and **glucose intolerance**.[30] Combining a moderate amount of high-glycemic foods with low-glycemic index foods or with some fat and protein, however, can bring the average index down.

Syndrome X

As the cells resist insulin's action, the pancreas releases even more insulin in an attempt to keep blood glucose from rising. A chronic rise in insulin appears to trigger a series of abnormalities referred to as **syndrome X** or **metabolic syndrome**.[31] These abnormal conditions include low HDL-cholesterol, high triglycerides, and an increased blood clotting mechanism. Many individuals with syndrome X also have high blood pressure. All of these conditions increase the risk for CHD and other diabetic-related conditions (blindness, infection, nerve damage, and kidney failure). Approximately 70 million Americans are afflicted by this condition.

People who suffer from syndrome X have an abnormal insulin response to carbohydrates, in particular high-glycemic foods. In contrast with the American Heart Association dietary guidelines, syndrome X researchers indicate that the current low-fat, high-carbohydrate diet may not be the best

DIAGNOSIS OF SYNDROME X

Fasting triglycerides	≥200 mg/dl
Fasting HDL-cholesterol	≤35 mg/dl
Blood pressure	≥145/90
Fasting blood glucose	≥110 mg/dl
Being overweight by	≥15 lb

Source: G. M. Reaven, "Syndrome X: The Little Known Cause of Many Heart Attacks," *Bottom Line / Personal Health* 14 (June 2000).

unfit and having low blood pressure (see Figure 12.10). The death rates for unfit individuals with low systolic blood pressure are much higher than for highly fit people with high systolic blood pressure.

Moderate-intensity exercise lowers high blood pressure more effectively than high-intensity exercise.

Most important is a preventive approach. Keeping blood pressure under control is easier than trying to bring it down once it is high. Regardless of your blood pressure history, high or low, you should have it checked routinely. To keep your blood pressure as low as possible, exercise regularly; lose excess weight; eat less salt and sodium-containing foods; do not smoke; practice stress management; do not consume more than two alcoholic beverages a day if you are a man, one if you are a woman; and consume more potassium-rich foods such as potatoes, bananas, orange juice, cantaloupe, tomatoes, and beans (see "Guidelines to Stop Hypertension"). The Dietary Approach to Stop Hypertension (DASH)—which emphasizes fruits, vegetables, grains, and dairy products—has shown to lower systolic blood pressure by 11 points and diastolic by 5.5 points.[40]

Those who are taking medication for hypertension should not stop unless the prescribing physician gives the go-ahead. If it is not treated properly, high blood pressure can kill. By combining medication with the other treatments, drug therapy eventually may be reduced or completely eliminated.

Excessive Body Fat

Body composition refers to the ratio of lean body weight to fat weight. If the body contains too much fat, the person is considered overweight or obese (see Table 4.9, page 104).

Although some experts recognize obesity as an independent risk factor for CHD, the risks attributed to obesity actually may be augmented by other risk factors that usually accompany excessive body fat. Risk factors such as high blood lipids, hypertension, and diabetes usually improve with increased physical activity. As discussed in Chapter 5, overweight people who are physically active do not seem to be at increased risk for premature death.

Attaining recommended body composition helps improve some of the CHD risk factors and also helps to reach a better state of health and wellness. People who have a weight problem and want to get down to recommended weight must implement the following:

1. Increase daily physical activity and participate in aerobic and strength-training programs.

GUIDELINES TO STOP HYPERTENSION

- Participate in moderate-intensity aerobic exercise program (50% intensity) for 30 to 45 minutes 5 to 7 times per week.
- Participate in a moderate-resistance strength-training program (use 12 to 15 repetitions to near-fatigue on each set) two times per week (seek your physician's approval and advice for this program).
- Lose weight if you are above recommended body weight.
- Eat less salt and sodium-containing foods.
- Do not smoke cigarettes or use tobacco in any other form.
- Practice stress management.
- Do not consume more than two alcoholic beverages a day if you are a man or one if you are a woman.
- Consume more potassium-rich foods.
- Follow the Dietary Approach to Stop Hypertension (DASH Diet):
  - Seven or eight daily servings of grains, bread, cereal, or pasta
  - Eight to ten daily servings of fruits and vegetables.
  - Two or three daily servings of nonfat/low-fat dairy products.
  - Two or less daily servings of meat, poultry, or fish (less than 3 ounces per serving).
  - Four or five servings *per week* of beans, peas, nuts, or seeds.

2. Follow a diet low in fat and refined sugars and high in complex carbohydrates and fiber.
3. Reduce total caloric intake moderately while getting the necessary nutrients to sustain normal body functions.

Additional recommendations for weight reduction and weight control are discussed in Chapter 5.

Smoking

More than 47 million adults and 3.5 million adolescents in the United States smoke cigarettes. Smoking is the single largest preventable cause of illness and premature death in the United States. Smoking has been linked to cardiovascular disease, cancer, bronchitis, emphysema, and peptic ulcers. In relation to coronary disease, not only does smoking speed up the process of atherosclerosis, but it also carries a threefold increase in the risk of sudden death following a myocardial infarction.

Smoking prompts the release of nicotine and some other 1,200 toxic compounds into the bloodstream. Similar to hypertension, many of these

substances are destructive to the inner membrane that protects the walls of the arteries. Once the lining is damaged, cholesterol and triglycerides can be deposited readily in the arterial wall. As the plaque builds up, it obstructs blood flow through the arteries (Figure 12.11).

Furthermore, smoking encourages the formation of blood clots, which can completely block an artery already narrowed by atherosclerosis. In addition, carbon monoxide, a byproduct of cigarette smoke, decreases the blood's oxygen-carrying capacity. A combination of obstructed arteries, less oxygen, and nicotine in the heart muscle heightens the risk for a serious heart problem.

Smoking also increases heart rate, raises blood pressure, and irritates the heart, which can trigger fatal cardiac arrhythmias. Another harmful effect is a decrease in HDL-cholesterol, the "good" type that helps control blood lipids. Smoking actually presents a much greater risk of death from heart disease than from lung disease.

Pipe and cigar smoking and chewing tobacco also increase the risk for heart disease. Even if the smoker inhales no smoke, he or she absorbs toxic substances through the membranes of the mouth, and these end up in the bloodstream. Individuals who use tobacco in any of these three forms also have a much greater risk for cancer of the oral cavity.

The risks for both cardiovascular disease and cancer start to decrease the moment you quit smoking. The risk decreases to that of a lifetime nonsmoker 10 years (for CHD) and 15 years (for cancer) after quitting. A more thorough discussion of the harmful effects of cigarette smoking, the benefits of quitting, and a complete program for quitting are detailed in Chapter 14.

Tension and Stress

Tension and stress have become a part of life. Everyone has to deal daily with goals, deadlines, responsibilities, pressures. Almost everything in life (whether positive or negative) can be a source of stress. The stressor itself is not what creates the health hazard but, rather, the individual's response to it.

The human body responds to stress by producing more **catecholamines** to prepare the body for "fight or flight." These hormones increase heart rate, blood pressure, and blood glucose levels, enabling the person to take action. If the person actually fights or flees, the higher levels of catecholamines are metabolized and the body is able to return to a normal state. If, however, a person is under constant stress and unable to take action (as in the death of a close relative or friend, loss of a job, trouble at work, or financial insecurity), the catecholamines remain elevated in the bloodstream.

People who are not able to relax have a constant low-level strain on the cardiovascular system that could manifest itself as heart disease. In addition, when a person is in a stressful situation, the coronary arteries that feed the heart muscle constrict, reducing the oxygen supply to the heart. If the blood vessels are largely blocked by atherosclerosis, **arrhythmias** or even a heart attack may follow.

Individuals who are under a lot of stress and do not cope well with it need to take measures to counteract the effects of stress in their lives. One way is to identify the sources of stress and learn how to cope with them. People need to take control of themselves, examine and act upon the things that are most important in their lives, and ignore less-meaningful details.

Figure 12.11

Comparison of a normal and an atherosclerotic artery at the base of the brain.

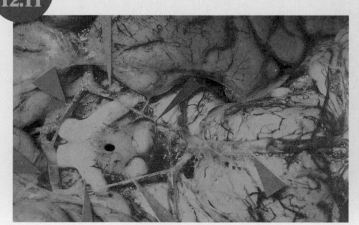

Healthy artery

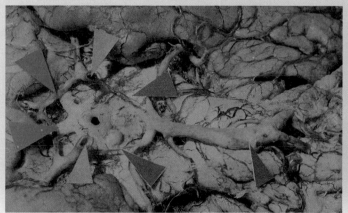

Obstruction of the same artery by fatty substances in a chronic smoker

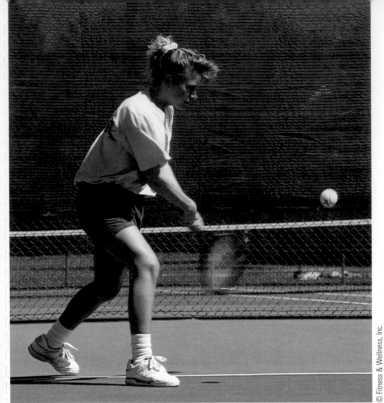

Physical activity, one of the best ways to relieve stress.

Physical activity is one of the best ways to relieve stress. When a person takes part in physical activity, the body metabolizes excess catecholamines and is able to return to a normal state. Exercise also steps up muscular activity, which contributes to muscular relaxation after completing the physical activity.

Many executives in large cities are choosing the evening hours for their physical activity programs, stopping after work at the health or fitness club. In doing this, they are able to "burn up" the excess tension accumulated during the day and enjoy the evening hours. This has proven to be one of the best stress management techniques. More information on stress management techniques is presented in Chapter 11.

Personal and Family History

Individuals who have had cardiovascular problems are at higher risk than those who have never had a problem. People with this history should control the other risk factors as much as they can. Most risk factors are reversible, so this will greatly decrease the risk for future problems. The more time that passes since the cardiovascular problem occurred, the lower the risk for recurrence.

Genetic predisposition toward heart disease has been demonstrated clearly. All other factors being equal, a person with blood relatives who now have or did have heart disease run a greater risk than someone with no such history. Premature CHD is defined as a heart attack before age 55 in a close male relative or before age 65 in a close female relative. The younger the age at which the cardiovascular incident happened to the relative, the greater the risk for the disease.

In some cases there is no way of knowing whether it was a person's genetic predisposition or simply poor lifestyle habits that led to a heart problem. A person may have been physically inactive, been overweight, smoked, and had bad dietary habits—all of which contributed to a heart attack. Regardless, blood relatives fall in the family history category. Because we have no reliable way to differentiate all the factors contributing to cardiovascular disease, a person with a family history should watch all other factors closely and maintain the lowest risk level possible. In addition, the person should have a blood chemistry analysis annually to make sure the body is handling blood lipids properly.

Age

Age is a risk factor because of the higher incidence of heart disease in older people. This tendency may be induced partly by other factors stemming from changes in lifestyle as we get older—less physical activity, poorer nutrition, obesity, and so on.

Young people should not think they are exempt from heart disease. The process begins early in life. Autopsies conducted on American soldiers killed at age 22 and younger revealed that approximately 70 percent had early stages of atherosclerosis. Other studies found elevated blood cholesterol levels in children as young as 10 years old.

Although the aging process cannot be stopped, it certainly can be slowed down. Physiological versus chronological age is important in preventing disease. Some individuals in their 60s or older have the body of a 20-year-old. And 20-year-olds often are in such poor condition and health that they almost seem to have the body of 60-year-olds. Risk factor management and positive lifestyle habits are the best means of slowing down the natural aging process.

Catecholamines "Fight-or-flight" hormones, including epinephrine and norepinephrine.

Arrhythmias Irregular heart rhythms.

Other Factors

Additional evidence points to a few other factors that may be linked to coronary heart disease. One of these factors is gum disease. The oral bacteria that builds up with dental plaque can enter the blood stream and contribute to blood vessel plaque formation, increase blood clots, and thus increase heart attack risk. Daily flossing for 1 to 2 minutes is the best way to prevent gum disease.

Loud snoring has also been linked to cardio-vascular disease. People who snore heavily may suffer from sleep apnea, a sleep disorder in which the throat closes for a brief moment, causing breathing to stop. In one study, individuals who snored heavily tripled their risk of a heart attack and quadrupled the risk of a stroke.[41]

A Final Word on Coronary Risk Reduction

Most of the risk factors for CHD are reversible and preventable. Having a family history of heart disease, and possibly some of the other risk factors because of neglect in lifestyle, does not mean that you are doomed. A healthier lifestyle—free of cardiovascular problems—is something over which you have much control. You are encouraged to be persistent. Willpower and commitment are required to develop patterns that eventually will turn into healthy habits contributing to total well-being.

Web Interactive

- The Heart: An Online Exploration. This interesting site, developed by the Franklin Institute of Science, provides an interactive multimedia tour of the heart, as well as statistical information, resources, and links. There is information on how to monitor your heart's health by becoming aware of your vital signs.

  http://www.fi.edu/biosci/heart.html

- Heart Information Network: Determining and Reducing Your Risk of Heart Attack. This site describes the symptoms and risk factors for coronary artery disease and provides information on how to reduce your risk. It also features information on several screening tests for heart disease, questions to ask your doctor, and provides tips on ways to reduce your risk. You can view diagrams and photographs of blocked arteries.

  http://www.heartinfo.com/detrisk.htm

- Improving Cardiovascular Health in African Americans. A series of seven brochures from the National Heart, Lung, and Blood Institute that you can download or read online. Topics include cholesterol, blood pressure, low sodium diet, weight loss, smoking cessation, and exercise.

  http://www.nhlbi.nih.gov/health/public/heart/other/chdblack/index.htm

Interactive Sites:

- Create a Diet to Lower your Cholesterol. This interactive site will provide personalized guidelines on how to eat healthy and decrease your risk of heart disease, based on your height, weight, age, gender, and activity level.

  http://www.nhlbisupport.com/chd1/create.htm

- Healthy Eating for a Healthy Heart. This site, sponsored by CyberDiet.com features information on healthy diets designed to decrease risk of atherosclerosis. The site features a personalized nutrition assessment, diet guidelines, meal planning tools, target foods, and tips when cooking or when dining out. There is also information regarding other risk factors for heart disease, including weight, smoking, stress, and exercise. There is also a ten question multiple choice quiz "Eating Smart for a Healthy Heart: Is Your Heart at Risk?"

  http://www.cyberdiet.com/modules/hd/outline.html

- Check Your Healthy Heart IQ: This site is sponsored by the National Heart, Lung, and Blood Institute. Test your knowledge about heart disease and its risks (high blood pressure, high blood cholesterol, smoking, lack of exercise, and overweight) and ways to reduce your risk.

  http://www.nhlbi.nih.gov/health/public/heart/other/hh_iq_ab.htm

Notes

1. American Heart Association, *Heart and Stroke Facts: 2000* (Statistical Supplement) (Dallas: AHA, 1999).

2. U.S. Department of Health and Human Services, Centers for Disease Control and Prevention, National Center for Health Statistics, National Vital Statistics System: *Deaths: Final Data for 1998* 48, no. 11 (July 24, 1998).

3. American Heart Association, *1999 Heart and Stroke Facts Statistical Update* (Dallas: AHA, 1998).

4. See note 3.

5. See note 2.

6. See note 3.

7. S. N. Blair, H. W. Kohl III, R. S. Paffenbarger, Jr., D. G. Clark, K. H. Cooper, and L. W. Gibbons, "Physical Fitness and All-Cause Mortality: A Prospective Study of Healthy Men and Women," *Journal of the American Medical Association* 262 (1989): 2395–2401.

8. R. S. Paffenbarger, Jr., R. T. Hyde, A. L. Wing, I. Lee, D. L. Jung, and J. B. Kampert, "The Association of Changes in Physical-Activity Level and Other Lifestyle Characteristics with Mortality Among Men," *New England Journal of Medicine* 328 (1993): 538–545.

9. "Lipid Research Clinics Program: The Lipid Research Clinic Coronary Primary Prevention Trial Results," *Journal of the American Medical Association* 251 (1984): 351–364.

10. See note 3.

11. W. P. Castelli and K. Anderson, "A Population at Risk: Prevalence of High Cholesterol Levels in Hypertensive Patients in the Framingham Study," *American Journal of Medicine* 80, Supplement 2A (1986): 23–32.

12. P. A. Romm, M. K. Hong, and C. E. Rackley, "High-Density-Lipoprotein Cholesterol and Risk of Coronary Heart Disease," *Practical Cardiology* 16 (1990): 28–40.

13. "HDL on the Rise," *HealthNews* (September 10, 1999).

14. C. J. Gluek, "Nonpharmacologic and Pharmacologic Alteration of High Density Lipoprotein Cholesterol: Therapeutic Approaches to Prevention of Atherosclerosis," *American Heart Journal* 110 (1985): 1107–1115.

15. J. M. Gaziano and C. H. Hennekens, "A New Look at What Can Unclog Your Arteries," *Executive Health Report* 27, no. 8 (1991): 16.

16. See note 15.

17. See note 12.

18. American Heart Association, *Heart and Stroke Facts* (Dallas: AHA, 1999).

19. M. L. Stefanick et al., "Effects of Diet in Men and Postmenopausal Women with Low Levels of HDL Cholesterol and High Levels of LDL Cholesterol," *New England Journal of Medicine* 339 (1998): 12–20.

20. E. B. Rimm, A. Ascherio, E. Giovannucci, D. Spiegelman, M. J. Stampfer, and W. C. Willett, "Vegetable, Fruit, and Cereal Fiber Intake and Risk of Coronary Heart Disease Among Men," *Journal of the American Medical Association* 275 (1996): 447–451.

21. R. J. Barnard, "Effects of Lifestyle Modification on Serum Lipids," *Archives of Internal Medicine* 151 (1991): 1389–1394.

22. W. Castelli, "Smart Heart Strategies: Best Ways to Beat Heart Disease," *Bottom Line / Personal Health* 19, no. 4 (1998): 1–3.

23. R. Superko, "Platelets and Lipid Interaction with a Vessel Wall," (presented in symposium at American College of Sports Medicine Annual Meeting, 1991).

24. O. Nygard, J. E. Nordreahaug, H. Refsum, P. M. Ueland, M. Farstad, and S. E. Vollset, "Plasma Homocysteine Levels and Mortality in Patients with Coronary Heart Disease," *New England Journal of Medicine* 337 (1997): 230–236.

25. "The Homocysteine-CVD Connection," *HealthNews* (October 25, 1999).

26. C. J. Boushey, S. A. A. Beresford, G. S. Omenn, and A. G. Motulsky, "A Quantitative Assessment of Plasma Homocysteine as a Risk Factor for Vascular Disease," *Journal of the American Medical Association* 274 (1995): 1049–1057.

27. "Diabetes: Weight Control and Exercise May Keep You Off the Road to High Blood Sugar," Medical Essay, supplement to *Mayo Clinic Health Letter* (February 1998).

28. S. P. Helmrich, D. R. Ragland, R. W. Leung, and R. S. Paffenbarger, "Physical Activity and Reduced Occurrences of Non-Insulin-Dependent Diabetes Mellitus," *New England Journal of Medicine* 325 (1991): 147–152.

29. E. J. Mayer et al., "Intensity and Amount of Physical Activity in Relation to Insulin Sensitivity," *Journal of the American Medical Association* 279 (1998): 669–674.

30. S. Liu et al., "A Prospective Study of Dietary Glycemic Load, Carbohydrate Intake, and Risk of Coronary Heart Disease in the U.S.," *American Journal of Clinical Nutrition* 71 (2000): 1455–1461.

31. G. M. Reaven, "Syndrome X: The Little Known Cause of Many Heart Attacks," *Bottom Line / Personal Health* 14 (June 2000).

32. See note 30.

33. G. M. Reaven, T. K. Strom, and B. Fox, *Syndrome X: Overcoming the Silent Killer That Can Give You a Heart Attack* (Simon & Schuster, 2000).

34. See note 33.

35. G. Kelley, "Dynamic Resistance Exercise and Resting Blood Pressure in Adults: A Meta-analysis," *Journal of Applied Physiology* 82 (1997): 1559–1565.

G. A. Kelley and Z. Tran, "Aerobic Exercise and Normotensive Adults: A Meta-analysis," *Medicine and Science in Sports and Exercise* 27 (1995): 1371–1377.

G. Kelley, and P. McClellan, "Antihypertensive Effects of Aerobic Exercise: A Brief Meta-analytic Review of Randomized Controlled Trials," *American Journal of Hypertension* 7 (1994): 115–119.

36. R. Collins et al., "Blood Pressure, Stroke, and Coronary Heart Disease; Part 2, Short-term Reductions in Blood Pressure: Overview of Randomized Drug Trials in Their Epidemiological Context," *Lancet* 335 (1990): 827–838.

37. S. N. Blair et al., "Influences of Cardiorespiratory Fitness and Other Precursors on Cardiovascular Disease and All-cause Mortality in Men and Women," *Journal of the American Medical Association* 276 (1996): 205–210.

38. G. A. Kelley and K. S. Kelley, "Progressive Resistance Exercise and Resting Blood Pressure: A Meta-Analysis of Randomized Controlled Trials," *Hypertension* 35 (2000): 838–843.

39. F. W. Kash, J. L. Boyer, S. P. Van Camp, L. S. Verity, and J. P. Wallace, "The Effect of Physical Activity on Aerobic Power in Older Men (A Longitudinal Study)," *Physician and Sports Medicine* 18, no. 4 (1990): 73–83.

40. S. G. Sheps, "High Blood Pressure Can Often Be Controlled Without Medication," *Bottom Line / Personal Health* (November, 1999).

41. "Checkup for the New Millennium," *Consumer Reports on Health* (December, 1999).

Suggested Readings

American Heart Association. *2000 Heart and Stroke Facts Statistical Update*. Dallas: AHA, 1999.

American Heart Association. *Heart and Stroke Facts*. Dallas: AHA, 1999.

Barnard, R. J. "A Carbohydrate Diet to Prevent and Control Coronary Heart Disease." *ACSM's Health and Fitness Journal* 3 (May/June 1999): 23–26.

Blair, S. N., et al. "Physical Activity, Nutrition, and Chronic Disease." *Medicine and Science in Sports and Exercise* 28 (1996): 335–349.

Gibbons, L. W., S. Blair, K. H. Cooper, and M. Smith. "Association Between Coronary Heart Disease Risk Factors and Physical Fitness in Healthy Adult Women." *Circulation* 5 (1993): 977–983.

Ornish, D. S., E. Brown, L. W. Scherwitz et al. "Can Lifestyle Changes Reverse Coronary Heart Disease? Lifestyle Heart Trial." *Lancet* 336 (1990): 129–133.

Superko, H. R. "New Aspects of Cardiovascular Risk Factors Including Small Dense LDL, Homocysteinemia, and Lp(a)." *Current Opinions in Cardiology* 10 (1995): 347–354.

Superko, H. R. "The Most Common Cause of Coronary Heart Disease Can Be Successfully Treated by the Least Expensive Therapy: Exercise." *Certified News* (1998): 1–5.

Superko, H. R., R. M. Kraus, and E. M. Alderman. "Diabetics Have Rapid Arteriographic Coronary Disease Progression but Also Arteriographic Benefit from Risk Reduction." *Circulation* 96 (1997): 4289.

Whaley, M. H., and S. N. Blair. "Epidemiology of Physical Activity, Physical Fitness and Coronary Heart Disease." *Certified News* 5, no. 2 (1995): 1–7.

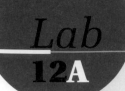

Lab 12A

SELF-EVALUATION OF CARDIOVASCULAR RISK AND BEHAVIOR MODIFICATION PROGRAM

Name: _____   Date: _____   Grade: _____

Instructor: _____   Course: _____   Section: _____

Necessary Lab Equipment

Basic lab equipment to repeat the body composition and blood pressure tests, and if possible, a blood chemistry analysis should be performed prior to this lab.

Objective

To assess your current risk for coronary heart disease (CHD) and develop a behavior modification program.

I. Self-Assessment: Coronary Heart Disease Risk Factor Analysis

Instructions The disease process for cardiovascular disease starts early in life, primarily as a result of poor lifestyle habits. Studies have shown beginning stages of atherosclerosis and elevated blood lipids in children as young as 10 years old. Consequently, the purpose of this lab is to establish a baseline CHD risk profile and to point out the "zero-risk" level for each coronary risk factor.

You may want to repeat the body composition and blood pressure tests to obtain current values for this lab experience. If time does not allow for reassessment of these parameters, use the results obtained in previous labs. In addition, if you have had a blood chemistry analysis performed recently that included total cholesterol, HDL-cholesterol, triglycerides, and glucose levels, you may use the results for this lab.

			Score
1. Physical Activity	Do you participate in a regular aerobic exercise program (brisk walking, jogging, swimming, bicycling, aerobics, etc.) for more than 20 minutes:		
	Once a week or less	8	
	Two times per week	3	
	Three or more times per week	0	

2. Resting and Stress Electrocardiograms (ECG)	Add scores for both ECGs				
	ECG	Resting	Stress		
	Normal	(0)	(0)	....	0
	Equivocal	(1)	(4)	....	1–5
	Abnormal	(3)	(8)	....	3–11

3. HDL-Cholesterol (If unknown, answer Question 6)	Men	Women		Score
	≥45	≥55	....	0
	35–44	45–54	....	3
	≤34	≤44	....	6

4. LDL-Cholesterol (If unknown, answer Question 6)			Score
	≤130	....	0
	131–159	....	3
	≥160	....	6

5. Triglycerides (If unknown, answer Question 6)			Score
	≤125	....	0
	126–499	....	1
	≥500	....	2

Subtotal Risk Score: _____

Subtotal Risk Score (from previous page): ☐

6. Diet (Do not answer if Questions 3, 4 and 5 have been answered)	Does your regular diet include (high score if all apply): One or more daily servings of red meat; 7 or more eggs/week; daily butter, cheese, whole milk, sweets and alcohol...	10–14
	Four to six servings of red meat/week, 4–6 eggs per week, margarine, 1% or 2% milk, some cheese, sweets, and alcohol	4–10
	Fish, poultry, red meat less than three times/week, fewer than 3 eggs/week, skim milk and skim milk products, moderate sweets and alcohol...............................	0–3 ☐

7. Homocysteine	Does your daily diet include: 2 and 3 servings of fruits and vegetables respectively ....0 Less than 2 and 3 servings of fruits and vegetables respectively..............4	☐

8. Diabetes/Glucose	≤120	0
	121–128	1
	129–136	1.5
	137–144	2
	145–149	2.5
	≥150	3
	Diabetics add another 3 points	3

9. Blood Pressure	Add scores for both readings (e.g., 144/88 score = 4)		
	Systolic	Diastolic	
	≤120............(0)	≤80 ....(0)	0
	121–130 ....(1)	81–90 ....(1)	1–2
	131–140 ....(2)	91–98 ....(2)	2–4
	141–150 ....(3)	99–106..........(3)	3–6
	≥151............(4)	≥107............(4)	4–8 ☐

10. Percent Body Fat	Men	Women	
	12–17%	18–22%	0
	18–22%	23–27%	1
	23–27%	28–32%	2
	≥28%	≥33%	3 ☐

11. Smoking	Lifetime nonsmoker	0
	Ex-smoker over 1 year	0
	Ex-smoker less than 1 year	1
	Smoke 1 cigarette/day or none	1
	Nonsmoker, but live or work in smoking environment	2
	Pipe or cigar smoker, or chew tobacco	3
	Smoke 1–9 cigarettes/day	3
	Smoke 10–19 cigarettes/day	4
	Smoke 20–29 cigarettes/day	5
	Smoke 30–39 cigarettes/day	6
	Smoke 40 or more cigarettes/day	8 ☐

Subtotal Risk Score: ☐

Subtotal Risk Score (from previous page):

12.	Tension and Stress	Are you:	
		Sometimes tense	0
		Often tense	1
		Nearly always tense	2
		Always tense	3

13.	Personal History	Have you ever had a heart attack, stroke, coronary disease, or any known heart problem:	
		During the last year	8
		1–2 years ago	5
		2–5 years ago	3
		More than 5 years ago	2
		Never had heart disease	0

14.	Family History	Have any of your blood relatives (parents, uncles, brothers, sisters, grandparents) had cardiovascular disease (heart attack, strokes, bypass surgery):	
		One or more before age 51	6
		One or more between 51 and 60	3
		One or more after age 60	1
		None had cardiovascular disease	0

15.	Age	29 or younger	0
		30–39	1
		40–49	2
		50–59	3
		$\geq$60	4

Total Risk Score:

How to Score

Risk Category	Total Risk Score
Very Low	5 or less points
Low	Between 6 and 15 points
Moderate	Between 16 and 25 points
High	Between 26 and 35 points
Very High	36 or more points

II. Stage of Change for Cardiovascular Disease Prevention

Using Figure 2.3 (page 40) and Table 2.3 (page 41), identify your current stage of change for participation in a cardiovascular disease risk-reduction program:

III. In a few sentences, discuss your family and personal risk for cardiovascular disease:

IV. Discuss lifestyle changes that you have already implemented in this course, as well as additional changes that you can make to decrease your own risk of developing cardiovascular disease in the future.

Chapter 13

Cancer Risk Management

Objectives

- Be able to define cancer and how it starts and spreads.

- Become acquainted with guidelines for preventing cancer.

- Become familiar with major risk factors that lead to specific types of cancer.

- Assess the risk for developing certain types of cancer.

The human body has approximately 100 trillion cells. Under normal conditions, these cells reproduce themselves in an orderly way. Cell growth (cell reproduction) takes place so old, worn-out tissue can be replaced and injuries can be repaired.

Cell growth is controlled by **deoxyribonucleic acid** (DNA) and **ribonucleic acid** (RNA), found in the nucleus of each cell. When nuclei lose their ability to regulate and control cell growth, cell division is disrupted and mutant cells can develop (see Figure 13.1). Some of these cells might grow uncontrollably and abnormally, forming a mass of tissue called a tumor, which can be either **benign** or **malignant**. Benign tumors do not invade other tissues. They can interfere with normal bodily functions, but they rarely cause death. A malignant tumor is a **cancer**. More than 100 types of cancer can develop in any tissue or organ of the human body.

The process of cancer actually begins with an alteration in DNA. Found within DNA are **oncogenes** and tumor **suppressor genes**, which normally work together to repair and replace cells. Defects in these genes—caused by external factors such as radiation, chemicals, and viruses, as well as internal factors such as immune conditions, hormones, and genetic mutations—ultimately allow the cell to grow into a tumor.

A healthy cell may duplicate as many as 100 times in its lifetime. Normally, the DNA molecule is duplicated perfectly during cell division. In the few cases when the DNA molecule is not replicated exactly, specialized enzymes make repairs quickly. Occasionally, however, cells with defective DNA keep dividing and ultimately form a small tumor. As more mutations occur, the altered cells continue to divide and can become malignant. A decade or more can pass between carcinogenic exposure or mutations and the time cancer is diagnosed.

The process of abnormal cell division is related indirectly to chromosome segments called **telomeres** (see Figure 13.2). Each time a cell divides, chromosomes lose some telomeres. After many cell divisions, chromosomes eventually run out of telomeres and the cell then invariably dies.

Scientists have discovered that human tumors make an enzyme known as **telomerase**. In cancer cells, telomerase keeps the chromosome from running out of telomeres entirely. The shortened strand of telomeres (see Figure 13.3) now allows cells to reproduce indefinitely.[1]

Telomerase seems to have another function that is still under investigation: After many cell divisions, by nature cancer cells grow old, but telomerase keeps them from dying. If scientists can confirm that

 Figure 13.1 Mutant (cancer) cells.

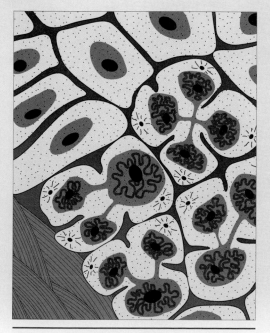

Illustration courtesy of American Cancer Society (contained in *Youth Looks at Cancer*. New York: American Cancer Society, 1982, p. 4).

Figure 13.2 Erosion of chromosome telomeres in normal cells.

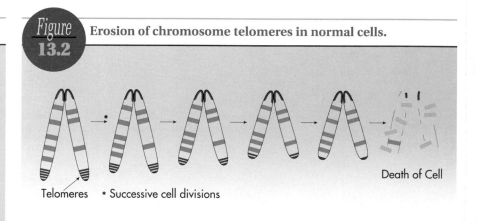

Telomeres   * Successive cell divisions

Death of Cell

Figure 13.3 Action of the enzyme telomerase.

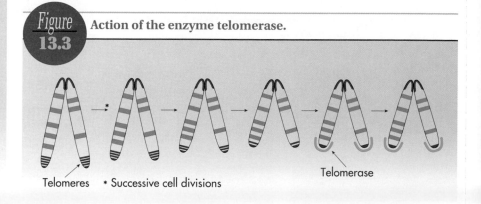

Telomeres   * Successive cell divisions

Telomerase

telomerase plays such a crucial role in the formation of tumors, research efforts will be directed to finding a way to block the action of telomerase, thereby making cancerous cells die.

Cancer starts with the abnormal growth of one cell, which then can multiply into billions of cancerous cells. A critical turning point in the development of cancer is when a tumor reaches about 1 million cells. At this stage, it is referred to as **carcinoma in situ**. Such an undetected tumor may go for months and years without any significant growth. While it remains encapsulated, it does not pose a serious threat to human health. However, to grow, the tumor requires more oxygen and nutrients. In time, a few of the cancer cells start producing chemicals that enhance **angiogenesis**, or capillary (blood vessel) formation into the tumor. Angiogenesis is the precursor of **metastasis**. Through the new vessels formed by angiogenesis, cancerous cells now can break away from a malignant tumor and migrate to other parts of the body, where they can cause new cancer (Figure 13.4).

Most adults have precancerous or cancerous cells in their bodies. By middle age, our bodies contain millions of precancerous cells. Although the immune system and the blood turbulence destroy most cancer cells, it takes only one abnormal cell lodging elsewhere to start a new cancer. These cells grow and multiply uncontrollably, invading and destroying normal tissue. The rate at which cancer cells grow varies from one type to another. Some types grow fast; others take years.

Once cancer cells metastasize, treatment becomes more difficult. Although therapy can kill

Deoxyribonucleic acid (DNA)   Genetic substance of which genes are made; molecule that bears cell's genetic code.

Ribonucleic acid (RNA)   Genetic material that guides the formation of cell proteins.

Benign   Noncancerous.

Malignant   Cancerous.

Cancer   Group of diseases characterized by uncontrolled growth and spread of abnormal cells into malignant tumors.

Oncogenes   Genes that initiate cell division.

Suppressor genes   Genes that deactivate the process of cell division.

Telomeres   A strand of molecules at both ends of a chromosome.

Telomerase   An enzyme that allows cells to reproduce indefinitely.

Carcinoma in situ   Encapsulated malignant tumor that has not spread.

Angiogenesis   Formation of blood vessels, or capillaries.

Metastasis   The movement of cells from one part of the body to another.

Figure 13.4

How cancer starts and spreads.

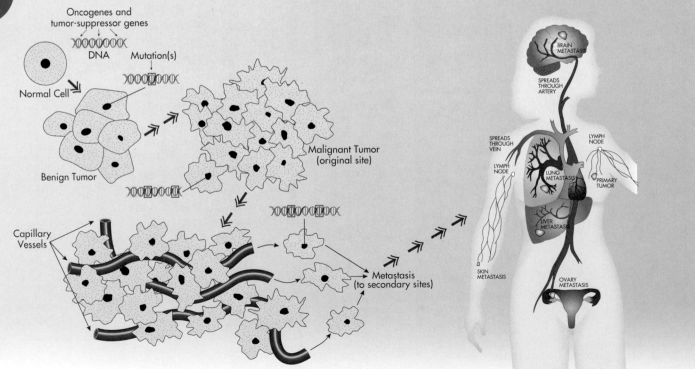

most cancer cells, a few cells might become resistant to treatment. These cells then can grow into a new tumor that will not respond to the same treatment.

Incidence of Cancer

According to the final mortality statistics for 1997 from the National Center for Health Statistics, cancer was the cause of 23.3 percent of all deaths in the United States. It is the second leading cause of death in the country and the leading cause in children between ages 1 and 14.

Cancer will develop in approximately 1 in 2 men and 1 in 3 women in the United States, striking approximately 3 of every 4 families. About 552,200 Americans died from cancer in 2000, and approximately 1,220,100 new cases were diagnosed that same year.[2]

The year 2000 statistical estimates of the incidence of cancer and deaths by sex and site are given in Figure 13.5. These estimates exclude **nonmelanoma skin cancer** and carcinoma in situ.

Like coronary heart disease, cancer is largely preventable. As much as 80 percent of all human cancer is related to lifestyle or environmental factors (including diet and obesity, tobacco use, sedentary lifestyle, excessive use of alcohol, and exposure to occupational hazards—see Figure 13.6).

Most of these cancers could be prevented through positive lifestyle habits.

Research sponsored by the American Cancer Society and the National Cancer Institute showed that individuals who have a healthy lifestyle have some of the lowest cancer mortality rates ever reported in scientific studies.[3] A group of about 10,000 members of the Church of Jesus Christ of Latter Day Saints (commonly referred to as the Mormon church) in California was reported to have only about one-third (men) to one-half (women) the rate of cancer mortality of the general white population (Figure 13.7). In this study the investigators looked at three general health habits in the participants: lifetime abstinence from smoking, regular physical activity, and sufficient sleep. In addition, healthy lifestyle guidelines encouraged by the church since 1833 include abstaining from all forms of tobacco, alcohol, caffeine, and drugs and adhering to a well-balanced diet based on grains, fruits, and vegetables, and moderate amounts of poultry and red meat.

Equally important is that more than 8.4 million Americans with a history of cancer were alive in 2000. Currently, 4 of 10 people diagnosed with cancer are expected to be alive 5 years after the initial diagnosis.[4]

Figure 13.5 Year 2001 estimated cancer incidence and deaths by site and sex.

Cancer Cases by Site and Sex*

Male	Female
Prostate 198,100	Breast 192,200
Lung & Bronchus 90,700	Lung & Bronchus 78,800
Colon & Rectum 67,300	Colon & Rectum 68,100
Urinary Bladder 39,200	Uterine Corpus 38,300
Non-Hodgkin's Lymphoma 31,100	Non-Hodgkin's Lymphoma 25,100
Melanoma of the Skin 29,000	Ovary 23,400
Oral Cavity 20,200	Melanoma of the skin 22,400
Kidney 18,700	Urinary Bladder 15,100
Leukemia 17,700	Pancreas 15,000
Pancreas 14,200	Thyroid 14,900
All Sites 643,000	All Sites 625,000

Cancer Deaths by Site and Sex*

Male	Female
Lung & Bronchus 90,100	Lung & Bronchus 67,300
Prostate 31,500	Breast 40,200
Colon & Rectum 27,700	Colon & Rectum 29,000
Pancreas 14,100	Pancreas 14,800
Non-Hodgkin's Lymphoma 13,800	Ovary 13,900
Leukemia 12,000	Non-Hodgkin's Lymphoma 12,500
Esophagus 9,500	Leukemia 9,500
Liver 8,900	Uterine Corpus 6,600
Urinary Bladder 8,300	Brain 5,900
Kidney 7,500	Stomach 5,400
All Sites 286,100	All Sites 267,300

*Excludes basal and squamous cell skin cancers and in situ carcinomas except urinary bladder.

Source: 2001 Cancer Facts and Figures. American Cancer Society (New York: ACS, 2001).

Figure 13.6

Estmate of the relative role of the major cancer-causing factors.

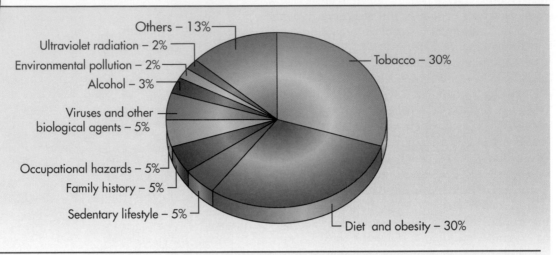

- Others – 13%
- Ultraviolet radiation – 2%
- Environmental pollution – 2%
- Alcohol – 3%
- Viruses and other biological agents – 5%
- Occupational hazards – 5%
- Family history – 5%
- Sedentary lifestyle – 5%
- Tobacco – 30%
- Diet and obesity – 30%

Source: Harvard Center for Cancer Prevention. *Causes of Human Cancer, Harvard Report on Cancer Prevention*, 1 (1996).

Figure 13.7

Effects of a healthy lifestyle on cancer mortality rate.

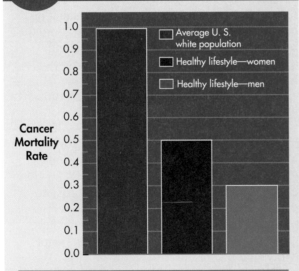

Cancer Mortality Rate

- ☐ Average U. S. white population
- ■ Healthy lifestyle—women
- ☐ Healthy lifestyle—men

Note: Healthy lifestyle factors include proper nutrition, abstinence from cigarette smoking, regular sleep (7–8 hours per night), and regular physical activity.

Source: "Health Practices and Cancer Mortality Among Active California Mormons," *Journal of the National Cancer Institute* 81 (1989): 1807–1814.

Guidelines for Preventing Cancer

The biggest factor in fighting cancer today is health education. People need to be informed about the risk factors for cancer and the guidelines for early detection. The most effective way to protect against cancer is to change negative lifestyle habits and behaviors. Following are some guidelines for preventing cancer.

Dietary Changes

The American Cancer Society estimates that one-third of all cancers in the United States are related to nutrition. A healthy diet, therefore, is crucial to decrease the risk for cancer. The diet should be predominately vegetarian, high in fiber, and low in fat (particularly from animal sources). **Cruciferous vegetables**, tea, soy products, calcium, and omega-3 fats are encouraged. Protein intake should be kept within the recommended nutrient guidelines. If alcohol is used, it should be used in moderation. Obesity should be avoided.

Green and dark yellow vegetables, cruciferous vegetables (cauliflower, broccoli, cabbage, Brussels sprouts, and kohlrabi), and beans (legumes) seem to protect against cancer. Folate, found naturally in dark green leafy vegetables, dried beans, and orange juice, may reduce the risk of colon and cervical cancers. Brightly colored fruits and vegetables also contain **carotenoids** and vitamin C. Lycopene, one

Nonmelanoma skin cancer Cancer that spreads or grows directly from the original site but does not metastasize to other regions of the body.

Cruciferous vegetables Plants that produce cross-shaped leaves (cauliflower, broccoli, cabbage, Brussels sprouts, and kohlrabi); seem to have a protective effect against cancer.

Carotenoids Pigment substances in plants that are often precursors to vitamin A. Over 600 carotenoids are found in nature and about 50 of them are precursors to vitamin A, the most potent one being beta-carotene.

of the many carotenoids (a phytochemical—see discussion below), has been linked to lower risk of cancers of the prostate, colon, and cervix. Lycopene is especially abundant in cooked tomato products.

Researchers believe the antioxidant effect of vitamins and the mineral selenium help protect the body from oxygen free radicals. As discussed in Chapter 3, during normal metabolism most of the oxygen in the human body is converted into stable forms of carbon dioxide and water. A small amount, however, ends up in an unstable form known as oxygen free radicals, which are thought to attack and damage the cell membrane and DNA, leading to the formation of cancers. Antioxidants absorb free radicals before they can cause damage and also interrupt the sequence of reactions once damage has begun.

A promising horizon in cancer prevention is the discovery of **phytochemicals**. These compounds, found in abundance in fruits and vegetables, seem to prevent cancer by blocking the formation of cancerous tumors and disrupting the process at almost every step of the way. Phytochemicals exert their protective action in all of the following ways:[5]

- Removing **carcinogens** from cells before they cause damage.
- Activating enzymes that detoxify cancer-causing agents.
- Keeping carcinogens from locking onto cells.
- Preventing carcinogens from binding to DNA.
- Breaking up cancer-causing precursors to benign forms.
- Disrupting the chemical combination of cell molecules that can produce carcinogens.
- Keeping small tumors from accessing capillaries (small blood vessels) to get oxygen and nutrients.

Examples of phytochemicals and their effects are found in Table 13.1.

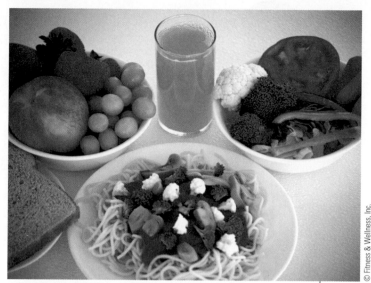

Nutrition guidelines for a cancer-prevention program include a diet low in fat and high in fiber, with ample amounts of fruits and vegetables.

Although one recent study failed to show an association, many studies have linked low intake of fiber to increased risk for colon cancer. Fiber binds to bile acids in the intestine for excretion from the body in the stools. Bile acids' interaction with intestinal bacteria releases carcinogenic byproducts. Bile-acid production increases with higher fat content in the small intestine (created, of course, by higher fat content in the diet).

Daily consumption of 25 to 35 grams of fiber is recommended. Grains are high in fiber and contain vitamins and minerals (folate, selenium, and calcium), which seem to decrease the risk for colon cancer. Selenium also protects against prostate cancer and, possibly, lung cancer. Calcium may also protect against colon cancer by preventing rapid growth of cells in the colon, especially in people with colon polyps.

Polyphenols (phytochemicals) are potent cancer-fighting antioxidants found in fresh fruits and vegetables, many grains, and regular teas. Green, black, and red tea all appear to provide protection. Evidence also points to certain components in tea that can block the spread of cancers to other parts of the body.

The antioxidant effect of one of the polyphenols in green tea, epigallocatechin gallate, or EGCG, is at least 25 times more effective than vitamin E and 100 times more effective than vitamin C at protecting cells and the DNA from damage believed to cause cancer, heart disease, and other diseases associated with free radicals.[6] EGCG is also twice as strong as the red wine antioxidant resveratrol in helping prevent heart disease. Other research indicates that phytochemicals in green tea induce cancer cells to

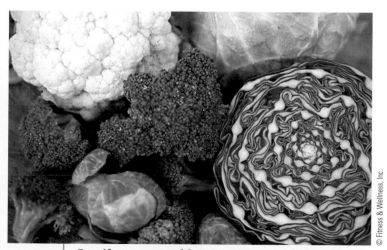

Cruciferous vegetables are recommended in a cancer-prevention diet.

Table 13.1 Selected Phytochemicals, Their Effects, and Sources

Phytochemical	Effect	Good Sources
Sulforaphane	Removes carcinogens from cells	Broccoli
PEITC	Keeps carcinogens from binding to DNA	Broccoli
Genistein	Prevents small tumors from accessing capillaries to get oxygen and nutrients	Soybeans
Flavonoids	Helps keep cancer-causing hormones from locking onto cells	Most fruits and vegetables
p-coumaric and chlorogenic acids	Disrupts the chemical combination of cell molecules that can produce carcinogens	Strawberries, green peppers, tomatoes, pineapple
Capsaicin	Keeps carcinogens from binding to DNA	Hot chili peppers

self-destruct.[7] Polyphenols are known to block the formation of nitrosamines and quell the activation of carcinogens. Both green and black tea have similar amounts of polyphenols. Herbal teas do not provide the same benefits as regular tea.[8]

Polyphenols are also thought to fight cancer by shutting off the formation of cancer cells, turning up the body's natural detoxification defenses and thereby suppressing progression of the disease. Green tea seems to be especially helpful in preventing gastrointestinal cancers, including those of the stomach, small intestines, pancreas, and colon. Consumption of green tea also has been linked to a lower incidence of lung, esophageal, and estrogen-related cancers, including most breast cancers. In Japan, where people drink green tea regularly but smoke twice as much as do people in the United States, the incidence of lung cancer is half that of the United States. A cancer-prevention diet recommends drinking 2 or more cups of green tea daily.

High fat intake may promote cancer and excessive weight. Some experts recommend that total fat intake should be limited to less than 20 percent of total daily calories.[9] Fat intake should be primarily monounsaturated and omega-3 fats. Omega 3-fats (found in many types of fish, flaxseeds, and flaxseed oil) seem to offer protection against colorectal, pancreatic, breast, oral, esophageal, and stomach cancers. Omega 3-fats block the synthesis of prostaglandins, bodily compounds that promote tumor growth.

Foods high in vitamin C may deter some cancers. Salt-cured, smoked, and nitrite-cured foods have been associated with cancer of the esophagus and stomach.

> *A cancer-prevention diet should limit fat intake to less than 20 percent of total daily calories.*

Processed meats should be consumed sparingly and always with orange juice or other vitamin C–rich foods. Vitamin C seems to discourage the formation of **nitrosamines**. These potentially cancer-causing compounds are formed when nitrites and nitrates, which are used to prevent the growth of harmful bacteria in processed meats, combine with other chemicals in the stomach.

Nutritional guidelines also discourage excessive intake of protein. The daily protein intake for some people is almost twice the amount the human body needs. Too much animal protein seems to decrease blood enzymes that prevent precancerous cells from developing into tumors.

Some research suggests that grilling protein (fat or lean) at high temperatures for a long time increases the formation of carcinogenic substances on the skin or surface of the meat. Microwaving the meat for a couple of minutes before barbecuing decreases the risk, as long as the fluid released by the meat is discarded. Most of the potential carcinogens collect in this solution. Removing the skin before serving and cooking at lower heat to "medium" rather than "well done" also seem to lower the risk.[10] Soy protein also seems to decrease the formation of carcinogens during cooking of meats.[11]

Soy foods may help because soy contains chemicals that prevent cancer. Although further research is merited, isoflavones (phytochemicals)

Phytochemicals Compounds found in fruits and vegetables that block the formation of cancerous tumors and disrupt the process of cancer.

Carcinogens Substances that contribute to the formation of cancers.

Nitrosamines Potentially cancer-causing compounds formed when nitrites and nitrates, which are used to prevent the growth of harmful bacteria in processed meats, combine with other chemicals in the stomach.

TIPS FOR A HEALTHY CANCER-FIGHTING DIET

Increase intake of phytochemicals, fiber, cruciferous vegetables, and more antioxidants by

- Eating a predominantly vegetarian diet
- Eating more fruits and vegetables every day (six to eight servings per day maximize anticancer benefits)
- Increasing the consumption of broccoli, cauliflower, kale, turnips, cabbage, kohlrabi, Brussels sprouts, hot chili peppers, red and green peppers, carrots, sweet potatoes, winter squash, spinach, garlic, onions, strawberries, tomatoes, pineapple, and citrus fruits in your regular diet
- Eating vegetables raw or quickly cooked by steaming or stir-frying
- Substituting tea, fruit, and vegetable juices for coffee and soda
- Eating whole grain breads
- Including calcium in the diet (or from a supplement)
- Including soy products in the diet
- Using whole wheat flour instead of refined white flour in baking
- Using brown (unpolished) rice instead of white (polished) rice

Decrease daily fat intake to 20% of total caloric intake by

- Limiting consumption of beef, poultry, or fish to no more 3 to 6 ounces (about the size of a deck of cards) once or twice a week
- Trimming all visible fat from meat and removing skin from poultry prior to cooking
- Decreasing the amount of fat and oils used in cooking
- Substituting low-fat for high-fat dairy products
- Using salad dressings sparingly
- Using only half to three-quarters the amount of fat required in baking recipes
- Limiting fat intake to mostly monounsaturated (olive oil, canola oil, nuts, and seeds) and omega-3 fats (fish, flaxseed, and flaxseed oil)
- Eating fish once or twice a week
- Including flaxseed oil (or flaxseeds) in the diet

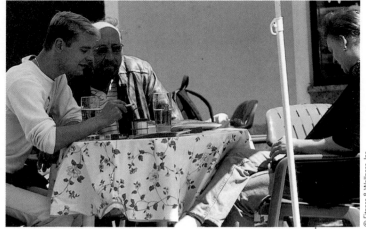

Heavy drinking and smoking greatly increase the risk of oral cancer.

found in soy are structurally similar to estrogen and may prevent breast, prostate, lung, and colon cancers. These isoflavones are frequently referred to as "phytoestrogens" or "plant estrogens." Isoflavones also block angiogenesis. Presently, it is not known if the health benefits of soy are derived from iso-flavones by themselves or in combination with other nutrients found in soy.

One drawback of soy was found in animal studies wherein animals with tumors were given very large amounts of soy: The estrogen-like activity of soy isoflavones actually led to the growth of estrogen-dependent tumors. Experts, therefore, caution women with breast cancer or a history of this disease to limit soy intake because it may stimulate cancer cells by closely imitating estrogen's actions.

No specific recommendations are presently available as to the amount of daily soy protein intake for cancer prevention. The FDA allows the health claim that 25 grams per day in conjunction with a diet low in saturated fat and cholesterol lowers the risk for cardiovascular disease (see Chapter 12). Based on the traditional diets of people (including children) in China and Japan who regularly consume soy foods, there doesn't appear to be an unsafe natural level of consumption. Soy protein powder supplementation, however, may elevate soy protein intake to an unnatural (and perhaps unsafe) level.[12]

Alcohol should be consumed in moderation, because too much alcohol raises the risk for developing certain cancers, especially when it is combined with tobacco smoking or smokeless tobacco. In combination, these substances significantly increase the risk for cancers of the mouth, larynx, throat, esophagus, and liver. Approximately 17,000 deaths from cancer yearly are attributed to excessive use of alcohol, often in combination with smoking. The combined action of heavy alcohol and tobacco use can increase odds of developing cancer of the oral cavity fifteenfold.

Maintaining recommended body weight also is encouraged. Obesity may be associated with cancers of the colon, rectum, breast, prostate, endometrium, and kidney.

Abstaining from Tobacco

Cigarette smoking by itself is a major health hazard. If we include all related deaths, smoking

is responsible for more than 400,000 unnecessary deaths in the United States each year. The World Health Organization estimates that smoking causes 3 million deaths worldwide annually. The average life expectancy for a chronic smoker is about 15 years shorter than for a nonsmoker.[13]

The biggest carcinogenic exposure in the workplace is cigarette smoke. Of all cancers, at least 28 percent are tied to smoking, and 87 percent of lung cancers are tied to smoking. Use of smokeless tobacco also can lead to nicotine addiction and dependence as well as increased risk for mouth, larynx, throat, and esophageal cancers.[14]

Avoiding Excessive Sun Exposure

Too much exposure to ultraviolet radiation (both UVB and UVA rays) is a major contributor to skin cancer. The most common sites of skin cancer are those areas exposed to the sun most often (face, neck, and back of the hands).

The three types of skin cancer are

1. Basal cell carcinoma
2. Squamous cell carcinoma
3. Malignant melanoma

Nearly 90 percent of the almost 1 million cases of basal cell or squamous cell skin cancers reported yearly in the United States could have been prevented by protecting the skin from the sun's rays.

> *Tanning of the skin is the body's natural reaction to permanent and irreversible damage from too much exposure to the sun.*

Melanoma is the most deadly, causing approximately 7,700 deaths in 2000. One in every six Americans will develop some type of skin cancer eventually. Nothing is healthy about a "healthy tan." Tanning of the skin is the body's natural reaction to permanent and irreversible damage from too much exposure to the sun. Even small doses of sunlight add up to a greater risk for skin cancer and premature aging. The tan fades at the end of the summer season, but the underlying skin damage does not disappear. People with sensitive skin in particular should avoid sun exposure between 10:00 A.M. and 4:00 P.M.

The stinging sunburn comes from **ultraviolet B rays** (UVB), which also are thought to be the main cause of premature wrinkling and skin aging, roughened/leathery/sagging skin, and skin cancer. Unfortunately, the damage may not become evident until up to 20 years later. In comparison, skin that has not been overexposed to the sun remains

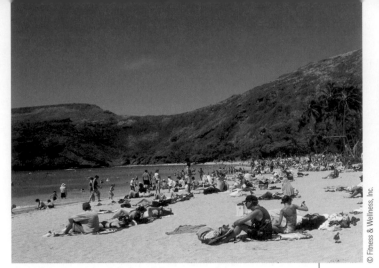

Tanning poses a risk for skin cancer from overexposure to ultraviolet rays.

smooth and unblemished, and, over time, shows less evidence of aging.

Sun lamps and tanning parlors provide mainly ultraviolet A rays (UVA). Once thought to be safe, they are now known to be damaging and have been linked to melanoma, the most serious form of skin cancer. As little as 15 to 30 minutes of exposure to UVA can be as dangerous as a day spent in the sun.[15]

Sunscreen lotion should be applied about 30 minutes before lengthy exposure to the sun because the skin takes that long to absorb the protective ingredients. A **sun protection factor** (SPF) of at least 15 is recommended. SPF 15 means that the skin takes 15 times longer to burn than with no lotion. If you ordinarily get a mild sunburn after 20 minutes of noonday sun, an SPF 15 allows you to remain in the sun about 300 minutes before burning. The higher the number, the stronger the protection. When swimming or sweating, you should reapply waterproof sunscreens more often because all sunscreens lose strength when they are diluted.

Monitoring Estrogen, Radiation Exposure, and Potential Occupational Hazards

Intake of estrogen has been linked to endometrial cancer in some studies, but other evidence contradicts those findings. And, although exposure to

---

Melanoma   The most virulent, rapidly spreading form of skin cancer.

Ultraviolet B rays (UVB)   Portion of sunlight that causes sunburn and encourages skin cancers.

Sun protection factor (SPF)   Degree of protection offered by ingredients in sunscreen lotion; at least SPF 15 is recommended.

radiation increases the risk for cancer, the benefits of X rays may outweigh the risk involved, and most medical facilities use the lowest dose possible to keep the risk to a minimum. Occupational hazards —such as asbestos fibers, nickel and uranium dusts, chromium compounds, vinyl chloride, and bischlormethyl ether—increase the risk for cancer. Cigarette smoking magnifies the risk from occupational hazards.

Engaging in Physical Activity

An active lifestyle seems to have a protective effect against cancer. Although the mechanism is not clear, physical fitness and cancer mortality in men and women may have a graded and consistent inverse relationship[16] (see Figure 13.8). A daily 30-minute moderate-intensity exercise program lowers the risk for colon cancer and may lower the risk for cancers of the breast and reproductive system. Research has shown that regular exercise lowers the risk for breast cancer in women by 20 to 30 percent. In addition, growing evidence suggests that the body's auto-immune system may play a role in preventing cancer. Moderate exercise improves the auto-immune system.[17]

Early Detection

Fortunately, many cancers can be controlled or cured through early detection. The real problem

CANCER PROMOTERS

- Physical inactivity
- Being more than 10 pounds overweight
- Frequent consumption of red meat
- A diet high in fat
- Charred/burned foods
- Frequent consumption of nitrate/nitrite-cured, salt-cured, or smoked foods
- Alcohol consumption
- Excessive sun exposure

comes when cancerous cells spread, because they become more difficult to destroy. Therefore, effective prevention, or at least early detection, is crucial. Herein lies the importance of periodic screening. Once a month, women should practice breast self-examination (BSE) (see Figure 13.11, page 348) and men testicular self-examination (TSE) (see Figure 13.12, page 350). Men should pick a regular day each month (for example, the first day of each month) to practice TSE, and women should perform BSE 2 or 3 days after the menstrual period is over.

Other Factors

The contribution of many of the other much-publicized factors is not as significant as those just

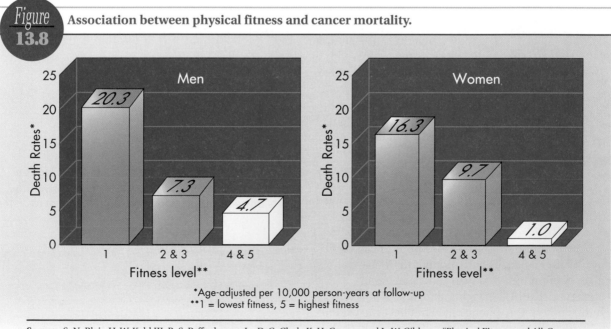

Figure 13.8 Association between physical fitness and cancer mortality.

*Age-adjusted per 10,000 person-years at follow-up
**1 = lowest fitness, 5 = highest fitness

Source: S. N. Blair, H. W. Kohl III, R. S. Paffenbarger, Jr., D. G. Clark, K. H. Cooper, and L. W. Gibbons, "Physical Fitness and All-Cause Mortality: A Prospective Study of Healthy Men and Women," *Journal of the American Medical Association* 262 (1989): 2395–2401.

pointed out. Intentional food additives, saccharin, processing agents, pesticides, and packaging materials currently used in the United States and other developed countries seem to have minimal consequences. High levels of tension and stress and poor coping may affect the autoimmune system negatively and render the body less effective in dealing with the various cancers.

Genetics plays a role in susceptibility in about 10 percent of all cancers. Most of the effect is seen in the early childhood years. Some cancers are a combination of genetic and environmental liability: Genetics may add to the environmental risk of certain types of cancers. The biggest carcinogenic exposure in the workplace is cigarette smoke. "Environment," however, means more than pollution and smoke. It incorporates diet, lifestyle-related events, viruses, and physical agents such as X rays and exposure to the sun.

Warning Signals of Cancer

Everyone should become familiar with the following seven warning signals for cancer and bring them to a physician's attention if any are present:

1. Change in bowel or bladder habits.
2. Sore that does not heal.
3. Unusual bleeding or discharge.
4. Thickening or lump in breast or elsewhere.
5. Indigestion or difficulty in swallowing.
6. Obvious change in wart or mole.
7. Nagging cough or hoarseness.

The recommendations for early detection of cancer in asymptomatic people by the American Cancer Society, outlined in Table 13.2, should be heeded in regular physical examinations as part of a cancer-prevention program. In Lab 13A you will be

Table 13.2 — Summary of Recommendations for Early Detection of Cancer in Asymptomatic People

Cancer-related Checkup	A cancer-related checkup is recommended every 3 years for people aged 20–40 and every year for people age 40 and older. This exam should include health counseling and depending on a person's age, might include examinations for cancers of the thyroid, oral cavity, skin, lymph nodes, testes, and ovaries, as well as for some nonmalignant diseases.
Breast	Women 40 and older should have an annual mammogram, an annual clinical breast examination (CBE) by a health-care professional, and should perform monthly breast self-examination (BSE). The CBE should be conducted close to and preferably before the scheduled mammogram.
	Women aged 20–39 should have a clinical breast examination by a health-care professional every three years and should perform monthly BSE.
Colon & Rectum	Beginning at age 50, men and women at average risk should follow one of the examination schedules below: ■ Fecal occult blood test (FOBT) every year, or ■ Flexible sigmoidoscopy every five years,* or ■ FOBT every year and flexible sigmoidoscopy every 5 years,* or ■ Double-contrast barium enema every 5 years,* or ■ Colonoscopy every 10 years.* }Of these 3 options, the American Cancer Society prefers the third option, annual FOBT and flexible sigmoidoscopy every 5 years. * A digital rectal exam should be done at the same time as sigmoidoscopy, colonoscopy, or double-contrast barium enema. People who are at increased or high risk for colorectal cancer should talk with a doctor about a different testing schedule.
Prostate	Beginning at age 50, the prostate-specific antigen (PSA) test and the digital rectal exam should be offered annually to men who have a life expectancy of at least 10 years. Men at high risk (African-American men and men who have a first-degree relative who was diagnosed with prostate cancer at a young age) should begin testing at age 45. Patients should be given information about the benefits and limitations of tests so they can make an informed decision.
Uterus	**Cervix:** All women who are or have been sexually active or who are 18 and older should have an annual Pap test and pelvic examination. After three or more consecutive satisfactory examinations with normal findings, the Pap test may be performed less frequently. Discuss the matter with your physician.
	Endometrium: Beginning at age 35, women with or at risk for hereditary non-polyposis colon cancer should be offered endometrial biopsy annually to screen for endometrial cancer.

Cancer Facts and Figures. © 2001, American Cancer Society, Inc. Used by permission.

able to determine how well you are doing in terms of cancer prevention and also respond to a questionnaire developed by the American Medical Association to alert people to symptoms that may indicate a serious health problem. Although in most cases nothing serious will be found, any of the symptoms calls for a physician's attention as soon as possible. Scientific evidence and testing procedures for prevention and early detection of cancer do change. Studies continue to provide new information. The intent of cancer-prevention programs is to educate and guide individuals toward a lifestyle that will help prevent cancer and enable early detection of malignancy.

Treatment of cancer always should be left to specialized physicians and cancer clinics. Current treatment modalities include surgery, radiation, radioactive substances, chemotherapy, hormones, and immunotherapy.

Cancer Questionnaire: Assessing Your Risks

The Texas Division of the American Cancer Society designed a simple self-testing questionnaire, shown in Figure 13.9, to help people assess their risk for cancer. These are the major risk factors for specific cancer sites and by no means represent the only ones that might be involved. Both men and women should complete the questions for lung, colon-rectum, and skin cancer. Three additional cancer types are included for women: breast, cervical, and endometrial.

Check your status against the factors contained in this questionnaire, total your scores, and then locate your "Total Risk" in the sections below. Individual numbers for specific questions are not to be interpreted as a precise measure of relative risk, but the totals for a given site should give you a general indication of your risk. Explanations of the risk factors for each type of cancer follows. If you are at higher risk, you are advised to discuss the results with your physician.

To assess your own risk levels, fill out the questionnaire in Figure 13.9, total the points, and then locate your risk levels in the following section. Record your risk level totals for each cancer site in Lab 13B.

The potential risks for cancer are based on individual lifestyle and medical history.

Lung Cancer

Risk Factors

1. *Sex.* Men have a higher risk for developing lung cancer than women do, equating them for type,

amount, and duration of smoking. However, because more women are smoking cigarettes for a longer duration than previously, their incidence of lung and upper respiratory tract (mouth, tongue, and larynx) cancer is increasing. Lung cancer is now number one in mortality for women by type of cancer.

2. *Age.* The occurrence of lung and upper respiratory tract cancers increases with age.

3. *Smoking status.* Cigarette smokers have up to 20 times or even greater risk than nonsmokers. The rates of ex-smokers who have not smoked for 10 years, however, approach those of nonsmokers.

4. *Type of smoking.* Pipe and cigar smokers are at a higher risk for lung cancer than nonsmokers. Cigarette smokers are at a much higher risk than nonsmokers or pipe and cigar smokers. All forms of tobacco, including chewing, markedly increase the user's risk of developing cancer of the mouth.

5. *Number of cigarettes smoked per day.* Male smokers of less than one-half pack per day have 5 times higher lung cancer rates than nonsmokers. Male smokers of one to two packs per day have 15 times higher lung cancer rates than nonsmokers. Smokers of more than two packs per day are 20 times more likely to develop lung cancer than nonsmokers.

6. *Type of cigarette.* Smokers of low-tar/nicotine cigarettes have slightly lower lung cancer rates.

7. *Duration of smoking.* The frequency of lung and upper respiratory tract cancer increases with the length of time people have smoked.

8. *Type of industrial work.* Exposure to materials used in the industries mentioned in Figure 13.9 (Question 8) have been demonstrated to be associated with lung cancer. Exposure to materials in other industries also carry a higher risk. Smokers who work in these industries have greatly increased risks. Exposure to arsenic, radon, radiation from occupational/medical/environmental sources, and air pollution increase the risk of lung cancer.

Total Risk

24 or less	You have a low risk for lung cancer (low-risk category).
25–49	You may be a light smoker and would have a good chance of kicking the habit (light risk).
50–74	As a moderate smoker, your risks of lung and upper respiratory tract cancers are increased. If you stop smoking now, these risks will decrease (moderate risk).
75 or over	As a heavy cigarette smoker, your chances of getting cancer of the lung

Figure 13.9   Cancer questionnaire: Assessing your risks.

Assessing Your Risks for Cancer

Read each question concerning each site and its specific risk factors. Be honest in your responses. Place the number in parentheses (risk points) in the box provided to the left of each question. For example, Question #2 on lung cancer: If you are 53 years old (age 50 to 59), then enter 5 (risk points) as your score on the left. At the end of each site, total your number of points for that site. Record the final number of points in Lab 13A, page 355.

Lung Cancer

1. Sex
   a. Male (2)
   b. Female (1)

2. Age
   a. 39 or less (1)
   b. 40–49 (2)
   c. 50–59 (5)
   d. 60+ (7)

3. Smoking status
   a. Smoker (8)
   b. Nonsmoker (1)

4. Type of smoking
   a. Current cigarettes or little cigars (10)
   b. Pipe and/or cigar, but not cigarettes (3)
   c. Ex-cigarette smoker (2)

5. Amount of cigarettes smoked per day
   a. 0 cigarettes (1)
   b. Less than 1 pack per day (5)
   c. 1 pack (9)
   d. 1–2 packs (15)
   e. 2+ packs (20)

6. Type of cigarette
   a. High tar/nicotine (10)*
   b. Medium T/N (9)
   c. Low T/N (7)
   d. Nonsmoker (1)

7. Duration of smoking
   a. Never smoked (1)
   b. Ex-smoker (3)
   c. Up to 15 years (5)
   d. 15–25 years (10)
   e. 25+ years (20)

8. Type of industrial work
   a. Mining (3)
   b. Asbestos (7)
   c. Uranium and radioactive products (5)

Total

Colon-Rectum Cancer

1. Age
   a. 39 or less (10)
   b. 40–59 (20)
   c. 60+ (50)

2. Has anyone in your immediate family ever had
   a. Colon cancer (20)
   b. One or more polyps of the colon (10)
   c. Neither (1)

3. Have you ever had
   a. Colon cancer (100)
   b. One or more polyps of the colon (40)
   c. Ulcerative colitis (20)
   d. Cancer of the breast or uterus (10)
   e. None (1)

4. Bleeding from the rectum (other than obvious hemorrhoids or piles)
   a. Yes (75)
   b. No (1)

Total

Skin Cancer

1. Frequent work or play in the sun:
   a. Yes (10)
   b. No (1)

2. Work in mines, around coal tars, or around radioactivity:
   a. Yes (10)
   b. No (1)

3. Complexion—fair and/or light skin:
   a. Yes (10)
   b. No (1)

Total

Source: Adapted from the Texas Division of the American Cancer Society. Reproduced with permission. (NOTE: This questionnaire is not available nationwide; distribution is limited to Texas residents only.)

Figure 13.9

Cancer questionnaire: Assessing your risks (continued)

Breast Cancer

1. Age group
   a. 20–34 (10)
   b. 35–49 (40)
   c. 50+ (90)

2. Race group
   a. Oriental (5)
   b. African American (20)
   c. White (25)
   d. Hispanic American (10)

3. Family history
   a. Mother, sister, aunt, or grandmother with breast cancer (30)
   b. None (10)

4. Your history
   a. Previous lumps or cysts (25)
   b. No breast disease (10)
   c. Previous breast cancer (100)

5. Maternity
   a. First pregnancy before 25 (10)
   b. First pregnancy after 25 (15)
   c. No pregnancies (20)

   Total

Cervical Cancer

(Lower portion of uterus. These questions do not apply to a woman who has had a total hysterectomy.)

1. Age group
   a. Less than 25 (10)
   b. 25–39 (20)
   c. 40–54 (30)
   d. 55+ (30)

2. Race
   a. Oriental (10)
   b. Puerto Rican (20)
   c. African American (20)
   d. White (10)
   e. Hispanic American (20)

3. Number of pregnancies
   a. 0 (10)
   b. 1–3 (20)
   c. 4 and over (30)

4. Viral infections
   a. Herpes and other viral infections or ulcer formations on the vagina (10)
   b. Never (1)

5. Age at first intercourse
   a. Before 15 (40)
   b. 15–19 (30)
   c. 20–24 (20)
   d. 25 and over (10)
   e. Never (5)

6. Bleeding between periods or after intercourse
   a. Yes (40)
   b. No (1)

   Total

Endometrial Cancer

(Body of uterus. These questions do not apply to a woman who has had a total hysterectomy.)

1. Age group
   a. 39 or less (5)
   b. 40–49 (20)
   c. 50+ (60)

2. Race
   a. Oriental (10)
   b. African American (10)
   c. White (20)
   d. Hispanic American (10)

3. Births
   a. None (15)
   b. 1 to 4 (7)
   c. 5 or more (5)

4. Weight
   a. 50 or more pounds overweight (50)
   b. 20–49 pounds overweight (15)
   c. Underweight for height (10)
   d. Normal (10)

5. Diabetes (elevated blood sugar)
   a. Yes (3)
   b. No (1)

6. Estrogen hormone intake
   a. Yes, regularly (15)
   b. Yes, occasionally (12)
   c. None (10)

7. Abnormal uterine bleeding
   a. Yes (40)
   b. No (1)

8. Hypertension (high blood pressure)
   a. Yes (3)
   b. No (1)

   Total

and upper respiratory tract are greatly increased. Your best bet is to stop smoking now—for the health of it. See your doctor if you have a nagging cough, hoarseness, persistent pain, or a sore in the mouth or throat (high risk).

Colon/Rectum Cancer

Risk Factors

1. *Age.* Colon cancer occurs more frequently after 50 years of age.
2. *Family predisposition.* Colon cancer is more common in families that have a previous history of this disease.
3. *Personal history.* Polyps and bowel diseases are associated with colon cancer.
4. *Rectal bleeding.* Rectal bleeding may be a sign of colorectal cancer.

Total Risk:

29 or less	You are at low risk for colon/rectum cancer.
30–69	This is a moderate-risk category. Testing by your physician may be indicated.
70 or over	This is a high-risk category. You should see your physician for the following tests: digital rectal exam, guaiac (stool) slide test, and proctoscopic exam.

In addition to the risk factors mentioned in the questionnaire, a diet high in fat and low in fiber, inadequate consumption of fruits and vegetables, physical inactivity, a history of breast or endometrial cancer, and inflammatory bowel disease also increase the risk for colon/rectum cancer.

Skin Cancer

Risk Factors

1. *Sun exposure.* Excessive ultraviolet light is a culprit in skin cancer. Protect yourself with a sunscreen medication.
2. *Work environment.* Working in mines, around coal tar, or around radioactive materials can cause cancer of the skin.
3. *Complexion.* Individuals with light complexions need more protection than others.

Total Risk:

Numerical risks for skin cancer are difficult to state. For instance, a person with a dark complexion can work longer in the sun and be less likely to develop cancer than a light-skinned person. Furthermore, a person wearing a long sleeved shirt and a wide-brimmed hat who works in the sun has less risk than a person who wears a bathing suit for only a short period. The risk increases greatly with age, and family history also plays a role.

If you answer "yes" to any question, you need to protect your skin from the sun or any other toxic material. Changes in moles, warts, or skin sores are important and should be evaluated by your doctor (see Figure 13.10).

Breast Cancer

Risk Factors

1. *Age.* The risk for breast cancer significantly increases after 50 years of age.
2. *Race.* Breast cancer occurs more frequently in white women than any other group.
3. *Family history.* The risk for breast cancer is higher in women with a family history of this type of cancer. The risk is even higher if more than one family member has developed breast cancer and is further enhanced by the closeness of the relationship of family member(s) (e.g., a mother or sister with breast cancer indicates a higher risk than a cousin with breast cancer).
4. *Personal history.* A previous history of breast or ovarian cancer would indicate a greater risk.

Figure 13.10 **Warning signs of melanoma: ABCD Rule.**

A. *Asymmetry:* One half of a mole or lesion doesn't look like the other half.

B. *Border:* A mole has an irregular, scalloped, or not clearly defined border.

C. *Color:* The color varies or is not uniform from one area of a mole or lesion to another, whether the color is tan, brown, black, white, red, or blue.

D. *Diameter:* The lesion is larger than 6 millimeters (¼ inch) or larger than a pencil eraser.

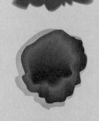

Adapted from *FDA Consumer*, May 1991.

5. *Maternity.* The risk is higher in women who never have had children and in women who bear children after 30 years of age.

Total Risk:

Under 100	Low-risk women should practice monthly breast self-examination (BSE —see Figure 13.11) and have their breasts examined by a doctor as a part of a cancer-related check-up.
100–199	Moderate-risk women should practice monthly BSE and have their breasts examined by a doctor as part of a cancer-related check-up. Periodic **mammograms** (see below) should be included as recommended.
200 or over	High-risk women should practice monthly BSE and have the above examinations more often. See your doctor for

the recommended (frequency of breast physical examinations and mammograms) examinations related to you.

Clinical breast exams by a physician are recommended every three years for women between ages 20 and 40 and every year for women over 40. The American Cancer Society also recommends an annual mammogram for women over 40. The latter is still an area of debate among health care practitioners, and personal risk factors should be considered to determine the frequency of mammograms.

Other possible risk factors for breast cancer not listed in the questionnaire are a long menstrual history (onset of menstruation prior to age 13 and ending later in life), recent use of oral contraceptives or postmenopausal estrogens, drinking two or more alcoholic beverages per day, chronic cystic disease, and ionizing radiation. A diet high in fat has also

---

Figure 13.11 **Breast self-examination.**

Why do the breast self-exam?

There are many good reasons for doing a breast self-exam each month. One reason is that it is easy to do and the more you do it, the better you will get at it. When you get to know how your breasts normally feel, you will quickly be able to feel any change, and early detection is the key to successful treatment.

Remember: A breast self-exam could save your breast—and save your life. Most breast lumps are found by women themselves, but in fact, most lumps in the breast are not cancer. Be safe, be sure.

When to do breast self-exam

The best time to do breast self-exam is right after your period, when breasts are not tender or swollen. If you do not have regular periods or sometimes skip a month, do it on the same day every month.

How to do breast self-exam

1. Lie down and put a pillow under your right shoulder. Place your right arm behind your head.
2. Use the finger pads of your three middle fingers on your left hand to feel for lumps or thickening. Your finger pads are the top third of each finger.
3. Press firmly enough to know how your breast feels. If you're not sure how hard to press, ask your health care provider. Or try to copy the way your health care provider uses the finger pads during a breast exam. Learn what your breast feels like most of the time. A firm ridge in the lower curve of each breast is normal.
4. Move around the breast in a set way. You can choose either the circle (A), the up and down (B), or the wedge (C). Do it the same way every time. It will help you to make sure that you've gone over the entire breast area, and to remember how your breast feels.
5. Now examine your left breast using right-hand finger pads.
6. Repeat the examination of both breasts while standing, with one arm behind your head. The upright position makes it easier to check the upper and outer part of the breasts (toward your armpit). You may want to do the standing part of the BSE while you are in the shower. Some breast changes can be felt more easily when your skin is wet and soapy.

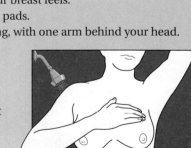

For added safety, you can also check your breasts for any dimpling of the skin, changes in the nipple, redness, or swelling while standing in front of a mirror right after your BSE each month.

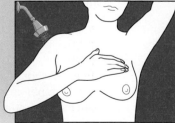

A   B   C

been viewed as a predisposing factor, although recent research has questioned its link to breast cancer.

Cervical Cancer

Risk Factors

1. *Age.* The highest occurrence is in the 40 and over age group. The score numbers in the questionnaire represent the relative rates of cancer for different age groups—that is, a 45-year-old woman has a risk 3 times greater than a 20-year-old.
2. *Race.* Puerto Ricans, African Americans, and Hispanic Americans have higher rates of cervical cancer.
3. *Number of pregnancies.* Women who have delivered more children have a higher occurrence.
4. *Viral infections.* Viral infections of the cervix and vagina are associated with cervical cancer.
5. *Age at first intercourse.* Women with earlier intercourse and with more sexual partners are at a higher risk.
6. *Bleeding.* Irregular bleeding may be a sign of uterine cancer.

Total Risk:

40–69	This is a low-risk group. Ask your doctor for a Pap test. You will be advised how often you should be tested after your first test.
70–99	In this moderate-risk group, more frequent Pap tests may be required.
100 or over	You are in a high-risk group and should have a Pap test (and pelvic exam) as advised by your doctor.

Early detection through a Pap test during a pelvic exam should be performed annually in women who are or have been sexually active or who have reached the age of 18. Following three normal tests during three consecutive years, the Pap test may be done less frequently, at the discretion of the physician.

Endometrial Cancer

Risk Factors

1. *Age.* Endometrial cancer is seen in older age groups. The scoring numbers by the age groups represent relative rates of endometrial cancer at different ages—that is, a 50-year-old woman has a risk 12 times higher than that of a 35-year-old woman.
2. *Race.* White women have a higher occurrence.
3. *Births.* The fewer children one has delivered, the greater is the risk of endometrial cancer.

4. *Weight.* Women who are overweight are at greater risk.
5. *Diabetes.* Cancer of the endometrium is associated with diabetes.
6. *Estrogen use.* Cancer of the endometrium may be associated with prolonged continuous estrogen hormone intake. This occurs in only a small number of women. Hormone replacement therapy (progesterone plus estrogen) is thought to offset the increased risk related to estrogen use. You should consult your physician before starting or stopping any estrogen medication.
7. *Abnormal bleeding.* Women who do not have cyclic menstrual periods are at greater risk.
8. *Hypertension.* Cancer of the endometrium is associated with high blood pressure.

Total Risk:

49–59	You are at low risk for developing endometrial cancer.
60–99	Your risks are slightly higher (moderate risk). Report any abnormal bleeding immediately to your doctor. Tissue sampling at menopause is recommended.
100 or over	Your risks are much greater (high risk). See your doctor for tests as appropriate.

Additional risk factors that may be associated with endometrial cancer, not included in the questionnaire, are infertility, a prolonged history of failure to ovulate, and menopause after age 55. Women over 40 should have a yearly pelvic exam by a physician.

Other Cancer Sites

Following are other types of cancers whose risk factors are not as clearly defined as those in Figure 13.9. Risk factors and prevention techniques for these types of cancer have been outlined in *The Causes of Cancer*,[18] published by the American Cancer Society, as well as in a series of pamphlets titled "Facts on Cancer," also available at the American Cancer Society. These types of cancer are presented with the risk factors associated with each type and preventive techniques to decrease risk. No numeric weights for the different risk factors have been assigned. As you read the information, however, rate yourself on a scale from 1 to 3 (1 for low risk, 2 for moderate risk, 3 for high risk) for each cancer site and record your results in Lab 13B.

Mammogram Low-dose X rays of the breasts used as a screening technique for the early detection of breast cancer.

Prostate Cancer

The prostate gland is actually a cluster of smaller glands that encircles the top section of the urethra (urinary channel) at the point where it leaves the bladder. Although the function of the prostate is not entirely clear, the muscles of these small glands help squeeze prostatic secretions into the urethra.

Risk Factors

1. *Advancing age.* The highest incidence of prostate cancer is found in men over 65 (75 percent of cases). The incidence is also higher among Blacks than Whites, and more married men than single men develop this type of cancer.
2. *A family history.*
3. *Race.* African Americans have the highest rate in the world.
4. *Diet.* A diet high in fat.

Prevention and Warning Signals

Prostate cancer is difficult to detect and control because the causes are not known. Death rates can be lowered through early detection and awareness of the warning signals. Detection is done by a digital rectal exam of the gland and a prostate-specific antigen (PSA) blood test once a year after the age of 50. Possible warning signals include difficulties in urination (especially at night), painful urination, blood in the urine, and constant pain in the lower back or hip area.

Testicular Cancer

Testicular cancer accounts for only 1 percent of all male cancers, but it is the most common type of cancer seen in men between ages 25 and 35. The incidence is slightly higher in whites than in African Americans, and it is rarely seen in middle-aged and older men. The malignancy rate of testicular tumors is 96 percent, but if it is diagnosed early, this type of cancer is highly curable.

Risk Factors

1. Undescended testicle not corrected before age 6.
2. Atrophy of the testicle following mumps or virus infection.
3. Family history of testicular cancer.
4. Recurring injury to the testicle.
5. Abnormalities of the endocrine system (e.g., high hormone levels of pituitary gonadotropin or androgens).
6. Incomplete testicular development.

Prevention and Warning Signals

The incidence of testicular cancer is quite high in males born with an undescended testicle. Therefore, this condition should be corrected early in life. Parents of infant males need to make sure that the child is checked by a physician to ensure that the testes have descended into the scrotum. Testicular self-examination (TSE) once a month following a warm bath or shower (when the scrotal skin is relaxed) is recommended. Guidelines for performing a TSE are given in see Figure 13.12.

Some of the warning signs associated with testicular cancer are a small lump on the testicle, slight enlargement (usually painless) and change in consistency of the testis, sudden build-up of blood or fluid in the scrotum, pain in the groin and lower abdomen or discomfort accompanied by a sensation of dragging and heaviness, breast enlargement or tenderness, and enlarged lymph glands.

Early diagnosis of testicular cancer is essential, because this type of cancer spreads rapidly to other

---

Figure 13.12 Testicular self-examination.

How To Examine The Testicles

You can increase your chances of early detection of testicular cancer by regularly performing a testicular self examination (TSE). The following procedure is recommended:

■ Perform the self-exam once a month. Select an easy day to remember such as the first day or first Sunday of the month.

■ Learn how your testicle feels normally so that it will be easier to identify changes. A normal testicle should feel oval, smooth, and uniformly firm, like a hard-boiled egg.

■ Perform TSE following a warm shower or bath, when the scrotum is relaxed.

■ Gently roll each testicle between your thumb and the first three fingers until you have felt the entire surface. Pay particular attention to any lumps, change in size or texture, pain, or a dragging or heavy sensation since your last self-exam. Do not confuse the epididymis at the rear of the testicle for an abnormality.

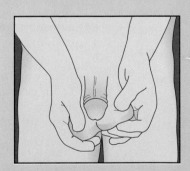

■ Bring any changes to the attention of your physician. A change does not necessarily indicate a malignancy, but only a physician is able to determine that.

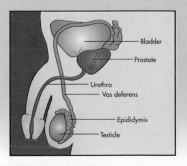

HEALTH QUESTIONNAIRES: CANCER PREVENTION AND EARLY WARNING SIGNS OF DISEASE

Name: _____   Date: _____   Grade: _____

Instructor: _____   Course: _____   Section: _____

Necessary Lab Equipment
None required.

Lab Preparation
None required.

Objective
To encourage healthy lifestyle practices that will help decrease the risk for cancer.

I. Cancer Prevention: Are You Taking Control?

Today, scientists think most cancers may be related to lifestyle and environment—what you eat and drink, whether you smoke, and where you work and play. The good news, then, is that you can help reduce your own cancer risk by taking control of things in your daily life.

10 Steps to a Healthier Life and Reduced Cancer Risk   Yes   No

1. **Are you eating more cabbage-family vegetables?**
   They include broccoli, cauliflower, Brussels sprouts, all cabbages, and kale.

2. **Are high-fiber foods included in your diet?**
   Fiber is found in whole grains, fruits, and vegetables including peaches, strawberries, potatoes, spinach, tomatoes, wheat and bran cereals, rice, popcorn, and whole-wheat bread.

3. **Do you choose foods with vitamin A?**
   Fresh foods with beta-carotene, including carrots, peaches, apricots, squash, and broccoli are the best source—not vitamin pills.

4. **Is vitamin C included in your diet?**
   You'll find it naturally in lots of fresh fruits and vegetables including grapefruit, cantaloupe, oranges, strawberries, red and green peppers, broccoli, and tomatoes.

5. **Do you exercise and monitor calorie intake to avoid weight gain?**
   Walking is ideal exercise for many people.

6. **Are you cutting overall fat intake?**
   This is done by eating lean meat, fish, skinned poultry, and low-fat dairy products.

7. **Do you limit salt-cured, smoked, nitrite-cured foods?**
   Choose bacon, ham, hot dogs or salt-cured fish only occasionally if you like them a lot.

8. **If you smoke, have you tried quitting?**

9. **If you drink alcohol, are you moderate in your intake?**

10. **Do you respect the sun's rays?**
    Protect yourself with sunscreen (at least SPE 15) and wear long sleeves and a hat, especially during midday hours—10 A.M. to 2 P.M.

11. **Do you have a family history of any type of cancer? If so, have you brought this to the attention of your personal physician?**

12. **Are you familiar with the seven warning signals for cancer?**

If you answered "yes" to most of these questions, **congratulations**. You are taking control of simple lifestyle factors that will help you feel better and reduce your risk for cancer.

Adapted from the American Cancer Society, Texas Division.

II. Early Warning Signs of Possible Serious Illness

Many serious illnesses begin with apparently minor or localized symptoms that, if recognized early, can alert you to act in time for the disease to be cured or controlled. In most cases, nothing is seriously wrong. **If you experience any of the following symptoms, discuss the problem with your physician without delay.** Check only conditions that apply.

- [ ] 1. Rapid loss of weight—more than about 4 kg (10 lbs) in 10 weeks—without apparent cause.

- [ ] 2. A sore, scab, or ulcer, either in the mouth or on the body, that fails to heal within about 3 weeks.

- [ ] 3. A skin blemish or mole that begins to bleed or itch or that changes color, size, or shape.

- [ ] 4. Severe headaches that develop for no obvious reason.

- [ ] 5. Sudden attacks of vomiting, without preceding nausea.

- [ ] 6. Fainting spells for no apparent reason.

- [ ] 7. Visual problems such as seeing "haloes" around lights or intermittently blurred vision, especially in dim light.

- [ ] 8. Increasing difficulty with swallowing.

- [ ] 9. Hoarseness without apparent cause that lasts for a week or more.

- [ ] 10. A "smoker's cough" or any other nagging cough that has been getting worse.

- [ ] 11. Blood in coughed-up phlegm, or sputum.

- [ ] 12. Constantly swollen ankles.

- [ ] 13. A bluish tinge to the lips, the insides of the eyelids, or the nailbeds.

- [ ] 14. Extreme shortness of breath for no apparent reason.

- [ ] 15. Vomiting of blood or a substance that resembles coffee grounds.

- [ ] 16. Persistent indigestion or abdominal pain.

- [ ] 17. A marked change in normal bowel habits, such as alternating attacks of diarrhea and constipation.

- [ ] 18. Bowel movements that look black and tarry.

- [ ] 19. Rectal bleeding.

- [ ] 20. Unusually cloudy, pink, red, or smoky-looking urine.

- [ ] 21. In men, discomfort or difficulty when urinating.

- [ ] 22. In men, discharge from the tip of the penis.

- [ ] 23. In women, a lump or unusual thickening of a breast or any alteration in breast shape such as flattening, bulging, or puckering of skin.

- [ ] 24. In women, bleeding or unusual discharge from the nipple.

- [ ] 25. In women, vaginal bleeding or "spotting" that occurs between usual menstrual periods or after menopause.

Reproduced with permission from Family Medical Guide by American Medical Association (New York: Random House, 1982).

Name: _____ **Date:** _____ **Grade:** _____

Instructor: _____ **Course:** _____ **Section:** _____

Necessary Lab Equipment
None required.

Objective
To determine your risk for selected cancer sites.

I. Cancer Risk Profile

Instructions—Read the sections *Cancer Questionnaire: Assessing Your Risks* and *Other Cancer Sites* in Chapter 13 (pages 344–353) and complete the Cancer Questionnaire in Figure 13.9 (pages 345–346). Copy your scores from Figure 13.9 into the blanks for those sites below. For all other sites, rate yourself on a scale from 1 to 3 (1 = low risk, 2 = moderate risk, 3 = high risk) according to the risk factors provided for each site under the *Other Cancer Sites* section.

Cancer Site	Total Points		Risk Category
	Men	Women	
Lung			
Colon-Rectum			
Skin			
Breast			
Cervical			
Endometrial			
Prostate			
Testicular			
Pancreatic			
Kidney and Bladder			
Oral			
Esophageal and Stomach			
Ovarian			
Thyroid			
Liver			
Leukemia			
Lymphomas			

II. Stage of Change for Cancer Prevention

Using Figure 2.3 (page 40) and Table 2.3 (page 41), identify your current stage of change for participation in a cancer-prevention program:

III. Personal Interpretation

In the space provided below, discuss your results for the various cancer sites. State your feelings about cancer and comment on any experiences that you may have had with cancer patients.

IV. Cancer Prevention

Discuss lifestyle habits that you should eliminate and habits that you need to adopt to reduce your own risk of cancer. Also indicate how you can best implement and adhere to these changes.

Chapter 14

Addictive Behavior and Wellness

Objectives

- Address the detrimental effects of addictive substances, including marijuana, cocaine, methamphetamine, heroin, and alcohol.

- Understand the detrimental health effects of tobacco use in general.

- Recognize cigarette smoking as the largest preventable cause of premature illness and death in the United States.

- Learn the fundamental reasons people smoke.

- Understand the benefits and the significance of a smoking cessation program.

- Learn how to implement a smoking cessation program, either for yourself (if you smoke), or to help others go through the quitting process.

As we begin the 21st century, one of the most serious health problems that continues to afflict society is that of chemical dependency. Substance abuse is an extremely destructive behavior that has ruined and ended millions of lives. Perhaps more than with any other unhealthy behavior, education is critical when addictive behaviors are at issue. The time to make healthy choices is now. The information in this chapter will help you make informed decisions. Education concerning these subjects may assist in the search for answers, treatment, and a more productive and happier life.

Addiction

When people think of **addiction**, most probably think of dark and dirty alleys, an addict shooting drugs into the veins, or a wino passed out next to a garbage can after having spent an evening with alcohol. Jacquelyn Small, psychotherapist and author, has described addiction as a problem of imbalance or unease within the body and mind.

Almost anything can be addicting. Of the many types of addiction, some addictive behaviors are more detrimental than others. The most serious type of addiction is chemical dependency on drugs such as tobacco, coffee, alcohol, cocaine, methamphetamine, heroin, marijuana, and prescription drugs. Less serious addictions are to work, compulsive shopping, and even exercise.

People who are addicted to food eat to release stress or boredom or to reward themselves for every small personal achievement. Many people are addicted to television and the Internet. Others become so addicted to their jobs that all they think about is work. Although work may start out as an enjoyable activity, when it totally consumes a person's life, work can become an unhealthy behavior.

If you find that you are readily irritated, moody, grouchy, constantly tired, not as alert as you used to be, or making more mistakes than usual, you may be becoming a workaholic and need to slow down or take time off work.

Even though exercise has enhanced the health and quality of life of millions of people, a relatively small number become obsessed with exercise, which has the potential for overuse and addiction. Compulsive exercisers feel guilty and uncomfortable when they miss a day's workout. Often they continue to exercise even when they have injuries and sickness that require proper rest for adequate recovery. People who exceed the recommended guidelines for development and maintenance of fitness (see Chapters 7, 8, and 9) are exercising for reasons other than health—including addictive behavior.

Americans spend more than $100 billion annually on illegal drugs.

Addiction to caffeine can produce undesirable side effects. Caffeine doses in excess of 200 to 500 mg can produce an abnormally rapid heart rate, abnormal heart rhythms, higher blood pressure, higher body temperature, and increased secretion of gastric acids leading to stomach problems, as well as birth defects in offspring. It may also induce symptoms of anxiety, depression, nervousness, and dizziness. The caffeine content of drinks varies according to the product. In 6 ounces of coffee, for example, the content varies from 65 mg in instant coffee to as high as 180 mg in drip coffee. Soft drinks, mainly colas, range in caffeine content from about 30 to 70 mg per 12-ounce can.

The previous examples, as well as more serious forms of chemical dependency, are by no means the only types of addiction but are used here to illustrate addictive behaviors. Other addictions are gambling, pornography, sex, people, places, and on and on.

Recognizing that all forms of addiction are unhealthy, this chapter focuses on some of the most self-destructive addictive substances in our society: marijuana, cocaine, methamphetamine, heroin, alcohol, and tobacco. About a half a million Americans die each year from tobacco, alcohol, and illegal drug use.

Drugs and Dependence

A drug is any substance that alters the user's ability to function. Drugs encompass over-the-counter drugs, prescription medications, and illegal substances. Many drugs lead to physical and psychological dependence.

Any drug can be misused and abused. Drug misuse implies the intentional or inappropriate use of over-the-counter or prescribed medications.[1] Examples of drug misuse include the intake of a greater amount of a medication than prescribed, mixing drugs, not following prescription instructions, or discontinuing a drug prior to a physicians' approval.

Drug abuse is the intentional and inappropriate use of a drug resulting in physical, emotional, financial, intellectual, or social consequences for their use.[2] Many substances, if used in the wrong manner, can be abused.

When drugs are used regularly, they integrate into the body's chemistry, increasing tolerance to the drug and forcing the user to constantly increase the dosage to obtain similar results. Drug abuse leads to serious health problems, and more than half of all adolescent suicides are drug-related. Often, drug abuse also opens the gate to other illegal activities. According to U.S. Department of Justice, the

majority of convicted criminals—about 70 percent of federal inmates and 80 percent of state inmates—have abused drugs.

Approximately 60 percent of the world's production of illegal drugs is consumed in the United States. Each year Americans spend more than $100 billion on illegal drugs, an amount that surpasses the total dollars taken in from all crops by U. S. farmers. According to the U.S. Department of Education, today's drugs are stronger and more addictive, and they pose a greater risk than ever before. If you are uncertain about addictive behavior(s) in your life, the questionnaire "Could You Be an Addict?" in Lab 14A (page 381) can help you identify a potential problem. Some of the most commonly abused drugs in our society are discussed next.

Marijuana

Marijuana (pot or grass, as it is commonly called) is the most widely used illegal drug in the United States. Estimates by the Office of National Drug Control Policy indicate that 46 percent of Americans between ages 18 and 25 and 42 percent of those age 26 and older have smoked marijuana. Approximately 31 million people in the United States use marijuana regularly. Most users smoke loose marijuana that has been rolled in to a joint or packed into a pipe. A few users will bake it into foods such as brownies.

In small doses, marijuana has a sedative effect. Larger doses produce physical and psychic changes. Studies in the 1960s indicated that the potential effects of marijuana were exaggerated and that the drug was relatively harmless. The drug as it is used today, however, is as much as 10 times stronger than when the initial studies were conducted. Most of the research today shows marijuana to be dangerous and harmful.

The main, and most active, psychoactive and mind-altering ingredient in marijuana is thought to be delta-9-tetrahydrocannabinol (THC). In the 1960s, THC content in marijuana ranged from .02 to 2 percent. Users called the latter "real good grass." Today's THC content averages 4 to 6 percent, although it has been reported as high as 20 percent. The THC content in sinsemilla, a variety of high-potency marijuana grown from the seedless female cannabis plant, is approximately 6.66 percent THC.

THC reaches the brain within a few seconds after marijuana smoke is inhaled, and the psychic and physical changes reach their peak in about 2 or 3 minutes. THC then is metabolized in the liver to waste metabolites, but 30 percent of it remains in the body a week after the marijuana was smoked. THC is not completely eliminated until 30 days or

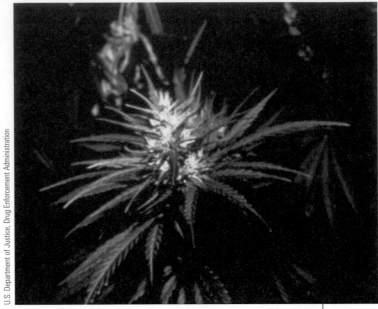

U.S. Department of Justice, Drug Enforcement Administration

The flowering top of *Cannabis sativa*.

longer after an initial dose of the drug. The drug always remains in the system of regular users.

Some of the short-term effects of marijuana are **tachycardia**, dryness of the mouth, reddened eyes, stronger appetite, decrease in coordination and tracking (following a moving stimulus), difficulty in concentration, intermittent confusion, impairment of short-term memory and continuity of speech, interference with the physical and mental learning process during periods of intoxication, and increased risk of a heart attack for a full day after smoking the drug. Another common effect is the **amotivational syndrome**. This syndrome persists after periods of intoxication but usually disappears a few weeks after the individual stops using the drug. Long-term harmful effects include atrophy of the brain (leading to irreversible brain damage), less resistance to infectious diseases, chronic bronchitis, lung cancer (marijuana smoke may contain as much as 50 percent more cancer-producing hydrocarbons than cigarette smoke), and possible sterility and impotence.

Addiction   Compulsive and uncontrollable behavior(s) or use of substance(s).

Marijuana   A psychoactive drug prepared from a mixture of crushed leaves, flowers, small branches, stems, and seeds from the hemp plant *cannabis sativa*.

Tachycardia   Faster-than-normal heart rate.

Amotivational syndrome   A condition characterized by loss of motivation, dullness, apathy, and no interest in the future.

One of the most common myths about marijuana use is that it is not addictive. This myth has grown recently among young people as lobbyists work to convince the federal government to legalize marijuana for medical purposes. Ample scientific evidence clearly shows that regular users of marijuana do develop physical and psychological dependence. As with cigarette smokers, when regular users go without the drug, they crave the substance, go through mood changes, are irritable and nervous, and develop an obsession to get more.

Cocaine

Similar to marijuana, **cocaine** was thought for many years to be relatively harmless. This misconception came to an abrupt halt in the mid-1980s when two well-known athletes (Len Bias—basketball, and Don Rogers—football), died suddenly following cocaine overdoses. Between 1 and 1.5 million Americans use cocaine, 96 percent of whom had used marijuana previously. Over the years it has been given several different names including, among others, coke, C, snow, blow, toot, flake, Peruvian lady, white girl, and happy dust. This drug can be sniffed or snorted, smoked, or injected.

> *Cocaine hallucinations include "coke bugs" or imaginary insects and snakes crawling on or underneath the skin.*

When cocaine is snorted, it is absorbed quickly through the mucous membranes of the nose into the bloodstream. The drug is usually arranged in fine powder lines 1 to 2 inches long. Each line stimulates the autonomic nervous system for about 30 minutes. When cocaine is injected intravenously, larger amounts of cocaine can enter the body in less time. The popularity of cocaine is based on the almost universal guarantee that users will find themselves in an immediate state of euphoria and well-being. An expensive drug, some users pay more than $4,800 per ounce for cocaine. Cocaine used in medical therapy sells for about $100 per ounce. The addiction begins with a desire to get high, often at social gatherings, and usually with the assurance that "occasional use is harmless." About 1 in 5 of these first-time users will continue to use the drug now and then, and for some it is the beginning of a lifetime nightmare.

Crack cocaine is a smokable form of cocaine that has become more popular in the past decade. It is many times more potent than cocaine and is highly addictive; two-thirds of users in the United States who are addicted to cocaine use crack. Because they are so potent, crack doses are smaller and therefore less expensive, at a price of $10 to $30 each, although users will still spend hundreds of dollars a day to support their addiction.

Crack is often made by boiling cocaine hydrochloride in a solution of baking soda, then letting the solution dry. The residue is then broken up to be smoked in a pipe. The high from crack comes within seconds, faster than the high from injected cocaine. The crack high lasts about 12 minutes, which is shorter than the high from snorted or injected cocaine. Choosing to use cocaine in this form heightens the risk for emphysema and heart attack.

Cocaine seems to alleviate fatigue and raise energy levels, as well as lessen the need for food and sleep. Following the high comes a "crash," a state of physiological and psychological depression, often leaving the user with the desire to get more. This can lead to a constant craving for the drug. Similar to alcoholics, cocaine users recover only by abstaining from the drug completely. A single "backslide" can result in renewed addiction.

Light-to-moderate cocaine use is commonly associated with feelings of pleasure and well-being. Sustained cocaine snorting can lead to a constant runny nose, nasal congestion and inflammation, and perforation of the nasal septum. Long-term consequences of cocaine use include loss of appetite, digestive disorders, weight loss, malnutrition, insomnia, confusion, anxiety, and cocaine psychosis, characterized by paranoia and hallucinations. In one type of hallucination, referred to as formication or "coke bugs," the chronic user perceives imaginary insects or snakes crawling on or underneath the skin.

High doses of cocaine can cause nervousness, dizziness, blurred vision, vomiting, tremors, seizures, strokes, angina, cardiac arrhythmias, and high blood pressure. As with smoking marijuana, the increased risk of having a heart attack following cocaine use is immediate. The user's risk may be 24 times higher than normal for up to 3 hours following cocaine use. Almost one-third of cocaine users who suffered a heart attack had no symptoms of heart disease prior to taking cocaine. Intravenous users are also at risk for hepatitis, HIV, and other infectious diseases.

Large overdoses of cocaine can precipitate sudden death from respiratory paralysis, cardiac arrhythmias, and severe convulsions. If individuals lack an enzyme used in metabolizing cocaine, as few as two to three lines of cocaine may be fatal.

Chronic users who constantly crave the drug often turn to crime, including murder, to sustain

their habit. Some users view suicide as the only solution to this sad syndrome.

Methamphetamine

Methamphetamine, or "meth," is a more potent form of **amphetamine** that has become the fastest-growing drug threat in the United States. Amphetamines in general are part of a large group of synthetic agents used to stimulate the central nervous system. Amphetamines were widely given to soldiers during World War II to help them overcome fatigue, improve endurance, enhance battlefield ferocity, heighten mood, and keep the soldiers going. During the Vietnam war, U.S. soldiers used a greater amount of amphetamines than soldiers from all countries combined during World War II.

Methamphetamine is a powerfully addictive drug. It falls under the same category of psycho-stimulant drugs as amphetamines and cocaine. Methamphetamine is typically a white, odorless, and bitter-tasting powder that dissolves readily in water or alcohol. The drug is a potent central nervous system stimulant that produces a general feeling of well-being, decreases appetite, increases motor activity, and decreases fatigue and the need for sleep.

Based on 1996 estimates by the National Institute on Drug Abuse (NIDA), 4.7 million Americans have tried methamphetamines. Unlike most other drugs, methamphetamine use reaches rural and urban populations alike. Young people especially prefer methamphetamines because of its low cost and the long-lasting effects of the drug, up to 12 hours following use.

Methamphetamine is easily manufactured with over-the-counter ingredients in clandestine "meth labs." These labs can be set up almost anywhere, including garages, basements, or hotel rooms. The abundance of potential meth lab sites makes it difficult for drug enforcement agencies to locate many of these facilities. The risk of injury in a meth lab, however, is high, because potentially explosive environmental contaminants are discarded during the production of the drug.

Methamphetamines can be snorted, swallowed, smoked, or injected. It is commonly referred to as speed or crystal when snorted or taken orally, ice or glass when smoked, and crank when injected. Depending on how it is taken, methamphetamines affect the body differently.

Smoked or injected methamphetamines provide an immediate intense, pleasurable rush that lasts only a few minutes. Negative effects, nonetheless, can continue for several hours. When the drug is snorted or taken orally, the user does not experience

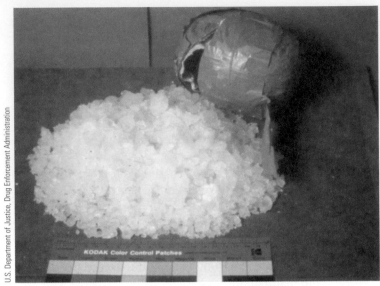

U.S. Department of Justice, Drug Enforcement Administration

"Ice," so named for its appearance, is a smokable form of methamphetamine.

a rush, but develops a feeling of euphoria that lasts up to 16 hours.

Methamphetamine users experience increases in body temperature, blood pressure, heart rate, and breathing rate; a decrease in appetite; hyperactivity; tremors; and violent behavior. High doses produce irritability, paranoia, irreversible damage to blood vessels in the brain (causing strokes), and risk of sudden death from hypothermia and convulsions if not treated at once.

Chronic abusers experience insomnia, confusion, hallucinations, inflammation to the heart lining, schizophrenia-like mental disorder, and brain-cell damage similar to that caused by strokes. Physical changes to the brain may last months or perhaps permanently. Over time, methamphetamine use may reduce brain levels of **dopamine**, which can lead to symptoms of Parkinson's disease. Additionally, users are frequently involved in violent crime, homicide, and suicide. Using methamphetamines during pregnancy may cause prenatal complications, premature delivery, and abnormal physical and emotional development of the child.

Cocaine   2-beta-carbomethoxy-3-betabenozoxytropane, the primary psychoactive ingredient derived from coca plant leaves.

Methamphetamine   A more potent form of amphetamine.

Amphetamine   Powerful central nervous system stimulants.

Dopamine   A neurotransmitter that affects emotional, mental, and motor functions.

Similar to other stimulants, methamphetamines are often used in a binge cycle. Addiction develops very quickly because tolerance to methamphetamines is developed within minutes of initial use. The high disappears long before drug blood levels drop significantly. The user then attempts to maintain the pleasurable feelings by taking in more of the drug, and a binge cycle ensues.

The binge cycle can last for a couple of weeks and consists of several stages. The initial "rush" lasts five to 30 minutes. During this stage heart rate, blood pressure, and metabolism increase along with a great sense of pleasure. The "high" follows for up to 16 hours; during this stage, users becomes aggressively smarter and more argumentative. The "binge" stage sets in next: It lasts between 2 and 14 days. Addicts continue to use the drug in an attempt to maintain the high for as long as possible.

When addicts can no longer achieve a satisfying high, they enter the "tweaking" stage, the most dangerous stage of the cycle. At this point users may have gone without food for several days and without sleep anywhere from 3 to 15 days. They become paranoid, irritable, and violent. Tweakers crave more of the drug, but no amount of amphetamines will restore the pleasurable/euphoric feelings achieved during the high. Thus the addicts become increasingly frustrated, unpredictable, and dangerous to those around them (including police officers, medical personnel, and even to themselves). Once they finally "crash," they are no longer dangerous. The user now becomes lethargic and sleeps for 1 to 3 days.

Following the crash, addicts fall into a 1- to 3-month period of "withdrawal." During this stage they can be paranoid, aggressive, fatigued, depressed, suicidal, and filled with an intense craving for another high. Reuse of the drug relieves these feelings, thus the incidence of relapse in users who seek treatment is high.

Heroin

For the first time in decades, **heroin** use is on the increase and its use is again being publicized by pop culture. Heroin started to make a comeback in 1991. It became increasingly stylish in 1995 following the arrests and deaths of prominent rock stars who abused the drug. According to the National Institute on Drug Abuse, some 600,000 Americans are currently addicted to heroin. Although the most common users are suburban middle-class people and lower-income populations, its use is starting to appear in more affluent communities as well.

Common nicknames for heroin include diesel, dope, dynamite, white death, nasty boy, china white, H. Harry, gumball, junk, brown sugar, smack, tootsie roll, black tar, and chasing the dragon. Heroin is classified as a narcotic drug. It is synthesized from morphine, a natural substance found in the seed pod of several types of poppy plants. In its purest form, heroin is a white powder, but on the streets it is typically available in yellow or brown powders. The latter colors are attained when pure heroin is combined with other drugs or substances such as sugar, cornstarch, chalk, brick dust, or laundry soap. Heroin is also sold in a hardened or solid form (black tar), which is usually dissolved with other liquids for use in injectable form. Many users combine heroin with cocaine, a risky process commonly referred to as "speedballing."

Today's heroin is more pure, powerful, and affordable than ever before. The average price has dropped by two-thirds over the last 10 years, which partially accounts for the increased popularity of the drug. For $100, drug users can get about 300 mg of heroin, an amount that will provide several "hits."

Heroin is a very dangerous drug. A significant health threat to users today is that they have no way of determining the strength of the drug purchased on the street, thus placing them at a constant risk for overdose and death. Based on a 1999 report from the Drug Abuse Warning Network, an estimated 15 percent of all drug-related hospital emergency room cases that year involved heroin use.

Heroin can be injected intravenously or intramuscularly, sniffed/snorted, or smoked. Although injection is the predominant method of heroin use, users are turning away from intravenous injections because of the risk for HIV infection. The availability of relatively low-priced, high-purity heroin further contributes to the number of people who smoke or snort the drug. Some users also have the misconception that heroin is less addictive when snorted or smoked. Whether injected, snorted, or smoked, heroin is an extremely addictive drug and both physical and psychological dependence develop very rapidly. Drug tolerance sets in quickly and, each time the drug is used, a higher dose is required to produce the same effects.

Heroin use induces a state of euphoria that comes within seconds of intravenous injection or within 5 to 15 minutes when other methods of administration are used. The drug is a sedative, so during the initial rush, the person has a sense of relaxation and does not feel any pain. In users who inhale the drug, however, the rush may be accompanied by nausea, vomiting, intense itching, and at times severe asthma attacks. As the rush wears off, users experience drowsiness, confusion, slowed cardiac function, and decreased breathing rate.

A heroin overdose can cause convulsions, coma, and death. During an overdose, heart rate,

breathing, blood pressure, and body temperature drop dramatically. These physiological responses can induce vomiting, tight muscles, and cause breathing to stop. Death is often the result of lack of oxygen or choking to death on vomit.

About 4 to 5 hours after the drug is taken, withdrawal sets in. Heroin withdrawal is painful and usually lasts up to 2 weeks—but could go on for several months.

Short-term use symptoms include red/raw nostrils; bone and muscle pains; muscle spasms and cramps; sweating; hot and cold flashes; runny nose and eyes; drowsiness; sluggishness; slurred speech; loss of appetite; nausea; diarrhea; restlessness and violent yawning. Heroin use can also kill a developing fetus or cause a spontaneous abortion.

Symptoms of long-term use of heroin include hallucinations, nightmares, constipation, sexual difficulties, impaired vision, reduced fertility, boils, collapsed veins, and a significantly elevated risk for lung, liver, and cardiovascular diseases, including bacterial infections in blood vessels and heart valves. The additives used in street heroin can clog vital blood vessels because they do not dissolve in the body, leading to infections and death of cells in vital organs. Sudden infant death syndrome (SIDS) is also more frequently seen in children born to addicted mothers.

Heroin addiction is treated with behavioral therapies and pharmaceutical agents. The use of medication helps suppress withdrawal symptoms, which makes it easier for patients to stop heroin use. The combination of these two treatment modalities helps the individual learn to lead a more stable, productive, and drug-free lifestyle.

Alcohol

Drinking **alcohol** has been a socially acceptable behavior for centuries. Alcohol is an accepted accompaniment at parties, ceremonies, dinners, sport contests, the establishment of kingdoms or governments, and the signing of treaties between nations. Alcohol also has been used for medical reasons as a mild sedative or as a painkiller for surgery.

For a short period of 14 years, from 1920 to 1933, by constitutional amendment, the sale and use of alcohol were declared illegal in the United States. This amendment was repealed because drinkers and nondrinkers alike questioned the right of government to pass judgment on individual moral standards. In addition, organized crime activities to smuggle and sell alcohol illegally expanded enormously during this period.

Alcohol is the cause of one of the most significant health-related drug problems in the United

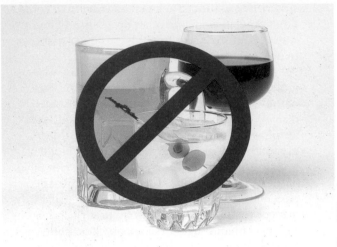

The sale of alcohol was illegal in the United States between 1920 and 1933.

States today. An estimated 6 in 10 adults—more than 100 million people 18 years and older—are drinkers. More than 13.8 million of them will develop a drinking problem, including **alcoholism**, in their lifetime. Another 10.4 million teenagers are thought to have a drinking problem.

The addiction to alcohol develops slowly. Most people think they are in control of their drinking habits and do not realize they have a problem until they become alcoholics, when they find themselves physically and emotionally dependent on the drug. This addiction is characterized by excessive use of and constant preoccupation with drinking. Alcohol abuse, in turn, leads to mental, emotional, physical, and social problems.

Alcohol intake impedes peripheral vision, lowers visual and hearing acuity, decreases reaction time, impairs concentration and motor performance (including increased swaying), and causes impaired judgment of distance and speed of moving objects. Further, it alleviates fear, increases risk-taking, stimulates urination, and induces sleep.

A single large dose of alcohol also may decrease sexual function. One of the most unpleasant, dangerous, and life-threatening effects of drinking is the **synergistic action** of alcohol when combined with other drugs, particularly central nervous

Heroin   A potent drug that is a derivative of opium.

Alcohol (ethyl alcohol)   A depressant drug that affects the brain and slows down central nervous system activity; has strong addictive properties.

Alcoholism   Disease in which an individual loses control over drinking alcoholic beverages.

system depressants. Each person reacts to a combination of alcohol and other drugs in a different way. The effects range from loss of consciousness to death.

Long-term effects of alcohol abuse are serious and often life-threatening (see Figure 14.1). Some of these detrimental effects are lower resistance to disease; **cirrhosis** of the liver; higher risk for oral, esophageal, stomach, and liver cancer; **cardiomyopathy**; irregular heartbeat; elevated blood pressure; greater risk for strokes; inflammation of the esophagus, stomach, small intestine, and pancreas; stomach ulcers; sexual impotence; birth defects; malnutrition; damage to brain cells leading to loss of memory; depression; psychosis; and hallucinations.

Alcohol on Campuses

Alcohol is the number-one drug problem among college students. According to national surveys, about 66 percent of college students reported using alcohol, and 43 percent of college students had engaged in binge drinking (5 or more drinks in a row) at least once in the 2 weeks preceding the survey. Alcohol is a factor in about 28 percent of all college dropouts, costing the federal government more than $3 billion in taxes. Today's student spends more on alcohol than on books.

Another survey involving 56,000 college students showed that grade point average (GPA) is related to average number of drinks per week (see Figure 14.2). Students with a "D" or "F" GPA reported a weekly consumption of almost 11 drinks. Students with "A" GPAs consumed about 3.5 drinks per week. Furthermore, 30 percent of all academic problems result from alcohol misuse. Of greater concern is that 36 percent of the surveyed students admitted driving while intoxicated. Of the 12 million college students in the United States, between 2 and 3 percent will die from alcohol-related causes. This represents more students than those who will receive advanced degrees (master's and doctorate degrees combined).

Another major concern is that more than half of college students participate in games that involve heavy drinking (6 to 10 drinks) in a short time. Often students take part because of peer pressure and fear of rejection. Up to 48 percent report getting drunk at least once a month. Excessive drinking can precipitate unplanned and unprotected sex (risking HIV infection) or date rape.

Long-term risks associated with alcohol abuse.

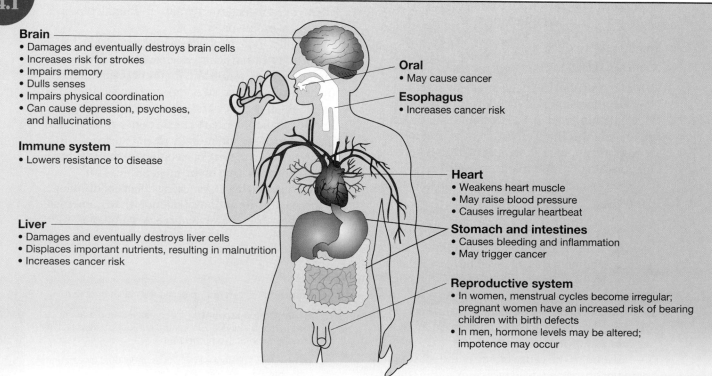

Brain
- Damages and eventually destroys brain cells
- Increases risk for strokes
- Impairs memory
- Dulls senses
- Impairs physical coordination
- Can cause depression, psychoses, and hallucinations

Immune system
- Lowers resistance to disease

Liver
- Damages and eventually destroys liver cells
- Displaces important nutrients, resulting in malnutrition
- Increases cancer risk

Oral
- May cause cancer

Esophagus
- Increases cancer risk

Heart
- Weakens heart muscle
- May raise blood pressure
- Causes irregular heartbeat

Stomach and intestines
- Causes bleeding and inflammation
- May trigger cancer

Reproductive system
- In women, menstrual cycles become irregular; pregnant women have an increased risk of bearing children with birth defects
- In men, hormone levels may be altered; impotence may occur

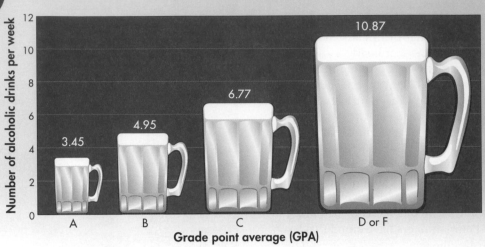

Figure 14.2 Average number of drinks by college students per week by GPA.

Number of alcoholic drinks per week

- A: 3.45
- B: 4.95
- C: 6.77
- D or F: 10.87

Grade point average (GPA)

How to Cut Down on Drinking

To find out if drinking is a problem in your life, refer to the questionnaire "Alcohol Abuse: Are You Drinking Too Much?," in Lab 14A, developed by the American Medical Association. If you respond "yes" twice or more on this questionnaire, you may be jeopardizing your health.

If a person is determined to control the problem, it is not that difficult. The first and most important step is to want to cut down. If you want to do this but you cannot, you had better accept the probability that alcohol is becoming a serious problem for you, and you should seek guidance from your physician or from an organization such as Alcoholics Anonymous. The next few suggestions also may help you cut down alcohol intake.

1. Set reasonable limits for yourself. Decide not to exceed a certain number of drinks on a given occasion and stick to your decision. No more than two beers or two cocktails a day is a reasonable limit. If you set a target such as this and consistently do not exceed it, you have proven to yourself that you can control your drinking.
2. Learn to say no. Many people have "just one more" drink because others in the group are doing this or because someone puts pressure on them, not because they really want a drink. When you reach the sensible limit you have set for yourself, politely but firmly refuse to exceed it. If you are being the generous host, pour yourself a glass of water or juice "on the rocks." Nobody will notice the difference.

Synergistic action The effect of mixing two or more drugs, which can be much greater than the sum of two or more drugs acting by themselves.

Cirrhosis A disease characterized by scarring of the liver.

Cardiomyopathy A disease affecting the heart muscle.

3. Drink slowly. Don't gulp down a drink. Choose your drinks for their flavor, not their "kick," and savor the taste of each sip.

4. Dilute your drinks. If you prefer cocktails to beer, try having "long" drinks. Instead of downing gin or whiskey neat or nearly so, drink it diluted with a mixer such as tonic water or soda water in a tall glass. That way you can enjoy both the flavor and the act of drinking but you will take longer to finish each drink. Also, you can make your two-drink limit last all evening or switch to the mixer by itself.

5. Do not drink on your own. Confine your drinking to social gatherings. You may have a hard time resisting the urge to pour yourself a relaxing drink at the end of a hard day, but many formerly heavy drinkers have found that a soft drink satisfies the need as well as alcohol did. What may help you really unwind, even with no drink at all, is a comfortable chair, loosened clothing, and perhaps a soothing audiotape, television program, or good book to read.

Treatment of Addiction

Recovery from alcoholism and other drug addictions is more likely to be successful with professional guidance and support. The first step is to recognize the reality of the problem. The questionnaire "Could You Be an Addict?" in Lab 14A will help you recognize possible addictive behavior in yourself or someone you know. If the answers to more than half of these questions are positive, a problem may exist—and you should contact a physician, your institution's counseling center, or the local mental health clinic for a referral (see the Yellow Pages in your phone book).

A person may also contact the National Center for Substance Abuse Treatment at 1-800-662-HELP (1-800-662-4357) for 24-hour substance abuse treatment centers in their local area. The national center also provides printed information on drug abuse and addictive behavior. All information discussed during a phone call to this center is kept strictly confidential.

About 5 million Americans have received treatment for addictive behavior.[3] An additional 7 million people are estimated to need treatment for substance abuse.[4] Treatment programs for addiction include a variety of intervention modalities, including psychotherapy, medical care, and behavior modification. If addiction is a problem in your life, you need to act upon it without delay. Addicts do not have to resign themselves to a lifetime of addiction. The sooner you start, and the longer you stay in treatment, the better the chances for recovery and a healthier and more productive life.

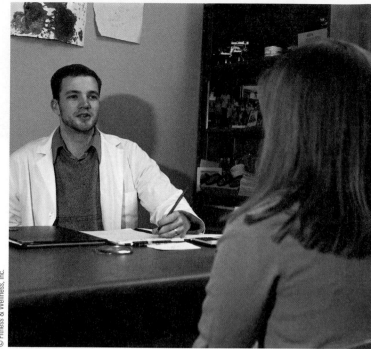

The sooner treatment for addiction is started, the longer the user stays in treatment, the better the chances for recovery and a more productive life.

Tobacco Use

People throughout the world have used tobacco for hundreds of years. Before the 18th century, they smoked tobacco primarily in the form of pipes or cigars. Cigarette smoking per se did not become popular until the mid-1800s, and its use started to increase dramatically in the 20th century.

In 1900, people in the United States consumed 2.5 billion cigarettes, compared to 640 billion in 1981. This figure dropped to 487 billion in 1995. Nonetheless, more than 47 million Americans over age 18 still smoked in 1995.

The harmful effects of cigarette smoking and tobacco use in general were not exactly known until the early 1960s, when research began to show a link between tobacco use and disease. In 1964, the U.S. Surgeon General issued the first major report presenting scientific evidence that cigarettes were indeed a major health hazard in our society.

Tobacco use in all its forms is considered a significant threat to life. World Health Organization estimates indicate that 10 percent of the 5 billion people presently living will die as a result of smoking-related illnesses, which kill approximately 4 million people each year. At the present rate of escalation, this figure is expected to climb to 10 million annual deaths by the year 2030. Tobacco will kill 150 million people in the first quarter of this century and another 300 million in the second quarter.

Morbidity and Mortality

Illegal drug overdoses kill about 17,500 people per year in the United States. Drug felonies and drug-related murders kill another 1,600 people each year. This brings drug-related deaths to a grand total of 19,100. Citizens and the government have mounted a tremendous campaign to eradicate illegal drug use in America. Cigarettes, however, a legal drug, kill about 26 times as many people as all illegal drugs combined.

Cigarette smoking is the largest preventable cause of illness and premature death in the United States. When considering all related deaths, smoking is responsible for about 430,000 unnecessary deaths each year—enough deaths to wipe out the entire population of Miami and Miami Beach in a single year.

Death rates from heart disease, cancer, stroke, aortic aneurysm, chronic bronchitis, emphysema, and peptic ulcers have increased. Figure 14.3 illustrates normal and diseased **alveoli**. Cigarette smoking by pregnant women has been linked to retarded fetal growth, higher risk for spontaneous abortion (miscarriage), and prenatal death. Smoking also is the most prevalent cause of injury and death from fire. The average life expectancy for a chronic smoker is as much as 18 years shorter than for a nonsmoker, and the death rate among chronic smokers during the most productive years of life, between ages 25 and 65, is twice the national average.

> *Cigarettes, a legal drug, kill about 26 times as many people as all illegal drugs combined.*

Based on a 1993 report by U.S. government physicians, each cigarette shortens life by 7 minutes. This figure represents 5 million years of potential life that Americans lose to smoking each year. According to estimates by the American Heart Association, more than 30 percent of fatal heart attacks—or 120,000 in the United States annually—result from smoking. The risk for heart attack is 50 to 100 percent higher for smokers than for nonsmokers. The mortality rate following heart attacks also is higher for smokers, because their attacks usually are more severe and their risk for deadly arrhythmias is much greater.

Cigarette smoking affects the cardiovascular system by increasing heart rate, blood pressure, and susceptibility to atherosclerosis, blood clots, coronary artery spasm, cardiac arrhythmia, and arteriosclerotic peripheral vascular disease. Evidence also indicates that smoking decreases high-density lipoprotein (HDL) cholesterol, the "good" cholesterol that lowers the risk for heart disease. Smoking further increases the amount of fatty acids, glucose, and various hormones in the blood. The carbon monoxide in smoke hinders the capacity of the blood to carry oxygen to body tissues. Both carbon monoxide and **nicotine** can damage the inner walls of the arteries and thus encourage the build-up of fat on these walls.

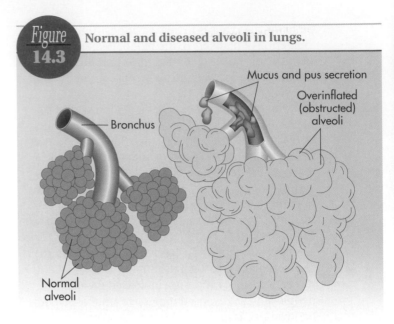

Figure 14.3 Normal and diseased alveoli in lungs.

Bronchus • Normal alveoli • Mucus and pus secretion • Overinflated (obstructed) alveoli

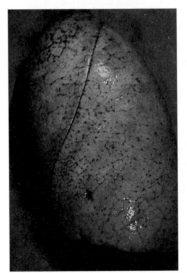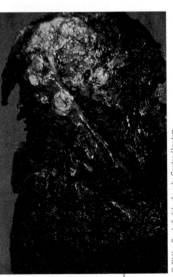

© "If You Smoke" slide show by Gordon Hewlett

Normal lung (left) is contrasted with diseased lung (right). The white growth near the top of the diseased lung is cancer; the dark appearance on the bottom half is emphysema.

Alveoli Air sacs in the lungs where gas exchange (oxygen and carbon dioxide) takes place.

Nicotine Addictive compound found in tobacco leaves.

Smoking also causes increased adhesiveness and clustering of platelets in the blood, decreases platelet survival and clotting time, and increases blood thickness. All of these effects can precipitate a heart attack.

The American Cancer Society reports that 87 percent of lung cancer is attributable to smoking. Lung cancer is the leading cancer killer, accounting for approximately 157,000 deaths in the United States in the year 2000, or about 28 percent of all deaths from cancer.[5] Cigarette smoking also leads to chronic obstructive pulmonary disease, the third leading cause of death in the United States (also see Chapter 1).

The most common carcinogenic exposure in the workplace is to cigarette smoke. Both fatal and nonfatal cardiac events are increased greatly in people who are exposed to passive smoke. Second-hand smoke is ranked behind active smoking and alcohol as the third leading preventable cause of death in the United States.[6] About 3,000 people die each year from lung cancer because of secondhand smoke. Passive smoke is also a significant risk factor for heart disease in children and adults alike. It causes an estimated 35,000 to 40,000 yearly deaths from heart disease in nonsmokers.[7]

Although half of all cancers are now curable, the 5-year survival rate for lung cancer is less than 13 percent. Cigarette smoking is also responsible for most cancers of the oral cavity, larynx, and esophagus (see Figure 14.4). Tobacco use also is related to the development of and deaths from bladder, pancreas, and kidney, and cervical cancers.

Even though many tobacco users are aware of the health consequences of cigarette smoking, they may fail to realize the risk of pipe smoking, cigar smoking, and tobacco chewing. As a group, pipe and cigar smokers have lower risks for heart disease and lung cancer. Nevertheless, blood nicotine levels in pipe and cigar smokers have been shown to approach those of cigarette smokers, because nicotine is still absorbed through the membranes of the mouth. Therefore, these tobacco users still have a higher risk for heart disease than nonsmokers do.

Cigarette smokers who substitute pipe or cigar smoking for cigarettes usually continue to inhale the smoke, which actually results in more nicotine and **tar** being brought into the lungs. Consequently, the risk for disease is even higher if pipe or cigar smoke is inhaled. The risk and mortality rates for lip, mouth,

Approximately 430,000 people die each year in the United States from smoking-related conditions.

Figure 14.4 The health effects of smoking.

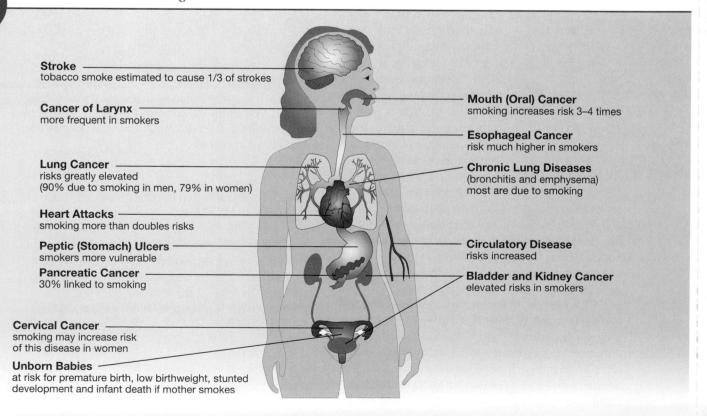

Stroke
tobacco smoke estimated to cause 1/3 of strokes

Cancer of Larynx
more frequent in smokers

Lung Cancer
risks greatly elevated
(90% due to smoking in men, 79% in women)

Heart Attacks
smoking more than doubles risks

Peptic (Stomach) Ulcers
smokers more vulnerable

Pancreatic Cancer
30% linked to smoking

Cervical Cancer
smoking may increase risk
of this disease in women

Unborn Babies
at risk for premature birth, low birthweight, stunted
development and infant death if mother smokes

Mouth (Oral) Cancer
smoking increases risk 3–4 times

Esophageal Cancer
risk much higher in smokers

Chronic Lung Diseases
(bronchitis and emphysema)
most are due to smoking

Circulatory Disease
risks increased

Bladder and Kidney Cancer
elevated risks in smokers

and larynx cancer for pipe smoking, cigar smoking, and tobacco chewing are actually higher than for cigarette smoking.

Economic Impact

The economic impact of cigarette smoking on the health-care system is staggering. In 1992, the Surgeon General calculated the lifetime excess medical care costs for smokers and former smokers at $501 billion above that of nonsmokers. Other estimates indicate that in the United States people pay more than $100 billion annually for tobacco-related health-care costs and lost productivity. Each pack of cigarettes sold represents about $3.90 in smoking-related expenses.[8]

Heavy smokers use the health-care system, especially hospitals, twice as much as nonsmokers do. The yearly cost to a given company has been estimated to be between $624 and $4,611 per smoking employee. These costs include employee health care, absenteeism, additional health insurance, morbidity/disability and early mortality, on-the-job time lost, property damage/maintenance and depreciation, worker compensation, and the impact of secondhand smoke.

Every day more than 1,200 Americans die from smoking-related illnesses. That is the equivalent of three fully loaded jumbo jets crashing each day with no survivors.[9] Imagine what the coverage and concern would be if 430,000 people each year were to die in the United States alone because of airplane accidents! People would not even consider flying any more. Most individuals would think of it as a form of suicide.

Smoking kills more Americans in a single year than those who died in battle during World War II and the Vietnam War combined. Think of the public outrage if 430,000 Americans were to die annually in a meaningless war. What if a single nonprescription drug caused more than 138,000 deaths from cancer and 120,000 fatal heart attacks each year? The U.S. public would not tolerate these situations. We probably would mount an intense fight to prevent the deaths.

Yet, are we not committing slow suicide by smoking cigarettes? Isn't tobacco a nonprescription drug available to almost anyone who wishes to smoke, killing more than 400,000 people each year? If cigarettes were invented today, the tobacco industry would be put on trial for mass murder.

Trends

The fight against all forms of tobacco use has been gaining momentum in the last few years. This was not always the case. It has been difficult to fight an industry that has as great a financial and political influence as the tobacco industry has in the United States. Tobacco is the sixth largest cash crop in the United States, producing 2.5 percent of the gross national product. It has influenced elections cleverly by emphasizing the individual's right to smoke, avoiding the fact that so many people die because of its use.

In 1990, Philip Morris, one of the largest tobacco-producing companies in the world, ranked seventh among Fortune 500 companies. Nearly 70 percent of its profits came from the sale of cigarettes. In 1992, Philip Morris donated about $17 million to several prominent organizations, so they no longer question the detrimental effects of tobacco use. Among the organizations receiving donations from Philip Morris in 1992 were United Way, YMCA, Salvation Army, Pediatric AIDS Foundation, Red Cross, Cystic Fibrosis Foundation, March of Dimes, Easter Seals, Muscular Dystrophy Association, Multiple Sclerosis Society, Hemophilia Foundation, United Cerebral Palsy, American Civil Liberties Union, American Bar Association, Task Force for Battered Women, Boy Scouts, Boys and Girls Club, and Big Brothers and Big Sisters. We call Colombian drug-runners unprincipled scum (responsible for about 19,100 illegal drug-related deaths per year), yet we welcome Philip Morris with glee and we call it civic pride.[10]

Tobacco was socially accepted for many years. In the 1980s, however, cigarette smoking no longer was acceptable in many social circles. Nonsmokers and ex-smokers alike are fighting for their rights to clean air and health. If every smoker were to give up cigarettes, in one year alone sick time would drop by approximately 90 million days, heart conditions would decrease by 280,000, chronic bronchitis and emphysema would number 1 million fewer cases, and total death rates from cardio-vascular disease, cancer, and peptic ulcers would fall off drastically.

Each cigarette smoked shortens a person's life by 7 minutes.

Many smokers are unaware of, or simply do not care to realize, how much cigarette smoke bothers nonsmokers. Smokers sometimes think that blowing the smoke off to the side is enough to get it out of the way. As a matter of fact, it is not enough. Smokers do not comprehend this until they quit and later find themselves in that situation. Suddenly, they realize

Tar Chemical compound that forms during the burning of tobacco leaves.

why cigarette smoke is so unpleasant and undesirable to most people.

In recent years, the Food and Drug Administration (FDA) Drug Abuse Advisory Committee has taken a strong stance against the use of all forms of tobacco products. Although the American Heart Association (AHA) commends the work initiated by the FDA, the AHA has further stated that the FDA and the federal government have an obligation to take regulatory action against the national problem of nicotine addiction to and abuse of cigarettes and tobacco products in general. In a 1992 statement before the FDA Drug Abuse Advisory Committee, the AHA indicated the following:

> It is a national health travesty that a product (tobacco), which accounts for over 430,000 deaths in the U.S. each year, has escaped regulation under every major health and safety law enacted by Congress to protect the public health.[11]

Smokeless Tobacco

Smokeless tobacco often is promoted as a safe alternative to cigarette smoking. According to the Advisory Committee to the U.S. Surgeon General, smokeless tobacco represents a significant health risk and is just as addictive as cigarette smoking.

Unlike smoking, the use of smokeless tobacco has increased during the last 15 years. Currently, some 15 million Americans use tobacco in this form. The greatest concern is the increase in use of "spit" tobacco, especially by young people. More than 2 million people under age 25 use spit tobacco, including nearly 20 percent of all males in grades 9 through 12. One-third of those who use spit tobacco started at age 5, and the average starting age was 9. Spit tobacco contains 2.5 times as much nicotine as a similarly priced pack of cigarettes.

Using smokeless tobacco can lead to gingivitis and periodontitis. It carries a fourfold increase in oral cancer, and in some cases even premature death. People who chew or dip also have a higher rate of cavities, sore gums, bad breath, and stained teeth. Their senses of smell and taste diminish; consequently, they tend to add more sugar and salt to food. These practices alone increase the risk for being overweight and having high blood pressure.

Nicotine addiction and its related health risks also hold true for smokeless tobacco users. Nicotine blood levels approach those of cigarette smokers, increasing the risk for diseases of the cardiovascular system. Further, research has revealed changes in heart rate and blood pressure similar to those of cigarette smokers.

Using tobacco in any form can be addictive and poses a serious threat to health and well-being.

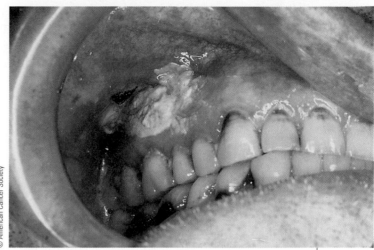

Smokeless tobacco can lead to gum and teeth damage as well as oral cancer (pictured).

Completely eliminating its use is the single most important lifestyle change a tobacco user can make to improve health, quality of life, and longevity.

Why People Smoke

People typically begin to smoke without realizing its detrimental effects on their health and life in general. Although people start to smoke for many different reasons, the three fundamental instigators are peer pressure, the desire to appear "grown up," and rebellion against authority. Smoking only three packs of cigarettes can lead to physiological addiction, turning smoking into a nasty habit that has become the most widespread example of drug dependency in the United States.

More than 1,200 toxic chemicals have been found in tobacco smoke.

When tobacco leaves are burned, hot air and gases containing tar (chemical compounds) and nicotine are released in the smoke. More than 1,200 toxic chemicals have been found in tobacco smoke. Tar contains about 60 chemical compounds that are proven carcinogens.

Smoking Addiction

The drug nicotine has strong addictive properties. Within seconds of inhalation, nicotine affects the central nervous system and can act simultaneously as a tranquilizer and a stimulant. The stimulating effect produces strong physiological and psychological dependency. The physical addiction to nicotine is six to eight times more powerful than the addiction to alcohol, and most likely greater than for some of the hard drugs currently used.

Smoking Dependency

The psychological dependency develops over a longer time. People smoke to help themselves relax, and they also gain a certain amount of pleasure from the ritual of smoking. Smokers automatically associate many activities of daily life with cigarettes. Typical associated activities are coffee drinking, alcohol drinking, being part of a social gathering, relaxing after a meal, talking on the telephone, driving, reading, watching television. In many cases the social rituals of smoking are the most difficult to eliminate. The dependency is so strong that, years after people have stopped smoking, they may still crave cigarettes when they engage in particular social activities.

Most of the remaining information in this chapter is written directly to smokers. Nonsmokers, however, will gain a better understanding of smokers by reading it. The following material also provides valuable information so you can help others implement a smoking cessation program.

"Why-Do-You-Smoke?" Test

Most people smoke for a variety of reasons. To find out why people smoke, the National Clearinghouse for Smoking and Health developed a simple "Why-Do-You-Smoke?" Test. This test, contained in Lab 14B, lists some statements by people describing what they get out of smoking cigarettes. Smokers are asked to indicate how often they have the feelings described in each statement when they are smoking.

The scores obtained on this test give an indication for each of six factors that describe people's feelings when they smoke. The first three highlight the positive feelings people derive from smoking. The fourth factor relates to reducing tension and relaxing. The fifth reveals the extent of dependence on cigarettes. The sixth factor differentiates habit smoking and purely automatic smoking. Each of the remaining factors fits one of the six reasons for smoking, discussed next. A score of 11 or above on any factor indicates that smoking is an important source of satisfaction for you. The higher you score (15 is the highest), the more important a given factor is in your smoking and the more useful the discussion of that factor can be in your attempt to quit.

If you do not score high on any of the six factors, chances are that you do not smoke much or have not been smoking for very many years. If so, giving up smoking, and staying off, should be fairly easy.

1. *Stimulation.* If you score high or fairly high on the stimulation factor, you are one of those smokers who is stimulated by the cigarette. You think it helps wake you up, organize your energies, and keep you going. If you try to give up smoking, you may want a safe substitute—a brisk walk or moderate exercise, for example—whenever you feel the urge to smoke.

2. *Handling.* Handling things can be satisfying, but you can keep your hands busy in many ways without lighting up or playing with a cigarette. Why not toy with a pen or pencil? Try doodling. Play with a coin, a piece of jewelry, or some other harmless object.

3. *Accentuation of pleasure/pleasurable relaxation.* Finding out whether you use the cigarette to feel good—get real, honest pleasure from smoking (Factor 3)—or to keep from feeling bad (Factor 4) is not always easy. About two-thirds of smokers score high or fairly high on accentuation of pleasure, and about half of those also score as high or higher on reduction of negative feelings. Those who do get real pleasure from smoking often find that honest consideration of the harmful effects of their habit is enough to help them quit. They substitute social and physical activities and find they do not seriously miss cigarettes.

4. *Reduction of negative feelings, or "crutch."* Many smokers use cigarettes as a kind of crutch during moments of stress or discomfort. Ironically, the heavy smoker—the person who tries to handle severe personal problems by smoking many times a day—is apt to discover that cigarettes do not help deal with problems effectively. This kind of smoker may stop smoking readily when everything is going well but may be tempted to start again in a time of crisis. Again, physical exertion or social activity may be a useful substitute for cigarettes, especially in times of tension.

5. *Craving or dependence.* Quitting smoking is difficult for people who score high on this factor. The craving for a cigarette begins to build the moment the previous cigarette is put out, so tapering off is not likely to work. This smoker must go **cold turkey**. If you are dependent on cigarettes, you may try smoking more than usual for a day or two to spoil your taste for cigarettes, then isolating yourself completely from cigarettes until the craving is gone.

6. *Habit.* If you are smoking from habit, you no longer get much satisfaction from the cigarettes. You light them frequently without even realizing you are doing it. You may have an easy time quitting and staying off if you can break the habitual patterns you have built up. Cutting down gradually may be effective if you change

---

Cold turkey Eliminating a negative behavior all at once.

the way you smoke cigarettes and the conditions under which you smoke them. The key to success is to become aware of each cigarette you smoke. You can do this by asking yourself, "Do I really want this cigarette?" You may be surprised at how many you do not want.

Smoking Cessation

If you are contemplating or preparing to stop cigarette smoking, you need to know that quitting smoking is not easy. Annually, only about 20 percent of smokers who try to quit the first time succeed. The addictive properties of nicotine and smoke make quitting difficult.

The American Psychiatric Association and the National Institute on Drug Abuse have indicated that nicotine is perhaps the most addictive drug known to humans. The 1988 Surgeon General's Report on Nicotine Addiction concluded that[12]

- Cigarettes and other forms of tobacco are addicting.
- Nicotine is the drug responsible for the addictive behavior.
- Pharmacologic and behavioral traits that determine addiction to tobacco are similar to those that determine addiction to drugs such as heroin and cocaine.

Smokers develop a tolerance to nicotine and smoke. They become dependent on both and get physical and psychological withdrawal symptoms when they stop smoking. Even though giving up smoking can be extremely difficult, it is by no means impossible, as attested by the many people who have quit.

During the last three decades, cigarette smoking in the United States has been declining gradually among smokers of all ages with the exception of young women. Surveys have shown that between 75 and 90 percent of all smokers would like to quit. Forty percent of the adult population—53 percent of men and 32 percent of women—smoked in 1964 when the U.S. Surgeon General first reported the link between smoking and increased risk for disease and mortality. By 1995, only 25 percent, or 47 million adults, smoked. Among men, 25 million (28.2 percent) were smokers, and 22 million (23.1 percent) women smoked. More than 38 million Americans have given up cigarettes. More than 40 percent of all adults who have ever smoked have quit since 1964.

More than 95 percent of successful ex-smokers have been able to do it on their

Nicotine is perhaps the most addictive drug known to humans.

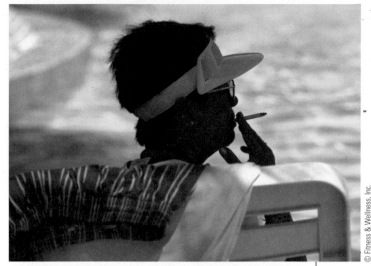

Cigarette smoking is the single largest preventable cause of illness and premature death in the United States.

© Fitness & Wellness, Inc.

own, either by quitting cold turkey or by using self-help kits available from organizations such as the American Cancer Society, the American Heart Association, and the American Lung Association. Only 3 percent of ex-smokers have done so as a result of formal cessation programs. Smokers' information and treatment centers are listed in the Yellow Pages of the telephone book.

"Do You Want To Quit?" Test

The most important factor in quitting cigarette smoking is the person's sincere desire to do so. Although some smokers can simply quit, this is not usually the case. Those who can quit easily are primarily light or casual smokers. They realize that the pleasure of an occasional cigarette is not worth the added risk of disease and premature death. For heavy smokers, quitting most likely will be a difficult battle. Even though many do not succeed the first time around, the odds of quitting are much better for those who try to stop repeatedly.

If you are a smoker and want to find your readiness to quit, the "Do You Want To Quit?" test contained in Lab 14B, developed by the National Clearinghouse for Smoking and Health, will measure your attitude toward the four primary reasons you want to quit smoking. The results give an indication of whether you are ready to start the program. On this test, the higher you score in any category, say the Health category, the more important that reason is to you. A score of 9 or above in one of these categories indicates that this is one of the most important reasons you may want to quit.

1. *Health*. Knowing the harmful consequences of cigarettes, many people have stopped smoking and many others are considering doing so. If your score on the Health factor is 9 or above, the health hazards of smoking may be enough to make you want to quit now. If your score on this factor is low (6 or below), consider the hazards of smoking. You may be lacking important information or may even have incorrect information. If so, health considerations are not playing the role they should be in your decision to keep smoking or to quit.

2. *Example*. Some people stop smoking because they want to set a good example for others. Parents quit to make it easier for their children to resist starting to smoke. Doctors quit to be role models for their patients. Teachers quit to discourage their students from smoking. Sports stars want to set an example for their young fans. Husbands quit to influence their wives to quit, and vice versa. Examples have a significant influence on our behavior. Surveys show that almost twice as many high school students smoke if both parents are smokers, compared with those whose parents are nonsmokers or former smokers.

    If your score is low (6 or lower), you might not be interested in giving up smoking to set an example for others. Perhaps you do not realize how important your example could be.

3. *Aesthetics*. People who score high (9 or above) in this category recognize and are disturbed by some of the unpleasant aspects of smoking. The smell of stale smoke on their clothing, bad breath, and stains on their fingers and teeth might be reason enough to consider quitting.

4. *Mastery*. If you score 9 or above on this factor, you are bothered by knowing that you cannot control your desire to smoke. You are not your own master. Awareness of this challenge to your self-control may make you want to quit.

Breaking the Habit

The following seven-step plan has been developed as a guide to help you quit smoking. The total program should be completed in 4 weeks or less. Steps One through Four combined should take no longer than 2 weeks. A maximum of 2 additional weeks is allowed for the rest of the program.

Step One

Decide positively that you want to quit. Avoid negative thoughts of how difficult this can be. Think positive. You can do it.

Now prepare a list of the reasons you smoke and why you want to quit (see Lab 14B, part IV). Make several copies of the list and keep them in places where you commonly smoke. Frequently review the reasons for quitting, because this will motivate and prepare you psychologically to quit.

When the reasons for quitting outweigh the reasons for smoking, you will have an easier time quitting. Try to read as much information as possible on the detrimental effects of tobacco and the benefits of quitting.

Step Two

Initiate a personal diet and exercise program. About one-third of the people who quit smoking gain weight. This could be caused by one or a combination of the following reasons:

1. Food becomes a substitute for cigarettes.
2. Appetite increases.
3. Basal metabolism may slow down.

If you start an exercise and weight-control program prior to quitting smoking, weight gain should not be a problem. If anything, exercise and lower body weight create more awareness of healthy living and strengthen the motivation for giving up cigarettes.

Even if you gain some weight, the harmful effects of cigarette smoking are much more

Giving up one pack of cigarettes a day is the equivalent of losing between 50 and 75 pounds of excess body fat!

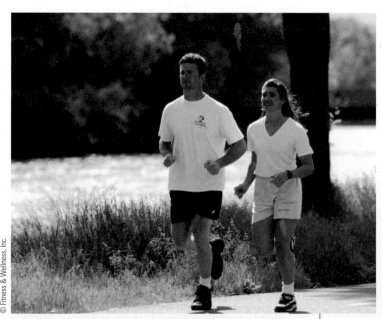

© Fitness & Wellness, Inc.

Starting an exercise program prior to giving up cigarettes encourages cessation and helps with weight control during the process.

detrimental to human health than a few extra pounds of body weight. Experts have indicated that, as far as the extra load on the heart is concerned, giving up one pack of cigarettes a day is the equivalent of losing between 50 and 75 pounds of excess body fat!

Step Three

Decide on the approach you will use to stop smoking. You may quit cold turkey or gradually cut down the number of cigarettes you smoke daily. Base your decision on your scores obtained on the "Why Do You Smoke?" test. If you scored 11 points or higher in either the "Crutch: Tension Reduction" or the "Craving: Psychological Addiction" categories, your best chance for success is quitting cold turkey. For any of the other four categories, you may choose either approach.

People still argue about which approach is more effective. Quitting cold turkey may cause fewer withdrawal symptoms than tapering off gradually. When you are cutting down slowly, the fewer the cigarettes you smoke, the more important each one becomes. Therefore, you have a greater chance for relapse and returning to the original number of cigarettes smoked. However, when the cutting-down approach is accompanied by a definite target date for quitting, the technique has been shown to be quite effective. Smokers who taper off without a target date for quitting are the most likely to relapse.

Step Four

Keep a daily log of your smoking habit for a few days. This will help you understand the situations in which you smoke. To assist you in doing this, make copies of part V, Lab 14B, or develop your own form. Keep this form with you and, every time you smoke, record the required information. Keep track of the number of cigarettes you smoke, times of day you smoke them, events associated with smoking, amount of each cigarette smoked, and a rating of how badly you needed that cigarette. Rate each cigarette from 1 to 3. A 1 means "desperately needed," a 2 means "moderately needed," and a 3 means "no real need." This daily log will assist you in three ways:

1. You will get to know your habit.
2. It will help you eliminate cigarettes you really do not crave.
3. It will help you find positive substitutes for situations that trigger your desire to smoke.

Step Five

Set the target date for quitting. If you are going to taper off gradually, read the instructions under the "Cutting Down Gradually" discussion before you proceed to Step Six. In setting the target date, a special date may add a little extra incentive. An upcoming birthday, anniversary, vacation, graduation, family reunion—all are examples of good dates to free yourself from smoking. Dates when you are going to be away from events and environments that trigger your desire to smoke may be especially helpful. Once you have set the date, do not change it. Do not let anyone or anything interfere with this date.

Let your friends and relatives know of your intentions, and ask for their support. Consider asking someone else to quit with you. That way, you can support each other in your efforts to stop. Avoid anyone who will not support you in your effort to quit. When you are attempting to quit, other people can be a prime obstacle. Many smokers are intolerable when they first stop smoking, so some friends and relatives prefer that the person continue to smoke.

Step Six

Stock up on low-calorie foods—carrots, broccoli, cauliflower, celery, popcorn (butter- and salt-free), fruits, sunflower seeds (in the shell), sugarless gum—and drink plenty of water. Keep the food handy on the day you stop and the first few days following cessation. Substitute this food for a cigarette when you want one.

Step Seven

On your quit day and the first few days thereafter, do not keep cigarettes handy. Stay away from friends and events that trigger your desire to smoke, and drink a lot of water and fruit juices. To replace the old behavior with new behavior, replace smoking time with new, positive substitutes that will make smoking difficult or impossible.

When you want a cigarette, take a few deep breaths and then occupy yourself by doing any of a number of things such as talking to someone else, washing your hands, brushing your teeth, eating a healthy snack, chewing on a straw, doing dishes, playing sports, going for a walk or a bike ride, going swimming, and so on. Engage in activities that require the use of your hands. Try gardening, sewing, writing letters, drawing, doing household chores, or washing the car. Visit nonsmoking places such as libraries, museums, stores, and theaters. Plan an outing or a trip away from home. Any of these activities can keep your mind off cigarettes. Record your choice of activity or substitute under the Remarks/Substitutes column in part V of Lab 14B.

Quitting Cold Turkey

Many people have found that quitting all at once is the easiest way to do it. Most smokers have tried this approach at least once. Even though it might not work the first time, they do not allow themselves to get discouraged, and they eventually succeed.

Many times after several attempts, all of a sudden they are able to overcome smoking without too much difficulty.

On the average, as few as three smokeless days are sufficient to break the physiological addiction to nicotine. The psychological addiction may linger for years but will get weaker as time goes by.

Cutting Down Gradually

Tapering off cigarettes can be done in several ways.

1. Eliminate cigarettes you do not strongly crave (those ranked numbers 3 and 2 on your daily log).
2. Switch to a brand lower in nicotine/tar every few days.
3. Smoke less of each cigarette.
4. Smoke fewer cigarettes each day.

Most people prefer a combination of these four suggestions.

Before you start cutting down, set a target date for quitting. Once the date is set, don't change it. The total time until your quit date should be no longer than 2 weeks. Reduce the total number of cigarettes you smoke each day by 10 to 25 percent. As you smoke less, be careful not to take more puffs or inhale more deeply as you smoke, because this would offset the principle of cutting down.

As an aid in tapering off, make several copies of part V, Lab 14B. (By now you should have already completed the first daily log of your smoking habit—see Step Four under "Breaking the Habit" on page 376.) Start a new daily log and, every night, review your data and set goals for the following day.

Decide which cigarettes will be easiest to give up, what brand you will smoke, the total number of cigarettes to be smoked, and how much of each you will smoke. Write down any comments or situations you want to avoid, as well as any substitutes you could use to help you in the program. For example, if you always smoke while drinking coffee, substitute juice for coffee. If you smoke while driving, arrange for a ride or take a bus to work. If you smoke with a certain friend at lunch, avoid having lunch with that friend for a week or so. Continue using this log until you have stopped smoking completely.

Nicotine Substitution Products

Nicotine substitution drug products such as nicotine transdermal patches and nicotine gum have been developed to help people kick the tobacco habit. These products are most effective when they are used in a physician-supervised cessation program. As with tapering off, these products gradually decrease amount of nicotine used until the person no longer craves the drug.

Nicotine patches are used to supply a steady dose of nicotine through the skin. These patches are available in various dosages, delivering anywhere from about 5 to 21 mg of nicotine in a 24-hour period. A typical program lasts between 3 and 10 weeks with an average weekly cost to the consumer of about $35. Sales of nicotine patches approximate $1 billion per year.

> *About three smokeless days are sufficient to break the physiological addiction to nicotine.*

Public safety concerns regarding the use of nicotine patches, including indications, precautions, warnings, contraindications, potential abuse, and marketing and labeling issues are monitored and regulated by the FDA. People contemplating their use should pay careful attention to contraindications and potential side effects. Pregnant and lactating women and people with heart disease, high blood pressure, or who have had a recent heart attack should check with their physician prior to using nicotine substitution products. Skin redness, swelling, or rashes are sometimes associated with the use of nicotine patches. Other undesirable side effects are listed on the label and should be monitored closely.

Life After Cigarettes

When you first quit smoking, you can expect a series of withdrawal symptoms during the first few days; among them are lower heart rate and blood pressure, headaches, gastrointestinal discomfort, mood changes, irritability, aggressiveness, and difficulty sleeping.

The physiological addiction to nicotine is broken only 3 days following your last cigarette. Thereafter, you should not crave cigarettes as much. For the habitual smoker, the psychological dependency could be the most difficult to break. The first few days probably will not be as difficult as the first few months. Any of the activities of daily life that have been associated with smoking—either stress or relaxation, joy or unhappiness—may trigger a relapse even months, or at times years, after quitting.

Ex-smokers should realize that, even though some harm may have been done already, it is never too late to quit. The greatest early benefit is a lower risk for sudden death. Furthermore, the risk for illness starts to decrease the moment you stop smoking. You will have fewer sore throats and sores in the mouth, less hoarseness, no more cigarette cough, and lower risk for peptic ulcers.

Circulation to the hands and feet will improve, as will gastrointestinal and kidney and bladder functions. Everything will taste and smell better. You will have more energy, and you will gain a sense of freedom, pride, and well-being. You no longer will have to worry whether you have enough cigarettes to last through a day, a party, a meeting, a weekend, a trip.

When you first quit and you think how tough it is and how miserable you feel because you cannot have a cigarette, try the opposite: Think of the benefits and how great it is not to smoke! The ex-smoker's risk for heart disease approaches that of a lifetime nonsmoker 10 years following cessation, and for cancer, 15 years after cessation.

If you have been successful and stopped smoking, a lot of events can still trigger your urge to smoke. When confronted with these events, some people rationalize and think, "One cigarette won't hurt. I've been off for months (years in some cases)" or, "I can handle it. I'll smoke just today." It won't work! Before you know it, you will be back to the regular nasty habit. Be prepared to take action in those situations. Find substitutes. In addition to the many things that have been discussed in this chapter, the tips given in Figure 14.5 should help you retrain yourself to live without cigarettes.

Start thinking of yourself as a nonsmoker—no "butts" about it. Remind yourself how difficult it has been and how long it has taken you to get to this point. If you have come this far, you certainly can resist brief moments of temptation. It will get easier rather than harder as time goes on.

Figure 14.5 **Tips to help stop smoking.**

The following are different ways smokers retrained themselves to live without cigarettes. Any one or several of these methods in combination might be helpful to you. Check the ones you like and, from these, develop your own retraining program.

☐ Before you quit smoking, try wrapping your cigarettes with a sheet of paper like a Christmas present. Every time you want a cigarette, unwrap the pack and write down what you are doing, how you feel, and how important this cigarette is to you. Do this for 2 weeks and you'll have cut down as well as developed new insights into your smoking.

☐ If cigarettes give you an energy boost, try gum, modest exercise, a brisk walk, or a new hobby. Avoid eating new foods that are high in calories.

☐ If cigarettes help you relax, try eating, drinking new beverages, or joining social activities within reasonable bounds.

☐ Try smoking an excess of cigarettes for a day or two before you quit so the taste of cigarettes is spoiled. Another opportune time to quit is when you are ill with a cold or flu and have lost your taste for cigarettes.

☐ On a 3" × 5" card, list what you like and dislike about smoking. Add to it and read it daily.

☐ Make up a short list of luxuries you have wanted or items you would like to purchase for a loved one. Next to each item, write down the cost. Now convert the cost to "packs of cigarettes." If you save the money each day from packs of cigarettes, you will be able to purchase these items. Use a special "piggy bank" for saving your money, or start a "Christmas Club" account at your bank.

☐ Don't smoke after you get a craving for a cigarette until 3 minutes have passed since you got the urge. During those 3 minutes, change your thinking or activity.

☐ Telephone an ex-smoker or somebody you can talk to until the craving subsides.

☐ Plan a memorable day for stopping. You might choose your vacation, New Year's Day, your birthday, a holiday, the birthday of your child, your anniversary. But don't make the date so distant that you lose momentum.

☐ If you smoke under stress at work, pick a date for stopping when you will be away from your work.

☐ Decide whether you are going to stop suddenly or gradually. If it is to be gradual, work out a tapering system so you have intermediate goals.

☐ Don't store cigarettes. Never buy a carton. Wait until one pack is finished before you buy another.

☐ Never carry cigarettes with you at home or at work. Keep your cigarettes as far from you as possible. Leave them with someone or lock them up.

☐ Until you quit, make yourself a "smoking corner" that is far from anything interesting. If you like to smoke with others, always smoke alone. If you like to smoke alone, always smoke with others, preferably if they are nonsmokers. Never smoke while watching television.

☐ Never carry matches or a lighter with you.

☐ Put away your ashtrays or fill them with objects so they cannot be used for ashes. Plant flowers in them or fill them with walnuts. The latter will give you something to do with your hands.

☐ Change your brand of cigarettes weekly so you always are smoking a brand of lower tar and nicotine content than the week before.

☐ Never say, "I quit smoking," because your resolution is broken if you have a cigarette. Better to say, "I don't want to smoke." This way you maintain your resolution even if you accidentally have a cigarette.

☐ Try to help someone else quit smoking, particularly your mate.

☐ Always ask yourself, "Do I need this cigarette or is this just a reflex?"

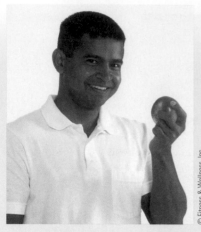

The simple pleasures of life, such as taste and smell, improve with smoking cessation.

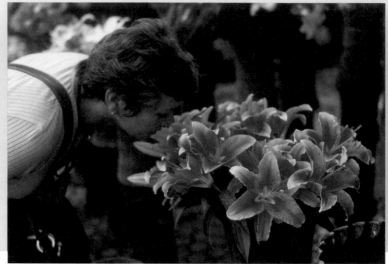

☐ Each day try to put off lighting your first cigarette.

☐ Decide arbitrarily that you will smoke only on even- or odd-numbered hours of the clock.

☐ Try going to bed early and rising a half hour earlier than usual to avoid hurrying through breakfast and rushing to work.

☐ Keep your hands occupied. Try playing a musical instrument, knitting, or fiddling with hand puzzles.

☐ Take a shower. You cannot smoke in the shower.

☐ Brush your teeth frequently to get rid of the tobacco taste and stains.

☐ If you have a sudden craving for a cigarette, take 10 deep breaths, holding the last breath while you strike a match. Exhale slowly, blowing out the match. Pretend the match was a cigarette by crushing it out in an ashtray. Now immediately get busy on some work or activity.

☐ Smoke only half a cigarette.

☐ After you quit, start using your lungs. Increase your activities and indulge in moderate exercise, such as short walks before or after a meal.

☐ Bet with someone that you can quit. Put the cigarette money in a jar each morning and forfeit it if you smoke. Keep the money if you don't smoke by the end of the week. Try to extend this period for a month.

☐ If you gain weight because you are not smoking, wait until you get over the craving before you diet. Dieting is easier then.

☐ If you are depressed or have physical symptoms that might be related to your smoking, relieve your mind by discussing this with your physician. It is easier to quit when you know your health status.

☐ After you quit, visit your dentist and have your teeth cleaned to get rid of the tobacco stains.

☐ If the cost of cigarettes is your motivation for quitting, purchase a money order equivalent to a year's supply of cigarettes. Give it to a friend. If you smoke in the next year, he or she cashes the money order and keeps the money. If you don't smoke, he or she gives back the money order at the end of the year.

☐ After you quit, redirect the temptation to smoke by calling or visiting someone.

☐ When you feel irritable or tense, shut your eyes and count backward from ten to zero as you imagine yourself descending a flight of stairs, or imagine that you are looking at the horizon as the sun sets in the west.

☐ Get out of your old habits. Seek new activities or perform old activities in a new way. Don't rely on the old ways of solving problems. Do things differently.

☐ If you are a "kitchen smoker" in the morning, volunteer your services to a school or nonprofit organization to get you out of the house.

☐ Stock up on light reading materials, crossword puzzles, and vacation brochures that you can read during your coffee breaks.

☐ Frequent places where you can't smoke, such as libraries, buses, theaters, swimming pools, department stores.

☐ Give yourself time to think and get fit by walking one-half hour each day. If you have a dog, take it for a walk with you.

Excerpted from *TIPS*, American Cancer Society, Texas Division. Used by permission.

Web Interactive

- Web of Addictions. This site features comprehensive and factual information on a variety of addictions, including alcohol and other drug abuse.

  http://www.well.com/user/woa

- CDC Page on Smoking and Health: Tobacco Information and Prevention Source. A comprehensive site featuring educational information, research, report from the U.S. Surgeon General, tips on how to quit, and much more.

  http://www.cdc.gov/tobacco

- Drugs of Abuse Table arranged by drug classification. Information from the National Clearinghouse for Alcohol and Drug Information features factual information regarding descriptions, effects, symptoms of overdose, withdrawal, symptoms and indications of misuse.

  http://www.health.org/pubs/catalog/RP0s.htm

- Binge Drinking Assessment. This tool sponsored by the Higher Education Center for Alcohol and Other Drug Prevention of the U.S. Department of Education provides rates of binge drinking at colleges and universities in the U.S. based on a school's demographics. Data come from the Harvard College Alcohol Study conducted in 1993 by Henry Wechsler, Ph.D., Harvard School of Public Health.

  http://www.edc.org/hec/other/binge-app1.htm

Interactive Sites:

- Why Do I Smoke? Quiz. An Interactive Self-assessment from the American Family Physician journal.

  http://familydoctor.org/handouts/296.html

- Alcohol: An Interactive Assessment for you and someone else. Sponsored by the Mayo Clinic.

  http://mayohealth.org/mayo/9707/htm/alcohol.htm

- Facts On Tap: Alcohol and Your College Experience: This excellent site is geared to college students, featuring links to the following topics, and more:

  Risky Relationship: Alcohol and Sex
  College Experience: Alcohol and Student Life
  The Naked Truth: Alcohol and Your Body
  When Someone Else's Drinking Gives You a Hangover

  http://www.factsontap.org

Notes

1. R. Goldberg, *Drugs Across the Spectrum* (Belmont, CA: Wadsworth/Thomson Learning, 2000).

2. See note 1.

3. *National Drug Control Strategy* (Washington, DC: U.S. Government Printing Office, 1998).

4. Join Together, *Results of the Fourth National Survey on Community Efforts to Reduce Substance Abuse and Gun Violence* (Boston: Join Together, 1999).

5. American Cancer Society, *Cancer Facts & Figures—2000* (New York: ACS, 2000).

6. S. A. Glantz and W. W. Parmley, "Passive Smoking and Heart Disease," *Journal of the American Medical Association* 273 (1995): 1047–1053.

7. See note 5.

8. See note 5.

9. "Wellness Facts," *University of California Berkeley Wellness Letter* 14 (1998): 1.

10. American Cancer Society, World Smoking & Health (Atlanta: ACS, 1993).

11. American Heart Association, AHA Public Affairs/Coalition on Smoking: Health Position (Dallas: AHA, 1996).

12. U.S. Department of Health and Human Services, *Nicotine Addiction, A Report of the Surgeon General* (Atlanta: U.S. Department of Health and Human Services, Centers for Disease Control and Prevention, National Center for Chronic Disease Prevention and Health Promotion, 1988).

Suggested Readings

American Cancer Society. *Fifty Most Often Asked Questions About Smoking and Health and the Answers*. New York: ACS, 1982.

American Cancer Society. *1998 Cancer Facts & Figures*. New York: ACS, 1998.

American Heart Association. *The Good Life: A Guide to Becoming a Nonsmoker*. Dallas: AHA, 1984.

American Heart Association. *How to Quit*. Dallas: AHA, 1984.

Goldberg, R. *Drugs Across the Spectrum*. Belmont, CA: Wadsworth/Thomson Learning, 2000.

Hodgson, R. J., and P. Miller. *Self-Watching: Addictions, Habits, Compulsions—What to Do*. New York: Facts on File, 1982.

U.S. Public Health Service. *Smoking Tobacco and Health: A Fact Book*. Rockville, MD: U.S. Department of Health and Human Services, 1981.

U.S. Public Health Service. *Why People Smoke Cigarettes*. Rockville, MD: U.S. Department of Health and Human Services, 1982.

U.S. Public Health Service. *A Self-Test for Smokers*. Rockville, MD: U.S. Department of Health and Human Services, 1983.

U.S. Public Health Service. *Chronic Obstructive Lung Disease: A Report of the Surgeon General*. Rockville, MD: U.S. Department of Health and Human Services, 1984.

U.S. Office on Smoking and Health. *Smoking and Health: A Report of the Surgeon General*. Washington, DC: U.S. Department of Health, Education and Welfare, 1979.

ADDICTIVE BEHAVIOR QUESTIONNAIRES

Name:	Date:	Grade:
Instructor:	Course:	Section:

Necessary Lab Equipment
None required.

Objective
To determine possible addictive behavior.

Instruction
The following questionnaires are for your own personal information. Answer all questions on a separate sheet of paper and keep that sheet for yourself. Turn in only this page to your instructor as proof that you have read and completed the questionnaire. If you wish to do so, you may personally discuss the results of these questionnaires with your course instructor.

Stage of Change for Addictive Behavior

If chemical dependency is a problem in your life, use Figure 2.3 (page 40) and Table 2.3 (page 41) and identify your current stage of change for participation in a treatment program for addictive behavior.

I. Addictive Behavior: Could You Be An Addict?

The following test, designed by Dr. Lawrence J. Hatterer, is not a way to diagnose whether you are in the early, middle, or chronic stage of addictive disease. It is merely meant to help you understand addictive behavior better so you can recognize it in yourself or perhaps in people you know.

1. I am a person of excesses. I can't regulate what I do for pleasure and often use a substance or indulge in an activity heavily, in order to get high.

2. I am an extremely self-involved person. People tell me that I am into myself too much.

3. I am compulsive. I must have what I want when I want it, regardless of the consequences.

4. I am excessively dependent on or independent of others.

5. I am preoccupied. I spend a lot of time thinking or fantasizing about a particular activity or substance. Also, I will work my day around doing it or go to pains to make sure it's available.

6. I deny that I do this and lie about it when others ask me.

7. I have been involved in this behavior for at least one year.

8. I've told myself I could easily stop, even though I've shown no signs of slowing down.

9. Once I start indulging in this behavior or substance, I find I have trouble stopping.

10. One or more members of my family are also involved in some kind of excessive behavior or substance abuse.

11. I find I gravitate mostly toward people who have the same behavior or take the same substance as I.

12. I seem to be developing a tolerance of the behavior or substance. I have had a need to steadily increase the amounts I take or the time I spend doing it.

13. I have found that my excessive use of highs has, in fact, only made my problems worse.

14. If someone tries to keep me from obtaining the substance or practicing the activity, I get angry and reject or abuse them.

15. I experience withdrawal symptoms if I cannot indulge in the substance or activity.

16. This has gotten in the way of my functioning. I have missed something important—days at work or time with my friends, family, children—because of it.

17. The substance/activity is destroying my home life. I know I am hurting those closest to me.

18. I have failed in many goals in life, lost money, given up many social and occupational contacts, all because of my excessive behavior.

19. I have tried to stop or cut down on my excesses but have been unsuccessful.

20. I have physically endangered myself or others in accidents that were a direct result of my excessive behavior.

How To Score

If you answer "yes" to half or more of the questions, you may have a problem with addictive disease and should seek immediate professional help. For a referral, contact your local mental health clinic (look in the Yellow Pages) or speak to your doctor.

Reprinted with permission from *McCall's Magazine*, November 1986.

II. Alcohol Abuse: Are You Drinking Too Much?

Using a separate sheet of paper, specifically indicate the steps that you are going to take to correct addictive behavior(s) and identify people or organizations that you will contact to help you get started.

1. When you are holding an empty glass at a party, do you always actively look for a refill instead of waiting to be offered one?

2. If given the chance, do you frequently pour out a more generous drink for yourself than seems to be the "going" amount for others?

3. Do you often have a drink or two when you are alone, either at home or in a bar?

4. Is your drinking ever the direct cause of a family quarrel, or do quarrels often seem to occur, if only by coincidence, after you have had a drink or two?

5. Do you feel that you must have a drink at a specific time every day—right after work, for instance?

6. When worried or under unusual stress, do you almost automatically take a stiff drink to "settle your nerves"?

7. Are you untruthful about how much you have had to drink when questioned on the subject?

8. Does drinking ever cause you to take time off work or to miss scheduled meetings or appointments?

9. Do you feel physically deprived if you cannot have at least one drink every day?

10. Do you sometimes crave a drink in the morning?

11. Do you sometimes have "mornings after" when you cannot remember what happened the night before?

How to Score

You should regard a "yes" answer to any one of the above questions as a warning sign. Do not increase your consumption of alcohol. Two "yes" answers suggest that you already may be becoming dependent on alcohol. Three or more "yes" answers indicate that you may have a serious problem and you should get professional help. Also refer to Chapter 14 (page 367) for general guidelines to cut down your drinking.

Reproduced with permission from *Family Medical Guide* by The American Medical Association (New York: Random House, 1982).

III. Changing Addictive Behavior

Using a separate sheet of paper, specifically indicate the steps that you are going to take to correct addictive behavior(s) and identify people or organizations that you will contact to help you get started.

Lab 14B

SMOKING CESSATION QUESTIONNAIRES

Name:		Date:		Grade:	
Instructor:		Course:		Section:	

Necessary Lab Equipment
None required.

Objective
To develop a smoking cessation program either for yourself or for friends and relatives.

I. Introduction

The forms provided in this lab have been designed to help smokers identify reasons why they smoke and their readiness to initiate a smoking cessation program. These forms should be filled out prior to initiating a smoking cessation program. Interpretation of the results are given in this chapter (pages 374–375). The daily cigarette smoking log, Part V of this lab, has been developed to help smokers get to know their habit, cut down on cigarettes not really needed, and find positive substitutes when confronted with situations that trigger their desire to smoke.

II. "Why Do You Smoke?" Test

		Always	Fre-quently	Occa-sionally	Seldom	Never
A.	I smoke cigarettes to keep myself from slowing down.	5	4	3	2	1
B	Handling a cigarette is part of the enjoyment of smoking it.	5	4	3	2	1
C.	Smoking cigarettes is pleasant and relaxing.	5	4	3	2	1
D.	I light up a cigarette when I feel angry about something.	5	4	3	2	1
E.	When I have run out of cigarettes, I find it almost unbearable until I can get them.	5	4	3	2	1
F.	I smoke cigarettes automatically without even being aware of it.	5	4	3	2	1
G.	I smoke cigarettes for stimulation, to perk myself up.	5	4	3	2	1
H.	Part of the enjoyment of smoking a cigarette comes from the steps I take to light up.	5	4	3	2	1
I.	I find cigarettes pleasurable.	5	4	3	2	1
J.	When I feel uncomfortable or upset about something, I light up a cigarette.	5	4	3	2	1
K.	I am very much aware of the fact when I am not smoking a cigarette.	5	4	3	2	1
L.	I light up a cigarette without realizing I still have one burning in the ashtray.	5	4	3	2	1
M.	I smoke cigarettes to give me a "lift."	5	4	3	2	1
N.	When I smoke a cigarette, part of the enjoyment is watching the smoke as I exhale it.	5	4	3	2	1
O.	I want a cigarette most when I am comfortable and relaxed.	5	4	3	2	1
P.	When I feel "blue" or want to take my mind off cares and worries, I smoke cigarettes.	5	4	3	2	1
Q.	I get a real gnawing hunger for a cigarette when I haven't smoked for a while.	5	4	3	2	1
R.	I've found a cigarette in my mouth and didn't remember putting it there.	5	4	3	2	1

How to Score: (See pages 374–375 to interpret your test results.)

Enter the numbers you have circled on the test questions in the spaces provided below, putting the number you have circled to question A on line A, to question B on line B, and so on. Add the three scores on each line to get a total for each factor. For example, the sum of your scores over lines A, G, and M gives you your score on "Stimulation"; lines B, H, and N give the score on "Handling." Scores can vary from 3 to 15. Any score 11 and above is high; any score 7 and below is low.

A		+ G		+ M		=		Stimulation
B		+ H		+ N		=		Handling
C		+ I		+ O		=		Pleasure Relaxation
D		+ J		+ P		=		Crutch: Tension Reduction
E		+ K		+ Q		=		Craving: Psychological Addiction
F		+ L		+ R		=		Habit

From *A Self-Test for Smokers*, U.S. Department of Health and Human Services, 1983.

III. "Do You Want to Quit" Test

	Strongly Agree	Mildly Agree	Mildly Disagree	Strongly Disagree
A. Cigarette smoking might give me a serious illness.	4	3	2	1
B. My cigarette smoking sets a bad example for others.	4	3	2	1
C. I find cigarette smoking to be a messy kind of habit.	4	3	2	1
D. Controlling my cigarette smoking is a challenge to me.	4	3	2	1
E. Smoking causes shortness of breath.	4	3	2	1
F. If I quit smoking cigarettes, it might influence others to stop.	4	3	2	1
G. Cigarettes cause damage to clothing and other personal property.	4	3	2	1
H. Quitting smoking would show that I have willpower.	4	3	2	1
I. My cigarette smoking will have a harmful effect on my health.	4	3	2	1
J. My cigarette smoking influences others close to me to take up or continue smoking.	4	3	2	1
K. If I quit smoking, my sense of taste or smell will improve.	4	3	2	1
L. I do not like the idea of feeling dependent on smoking.	4	3	2	1

How to Score (See pages 375–375) to interpret your test results.)

Write the number you have circled after each statement on the test in the corresponding space to the right. Add the scores on each line to get your totals. For example, the sum of your scores A, E, and I gives you your score for the Health factor. Scores can vary from 3 to 12. Any score of 9 or over is high; any score 6 or under is low.

A	+ E	+ I	=	Health
B	+ F	+ J	=	Example
C	+ G	+ K	=	Aesthetics
D	+ H	+ L	=	Mastery

From *A Self-Test for Smokers*, U.S. Department of Health and Human Services, 1983.

IV. Reasons to Smoke, Reasons to Quit

Reasons to Smoke Cigarettes

1. _____
2. _____
3. _____
4. _____
5. _____

Reasons to Quit Cigarette Smoking

1. _____
2. _____
3. _____
4. _____
5. _____

V. Daily Cigarette Smoking Log

Today's Date: _____ Quit Date: _____ Decision Date: _____

Cigarettes to be smoked today: _____ Brand: _____

No.	Time	Activity	Rating[a]	Amount Smoked[b]	Remarks/Substitutes
1.					
2.					
3.					
4.					
5.					
6.					
7.					
8.					
9.					
10.					
11.					
12.					
13.					
14.					
15.					
16.					
17.					
18.					
19.					
20.					

[a]Rating: 1 = desperately needed, 2 = moderately needed, 3 = no real need
[b]Amount Smoked: entire cigarette, two-thirds, half, etc.

Additional comments, list of friends and/or activities to avoid

_____
_____
_____
_____
_____
_____

VI. Conclusion

In a few sentences, indicate your feelings about cigarette smoking and what you have learned from the previous questionnaires.

Preventing Sexually Transmitted Diseases

Objectives

- Address the detrimental effects of addictive substances, including marijuana, cocaine, and alcohol.

- Describe the most common sexually transmitted diseases.

- Outline the health consequences of sexually transmitted diseases.

- Define the difference between HIV and AIDS.

- Be aware of ways to prevent sexually transmitted diseases.

Sexually transmitted diseases (STDs) have reached epidemic proportions in the United States. Of the more than 25 known STDs, some are still incurable. The American Social Health Association stated that 25 percent of all Americans will acquire at least one STD in their lifetime. Each year, more than 15 million people in the United States are newly infected with STDs, and more than 68 million Americans have an incurable STD.[1] Based on estimates by the World Health Organization, world wide, 1 million people are infected daily with STDs not including HIV. These infections include more than 4 million cases of chlamydia, 800,000 cases of gonorrhea, between one-half and 1 million cases of genital warts, half a million cases of herpes, and nearly 15,000 cases of syphilis. Attracting most of the attention because of its life-threatening potential is HIV infection, which leads to AIDS.

Chlamydia

Chlamydia is a bacterial infection that spreads during vaginal, anal, or oral sex, or from the vagina to a newborn baby during childbirth. Chlamydia can damage the reproductive system seriously. This disease is considered to be a major factor in male and female infertility. Because it may have no symptoms, 3 of 4 people don't have any symptoms until the infection has become quite serious. Each year, 3 million new cases of chlamydia are reported in the United States.[2] Furthermore, according to the U.S. Centers for Disease Control and Prevention (CDC), 15- to 19-year-old girls represent 46 percent of infections and 20- to 24-year-old women represent another 33 percent.[3]

When symptoms are present, they tend to mimic other STDs, so the disease can be mistreated. Symptoms of serious infection include abdominal pain, fever, nausea, vaginal bleeding, and arthritis. Chlamydia can be treated successfully with oral antibiotics, but its damage to the reproductive system is irreversible.

Gonorrhea

One of the oldest STDs, **gonorrhea** is also caused by a bacterial infection. Gonorrhea is transmitted through vaginal, anal, and oral sex.

Typical symptoms in men include a pus-like secretion from the penis and painful urination. Most infected women don't have any symptoms until the infection has become fairly serious. At this stage, women develop fever, severe abdominal pain, and pelvic inflammatory disease (see below).

If untreated, gonorrhea can produce infertility, widespread bacterial infection, heart damage, and arthritis in men and women and blindness in children born to infected women. Gonorrhea is

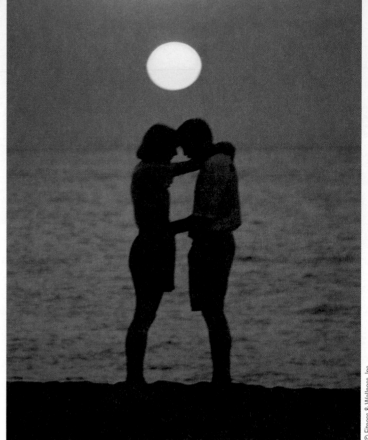

More than 25 diseases are spread through sexual contact. About 1 in 4 adults in the United States has a sexually transmitted disease.

treated successfully with penicillin and other antibiotics.

Pelvic Inflammatory Disease

Each year more than 1 million women in the United States develop a condition known under the umbrella term **pelvic inflammatory disease (PID)**.[4] It usually results from chlamydia or gonorrhea infection.

Typical symptoms of PID are fever, nausea, vomiting, chills, spotting between menstrual periods, heavy bleeding during periods, and pain in the lower abdomen during sexual intercourse, between menstrual periods, or urination. However, many women do not know they have PID because these symptoms are not always present.

PID often develops when the STD spreads to the fallopian tubes, uterus, and ovaries. If the woman becomes pregnant, she could have an ectopic (or tubal) pregnancy, which destroys the embryo and can kill the woman.

PID is treated with antibiotics, bed rest, and sexual abstinence. Further, surgery may be required to remove infected or scarred tissue or to repair or remove the fallopian tubes or uterus.

Genital Warts

Genital warts are caused by viral infection. They show up anywhere from 1 to 8 months after exposure. These warts may be flat or raised and usually are found on the penis or around the vulva and the vagina. They also can appear in the mouth, throat, rectum, on the cervix, or around the anus.

Based on data from the CDC, as many as one million new cases of this STD are diagnosed in the United States each year. In some cities, nearly half of all sexually active teenagers have genital warts. Similar to chlamydia, the virus is spread through vaginal, anal, or oral sex, or from the vagina to a newborn baby.

Health problems associated with genital warts include increased risk for cancers of the cervix, vulva, and penis, and enlargement and spread of the warts, leading to obstruction of the urethra, vagina, and anus. Babies born to infected mothers commonly develop warts over their bodies; therefore, Cesarean sections are recommended.

Treatment requires completely removing all warts. This can be done by freezing them with liquid nitrogen, dissolving them with chemicals, or removing them through electrosurgery or laser surgery. Infected patients may have to be treated more than once, because genital warts can recur.

Genital Herpes

Genital herpes, one of the most common STDs, is caused by the herpes simplex virus (HSV). The several types of HSV produce different ailments, including genital herpes, oral (lip) herpes, shingles, and chicken pox. The two most common forms of HSV are Types I and II. Type I is the HSV most often known to cause oral herpes—cold sores or fever blisters that appear on the lips and mouth. HSV Type II is better known as the virus that causes genital herpes.

HSV is a highly contagious virus. Victims are most contagious during an outbreak, and HSV spreads by contact with an active sore. The disease can also be spread through virus-containing secretions from the vagina or penis. A few days following infection, sores appear on the infected areas, most notably the mouth, genitals, and rectum, but may also surface on other parts of the body. In conjunction with the sores, victims usually have mild fever, swollen glands, and headaches. The symptoms usually disappear within a few weeks, causing some people to believe they are cured. Herpes is presently incurable, though, and its victims do remain infected. The virus can remain dormant for extended periods of time, but repeated outbreaks are common. Excessive stress and illness can precipitate new outbreaks.

Both HSV Type I and II can cause oral and genital sores. People who have an outbreak of oral herpes should not touch their genitals or someone else's after touching the oral cold sores; doing so can lead to herpes infection of the genitals. Oral sex can also cause transmission of the HSV from the lips to the genitals and vice versa. People with cold sores on the lips or mouth should exercise care not to touch these sores. Hands should be carefully washed with soap following contact with cold or herpes sores.

Syphilis

Another common type of STD, also caused by bacterial infection, is **syphilis**. Approximately 3 weeks after infection, a painless sore appears where the bacteria entered the body. This sore disappears on its own in a few weeks. If untreated, more sores may appear within 6 months of the initial outbreak but again will disappear by themselves.

A latent stage, during which the victim is not contagious, may last up to 30 years, lulling victims into thinking they are healed. During the last stage of the disease, some people develop paralysis, crippling, blindness, heart disease, brain damage and insanity, and they even can die as a direct result of the disease. One of the oldest known STDs, syphilis once killed its victims. Penicillin and other antibiotics now are used to treat it.

HIV and AIDS

AIDS is the most frightening of all STDs because it is fatal and has no known cure. AIDS—which stands for **acquired immunodeficiency syndrome (AIDS)**

Sexually transmitted diseases (STDs)   Communicable diseases spread through sexual contact.

Chlamydia   A sexually transmitted disease, caused by a bacterial infection, that can cause significant damage to the reproductive system.

Gonorrhea   Sexually transmitted disease caused by a bacterial infection.

Pelvic inflammatory disease (PID)   An overall designation referring to the effects of other STDs, primarily chlamydia and gonorrhea.

Genital warts   A sexually transmitted disease caused by a viral infection.

Genital herpes   A sexually transmitted disease caused by a viral infection of the herpes simplex virus Types I and II. The virus can attack different areas of the body, but commonly causes blisters on the genitals.

Syphilis   A sexually transmitted disease caused by a bacterial infection.

Acquired immunodeficiency syndrome (AIDS)   Any of a number of diseases that arise when the body's immune system is compromised by HIV.

—is the end stage of infection by the **human immunodeficiency virus (HIV)**. In Lab 15A you will have the opportunity to evaluate your basic understanding of HIV and AIDS.

HIV is a chronic infectious disease that spreads among individuals who engage in risky behavior such as having unprotected sex or sharing hypodermic needles. When a person becomes infected with HIV, the virus multiplies and attacks and destroys white blood cells. These cells are part of the immune system, and their function is to fight off infections and diseases in the body.

As the number of white blood cells killed increases, the body's immune system gradually breaks down or may be destroyed completely. Without the immune system, a person becomes susceptible to various **opportunistic diseases** and to cancers.

HIV is a progressive disease. At first, people who become infected with HIV might not know they are infected. An incubation period of weeks, months, or years may pass during which no symptoms appear. The virus may live in the body 10 years or longer before symptoms emerge.

As the infection progresses to the point at which certain diseases develop, the person is said to have AIDS. HIV itself doesn't kill. Nor do people die of AIDS. "AIDS" is the term designating the final stage of HIV infection. Death is caused by a weakened immune system that is unable to fight off these opportunistic diseases.

Earliest symptoms of AIDS include unexplained weight loss, constant fatigue, mild fever, swollen lymph glands, diarrhea, and sore throat. Advanced symptoms include loss of appetite, skin diseases, night sweats, and deterioration of mucous membranes.

Most of the illnesses that AIDS patients develop are harmless and rare in the general population but are fatal to AIDS victims. The two most common fatal conditions in AIDS patients are pneumocystis carinii pneumonia (a parasitic infection of the lungs) and Kaposi's sarcoma (a type of skin cancer). The AIDS virus also may attack the nervous system, causing damage to the brain and spinal cord.

On the average, the individual develops the symptoms that fit the case definition of AIDS about 9 to 10 years following infection. From that point on, the person might live another 3 years or so. In essence, from the point of infection, the individual might endure a chronic disease for about 12 years.

The only means to determine whether someone has HIV is through an HIV antibody test. Being HIV-positive does not necessarily mean the person has AIDS. Several years can go by before the person develops the diseases that fit the case definition of AIDS.

Upon HIV infection, the immune system forms antibodies that bind to the virus. HIV antibodies can be detected in the blood as early as 25 days following infection. According to the CDC, all except 5 percent of infected individuals will show these antibodies within 12 to 14 weeks of infection. In some cases, they are not detectable until after 6 months or longer.

If HIV infection is suspected, a person should wait 6 months to be tested, when the test is believed to be almost 100 percent accurate. During this time, and from then on, individuals should refrain from further endangering themselves and others through risky behaviors. Some people are tested to reassure themselves that their risky behaviors are acceptable. Even if the test turns up negative for HIV, this does not represent a "license" to continue risky behaviors.

No one has to become infected with HIV. At present, once infected, a person cannot become uninfected. There is no second chance. Everyone must protect himself or herself against this chronic disease. People who are so ignorant as to believe that it can never happen to them are putting themselves and their partners at risk.

New therapies are preventing AIDS from developing in a growing number of HIV-infected persons. Professionals, however, disagree as to how many HIV carriers actually will develop AIDS. Even if individuals have not developed AIDS, they can pass on the virus to others, who easily could then develop AIDS.

Transmission of HIV

HIV is transmitted by the exchange of cellular body fluids including blood, semen, vaginal secretions, and maternal milk. These fluids can be exchanged during sexual intercourse, by using hypodermic needles that infected individuals have used previously, between a pregnant woman and her developing fetus, by infection of babies from the mother during childbirth, less frequently during breast feeding, and, rarely, from a blood transfusion or organ transplant. The primary modes of HIV transmission in reported U.S. AIDS cases are presented in Table 15.1.

Today, the risk of being infected with HIV from a blood transfusion is slight. Prior to 1985, several cases of HIV infection came from blood transfusions because the blood was donated by HIV-infected individuals. Now, all individuals who donate blood are first tested for HIV. To be absolutely safe, people who are planning to have surgery might consider storing their own blood in advance so safe blood will be available if a transfusion becomes necessary.

A myth regarding HIV is that it can be transmitted by donating blood. People cannot get HIV

Table 15.1	Primary Modes of HIV Transmission in Adults Based on Reported U.S. and Estimated Worldwide AIDS Cases		
	U.S. Men	U.S. Women	Worldwide
Same-gender sexual contact	45%		10%
Heterosexual contact	7	38%	75
Sharing hypodermic needles	21	29	10
Unidentified cause	20	32	
Blood transfusion		1	5

Sources: "The HIV/AIDS Epidemic in the U.S." Kaiser Family Foundation, June 1999. UNAIDS: Joint United Nations Programme on HIV/AIDS, United Nations, 2000.

from giving blood. Health professionals use a brand-new needle every time they withdraw blood from a person. They use these needles only once and destroy them immediately after each person has donated blood.

People do not get HIV because of who they are but, rather, because of what they do. HIV and AIDS can threaten anyone, anywhere: men, women, children, teenagers, young people, older adults, whites, African Americans, Hispanic Americans, Asian Americans, Native Americans, Africans, Europeans, homosexuals, heterosexuals, bisexuals, druggies. Nobody is immune to HIV.

HIV can be transmitted between males, between females, from male to female, or from female to male. Although HIV and AIDS are preventable, almost all of the people who get HIV do so because they engage in risky behaviors.

Risky Behaviors

You cannot tell if people are infected with HIV or have AIDS by simply looking at them or taking their word. Not you, not a nurse, not even a doctor can tell without an HIV antibody test. Therefore, every time you engage in risky behavior, you run the risk of contracting HIV. The two most basic risky behaviors are the following:

1. Having unprotected vaginal, anal, or oral sex with an HIV-infected person. Unprotected sex means having sex without using a condom properly. A person should select only latex (rubber or prophylactic) condoms that state "disease prevention" on the package. Although you might have unprotected sex with an infected person and not get the virus, you also can get it by having unprotected sex only once with an infected individual.

Rubbing during sexual intercourse often damages mucous membranes and causes unseen bleeding (even in the mouth). During vaginal, anal, or oral sexual contact, infected blood, semen, or vaginal fluids can penetrate the mucous membranes that line the vagina, the penis, the rectum, the mouth, or the throat. From the membrane, HIV then travels into the previously uninfected person's blood.

Health experts believe that unprotected anal sex is the riskiest type of sex. Even though bleeding is not visible in most cases, anal sex almost always causes tiny tears and bleeding in the rectum. This happens because the rectum does not stretch easily, the mucous membrane is quite thin, and small blood vessels lie directly beneath the membrane. Condoms also are more likely to break during anal intercourse because of the greater friction produced in a smaller cavity. All of these factors greatly enhance the risk of transmitting HIV.

Although latex condoms, if used correctly, provide for "safer" sex, they are not 100 percent foolproof. Abstaining from sex is the only 100 percent sure way to protect yourself from HIV infection and other STDs.

2. Sharing hypodermic needles or other drug paraphernalia with someone who is infected. Following an injection, a small amount of blood remains in the needle, and sometimes in the syringe itself. If the person who used the syringe is infected with HIV and someone else uses that same syringe to shoot up, regardless of the drug used (legal or illegal), that small amount of blood is sufficient to spread the virus. All used syringes should be destroyed and disposed of immediately.

People do not get HIV because of who they are, but, rather, because of what they do.

In addition, a person must be cautious when getting acupuncture, getting a tattoo, or having the ears or other body parts pierced. If the needle used was used previously on

Human immunodeficiency virus (HIV) Virus that leads to acquired immunodeficiency syndrome (AIDS).

Opportunistic diseases Diseases that arise in the absence of a healthy immune system, which would fight them off in healthy people.

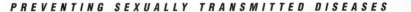

someone who is HIV-infected and the needle was not disinfected properly, the person risks getting HIV.

Otherwise prudent people often act irrationally and engage in risky behaviors when they are under the influence of drugs. Getting high can make you willing to have sex when you really didn't plan to—thereby running the risk of contracting HIV.

Small concentrations of the virus have been found in saliva and teardrops. In principle, if both people have open cuts in the lips, mouth, or gums, HIV could be transmitted through open-mouthed kissing, but these cases are rare.

The virus cannot be transmitted through perspiration. Sporting activities with no physical contact pose no risk to uninfected individuals unless they both have open wounds through which blood from an infected person can come in direct contact with the open wound of the uninfected person. The skin is an excellent line of defense against HIV. Blood from an infected person cannot penetrate the skin except through an opening in the skin. As an extra precaution, a person should use vinyl or latex gloves when performing work that requires direct contact with someone else's blood or open wound.

Some people fear getting HIV from health-care professionals. The chances of getting infected during physical or medical procedures are practically nil. Health-care workers take extra care to protect themselves and their patients from HIV.

With the advent of the Internet, people now search for sex partners online. Use of the Internet to find sexual partners may further increase the risk of contracting an STD. A recent study showed that those who seek sex partners over the Internet are at a greater risk of contracting an STD. Such people are also are more likely to have characteristics that increase the chance of transmitting STDs.[5]

HIV is not transmitted through casual contact. HIV cannot be caught by spending time with, shaking hands with, or hugging an infected person; from a toilet seat, dishes, or silverware used by an HIV patient; or by sharing a drink, food, a towel, or clothes with a person who has HIV.

What about dating? Dating and getting to know other people are normal aspects of life. Dating, however, does not mean the same thing as having sex. Sexual intercourse as a part of dating can be risky, and one of the risks is AIDS. You can't tell if someone you are dating or would like to date has been exposed to HIV. The good news is that as long as you avoid sexual activity and don't share drug needles, it doesn't matter whom you date.

Another myth regarding HIV transmission is that you can get it from insects or animals. The H in HIV stands for "human." You cannot catch HIV

VANESSA WAS IN A FATAL CAR ACCIDENT LAST NIGHT. ONLY SHE DOESN'T KNOW IT YET.

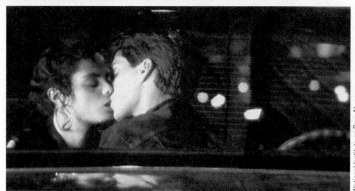

Drugs and alcohol use can make people more willing to have unplanned and unprotected sex, thereby risking HIV infection.

from insects or animals. Animals do not get infected with HIV.

HIV and AIDS Statistics

Based on estimates by the National Institute on Drug Abuse, around the world more than 34.3 million people are infected with HIV, and about 18.8 million have died from AIDS since the epidemic began. Estimates by the CDC indicate that between 300,000 and 900,000 people in the United States are infected with HIV. One in every 300 Americans is presently infected, and about 23 percent of the newly reported cases are women. Through the end of 1998, a cumulative total of 688,200 AIDS cases had been diagnosed in the United States (see Figure 15.1), and 410,800 people had died from the diseases caused by HIV. Most of the people who die (71.6 percent) are in the 25- to 44-year-old age group.

Although initially more than half of all AIDS cases in the United States occurred in homosexual or bisexual men, HIV infection is now is spreading at a faster rate in heterosexuals. Many heterosexuals practice unprotected sex because they don't believe it can happen to their segment of the population. HIV is an epidemic that does not discriminate by sexual orientation. Worldwide, up to 80 percent of the AIDS cases have been reported in heterosexuals.[6]

AIDS experts are turning their attention to the population of sub-Saharan Africa, where 70 percent of the world's HIV victims live. Within 10 years, life expectancy is predicted to hit its lowest point in a century in this part of the world, and the number of AIDS orphans will accelerate dramatically. The AIDS epidemic could also ruin the economies of these already impoverished countries. The medications

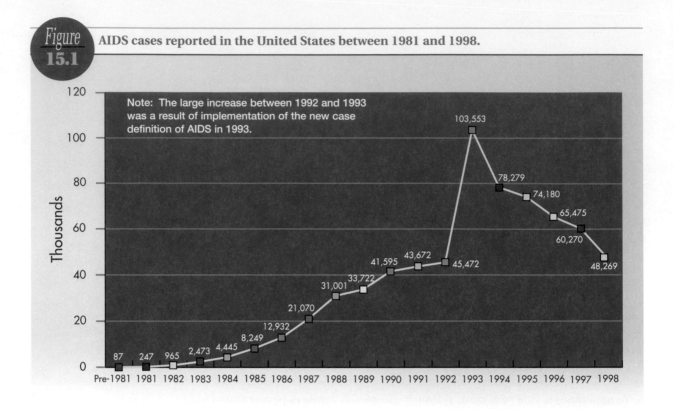

Figure 15.1 AIDS cases reported in the United States between 1981 and 1998.

Note: The large increase between 1992 and 1993 was a result of implementation of the new case definition of AIDS in 1993.

used to treat victims in Western countries are unaffordable in sub-Saharan Africa. Public-awareness programs may be the only answer to the HIV epidemic there.

As with any other serious illness, HIV infected people and AIDS patients deserve respect, understanding, and support. Rejection and discrimination are traits of immature, hateful, and ignorant people. Education, knowledge, and responsible behaviors are the best ways to minimize fear and discrimination.

HIV Testing

A person can be tested for HIV in several ways. You may look up your local Public Health Department or AIDS Information Service (or related names) in the phone book. Testing is usually free of charge, and the results are kept confidential.

Many states also conduct anonymous testing. Your name is never recorded. You can call several toll-free hotlines for more information on anonymous testing, treatment programs, support services, HIV and AIDS information, and STDs in general. All information discussed during a phone call to these hotlines is kept strictly confidential. The numbers to call are

■ National AIDS Hotline: 1-800-342-AIDS (1-800-342-2437) or La Linea Nacional de

SIDA: 1-800-344-SIDA (1-800-344-7432), for Spanish-speaking people.
■ STD Hotline: 1-800-227-8922.

HIV Treatment

Even though several drugs are being tested to treat and slow the disease process, AIDS has no known cure. Approximately 40 different approaches to an AIDS vaccine are being explored. The best advice at this point is to take a preventive approach.

Although HIV has no cure, medications are available that delay the progress of infection, allow HIV-infected patients to live longer, and even keep some people from developing AIDS. The sooner the treatment is initiated, the better the prognosis for a longer life.

Developing a vaccine to prevent HIV infection or AIDS seems highly unlikely within the decade. People should not expect a medical breakthrough. Treatment modalities, however, should continue to improve and allow HIV-infected persons and AIDS patients to live longer and more productive lives.

Presently, several AIDS clinical trials are available in the United States. These projects are co-sponsored by the CDC, the Food and Drug Administration, the National Institute of Allergy and Infectious Diseases, the National Library of Medicine, and the National Institute of Health.

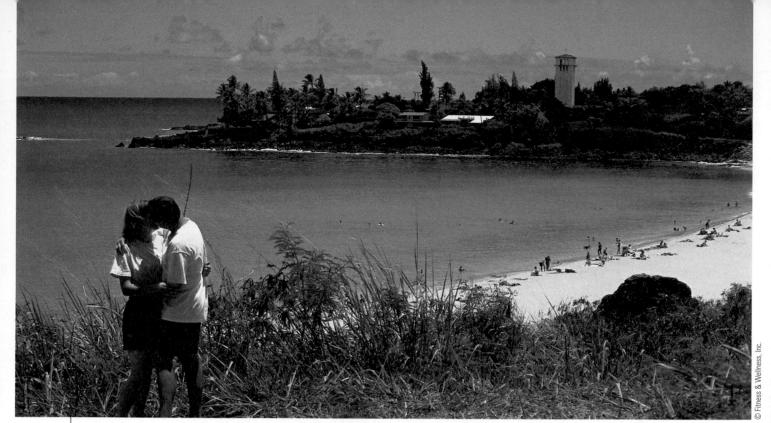

A monogamous sexual relationship almost completely removes people from risking HIV infection and the danger of developing other sexually transmitted diseases.

The purpose of AIDS clinical trials is to evaluate experimental drugs and various therapies for people at all stages of HIV infection. Interested individuals can call 1-800-TRIALS-A. As with all HIV testing, calls are completely confidential. Eligibility to participate in an AIDS clinical trial varies, and all applicants are evaluated individually. By calling the telephone number given, an interested person will receive information on the purpose and location of the trials (studies) that are open, eligibility requirements and exclusion criteria, and names and telephone numbers of persons to contact.

Economic Impact of HIV and AIDS

Federal government spending for AIDS-related projects gradually increased to more than $900 million between 1982 and 1988. Costs continued to escalate to $1.3 billion in 1989, $4.3 billion in 1992, $5.7 billion in 1997, and $9.7 billion in 1999. The CDC National Aids Clearinghouse estimates the direct-treatment cost per AIDS victim at about $133,500 over 8.3 years of life. This represents more than $41.2 billion to treat the 308,933 AIDS cases reported as of June 1999.

If the estimated 1 million people infected with HIV in the United States develop AIDS, direct health-care costs for the disease will equal $121.383 billion. To place this figure in perspective, a person would have to spend $1 million per day for the next 332.5 years to spend the $121.383 billion—a sobering amount for a preventable disease. Everyone in the United States will help pay for these costs through taxes and a more expensive health-care system.

Guidelines for Preventing Sexually Transmitted Diseases

The good news is that you can do things to prevent the spread of STDs and take precautions to keep yourself from becoming a victim. The facts are in: The best prevention technique is a mutually **monogamous** sexual relationship. This one behavior will remove you almost completely from any risk for developing an STD.

Unfortunately, in today's society, trust is elusive. You may be led to believe you are in a monogamous relationship when your partner actually (a) may cheat on you and get infected, (b) has a one-night stand with someone who is infected, (c) got the virus several years ago before the current relationship and still doesn't know about the infection, (d) may choose not to tell you about the infection, or (e) shoots up drugs and becomes infected. In any of these cases, HIV can be passed on to you.

Because your future and your life are at stake, and because you may never know if your partner is infected, you should give serious and careful consideration to postponing sex until you believe you have found an uninfected person with whom you can have a lifetime monogamous relationship. In doing so, you will not have to live with the fear of catching HIV or other STDs or deal with an unplanned pregnancy.

As strange as this may seem to some, many people postpone sexual activity until they are married. This is the best guarantee against HIV. Young people should understand that married life will provide plenty of time for fulfilling and rewarding sex.

If you choose to delay sex, do not let peers pressure you into having sex. Some people would have you believe that you are not a "real" man or woman if you don't have sex. Manhood and womanhood are not proven during sexual intercourse but, instead, through mature, responsible, and healthy choices.

Other people lead you to believe that love doesn't exist without sex. Sex in the early stages of a relationship is not the product of love. It is simply the fulfillment of a physical, and often selfish, drive. A loving relationship develops over a long time with mutual respect for each other.

Teenagers are especially susceptible to peer pressure leading to premature sexual intercourse. The result: more than a million teen pregnancies per year and a 43 percent pregnancy rate for all girls at least once as a teenager. Presently, the U.S. teen pregnancy rate is the highest of any industrialized nation. Too many young people wish they had postponed sex and silently admire those who do.

Sex lasts only a few minutes. The consequences of irresponsible sex may last a lifetime. And in some cases, they are fatal!

Sex lasts a few minutes, parenthood lasts a lifetime.

Then there are those who enjoy bragging about their sexual conquests and mock people who choose to wait. Many of these conquests are only fantasies expounded in an attempt to gain popularity with peers.

Sexual promiscuity never leads to a trusting, loving, and lasting relationship. Mature people respect others' choices. If someone does not respect your choice to wait, he or she certainly does not deserve your friendship or, for that matter, anything else.

There is no greater sex than that between two loving and responsible individuals who mutually trust, admire, and love each other. Contrary to many beliefs, these relationships are possible. They are built upon unselfish attitudes and behaviors.

As you look around, you will find that many people hold these values. Seek them out and build your friendships and future around people who respect you for who you are and what you believe. You don't have to compromise your choices or values. In the end, you will reap the greater rewards of a lasting relationship free of AIDS and other STDs.

Also, be prepared so that you will know your course of action before you get into an intimate situation. Look for common interests and work together toward them. Express your feelings openly: "I'm not ready for sex; I just want to have fun, and kissing is fine with me." If your friend does not accept your answer and is not willing to stop the advances, be prepared with a strong response. Statements like "Please stop" or "Don't!" are for the most part ineffective. Use a firm statement such as, "No, I'm not willing to have sex" or "I've already thought about this and I'm not going to have sex." If this still does not work, label the behavior as rape and say: "This is rape, and I'm going to call the police."

Reducing the Risk for STDs

What about those who do not have—or do not desire—a monogamous relationship? Some other things can be done to lower, but not completely eliminate, the risk for developing STDs in general:

1. Plan before you get into a sexual situation. Determine the conditions under which you will allow sex to take place. Take a few moments now and ask yourself: "Am I willing to have sex with this person?" If you decide to have sex, practice safer sex. There is no reason to accept anything else. You will feel better about yourself.
2. Know your partner. The days are gone when anonymous bathhouse or singles-bar sex is safe. Limit your sexual relationships and always practice safer sex.
3. Discuss STDs with the person you are contemplating having sex with before you do so. Even though talking about STDs might be awkward, the short-lived embarrassment of addressing intimate questions can keep you from contracting or spreading disease. If you do not know the person well enough to address this issue or you are uncertain about the answers, do not have sex with this individual.

Monogamous   A sexual relationship in which two people have sexual relations only with each other.

4. Limit the number of sexual partners you have. Having one partner lowers your chances of becoming infected. The more partners you have, the greater your chance for infection.

5. If you are sexually promiscuous, consider having periodic physical check-ups. You can easily get exposed to an STD from a person who does not have any symptoms and who is unaware of the infection. Sexually promiscuous men and women between ages 15 and 35 are considered a particularly high-risk group for developing STDs.

6. Use "barrier" methods of contraception to help prevent the disease from spreading. Condoms, diaphragms, and spermicidal suppositories, foams, and jellies can all deter the spread of certain STDs. Spermicidal agents may act as a disinfectant as well. Many physicians are encouraging promiscuous teenagers especially to use condoms. Traditionally, teenagers do not use birth-control methods at all and remain at high risk for STDs. Take a few minutes at this time and list at least three ways you might bring up the subject of condom use with your partner. Also, think of ways you might convince a person to use one. If your partner refuses to use a condom, your answer should be quite simple: "No condom, no sex."

7. Negotiate safer sex. Focus on the problem and not the person. Describe your feelings about the problem, using "I" instead of "you." For example, you might say, "I'm feeling awkward and uncomfortable. The only way I can feel comfortable is by using a condom." You also can offer options and provide alternative solutions to your partner. You might indicate: "We can work this out together. Let's go for a drive and get a condom with a spermicide agent. We'll feel better about what we're doing."

8. Be responsible enough to abstain from sexual activity if you know you have an infection. Go to a physician or a clinic for treatment, and ask your doctor when you can safely resume sexual activity. Abstain until it is safe. Just as you want to be protected in a sexual relationship, you should want to protect your partner as well.

   If you are diagnosed with an STD and you believe you know the person who gave it to you, think of ways you could bring up the subject of STDs with this person. You need to take responsibility and discuss this matter with your partner. As a result of your conversation, medical treatment can be initiated, and other people can be protected from infection as well.

9. Urinate immediately following sexual intercourse. Although this is not an entirely reliable method, it may help flush bacteria and viruses from the urinary tract.

10. Thoroughly wash immediately after sexual activity. Although washing with hot, soapy water will not guarantee safety against STDs, it can prevent you from spreading certain germs on your fingers and may wash away bacteria and viruses that have not entered the body yet.

11. If you suspect that your partner is infected with an STD, ask. He or she may not even be aware of the infection, so look for signs of infection, such as sores, redness, inflammation, a rash, growths, warts, or a discharge. If you are unsure, abstain.

12. Consider abstaining from sexual relations if you have any kind of an illness or disease, even a common cold. Any kind of illness makes you more susceptible to other illnesses, and lower immunity can make you more vulnerable to STDs. The same holds true for times when you are under extreme stress, when you are fatigued, and when you are overworked. Drugs and alcohol also can lower your resistance to disease.

13. Wear loose-fitting clothes made from natural fibers. Tight-fitting clothing made from synthetic fibers (especially underwear and nylon pantyhose) can create conditions that encourage the growth of bacteria and actually can aggravate STDs.

Reducing the Risks for HIV

Based upon recommendations from health experts, observing the following precautions can reduce your risk for getting HIV and, subsequently, AIDS:

1. Postpone sex until you and your uninfected partner are prepared to enter into a lifetime monogamous relationship.

2. Unless you are in a monogamous relationship and you know your partner is not infected (which you may never know for sure), practice safer sex every time you have sex. This means you should use a latex condom from start to finish for each sexual act. If you think your partner should use a condom but refuses to do so, say "No" to sex with that person.

   Many experts believe that greater protection can be obtained by placing a small amount of the spermicide nonoxynol-9 inside the condom at its tip and then lubricating the outside with additional spermicide. Nonoxynol-9 is used to kill the man's sperm for birth-control purposes. In test tubes, it has been shown to kill STD germs and HIV. This spermicide, however, should not be used in place of a condom, because it will not offer the same protection as the condom does by itself.

3. Don't have multiple and anonymous sexual partners. Keep in mind that anyone you have sex with could be infected with HIV.
4. Don't have sexual contact with anyone who doesn't practice safer sex.
5. Avoid sexual contact with anyone who has had sex with people at risk for getting HIV, even if they are now practicing safer sex.
6. Don't have sex with prostitutes.
7. If you do have sex with someone who might be infected with HIV or whose history is unknown to you, avoid exchange of body fluids.
8. Don't share toothbrushes, razors, or other implements that could become contaminated with blood with anyone who is, or who might be, infected with HIV.
9. Be cautious regarding procedures (such as acupuncture, tattooing, and ear piercing) in which needles or other nonsterile instruments may be used again and again to pierce the skin or mucous membranes. These procedures are safe if proper sterilization methods or disposable needles are followed. Before undergoing the procedure, ask what precautions are being taken.

10. If you are planning to undergo artificial insemination, insist on frozen sperm obtained from a laboratory that tests all donors for infection with HIV. Donors should be tested twice before the lab accepts the sperm—once at the time of donation and again a few months later.
11. If you know you will be having surgery in the near future, and if you are able, consider donating blood for your own use. This will eliminate completely the already small risk of contracting HIV through a blood transfusion. It also will eliminate the more substantial risk for contracting other bloodborne diseases, such as hepatitis, from a transfusion.

Avoiding risky behaviors that destroy quality of life and life itself is crucial to a healthy lifestyle. Learning the facts and acting upon your personal values, so you can make responsible choices, can protect you and those around you from painful, embarrassing, startling, unexpected, or fatal conditions.

Web Interactive

- Condoms: A User's Guide. This Mayo Clinic site features an outline of important information regarding proper condom use.

  http://mayohealth.org./mayo/9702/htm/condom_g.htm

- The Body: Safer Sex and Prevention: This site features information for consumers, gay men, and health care professionals on a variety of prevention issues, including safer sex and general prevention measures, condoms, sexual communication skills, sexual and non-sexual prevention, effective educational programs, treatment, and research.

  http://www.thebody.com/safesex.html

- The Johns Hopkins University STD Page. This comprehensive site stresses patient education and features information on a variety of sexually transmitted diseases as well as information concerning current research.

  http://www.med.jhu.edu/jhustd

- CDC National Center for HIV, STD, and TB Prevention. This comprehensive site features a variety of links to information regarding HIV/AIDS prevention, including the latest statistics.

  http://www.cdc.gov/hiv/dhap.htm

- Sexual Communication. This site written by Duke University Student Health Service provides excellent guidelines to help discuss sex (or abstinence) with your partner, as well as information about, sexual dysfunction, rape and sexual assault, as well as information concerning gay, lesbian, and

bisexual issues. There is also a link of 101 ways to please your lover without doing it.

http://healthydevil.stuaff.duke.edu/info/sex/sex.html

Interactive Sites:

- Assess Your Risk for HIV and Other Sexually Transmitted Diseases. By completing this simple 24-question multiple choice questionnaire, you will obtain an accurate portrayal of your personal risk for acquiring HIV and other types of sexually transmitted diseases.

  http://www.thebody.com/surveys/sexsurvey.html

- Contraceptive Choices: This site from Thriveonline features a variety of interesting topics, including information regarding the various forms of contraception, a birth control IQ test, an ovulation calculator, emergency contraception, chat rooms, message boards, ask the experts link, and an interactive personalized assessment of your contraceptive options, based on your preferences, health risks, cost, and safety.

  http://www.thriveonline.com/sex/contraceptive_choices

- Sexually Transmitted Diseases – A quiz. Take this ten question multiple choice quiz to test your knowledge of STDs, and learn more about their symptoms, prevention, and treatment.

  http://www.unspeakable.com/nph-survey.cgi?tag=std

Notes

1. Tanne, J. H., "US Has Epidemic of Sexually Transmitted Disease," *British Medical Journal* 317 (1998): 1616.

2. See note 2.

3. Unless otherwise indicated, all the statistics regarding STDs are from the U.S. Centers for Disease Control and Prevention, Atlanta.

4. Igra, V., "Pelvic Inflammatory Disease in Adolescents," *AIDS Patient Care & STDs* (February 1998): 109–124.

5. McFarlane, M., S. S. Bull, and C. A. Rietmeijer, "The Internet as a Newly Emerging Risk Environment for Sexually Transmitted Diseases," *Journal of the American Medical Association* 284 (2000): 443–446.

6. Philpott, P., "Heterosexual Transmission Studies," *Reappraising AIDS* 6, no. 1 (1998): 1.

Suggested Readings

W. W. K. Hoeger, L. W. Turner, and B. Q. Hafen. *Wellness: Guidelines for a Healthy Lifestyle*. Belmont, CA: Wadsworth/Thomson Learning, 2002.

Institute of Medicine. *The Hidden Epidemic: Confronting Sexually Transmitted Diseases*. Washington, D. C.: National Academy Press, 1997.

SELF-QUIZ ON HIV AND AIDS

Name: _____ Date: _____ Grade: _____

Instructor: _____ Course: _____ Section: _____

Necessary Lab Equipment
None required.

Instruction
Please answer all of the following questions.

Objective
To evaluate basic understanding of HIV and AIDS.

	Yes	No
1. AIDS—acquired immunodeficiency syndrome—is the end stage of infection caused by the human immunodeficiency virus, HIV.	☐	☐
2. HIV is a chronic infectious disease that spreads among individuals who choose to engage in risky behavior such as unprotected sex or the sharing of hypodermic needles.	☐	☐
3. There is a cure for AIDS.	☐	☐
4. Abstaining from sex is the only 100 percent sure way to protect yourself from HIV infection.	☐	☐
5. Using drugs and alcohol can make you willing to have sex when you really don't plan to.	☐	☐
6. Condoms are 100 percent effective in protecting you against HIV infection.	☐	☐
7. Using drugs and alcohol makes a person less likely to use a condom and use it correctly.	☐	☐
8. If you're sexually active, latex condoms provide the best protection against HIV infection.	☐	☐
9. Using drugs and alcohol can make you more likely to have unplanned and unprotected sex.	☐	☐
10. Each year more and more teens are infected with HIV.	☐	☐
11. You can become HIV-infected by donating blood.	☐	☐
12. You can tell by looking at someone if he/she is HIV-infected.	☐	☐
13. The only means to determine whether someone has HIV is through an HIV antibody test.	☐	☐
14. HIV can completely destroy the immune system.	☐	☐
15. The HIV virus may live in the body 10 years or longer before AIDS symptoms develop.	☐	☐
16. People infected with HIV have AIDS.	☐	☐
17. Once infected with HIV, a person never becomes uninfected.	☐	☐
18. HIV infection is preventable.	☐	☐

Selected items on this questionnaire are adapted from *Test Your Survival Smarts: Self-Quiz on Drugs and AIDS*, National Institute on Drug Abuse, U.S. Department of Health & Human Services.

Answers:

1. Yes. AIDS is the term used to define the manifestation of opportunistic diseases and cancers that occur as a result of HIV infection (also referred to as "HIV disease").
2. Yes. People do not get HIV because of who they are, but because of what they do. Almost all of the people who get HIV do so because they choose to engage in risky behaviors.
3. No. There is no cure for AIDS and there doesn't appear to be one in the foreseeable future.
4. Yes. Abstinence will protect you from HIV infection. But you may still get the disease by sharing hypodermic needles.
5. Yes. When you use alcohol or drugs, you can forget what you know about safer sex, and do things you normally wouldn't do. If you're drunk or high, you might have sex even though you really don't plan to.
6. No. Only abstaining from sex gives you 100 percent protection, but condoms are effective in protecting against HIV infection if they're used correctly.
7. Yes. Teens who are drunk or high are less likely to use condoms because, under the influence, they forget or feel that nothing "bad" can happen.
8. Yes. Proper use, however, is necessary to minimize the risk of infection.
9. Yes. Otherwise-prudent people often act irrationally and engage in risky behaviors when they are under the influence of drugs and alcohol.
10. Yes. In the early 1990s, the number of infected teens increased by 96 percent over a short span of 2 years. One reason for the increase may be that teens who are under the influence of drugs or alcohol often engage in risky sex. It is believed that about 20 percent of the AIDS patients today were infected as teenagers.
11. No. A myth regarding HIV is that it can be transmitted by donating blood. People cannot get HIV from giving blood. A brand new needle is used by health professionals every time blood is taken. These needles are only used once and are destroyed and thrown away immediately after each individual has donated blood.
12. No. The symptoms of AIDS are often not noticeable until several years after a person has been infected with HIV. That's why, no matter who your partner is, it's important to always protect yourself against HIV and the risk of developing AIDS—either by abstaining from sex or by using condoms if you decide to have sex.
13. Yes. Not you, not a nurse, not even a doctor can tell, unless an HIV antibody test is done. Upon HIV infection, the immune system's line of defense against the virus is the formation of antibodies that bind to the virus. On the average it takes 3 months for the body to manufacture enough antibodies to show positive in an HIV antibody test. Sometimes it takes 6 months or longer.
14. Yes. The virus multiplies, attacks, and destroys white blood cells. These cells are part of the immune system, and their function is to fight off infections and diseases in the body. As the number of white blood cells killed increases, the body's immune system gradually breaks down or may be completely destroyed.
15. Yes. Ten years or longer may go by before the person develops AIDS.
16. No. Being HIV-positive does not necessarily mean that the person has AIDS. It may be 10 years or longer following infection before the individual develops the symptoms that fit the case definition of AIDS. From that point on, the person may live another 2 to 3 years. In essence, from the point of infection, the individual may endure a chronic disease for about 12 or more years.
17. Yes. There is no second chance. Everyone must protect him- or herself against HIV infection.
18. Yes. The best prevention technique is abstaining from sex until the time comes for a mutually monogamous sexual relationship (two people having a sexual relationship only with each other). That one behavior will almost completely remove you from any risk of HIV infection or developing any other sexually transmitted disease.

Chapter 16

Healthy Lifestyle Issues and Wellness Guidelines for the Future

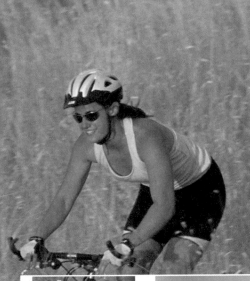

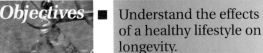

Objectives

- Understand the effects of a healthy lifestyle on longevity.

- Learn to differentiate between physiological and chronological age.

- Estimate your life expectancy and determine your real physiological age.

- Learn about complementary and alternative medicine practices.

- Learn guidelines for preventing consumer fraud.

- Understand factors to consider when selecting a health/fitness club.

- Know how to select appropriate exercise equipment.

- Review health/fitness accomplishments and chart a wellness program for the future.

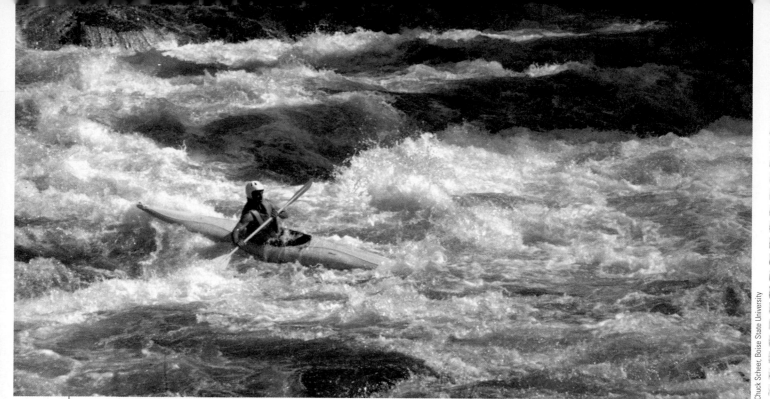

Good physical fitness provides freedom to enjoy many of life's recreational and leisure activities.

Better health, higher quality of life, and longevity are the three most important benefits derived from a lifetime fitness and wellness program. You have learned that physical fitness in itself does not always lower the risk for chronic diseases and ensure better health. Thus implementation of healthy behaviors is one means to attain your highest potential for complete well-being. The real challenge will come now that you are about to finish this course: a lifetime commitment to fitness and wellness. Adhering to a program in a structured setting is a lot easier, but from now on, you will be on your own.

This chapter will help you evaluate how well you are adhering to health-promoting behaviors and the impact that these behaviors may have on your **physiological age** and length of life. You will also learn how to chart a personal wellness program for the future.

Research data indicates that healthy (and unhealthy) lifestyle actions you take today will have an impact on health and quality of life in middle and advanced age. Whereas most young people don't seem to worry much about health and longevity, you may want to take a closer look at the quality of life of your parents or other middle-aged and older friends and relatives that you know. Though you may have a difficult time envisioning yourself at that age, their health status and functional capacity may help you determine how you would like to live when you reach your fourth, fifth, and sixth decade of life.

Although previous research has documented declines in physiologic function and motor capacity as a result of aging, no hard evidence at present proves that large declines in physical work capacity are related primarily to aging alone. Lack of physical activity—a common phenomenon seen in our society as people age—is accompanied by decreases in physical work capacity that are greater by far than the effects of aging itself.

Data on individuals who have taken part in systematic physical activity throughout life indicate that these people maintain a higher level of **functional capacity** and do not experience the typical declines in later years. From a functional point of view, typical sedentary people in the United States are about 25 years older than their **chronological age** indicates. Thus, an active 60-year-old person can have a physical work capacity similar to that of a sedentary 35-year-old person.

Sedentary people often stop living at age 60 but choose to be buried at age 70!

Unhealthy behaviors precipitate premature aging. For sedentary people, any type of physical activity is seriously impaired by age 40 and productive life ends before age 60. Most of these people hope to live to be age 65 or 70 and often must cope with serious physical ailments. These people "stop living at age 60 but choose to be buried at age 70" (see the theoretical model in Figure 16.1).

Scientists believe that a healthy lifestyle allows people to live a vibrant life—a physically,

Figure
16.1

Relationships between physical work capacity, aging, and lifestyle habits.

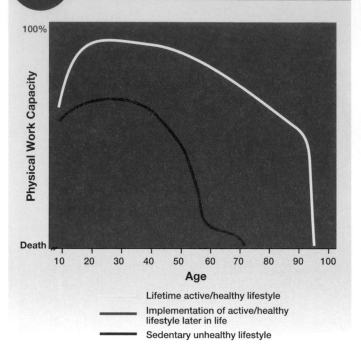

Lifetime active/healthy lifestyle

Implementation of active/healthy lifestyle later in life

Sedentary unhealthy lifestyle

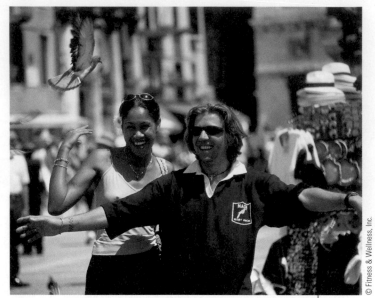

A healthy lifestyle enhances functional capacity and quality of life.

intellectually, emotionally, socially active, and functionally independent existence—to age 95. Such are the rewards of a wellness way of life. When death comes to active people, it usually is rather quick and not as a result of prolonged illness: In Figure 16.1, note the low, longer slope of the "unhealthy lifestyle" before death.

Life Expectancy and Physiological Age

Aging is a natural process, but some people seem to age better than others. Most likely you know someone who looks much younger than their chronological age indicates, or vice versa: They appear much older than their chronological age indicates. For example, you may have an instructor who you would have guessed was about 40, but in reality is 52 years old. On the other hand, you may have a relative who looks 60, but who is actually 50 years old. Why the differences?

During the aging process, natural biological changes occur within the body. Although no one measurement can predict how long you will live, the rate at which aging changes take place depends on a combination of genetic and lifestyle factors. Your lifestyle habits will determine to a great extent how your genes will affect your aging process. Hundreds of research studies now point to critical lifestyle

behaviors that will determine your statistical chances of dying at a younger age or living a longer life. Research also shows that lifestyle behaviors have a far greater impact on health and longevity than your genes alone.

Throughout this book, you have studied many of these factors. The question that you now need to ask yourself is: Are your lifestyle habits accelerating or decelerating the rate at which your body is aging? To help you determine how long and how well you may live the rest of your life, the **Life Expectancy** and Physiological Age Questionnaire, provided in Lab 16A, can help answer this question. By looking at 46 critical genetic and lifestyle factors, you will be able to estimate your life expectancy and your real physiological age. Of greater importance, most of these factors are under your own control and you can do something to make them work for you instead of against you.

As you fill out the questionnaire, you must be completely honest with yourself. Your life expectancy and physiological age prediction is based on your present lifestyle habits, should you continue

Physiological age The biological and functional capacity of the body.

Functional capacity The ability to perform ordinary and unusual demands of daily life without limitations and excessive fatigue or injury.

Chronological age Calendar age.

Life expectancy How many years a person is expected to live.

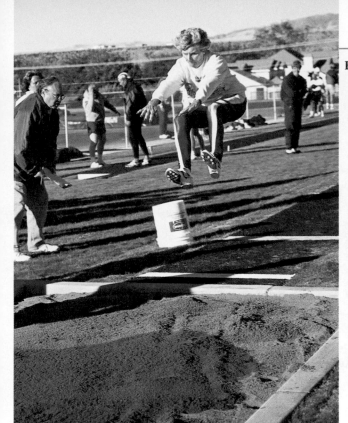

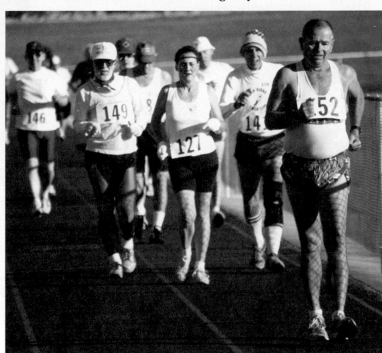

Exercise enhances health status and longevity.

Photos © Fitness & Wellness, Inc.

those habits for life. Using the questionnaire, you will review factors that you can modify or implement in daily living and that may add years and health to your life. Please note that the questionnaire is not a precise scientific instrument, but rather an estimated life expectancy analysis according to the impact of lifestyle factors on health and longevity. Also, the questionnaire is not intended as a substitute for advice and tests conducted by medical and health care practitioners.

Complementary and Alternative Medicine

Conventional Western medicine, also known as **allopathic medicine**, has seen major advances in care and treatment modalities during the last few decades. Conventional medicine is based on scientifically proven methods, wherein medical treatments are tested through rigorous scientific trials. In addition to a **primary care physician** (medical doctor), people seek advice from other practitioners of conventional medicine, including **osteopaths**, **dentists**, **oral surgeons**, **orthodontists**, **ophthalmologists**, **optometrists**, **physician assistants**, and **nurses**.

In spite of modern day technological and scientific advancements, many medical treatments either do not improve the patient's condition or create other ailments caused by the treatment itself. Only about 20 percent of conventional treatments have

been proven to be clinically effective in scientific trials.[1] Thus, millions of consumers are turning to **complementary** and **alternative medicine** (also called "unconventional" or "nonallopathic") in search of answers to their health problems.

The reasons for seeking complementary and alternative treatments are diverse. Lack of progress in curing illnesses and disease, frustration and dissatisfaction with physicians, lack of personal attention, testimonials about the effectiveness of alternative treatments, and rising health care costs are among the common reasons given by patients who seek unconventional treatments. **Unconventional medicine** is referred to as complementary and alternative medicine because patients use it to either augment their regular medical care or as a replacement to conventional practices. In 1997, over 46 percent of Americans used complementary and alternative medicine services. This figure represented about 629 million appointments with practitioners,[2] thereby surpassing the total number of visits to all U.S. primary care physicians.

The National Center for Complementary and Alternative Medicine (NCCAM), under the National Institutes of Health, was recently established to examine methods of healing that have previously been unexplored by science. The NCCAM defines complementary and alternative medicine as those treatments and health care practices not widely taught in medical schools, not generally used in hospitals, and not usually reimbursed by medical

insurance companies. Many physicians, nonetheless, now endorse complementary and alternative treatments, and an ever-increasing number of medical schools are offering courses in this area.

Alternative medicine practices have not gone through the same standard scrutiny as conventional medicine. Nonallopathic treatments are often based on theories that have not been scientifically proven. This does not imply that unconventional medicine practices do not help people. Many people have found relief from ailments or been cured through unconventional treatments. In due time, however, these theories will need to be investigated using scientific trials similar to those in conventional medicine.

Complementary and alternative medicine includes a wide range of healing philosophies, approaches, and therapies. The practices most often associated with **nonallopathic medicine** are **acupuncture, chiropractics, herbal medicine, homeopathy, naturopathic medicine, ayurveda, magnetic therapy,** and **massage therapy**. Each of these practices offers a different approach to treatments based on its beliefs about the body, some of which are hundreds or thousands of years old.

Many of these practitioners believe that their treatment modality aids the body as it performs its own natural healing process. Because of their approach, alternative treatments usually take longer than conventional allopathic medical care. Nonallopathic treatments are usually less harsh on the patient, and practitioners tend to avoid surgery and extensive use of medications.

Unconventional therapies are frequently viewed as "holistic," implying that the practitioner looks at all the dimensions of wellness when evaluating a person's condition. Practitioners often persuade patients to adopt healthier lifestyle habits that not only help to improve current conditions but prevent other ailments as well. Complementary and alternative medicine also allows patients to better understand treatments, and patients are often allowed to administer self-treatment.

Costs for complementary and alternative medicine practices are typically lower than conventional medicine costs. With the exception of acupuncture and chiropractic care, most nonallopathic treatments are not covered by health insurance. Typically, patients pay directly for these services. In 1997, a conservative estimate of $21.2 billion was spent on alternative medical treatments, with at least $12.2 billion paid out-of-pocket.[3] These costs exceeded the out-of-pocket expenses for all hospitalizations in the United States. If you are considering alternative medical therapies, consult with your health care insurance provider to determine which therapies are reimbursable.

Conventional Western medicine   Traditional medical practice based on methods that are tested through rigorous scientific trials.

Allopathic medicine   See conventional Western medicine.

Primary care physician   A medical practitioner who provides routine treatment of ailments; typically, the patient's first contact for health care.

Osteopath   A medical practitioner with specialized training in musculoskeletal problems who uses diagnostic and therapeutic methods of conventional medicine in addition to manipulative measures.

Dentist   Practitioner who specializes in diseases of the teeth, gums, and oral cavity.

Oral surgeon   A dentist who specializes in surgical procedures of the oral-facial complex.

Orthodontist   A dentist who specializes in the correction and prevention of teeth irregularities.

Ophthalmologist   Medical specialist concerned with diseases of the eye and prescription of corrective lenses.

Optometrist   Health care practitioner who specializes in the prescription and adaptation of lenses.

Physician assistant   A health care practitioner trained to treat most standard cases of care.

Nurse   Health care practitioner who assists in the diagnosis and treatment of health problems and provides many services to patients in a variety of settings.

Complementary and alternative medicine   A branch of medicine concerned with treatments and health care practices not widely taught in medical schools, not generally used in hospitals, and not usually reimbursed by medical insurance companies.

Unconventional medicine   See complementary and alternative medicine.

Nonallopathic medicine   See complementary and alternative medicine.

Acupuncture   Chinese medical system that requires body piercing with fine needles during therapy to relieve pain and treat ailments and diseases.

Chiropractics   Health care system that believes that many diseases and ailments are related to misalignments of the vertebrae and emphasizes the manipulation of the spinal column.

Herbal medicine   Unconventional system that uses herbs to treat ailments and disease.

Homeopathy   System of treatment based on the use of minute quantities of remedies that in large amounts produce effects similar to the disease being treated.

Naturopathic medicine   Unconventional system of medicine that relies exclusively on natural remedies to treat disease and ailments.

Ayurveda   Unconventional Hindu system of medicine based on herbs, diet, massage, meditation, and yoga to help the body boost its own natural healing.

Magnetic therapy   Unconventional treatment that relies on magnetic energy to promote healing.

Massage therapy   The rubbing or kneading of body parts to treat ailments.

Complementary and alternative medicine does have shortcomings. Many of the practitioners do not have the years of education given to conventional medical personnel and often know less about physiological responses that occur in the body. Some practices are completely void of science; hence, the practitioner can rarely explain the specific physiologic benefits of the treatment used. Much of the knowledge is based on experiences with previous patients.

The practice of complementary and alternative medicine is not regulated like that of conventional medicine. The training and certification of practitioners, malpractice liability, and evaluation of tests and methods used in treatments are not routinely standardized. Many states, however, license practitioners in the areas of chiropractic services, acupuncture, naturopathy, homeopathy, herbal therapy, and massage therapy. Other therapies, however, are unmonitored.

Another concern in unconventional medicine is the lack of regulation of natural and herbal products. The word "natural" does not imply that the product is safe. Many products, including some herbs, can be toxic in large doses. Additionally, an estimated 15 million Americans combine high-dose vitamins and/or herbal supplements with prescription drugs (about one-fifth of all prescription users).[4] Such combinations can yield undesirable side effects. Individuals should always let their health care practitioners know which medications and alternative (including vitamin and mineral) supplements are being taken in combination.

> *"Natural" does not imply that a product is safe. Many products, including some herbs, can be toxic in large doses.*

Increasingly, conventional health care providers can refer you to someone who is familiar with alternative treatments. But you need to be an informed consumer. Ask your primary care physician to obtain valid information regarding the safety and effectiveness of a particular treatment. At times, nonetheless, the medical community resists and rejects unconventional therapies. If your physician is unable or unwilling to provide you with this information, medical, college, or public libraries and popular bookstores are good places to search for this information. You need to educate yourself about the advantages and disadvantages of alternative treatments, risks, side effects, expected results, and length of therapy.

Information on a wide range of medical conditions or specific diseases can also be obtained by calling the National Institutes of Health (NIH) at (301) 496-4000. Ask the operator to direct you to the appropriate NIH office. The NCCAM office also provides a Web site (nccam.nih.gov) with access to over 180,000 bibliographic records of research published on complementary and alternative medicine during the last 35 years.

When selecting a primary care physician or a nonallopathic practitioner, local and state medical boards, other health regulatory boards and agencies, and consumer affairs departments can provide information about a given practitioner's education, accreditation, license, and complaints that may have been filed against this health care provider. Many of the unconventional medical fields also have a national organization that provides guidelines for practitioners and health consumers. These organizations can guide you to the appropriate regulatory agencies within your state where you can obtain information regarding a specific practitioner.

You may also talk to other individuals who have undergone similar therapies and learn about the confidence and competence of the practitioner in question. Keep in mind, however, that patient testimonials do not adequately assess the safety and effectiveness of alternative treatments. Whenever possible, search for results of controlled scientific trials of the therapy in question and use this information in your decision process.

When undergoing any type of treatment or therapy, always discuss this information with all of your health care providers, whether conventional or unconventional. Adequate health care management requires that health care providers be informed of all concurrent therapies, so they will have a complete picture of the treatment plan. Lack of knowledge by one health care provider regarding treatments by another provider can interfere with the healing process or even worsen a given condition.

Millions of Americans have benefited from complementary and alternative medicine practices. You may also benefit from such services, but you need to make careful and educated decisions about the available options. By finding well-trained (and preferably licensed) practitioners, you increase your chances for recovery from ailments and disease.

Quackery and Fraud

The rapid growth of the fitness and wellness industry during the last three decades has spurred the promotion of fraudulent products that deceive consumers into "miraculous," quick, and easy ways to achieve total well-being. **Quackery** and **fraud** have been defined as the conscious promotion of unproven claims for profit.

Today's market is saturated with "special" foods, diets, supplements, pills, cures, equipment, books,

and videos that promise quick, dramatic results. Advertisements for these products often are based on testimonials, unproven claims, secret research, half-truths, and quick-fix statements that the un-educated consumer wants to hear. In the meantime, the organization or enterprise making the claims stands to make a large profit from the consumers' willingness to pay for astonishing and spectacular solutions to problems related to their unhealthy lifestyle.

Television, magazine, and newspaper advertise-ments are not necessarily reliable. For instance, one piece of equipment sold through television and newspaper advertisements promised to "bust the gut" through 5 minutes of daily exercise that appeared to target the abdominal muscle group. This piece of equipment consisted of a metal spring attached to the feet on one end and held in the hands on the other end. According to handling and shipping distributors, the equipment was "selling like hotcakes," and companies could barely keep up with consumer demands.

Three problems became apparent to the educated consumer: First, there is no such thing as spot-reducing; therefore, the claims could not be true. Second, 5 minutes of daily exercise burn hardly any calories and, therefore, have no effect on weight loss. Third, the intended abdominal (gut) muscles were not really involved during the exercise. The exercise engaged mostly the gluteal and lower back muscles. This piece of equipment now can be found at garage sales for about a tenth of its original cost!

Although people in the United States tend to be firm believers in the benefits of physical activity and positive lifestyle habits as a means to promote better health, most do not reap these benefits because they simply do not know how to put into practice a sound fitness and wellness program that will give them the results they want. Unfortunately, many uneducated wellness consumers are targets of deception by organizations making fraudulent claims for their products.

If you have questions or concerns about a health product, you may write to the National Council for Reliable Health Information (NCRHI), P.O. Box 1276, Loma Linda, CA 92354. The purpose of this organization is to provide the consumer with responsible, reliable, evidence-driven health infor-mation. The organization also monitors deceitful advertising, investigates complaints, and offers public information regarding fraudulent health claims. You may also report any type of quackery on their Web site at http://www.ncahf.org/ The site also contains an updated list of reliable and unreliable health Web sites for the consumer.

Even though deceit is all around us, we can protect ourselves from consumer fraud. The first step, of course, is education. You have to be an informed consumer of the product you intend to purchase. If you do not have or cannot find the answers, seek the advice of a reputable professional. Ask someone who understands the product but does not stand to profit from the transaction. As examples, a physical educator or an exercise physi-ologist can advise you regarding exercise equipment; a registered dietitian can provide information on nutrition and weight control programs; a physician can offer advice on nutritive supplements. Also, be alert to those who bill themselves as "experts." Look for qualifications, degrees, professional experience, certifications, and reputation.

Another clue to possible fraud is that if it sounds too good to be true, it probably is. Quick-fix, miracu-lous, special, secret, mail-order only, money-back guarantee, and testimonials often are heard in advertisements of fraudulent promotions. When claims are made, ask where the claims are pub-lished. Newspapers, magazines, and trade books are apt to be unreliable sources of information; refereed scientific journals are the most reliable. When a researcher submits information for publication in a refereed journal, at least two qualified and reputable professionals in the field conduct blind reviews of the manuscript. A blind review means the author does not know who will review the manuscript and the reviewers do not know who submitted the manuscript. Acceptance for publication is based on this input and relevant changes.

Health/Fitness Club Memberships

As you follow a lifetime wellness program, you may want to consider joining a health/fitness facility. Or, if you have mastered the contents of this book and your choice of fitness activity is one you can pursue on your own (walking, jogging, cycling), you may not need to join a health club. Barring injuries, you may continue your exercise program outside the walls of a health club for the rest of your life. You also can conduct strength training and stretching programs in your own home (see Chapters 8 and 9).

To stay up-to-date on fitness and wellness developments, you probably should buy a reputable and updated fitness/wellness book every 4 to 5 years. You also may subscribe to a credible health, fitness, nutrition, or wellness newsletter to stay current. You can also surf the World Wide Web, but be sure that the sites you are searching are from credible and reliable organizations.

Quackery/Fraud The conscious promotion of unproven claims for profit.

RELIABLE SOURCES OF HEALTH, FITNESS, NUTRITION, AND WELLNESS INFORMATION

Newsletter	Approx. Yearly Issues	Annual Cost
Bottom Line / Personal Health P.O. Box 53408 Boulder, CO 80322–3408	12	$49
Consumer Reports Health Letter P.O. Box 56356 Boulder, CO 80323–2148	12	$24
HealthNews P.O. Box 8963 Waltham, MA 02254-9959	12	$29
Tufts University Diet & Nutrition Letter P.O. Box 57857 Boulder, CO 80322–7857	12	$28
University of California Berkeley *Wellness Letter* P.O. Box 420148 Palm Coast, FL 32142	12	$29

If you are contemplating membership in a fitness facility, do all of the following:

- Examine all exercise options in your community: health clubs/spas, YMCAs, gyms, colleges, schools, community centers, senior centers, and the like.
- Check to see if the facility's atmosphere is pleasurable and nonthreatening to you. Will you feel comfortable with the instructors and other people who go there? Is it clean and well kept up? If the answer is no, this may not be the right place for you.
- Analyze costs versus facilities, equipment, and programs. Take a look at your personal budget. Will you really use the facility? Will you exercise there regularly? Many people obtain memberships and permit dues to be withdrawn automatically from a local bank account, yet seldom attend the fitness center.
- Find out what types of facilities are available: walking/running track, basketball/tennis/racquetball courts, aerobic exercise room, strength training room, pool, locker rooms, saunas, hot tubs, handicapped access, and so on.

RELIABLE HEALTH WEB SITES

- American Cancer Society
  http://cancer.org/
- American Heart Association
  http://americanheart.org
- Clinical Trials Center
  http://www.med-library.com/medlibrary/
- Department of Health and Human Services
  http://www.healthfinder.gov
- HospitalWeb
  http://neuro-www.mgh.harvard.edu/hospitalweb.shtml
- National Cancer Institute
  http://cancernet.nci.nih.gov/
- National Center for Complementary and Alternative Medicine
  http://nccam.nih.gov/
- The National Library of Medicine
  http://www.nlm.nih.gov/
- The National Institutes of Health
  http://www.nih.gov/
- The Centers for Disease Control
  http://www.cdc.gov/
- The Global Health Network
  http://www.pitt.edu/HOME/GHNet/GHNet.html
- The Medical Matrix
  http://www.medmatrix.org/Index.asp
- The National Council for Reliable Health Information
  http://www.ncahf.org/
- The Annals of Internal Medicine
  http://www.acponline.org/index.html
- The Food and Drug Administration
  http://www.fda.gov/
- WebMD
  http://webmd.com/
- World Health Organization
  http://www.who.ch/

- Check the aerobic and strength-training equipment available. Does the facility have treadmills, bicycle ergometers, Stair Masters, cross-country skiing simulators, free weights, Universal Gym, Nautilus? Make sure the facilities and equipment meet your activity interests.
- Consider the location. Is the facility close, or do you have to travel several miles to get there? Distance often discourages participation

- Check on times the facility is accessible. Is it open during your preferred exercise time (for example, early morning or late evening)?
- Work out at the facility several times before becoming a member. Are people standing in line to use the equipment, or is it readily available during your exercise time?
- Inquire about the instructors' qualifications. Do the fitness instructors have college degrees or professional certifications from organizations such as the American College of Sports Medicine (ACSM) or the International Dance Exercise Association (IDEA)? These organizations have rigorous standards to ensure professional preparation and quality of instruction.
- Consider the approach to fitness (including all health-related components of fitness). Is it well-rounded? Do the instructors spend time with members, or do members have to seek them out constantly for help and instruction?
- Ask about supplementary services. Does the facility provide or contract out for regular health and fitness assessments (cardiovascular endurance, body composition, blood pressure, blood chemistry analysis)? Are wellness seminars (nutrition, weight control, stress management) offered? Do these have hidden costs?

Purchasing Exercise Equipment

A final consideration is that of purchasing your own exercise equipment. The first question you need to ask yourself is: Do I really need this piece of equipment? Most people buy on impulse because of television advertisements or because a salesperson convinced them it is a great piece of equipment that will do wonders for their health and fitness. With some creativity, you can implement an excellent and comprehensive exercise program with little, if any, equipment (see Chapters 7, 8, and 9).

Many people buy expensive equipment only to find they really do not enjoy that mode of activity. They do not remain regular users. Stationary bicycles (lower body only) and rowing ergometers were among the most popular pieces of equipment in the 1980s. Most of them now are seldom used and have become "fitness furniture" somewhere in the basement.

Exercise equipment does have its value for people who prefer to exercise indoors, especially during the winter months. It supports some people's motivation and adherence to exercise. The convenience of having equipment at home also allows for flexible scheduling. You can exercise before or after work or while you watch your favorite television show.

If you are going to purchase equipment, the best recommendation is to actually try it out several times before buying it. Ask yourself several questions: Did you enjoy the workout? Is the unit comfortable? Are you too short, tall, or heavy for it? Is it stable, sturdy, and strong? Do you have to assemble the machine? If so, how difficult is it to put together? How durable is it? Ask for references—people or clubs that have used the equipment extensively. Are they satisfied? Have they enjoyed using the equipment? Talk with professionals at colleges, sports-medicine clinics, or health clubs.

Another consideration is to look at used units for signs of wear and tear. Quality is important. Cheaper brands may not be durable, so your investment would be wasted.

Finally, watch out for expensive gadgets. Monitors that provide exercise heart rate, work output, caloric expenditure, speed, grade, and distance may help motivate you, but they are expensive, need repairs, and do not enhance the actual fitness benefits of the workout. Look at maintenance costs and check for service personnel in your community.

Self-Evaluation and Behavioral Objectives for the Future

The main objective of this book is to provide the information and experiences necessary to implement your personal fitness and wellness program. If you have implemented the programs in this book, including exercise, you should be convinced that a wellness lifestyle is the only way to attain a higher quality of life.

Most people who engage in a personal fitness and wellness program experience this new quality of life after only a few weeks of training and practicing healthy lifestyle patterns. In some instances, however—especially for individuals who have led a poor lifestyle for a long time—a few months may be required to establish positive habits and feelings of well-being. In the end, though, everyone who applies the principles of fitness and wellness will reap the desired benefits.

Self-Evaluation

Through various laboratory experiences, you have had an opportunity to assess your own fitness and wellness components and write behavioral objectives to improve your quality of life. You now should take the time to evaluate how well you have achieved your own objectives. Ideally, if time allows and facilities and technicians are available, you should reassess at least the health-related

components of physical fitness. If you are unable to reassess these components, determine subjectively how well you accomplished your objectives. You will find a self-evaluation form in part I of Lab 16B.

Behavioral Objectives for the Future

If you have not yet achieved all of your objectives during this course, or if you need to reach beyond your current achievements, a final assignment should be conducted to help you chart the future. To complete this assignment, fill out the Wellness Compass shown in part II of Lab 16B. This compass provides a list of various wellness components, each illustrating a scale from 5 to 1. A "5" indicates a low or poor rating; a "1" indicates an excellent or "wellness" rating for that component. Using the Wellness Compass, rate yourself for each component according to the following instructions:

1. Color in red a number from 5 to 1 to indicate where you stood on each component at the beginning of the semester. For example, if at the start of this course, you rated poor in cardiorespiratory endurance, color the number 5 in red.
2. Color in blue a second number from 5 to 1 to indicate where you stand on each component at the present time. If your level of cardiorespiratory endurance improved to average by the end of the semester, color the number 3 in blue. If you were not able to work on a given component, simply color in blue on top of the previous red.
3. Select one or two components you intend to work on in the next 2 months. Developing new behavioral patterns takes time and trying to work on too many components at once most likely will lower your chances for success.

Start with components in which you think you will have a high chance for success. Next, color in yellow the intended objective (number) to accomplish by the end of the 2 months. If your objective is to achieve a "good" level of cardiorespiratory endurance, color the number 2 in yellow. When you achieve this level, you may later color the number 1, also in yellow, to indicate your next objective.

Tips for Behavioral Change

After you have completed the previous exercise, write behavioral objectives for the two components you intend to work on during the next 2 months (use the form in part III of Lab 16B). As you write

and work on these objectives, keep in mind the following guidelines:

1. Set both general and specific objectives. The general objective is the ultimate goal you intend to achieve. The specific objectives are the steps required to reach this general objective. For example, a general objective might be to achieve recommended body weight. Several specific objectives could be to (a) lose an average of one pound (or one fat percentage point) per week, (b) monitor body weight before breakfast every morning, (c) assess body composition every 2 weeks, (d) limit fat intake to less than 25 percent of total calories, (e) eliminate all pastries from the diet during this time, or (f) exercise in the proper target zone for 45 minutes, five times per week.
2. Whenever possible, make objectives (general and specific) measurable. For example, "to lose weight" is not measurable. In the previous general objective, recommended body weight implies lowering your body weight (fat) to the recommended percent body fat standards given in Table 4.9 in Chapter 4. If this person is a 19-year-old female, the high fitness recommended fat percent would be in the range of 17 to 27 percent.

   To be more descriptive, the general objective could be reworded as "Reduce body weight to 22 percent body fat." The sample specific objectives given in Item 1 above also are measurable. For instance, you can figure out easily whether you are losing a pound or a percentage point per week, you can conduct a nutrient analysis to assess the average fat intake, or you can monitor your weekly exercise sessions to make sure you are meeting this specific objective.
3. Make objectives realistic. If you currently weigh 170 pounds and your target weight at 22 percent is 120 pounds, it would be unsound, if not impossible, to implement a weight loss program to lose 50 pounds in 2 months. This program would not allow implementation of adequate behavior modification techniques or ensure weight maintenance at the target weight.
4. Write either short-term or long-term objectives. If the general objective is to attain recommended body weight and you are 50 pounds overweight, setting a general short-term objective of losing 10 pounds and writing specific objectives to accomplish this goal is best. Then the task will not seem as overwhelming and will be easier to do.
5. Set a specific date to achieve your objective. To simply state "I will lose weight" is not

time-specific. With a deadline, a task is much easier to work toward.

6. Educate yourself about the objective you plan to work on. You cannot lose weight if you do not know the principles governing weight loss and maintenance. This is the reason only 3 in 10 individuals achieve the target weight loss and only 1 in those 3 is able to keep it off thereafter.

7. Think positive and reward yourself for your accomplishments. As difficult as some tasks may seem, where there's a will, there's a way. If you prepare a plan of action according to these guidelines, you should be able to achieve your objective. Reward yourself for your accomplishments. Buy yourself new clothing, exercise shoes, or something special you have wanted for some time.

8. Seek support from those around you. Losing weight is difficult if you share meal planning and cooking with a roommate who enjoys foods that are high in fat and sweets. It can be even worse if the roommate also has a weight problem and does not desire or have the willpower to lose weight. Surround yourself with people who will help and encourage you along the way. If necessary, plan and prepare your own meals.

9. Recognize that you will face obstacles and you will make mistakes. Making mistakes is human and does not mean failure. Failure comes only to those who give up. Use your mistakes and learn from them by creating a plan that will help you get around self-defeating behaviors in the future.

10. Monitor your progress regularly. You will not always meet the specific objectives. If you do not, you will need to evaluate your objectives and perhaps make changes in the general or the specific objectives, or both. People are different, and you may not be able to progress as fast as someone else. Be flexible with yourself, and reconsider your plan of action.

The Fitness/Wellness Experience and a Challenge for the Future

Patty Neavill is a typical example of someone who often tried to change her life but was unable to do so because she did not know how to implement a sound exercise and weight control program. At age 24 and at 240 pounds, she was discouraged with her weight, level of fitness, self-image, and quality of life in general. She had struggled with her weight most of her life. Like thousands of other people, she had made many unsuccessful attempts to lose weight.

Patty put her fears aside and decided to enroll in a fitness course. As part of the course requirement,

a battery of fitness tests was administered at the beginning of the semester. Patty's cardiovascular fitness and strength ratings were poor, her flexibility classification was average, and her percent body fat was 41.

Following the initial fitness assessment, Patty met with her course instructor, who prescribed an exercise and nutrition program like the one in this book. Patty fully committed to carry out the prescription. She walked/jogged five times a week. She enrolled in a weight training course that met twice a week. Her daily caloric intake was set in the range of 1,500 to 1,700 calories.

Determined to increase her level of activity further, Patty signed up for recreational volleyball and basketball courses. Besides being fun, these classes provided 4 additional hours of activity per week.

She took care to meet the minimum required servings from the basic food groups each day, which contributed about 1,200 calories to her diet. The remainder of the calories came primarily from complex carbohydrates.

At the end of the 16-week semester, Patty's cardiovascular fitness, strength, and flexibility ratings had all improved to the good category, she lost 50 pounds, and her percent body fat had decreased to 22.5!

Patty was tall. At 190 pounds, most people would have thought she was too heavy. Her percent body fat, however, was lower than the average for college female physical education major students (about 23 percent body fat).

A thank-you note from Patty to the course instructor at the end of the semester read:

Thank you for making me a new person. I truly appreciate the time you spent with me. Without your kindness and motivation, I would have never made it. It is great to be fit and trim. I've never had this feeling before, and I wish everyone could feel like this once in their life.
Thank you,
Your trim Patty!

Patty never had been taught the principles governing a sound weight loss program. In Patty's case, not only did she need this knowledge, but, like most Americans who never have experienced the process of becoming physically fit, she needed to be in a structured exercise setting to truly feel the joy of fitness.

Even more significant, Patty maintained her aerobic and strength-training programs. A year after ending her calorie-restricted diet, her weight increased by 10 pounds, but her body fat decreased from 22.5 to 21.2 percent. As you may recall from Chapter 5, this weight increase is related mostly to changes in lean tissue, lost during the weight-reduction phase.

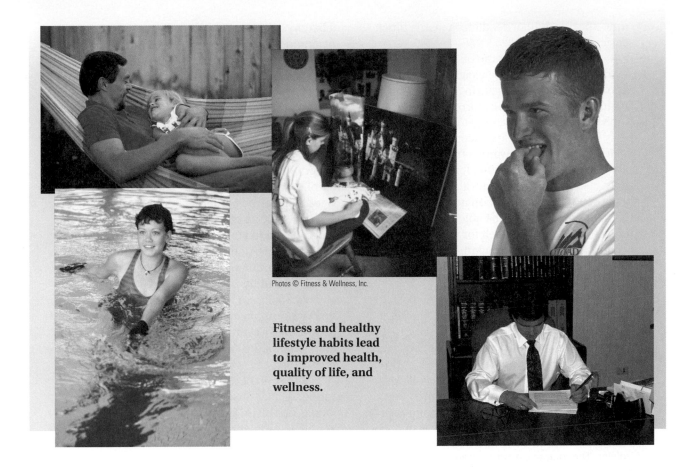

Photos © Fitness & Wellness, Inc.

Fitness and healthy lifestyle habits lead to improved health, quality of life, and wellness.

In spite of only a slight drop in weight during the second year following the calorie-restricted diet, the 2-year follow-up revealed a further decrease in body fat, to 19.5 percent. Patty understood the new quality of life reaped through a sound fitness program, and, at the same time, she finally learned how to apply the principles that regulate weight maintenance.

If you have read and successfully completed all of the assignments set out in this book, including a regular exercise program, you should be convinced of the value of exercise and healthy lifestyle habits in achieving a new quality of life.

Perhaps this new quality of life was explained best by the late Dr. George Sheehan, when he wrote:

> For every runner who tours the world running marathons, there are thousands who run to hear the leaves and listen to the rain, and look to the day when it is all suddenly as easy as a bird in flight. For them, sport is not a test but a therapy, not a trial but a reward, not a question but an answer.

The real challenge will come now: a lifetime commitment to fitness and wellness. To make the commitment easier, enjoy yourself and have fun along the way. Implement your program based on your interests and what you enjoy doing most. Then adhering to your new lifestyle will not be difficult.

Your activities over the last few weeks or months may have helped you develop "positive addictions" that will carry on throughout life. If you truly experience the feelings Dr. Sheehan expressed, there will be no looking back. If you don't get there, you won't know what it's like. Fitness and wellness is a process, and you need to put forth a constant and deliberate effort to achieve and maintain a higher quality of life. Improving the quality of your life, and most likely your longevity, is in your hands. Only you can take control of your lifestyle and thereby reap the benefits of wellness.

Web Interactive

- American College of Sports Medicine (ACSM). This site provides information on sport safety and research projects. This organization is committed to the practical application of sports medicine and exercise science to maintain and enhance physical fitness, health, and quality of life.

  http://www.acsm.org

- The Internet's Fitness Resource. This site features information on fitness products, sport-specific information, and health topics related to exercise. You can also ask a question to an online fitness trainer.

  http://sickbay.com/netsweat

- Fitness Basics—Developing Your Own Exercise Program— Information from the AMA featuring the benefits of exercise, planning and exercise program, exercise safety tips, as well as achieving specific fitness goals.

  http://www.ama-assn.org/insight/gen_hlth/fitness/fitness.htm

- Getting Started with an Exercise Program. This comprehensive site from the Department of Kinesiology and Health from Georgia State University features information on the benefits of exercise, how to choose a personal trainer, exercise safety and precautions, and lots more.

  http://www.gsu.edu/~wwwfit/getstart.html

- National Center for Complementary and Alternative Medicine. The comprehensive site features information about a variety of complementary therapies, geared for consumers, clinical practitioners, and investigators. The site also features a complementary medicine database, clinical trials information, and a list of resources.

  http://altmed.od.nih.gov

Interactive Sites:

- Cooper Fitness Interactive—What Kind of Shape Are You In? This comprehensive site features personalized fitness assessments in each of the following: cardiovascular, body fat, heart rates, strength, flexibility, and basal metabolic rate.

  http://www.cooperfitness.com/content/Profile/UpdateMenu.asp

- Health Calculators by Dr. Koop: Take all 21 quick health risk assessments to learn how to best manage your health and decrease risk factors. Some of the areas covered by these personal health calculators include: diabetes, pregnancy due date, fitness (BMI, target heart rate, calories burned by activity), diet and nutrition (various nutrients), smoking, sleep, stress, HIV risk, and heart disease risk.

  http://www.drkoop.com/tools/calculator

- Life Expectancy: The Longevity Game. This interactive site featuring a series of multiple choice questions related to your personal lifestyle and habits is sponsored by the Northwestern Mutual life Insurance Company.

  http://www.northwesternmutual.com/games/longevity

Notes

1. R. J. Donatelle and L. G. Davis, *Access to Health* (Boston: Allyn and Bacon, 2000).

2. D. M. Eisenberg et al., "Trends in Alternative Medicine Use in the United States, 1990–1997," *Journal of the American Medical Association* 280, no. 18 (1998): 1569–1575.

3. See note 2.

4. See note 2.

Suggested Readings

Roizen, M. F. *Real Age: Are You As Young As You Can Be?* New York: Cliff Street Books, 1999.

Name:	Date:	Grade:
Instructor:	Course:	Section:

Necessary Lab Equipment
None required.

Objective
To estimate the total number of years that you will live and your real physiological age based on your present lifestyle habits.

Instructions
Circle the points to the correct answer to each question. At the end of each page, obtain a net score for that page. Be completely honest with yourself. Your age prediction is based on your lifestyle habits, should you continue those habits for life. Using this questionnaire, you will learn about factors that you can modify or implement that can add years and health to your life. The scoring system is provided at the end of the questionnaire. Please note that the questionnaire is not a precise scientific instrument, but rather an estimated life expectancy analysis according to the impact of lifestyle factors on health and longevity. This questionnaire is not intended to substitute for advice and tests conducted by medical and health care practitioners.

I. Questionnaire

1. What is your current health status?
   A. Excellent   + 2
   B. Good   + 1
   C. Average   0
   D. Fair   − 1
   E. Poor   − 2
   F. Bad   − 3

2. How many days per week do you accumulate 30 minutes of moderate intensity physical activity (50 to 60% of heart rate reserve—see Chapter 7)?
   A. 6 to 7   + 3
   B. 3 to 5   + 1
   C. 1 to 2   0
   D. Less than once per week   − 3

3. How often do you participate in a high-intensity cardio-respiratory exercise (over 60% of heart rate reserve) for at least 20 minutes?
   A. 3 or more times per week   + 2
   B. 2 times per week   + 1
   C. Once a week   − 1
   D. Less than once per week   − 2

4. How often do you perform strength-training exercises per week (a minimum of 8 exercises using 8 to 12 repetitions to near-fatigue on each exercise)?
   A. 1–2 times   + 2
   B. Less than once or less than 8 exercises with 8 to 12 reps per session   0
   C. Do not strength-train   − 1

5. How many times per week do you perform flexibility exercises (at least 15 minutes per stretching session)?
   A. 3 or more   + 1
   B. 1 to 3 times   + .5
   C. Less than 1   0
   D. Do not perform flexibility exercises   − .5

6. How many servings of fruits and vegetables do you eat on a daily basis:
   A. 9 or more   + 3
   B. 6 to 8   + 2
   C. 5   + 1
   D. 3 to 4   0
   E. 2 or less   − 2

7. How many grams of fiber do you consume on an average day?
   A. 25 or over   + 1
   B. Between 13 and 24   0
   C. 10 to 12 or don't know   − 1
   D. Less than 10   − 2

8. As a percentage of total calories, what is your average fat intake on a daily basis?
   A. 20% to 30%   + 1
   B. 30%   0
   C. 30% to 35% or don't know   − 1
   D. Over 35%   − 2

9. As a percentage of total calories, what is your average saturated fat intake on a daily basis?
   A. 5% or less   + 1
   B. More than 5% but less than 10%   0
   C. Don't know   − 1
   D. Over 10%   − 2

10. How many servings of red meat (3 to 6 ounces) do you consume on a weekly basis?
    A. 1 or less   + 1
    B. 2 to 3   0
    C. 4 to 7   − 1
    D. More than 7   − 2

Page score:

*Source: Fitness & Wellness, Inc., Boise, Idaho, ©2000. Reproduced with permission.

11. How many servings of fish (3 to 6 ounces) do you consume on a weekly basis?
   A. 2 or more   + 1
   B. 1   0
   C. None   − 1

12. How many alcoholic drinks (a 12-ounce bottle of beer, a 4-ounce glass of wine, or a 1.5-ounce shot of 80 proof liquor) do you consume per day?
   A. Men 2 or less, women 1 or less   + 1
   B. None   0
   C. Men 3–4, women 2–4   − 1
   D. 5 or more   − 3

13. How many international units of vitamin E do you get from supplements on a daily basis?
   A. 400   + 2
   B. Over 200 but less than 400   + 1
   C. Between 50 and 200   0
   D. None   − 1

14. How many milligrams of vitamin C do you get from food on a daily basis?
   A. Between 250 and 500   + 1
   B. Over 90 but less than 250   +.5
   C. Less than 90   − 1

15. How many micrograms of selenium do you get on a daily basis (preferably from food)?
   A. Between 100 and 200   + 1
   B. Between 50 and 99   +.5
   C. Less than 50   − 1

16. How many milligrams of calcium and how many international units of vitamin D do you get from food and supplements on an average day?
   A. Calcium = 1,200, Vitamin D = 400 or more   + 1
   B. Calcium = 1,200, Vitamin D = unknown   +.5
   C. Calcium = 800 to 1,200, Vitamin D = less than 400   0
   D. Calcium = less than 800, Vitamin D = less than 400   − 1

17. How many times per week do you eat breakfast?
   A. 7   + 1
   B. 5 to 6   +.5
   C. 3 to 5   0
   D. Less than 3   −.5

18. How many cigarettes do you smoke each day?
   A. Never smoked cigarettes or more than 15 years since giving up cigarettes   + 2
   B. None for 5 to 15 years   + 1
   C. None for 1 to 5 years   0
   D. None for 0 to 1 year   − 1
   E. Smoker, less than 1 pack per day   − 3
   F. Smoker, 1 pack per day   − 5
   G. Smoker, up to 2 packs per day   − 7
   H. Smoker, more than 2 packs per day   − 10

19. Do you use tobacco products other than cigarettes?
   A. Never have   0
   B. Less than once per week   − 1
   C. Once per week   − 2
   D. 2 to 6 times per week   − 3
   E. More than 6 times per week   − 5

20. How often are you exposed to secondhand smoke or other environmental pollutants?
   A. Less than 1 hour per month   0
   B. Between 1 and 5 hours per month   − 1
   C. Between 5 and 29 hours per month   − 2
   D. Daily   − 3

21. Do you use addictive drugs, other than tobacco or alcohol?
   A. None   0
   B. 1   − 3
   C. 2 or more   − 5

22. What is the age of your parents (or how long did they live)?
   A. Both over 76   + 3
   B. Only one over 76   + 1
   C. Both are still alive and under 76   0
   D. Only one under 76   − 1
   E. Neither one lived past 76   − 3

23. What is your body composition category (see Table 4.9 in Chapter 4)?
   A. Excellent   + 2
   B. Good   + 1
   C. Average   0
   D. Overweight   − 1
   E. Significantly overweight   − 2

24. What is your blood pressure?
   A. 120/80 or less (both numbers)   + 2
   B. 120–140 or 80–90 (either number)   − 1
   C. Greater than 140/90 (either number)   − 3

25. What is your HDL-cholesterol?
   A. Men greater than 45, women over 55   + 2
   B. Men 35 to 44, women 45 to 54   0
   C. Don't know   − 1
   D. Men less than 35, women below 45   − 2

26. What is your LDL-cholesterol?
   A. Less than 130   + 2
   B. Don't know   − 1
   C. 130 to 159   − 1
   D. 160 or higher   − 2

27. Do you floss and brush your teeth regularly?
   A. Every day   +.5
   B. 3 to 6 days per week   0
   C. Less than 3 days per week   −.5

28. Are you a diabetic?
   A. No   0
   B. Yes, well-controlled   − 1
   C. Yes, poorly or not controlled   − 3

29. How often do you sunbathe (tan)?
   A. Not at all   + 1
   B. Between 1 and 3 times per year   −.5
   C. More than 3 times per year   − 1

30. How often do you wear a seat belt?
   A. All the time   + 1
   B. Most of the time   −.5
   C. Less than half the time   − 1

31. How fast do you drive?
   A. Always at or below the speed limit   0
   B. Up to 5 mph over the speed limit   −.5
   C. Between 5 and 10 mph over the speed limit   − 1
   D. More than 10 mph over the speed limit   − 2

Page score:

32. Do you drink and drive?
    A. Never   0
    B. Yes (even if only once)   − 5

33. In terms of your sexual activity:
    A. I am not sexually active
       or I am in a monogamous
       sexual relationship   + 1
    B. I have more than one
       sexual partner but I always
       practice safer sex   − 1
    C. I have multiple sexual
       partners and I do not
       practice safer sex
       techniques   − 3

34. What is your marital status?
    A. Happily married   + 1
    B. Single and happy   0
    C. Single and unhappy   −.5
    D. Divorced   − 1
    E. Widowed with a belief
       in life hereafter   − 1
    F. Widowed   − 2
    G. Married and unhappy   − 2

35. On the average, how many
    hours of sleep do you get
    each night?
    A. 7 to 8   + 1
    B. 7   0
    C. 6 to 7   − 1
    D. Less than 6   − 2

36. Your stress rating according
    to the Life Experiences Survey
    (see Lab 11A) is:
    A. Excellent   + 1
    B. Good   0
    C. Average   −.5
    D. Fair   − 1
    E. Poor   − 2

37. Your Type A behavior rating
    (see Lab 11A) is:
    A. Low   0
    B. Medium   − 1
    C. High   − 2

38. When under stress (distress),
    how often do you practice stress
    management techniques?
    A. Always   + 1
    B. Most of the time   +.5
    C. Not applicable (don't
       suffer from stress)   0
    D. Sometimes   − 1
    E. Never   − 2

39. Do you suffer from depression?
    A. Not at all   0
    B. Mild depression   − 1
    C. Severe depression   − 2

40. How often do you associate
    with people who have a
    positive attitude about life?
    A. Always   +.5
    B. Most of the time   0
    C. About half of the time   −.5
    D. Less than half the time   − 1

41. Do you have close family or
    personal relationships whom
    you can trust and rely on for
    help in times of need?
    A. Yes   + 1
    B. No   − 1

42. Do you feel loved and can
    you routinely give affection
    and love?
    A. Yes   + 1
    B. No   − 1

43. Do you have a good sense
    of humor?
    A. Yes   + 1
    B. No   − 1

44. How satisfied are you with
    your school work?
    A. Satisfied   +.5
    B. It's okay   0
    C. Not satisfied   −.5

45. How do you rate your
    present job satisfaction?
    A. Love it   + 1
    B. Like it   0
    C. It's okay   −.5
    D. Don't like it   − 1
    E. Hate it   − 2
    F. Not applicable   0

46. How do you rate yourself
    spiritually?
    A. Very spiritual   + 1
    B. Spiritual   0
    C. Somewhat spiritual   −.5
    D. Not spiritual at all   − 1

Page score:

Net score for all questions:

How To Score

To estimate the total number of years that you will live, (a) determine a net score by totaling the results from all 46 questions, (b) obtain an age change score by multiplying the net score by the age correction factor given below, and (c) add or subtract this number from your base life expectancy age (73 for men and 80 for women—the current life expectancies in the United States). For example, if you are a 20-year-old male and the net score from the answers to all questions was –16, your estimated life expectancy would be 68.2 years (age change score = –16 × .3 = –4.8, life expectancy = 73 – 4.8 = 68.2).

You can also determine your real physiological age by subtracting a positive age-change score or adding a negative age-change score to your current chronological (calendar) age. For instance, in the previous example, the real physiological age would be 24.8 years (20 + 4.8). If the age change score had been +4.8, the real physiological age would have been 16.2 years. Thus, a healthy lifestyle will always make your physiological age younger than your chronological age. Your real physiological age will have much greater significance in middle and older age, when it is not uncommon to see real-age reductions of 10 to 25 years in people who lead healthy lifestyles. Thus a 50-year-old person could easily have a real physiological age of 30.

Age Correction Factor (ACF)*

Age	ACF
≤30	.3
31–40	.4
41–50	.5
51–60	.6
61–70	.6
71–80	.5
81–90	.4
≥91	.3

*Adapted from: M. F. Roizen, *RealAge*, New York: Cliff Street Books, 1999.

Age Change Score (ACS) = _____ (net score) × _____ (ACF) = _____

Life expectancy

Men = 73 ± _____ (ACS) = _____ years

Women = 80 ± _____ (ACS) = _____ years

Real physiological Age**

Men = _____ (your age) ± _____ (ACS) = _____ years

Women = _____ (your age) ± _____ (ACS) = _____ years

**Subtract a positive ACS from, or add a negative ACS to, your current age.

State your feelings about the experience of taking this questionnaire, analyze your results, and list lifestyle factors that you can work on that will positively affect your health and longevity.

_____
_____
_____
_____
_____
_____
_____
_____
_____
_____
_____
_____
_____

Lab
16B

SELF-EVALUATION AND BEHAVIORAL OBJECTIVES FOR THE FUTURE

Name: _____   Date: _____   Grade: _____

Instructor: _____   Course: _____   Section: _____

Necessary Lab Equipment
None required unless fitness tests are repeated.

Objective
To conduct a self-evaluation of the goals achieved in this course and to write behavioral objectives for the future.

Lab Preparation
Read the section on self-evaluation and behavioral objectives for the future in this chapter (pp. 409–410). If time allows and technicians are available, repeat the assessments for the health-related components of fitness.

I. Fitness Evaluation

Conduct a self-evaluation of the fitness goals you accomplished in this course. Fill in the required information on the health-related fitness components below. If you were unable to repeat your fitness assessments, subjectively determine how well you reached your goals.

1. Did you accomplish your objective for:

    Cardiorespiratory Endurance (see Lab 6A)   ☐ Yes ☐ No

    Pre-assessment VO_{2max}: _____ ml/kg/min   Fitness Classification: _____

    Post-assessment VO_{2max}: _____ ml/kg/min   Fitness Classification: _____

    Body Composition (see Labs 4A and 4B)   ☐ Yes ☐ No

    Pre-assessment Percent Body Fat: _____   Body Composition Classification: _____

    Post-assessment Percent Body Fat: _____   Body Composition Classification: _____

    Muscular Strength and Endurance (see Lab 8A)   ☐ Yes ☐ No

    Pre-assessment Percentile Rank: _____   Fitness Classification: _____

    Post-assessment Percentile Rank: _____   Fitness Classification: _____

    Muscular Flexibility (see Lab 9A)   ☐ Yes ☐ No

    Pre-assessment Percentile Rank: _____   Fitness Classification: _____

    Post-assessment Percentile Rank: _____   Fitness Classification: _____

2. Explain the exercise program that you implemented in this course, indicate your feelings about the outcomes of this program, and evaluate how well you accomplished your fitness goals.

    _____
    _____
    _____
    _____
    _____
    _____
    _____

II. Wellness Evaluation

Using the Wellness Compass, rate yourself for each component and plan goals and objectives for the future according to the following instructions:

1. Color in red a number from 5 to 1 to indicate where you stood on each component at the beginning of the semester (5 = poor rating, 1 = excellent or ideal rating).
2. Color in blue a second number from 5 to 1 to indicate where you stand on each component at the present time.
3. Select one or two components that you intend to work on in the next 2 months. Start with components in which you think you will have a high chance for success. Color in yellow the intended objective (number) to accomplish by the end of the 2 months. Once you achieve your objective, you later may color another number, also in yellow, to indicate your next objective.

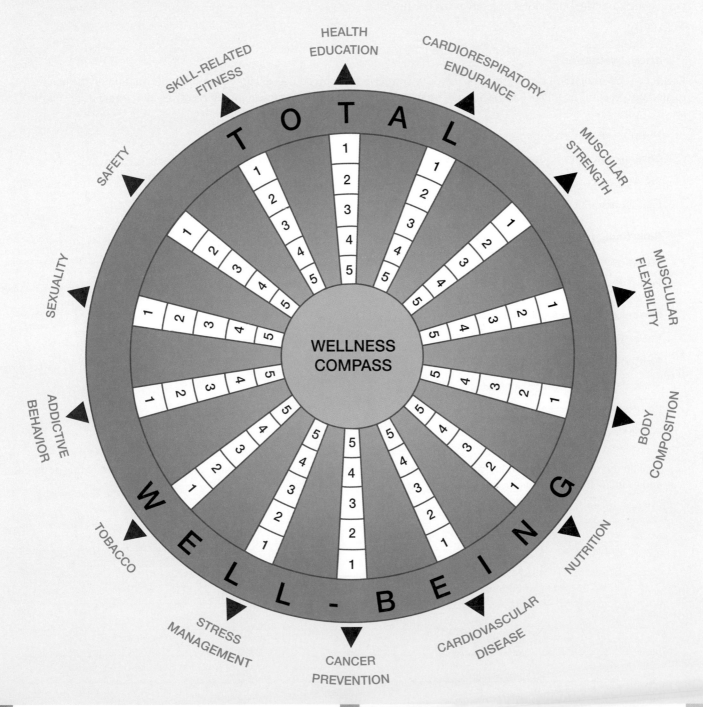

1. List nutritional or dietary changes that you were able to implement this term and the effects of these changes on your body composition and personal wellness.

_____
_____
_____
_____
_____
_____
_____
_____

2. List other lifestyle changes that you were able to make this term that may decrease your risk for disease. In a few sentences, explain how you feel about these changes and their impact on your overall well-being.

_____
_____
_____
_____
_____
_____
_____
_____
_____
_____
_____
_____
_____
_____
_____
_____
_____
_____

III. Behavioral Goals for the Future

Identify one or two goals you will work on during the next couple of months and write specific objectives that you will use to accomplish each goal (you may not need six objectives; write only as many as needed).

Goal: _____

Objectives:

1. _____
2. _____
3. _____
4. _____
5. _____
6. _____

Goal: _____

Objectives:

1. _____
2. _____
3. _____
4. _____
5. _____
6. _____

IV. This Course and Your Future Lifestyle

Briefly evaluate this course and its impact on your quality of life. Indicate what you feel will be needed for you to continue to adhere to an active and healthy lifestyle.

_____
_____
_____
_____
_____
_____
_____
_____
_____

Nutritive Value of Selected Foods

Food	Amount	Weight (g)	Calo-ries	Pro-tein (g)	Fat (g)	Sat. Fat (g)	Choles-terol (g)	Carbo-hydrate (g)	Fiber (g)	Cal-cium (mg)	Iron (mg)	Sodium (mg)	Vit A (IU)	Thia-min (Vit B₁) (mg)	Ribo-flavin (Vit B₂) (mg)	Niacin (mg)	Vit C (mg)	Folate (mcg)
Apples, fresh, w/peel, lrg	1 ea	150	88	0.3	1	0.1	0	23	4.1	10	0.3	0	80	0.03	0.02	0.1	9	4.2
Applesauce, swtnd, w/o salt, cnd	1 cup	255	194	0.5	0	0.1	0	51	3.1	10	0.9	8	28	0.03	0.07	0.5	4	1.53
Apricots, pitted, fresh, whole	3 ea	114	55	1.6	0	0	0	13	2.7	16	0.6	1	2978	0.03	0.05	0.7	11	9.8
Apricots, w/skin, in heavy syrup, cnd, whole	½ cup	120	100	0.6	0	0	0	26	1.9	11	0.4	5	1476	0.02	0.03	0.5	4	2.04
Asparagus, spears, ckd w/o salt	4 ea	60	14	1.6	0	0	0	3	1	12	0.4	7	323	0.07	0.08	0.6	6	87.6
Avocado, Calif, fresh	½ ea	120	212	2.5	21	3.1	0	8	5.9	13	1.4	14	734	0.13	0.15	2.3	9	78.6
Bagel, plain, 3½" diameter	1 ea	68	187	7.1	1	0.1	0	36	1.6	50	2.4	363	0	0.37	0.21	3.1	0	59.84
Banana, fresh, med	1 ea	140	129	1.4	1	0.3	0	33	3.4	8	0.4	1	113	0.06	0.14	0.8	13	26.74
Bar, granola, hard	1 ea	24	113	2.4	5	0.6	0	15	1.3	15	0.7	71	36	0.06	0.03	0.4	0	5.52
Beans, black, mature, ckd w/o salt	1 cup	172	227	15.2	1	0.2	0	41	15	46	3.6	2	10	0.42	0.1	0.9	0	255.9
Beans, chickpea/garbanzo, mature, ckd	1 cup	164	269	14.5	4	0.4	0	45	12.5	80	4.7	11	44	0.19	0.1	0.9	2	282.0
Beans, frijoles/refried, cnd	½ cup	145	136	8	2	0.7	12	23	7.7	51	2.4	434	0	0.04	0.02	0.5	9	15.95
Beans, green, snap/string, ckd	½ cup	65	23	1.2	2	0	0	5	2.1	30	0.8	2	433	0.05	0.06	0.4	6	21.64
Beans, kidney, red, mature, cnd	1 cup	185	157	9.7	1	0.1	0	29	11.8	44	2.3	631	0	0.19	0.16	0.8	2	93.61
Beans, lima, fordhook, immature, ckd f/fzn w/o salt, drained	½ cup	85	85	5.2	0	0.1	0	16	4.9	19	1.2	45	162	0.06	0.05	0.9	11	18.02
Beans, mung, mature, sprouted, raw	½ cup	52	16	1.6	0	0	0	3	0.9	7	0.5	3	11	0.04	0.06	0.4	7	31.62
Beans, pinto, mature, ckd w/o salt	1 cup	171	234	14	1	0.2	0	44	14.7	82	4.5	3	3	0.32	0.16	0.7	4	294.1
Beef, chuck arm pot roast, brsd, choice, ¼" trim	3 oz	85	296	22.9	22	8.6	84	0	0	8	2.6	50	0	0.06	0.2	2.7	0	7.65
Beef, corned, cnd	3 oz	85	212	23	13	5.3	73	0	0	10	1.8	855	0	0.02	0.12	2.1	0	7.65
Beef, ground, hamburger patty, brld, well done, 16% fat	3 oz	85	225	24.3	13	5.3	84	0	0	8	2.4	70	0	0.06	0.27	5	0	9.35
Beef, ground, hamburger patty, brld, well done, 18% fat	3 oz	85	238	24	15	5.9	86	0	0	10	2.1	76	0	0.05	0.2	5.1	0	9.35
Beef, liver, fried	3 oz	85	184	22.7	7	2.3	410	7	0	9	5.3	90	30689	0.18	3.52	12.3	20	187
Beef, T-bone steak, brld, choice, ¼" trim	3 oz	85	263	19.7	20	7.7	57	0	0	7	2.3	54	3	0.08	0.18	3.4	4	5.95
Beef, top sirloin steak, lean, brld, choice, ¼" trim	3 oz	85	172	25.8	7	2.6	76	0	0	9	2.9	56	0	0.11	0.25	3.6	0	8.5
Beer	12 fl-oz	360	148	1.1	0	0	0	13	0.7	18	0.1	18	0	0.02	0.09	1.6	0	21.6
Beer, light	12 fl-oz	354	99	0.7	0	0	0	5	0	18	0.1	11	0	0.03	0.11	1.4	0	14.51
Beets, cnd, drained, diced	½ cup	80	25	0.7	0	0	0	6	1.4	12	1.5	155	9	0.01	0.03	0.1	3	24.16
Biscuits, homemade	1 ea	35	124	2.5	6	1.5	1	16	0.5	82	1	203	29	0.12	0.11	1	0	21.35
Blueberries, fresh, bilberries	½ cup	73	41	0.5	0	0	0	13	2	4	0.1	4	73	0.04	0.04	0.3	9	4.67
Brandy, 86 proof	1 oz	28	70	0	0	0	0	0	0	0	0	0	0	0	0	0	0	0
Bread, banana, prep f/recipe w/veg shortening	1 pce	50	169	2.2	6	1.5	22	28	0.7	9	0.7	99	46	0.09	0.1	0.7	1	5.5
Bread, cracked wheat	1 pce	25	65	2.2	1	0.2	0	12	1.4	11	0.7	134	0	0.09	0.06	0.9	0	15.25
Bread, French	1 pce	35	96	3.1	1	0.2	0	18	1	26	0.9	213	0	0.18	0.12	1.7	0	33.25
Bread, mixed grain	1 pce	26	65	2.6	1	0.2	0	12	1.7	24	0.9	127	0	0.11	0.09	1.1	0	20.8
Bread, pita pocket, white	1 ea	60	165	5.5	1	0.1	0	33	1.3	52	1.6	322	0	0.36	0.2	2.8	0	57
Bread, pumpernickel	1 pce	32	80	2.8	1	0.1	0	15	2.1	22	0.9	215	0	0.1	0.1	1	0	25.6
Bread, rye	1 pce	25	65	2.1	1	0.2	0	12	1.5	18	0.7	165	2	0.11	0.08	1	0	21.5
Bread, white, f/recipe w/2% milk	1 pce	25	71	2	1	0.3	1	12	0.5	14	0.7	90	20	0.1	0.1	0.9	0	22.75
Bread, whole wheat	1 pce	25	62	2.4	1	0.2	0	12	1.7	18	0.8	132	0	0.09	0.05	1	0	12.5
Broccoli, med stalk, 8" long, ckd w/o add salt	1 ea	140	39	4.2	0	0.1	0	7	4.1	64	1.2	36	1943	0.08	0.16	0.8	104	70
Broccoli, spear, raw, 5" long	1 ea	114	32	3.4	0	0.1	0	6	3.4	55	1	31	1758	0.07	0.14	0.7	106	80.94
Brownie, chocolate, w/walnuts, prep f/rec	1 ea	20	93	1.2	6	1.5	15	10	0.4	11	0.4	69	153	0.03	0.04	0.2	0	5.8
Brussels Sprouts, ckd, drained	½ cup	78	30	2	0	0.1	0	7	2	28	0.9	16	561	0.08	0.06	0.5	48	46.8
Buns, hamburger	1 ea	40	114	3.4	2	0.5	0	20	1.1	56	1.3	224	0	0.19	0.12	1.6	0	38

Food	Amount	Weight (g)	Calo-ries	Pro-tein (g)	Fat (g)	Sat. Fat (g)	Choles-terol (g)	Carbo-hydrate (g)	Fiber (g)	Cal-cium (mg)	Iron (mg)	Sodium (mg)	Vit A (IU)	Thia-min (Vit B_1) (mg)	Ribo-flavin (Vit B_2) (mg)	Niacin (mg)	Vit C (mg)	Folate (mcg)
Buns, hot dog/frankfurter	1 ea	40	114	3.4	2	0.5	0	20	1.1	56	1.3	224	0	0.19	0.12	1.6	0	38
Burger/Patty, vegetarian, Gardenburger, original	1 ea	71	130	8	3	1	11	18	5	84	0	290	50	0.11	0.15	1.1	0	10.08
Burger/Patty, vegetarian, soy	1 ea	71	142	14.9	6	1	0	6	3.3	21	1.5	390	0	0.64	0.43	7.1	0	55.38
Butter, salted	1 Tbs	5	36	0	4	2.5	11	0	0	1	0	41	153	0	0	0	0	0.15
Buttermilk, skim, cultured	1 cup	245	99	8.1	2	1.3	9	12	0	285	0.1	257	81	0.08	0.38	0.1	2	12.25
Cabbage, ckd w/o add salt, drained, shredded	½ cup	85	19	0.9	0	0	0	4	2	26	0.1	7	112	0.05	0.05	0.2	17	17
Cabbage, raw, shredded	½ cup	45	11	0.6	0	0	0	2	1	21	0.3	8	60	0.02	0.02	0.1	14	19.35
Cake, angel food, cmrcl prep	1 pce	60	155	3.5	0	0.1	0	35	0.9	84	0.3	449	0	0.06	0.29	0.5	0	21
Cake, carrot, w/cream cheese icing	1 pce	96	419	4.4	25	4.7	52	45	1.2	24	1.2	236	3310	0.13	0.15	1	1	11.52
Cake, chocolate, w/chocolate icing, 1/8th	1 pce	69	253	2.8	11	3.3	29	38	1.9	30	1.5	230	59	0.02	0.09	0.4	0	11.73
Cake, devils food, marshmallow iced	1 pce	99	408	3.5	21	5.8	52	52	1.2	47	1.3	338	0				0	
Cake, pound, w/butter	1 pce	30	116	1.7	6	3.5	66	15	0.1	10	0.4	119	182	0.04	0.07	0.4	0	12.3
Cake, white, w/chocolate icing	1 pce	71	259	1.8	8	3.7	13	46	0.8	55	0.5	219	166	0.05	0.07	0.3	0	2.11
Calamari/Squid, fried, mixed species	1 cup	150	262	26.9	11	2.8	390	12	0	58	1.5	459	52	0.08	0.69	3.9	6	21
Candy Bar, Almond Joy, fun size	1½ oz	42	196	1.8	11	7.3	2	24	2	26	0.6	61	5	0.01	0.06	0.2	0	
Candy Bar, Mars almond	1 ea	50	234	4.1	12	3.6	8	31	1	84	0.6	85	94	0.02	0.16	0.5	0	9.5
Candy Bar, Milky Way, 2.1 oz bar	1 ea	60	254	2.7	10	4.7	8	43	1	78	0.5	144	65	0.02	0.13	0.2	1	6
Candy Bar, Special Dark sweet chocolate	1 ea	41	226	2	13	8.3	0	25	2	11	1	3	14	0.01	0.03	0.2	0	0.82
Candy, caramels, plain/chocolate	1 oz	28	107	1.3	2	1.8	2	22	0.3	39	0	69	9	0	0.05	0.1	0	1.4
Candy, hard, all flvrs	1 oz	28	110	0	0	0	0	27	0	1	0.1	11	0	0	0	0	0	0
Candy, Kisses, milk chocolate	1 oz	28	144	1.9	9	5.2	6	17	1	53	0.4	23	52	0.02	0.08	0.1	0	2.24
Candy, M & M's peanut chocolate	1 oz	28	144	2.7	7	2.9	3	17	1	28	0.3	13	26	0.03	0.05	1	0	9.8
Candy, M & M's plain chocolate	1 oz	28	138	1.2	6	3.7	4	20	0.7	29	0.3	17	57	0.02	0.06	0.1	0	1.68
Candy, milk chocolate, w/almonds	1 oz	28	147	2.5	10	4.8	5	15	1.7	63	0.5	21	21	0.02	0.12	0.2	0	3.36
Carrots, ckd w/o add salt, drained, slices	½ cup	73	33	0.8	0	0	0	8	2.4	23	0.5	48	17924	0.02	0.04	0.4	2	10.15
Carrots, raw, whole, 7½" long	1 ea	81	35	0.8	0	0	0	8	2.4	22	0.4	28	22784	0.08	0.05	0.8	8	11.34
Catsup/Ketchup	1 Tbs	15	16	0.2	0	0	0	4	0.2	3	0.1	178	152	0.01	0.01	0.2	2	2.25
Cauliflower, ckd, drained	½ cup	63	14	1.2	0	0	0	3	1.7	10	0.2	9	11	0.03	0.03	0.3	28	27.72
Celery, raw, med stalk, 8" long	1 ea	40	6	0.3	0	0	0	1	0.7	16	0.2	35	54	0.02	0.02	0.1	3	11.2
Cereal, 100% Bran, rte, dry	½ cup	33	89	4.1	2	0.3	0	24	9.8	23	4.1	229	0	0.79	0.89	10.5	31	23.43
Cereal, All-Bran, rte, dry	¼ cup	21	55	2.6	1	0.1	0	16	6.8	74	3.1	43	525	0.27	0.29	3.5	10	63
Cereal, Alpha-Bits, rte, dry	1 cup	28	110	2.2	1	0.1	0	24	1.2	8	2.7	178	1235	0.36	0.42	4.9	0	98.84
Cereal, bran flakes, rte, dry	¾ cup	30	96	2.8	1	0.1	0	24	5.3	17	8.1	220	750	0.38	0.43	5	0	99.9
Cereal, Cheerios	1 cup	23	84	2.4	1	0.3	0	18	2	42	6.2	218	958	0.29	0.33	3.8	12	76.59
Cereal, Chex, corn, rte, dry	1 cup	28	105	2	0	0.1	0	24	0.5	94	8.4	270	0	0.35	0	4.7	6	93.24
Cereal, Chex, wheat, rte, dry	1 cup	46	159	4.8	1	0.2	0	37	5.1	92	13.8	412	0	0.34	0.06	4.6	6	92
Cereal, corn flakes, rte, dry	1 cup	25	91	1.6	0	0.1	0	22	0.7	1	7.8	266	625	0.32	0.35	4.2	12	88.25
Cereal, Corn Pops, rte, dry	1 cup	28	107	1	0	0.1	0	26	0.4	2	1.7	111	700	0.36	0.39	4.7	14	98.84
Cereal, Cream of Wheat, quick, ckd w/water	1 cup	244	132	3.7	0	0.1	0	27	1.2	51	10.5	142	0	0.24	0	1.5	0	109.8
Cereal, Crispy Rice, rte, dry	¾ cup	22	87	1.4	0	0	0	19	0.3	4	0.6	161	971	0.41	0.46	5.4	12	108.6
Cereal, Frosted Flakes, rte, dry	1 cup	35	135	1.4	0	0.1	0	32	0.7	1	5.1	226	847	0.42	0.49	5.6	17	105
Cereal, Frosted Mini Wheats, rte, dry	1 cup	55	186	5.2	1	0.2	0	45	5.9	20	15.4	2	0	0.38	0.44	5.4	0	110
Cereal, granola, rte, dry	½ cup	57	257	6	10	1.3	0	38	3.6	43	1.8	92	0	0.18	0.06	0.6	0	8.55
Cereal, Grape Nuts, rte, dry	½ cup	57	205	6.2	1	0.2	0	46	5	19	15.9	348	737	0.37	0.42	4.9	0	98.04
Cereal, Honey Bran, rte, dry	½ cup	30	102	2.6	1	0.2	0	25	3.3	14	4.8	173	1323	0.39	0.45	5.3	16	20.1
Cereal, Life, plain, rte, dry	1 cup	44	167	4.3	2	0.3	0	35	2.8	134	12.3	240	16	0.55	0.62	7.3	0	146.9
Cereal, Mueslix, five grain muesli, rte, dry	1 cup	82	289	6.2	5	0.7	0	63	5.6	67	8.9	107	2488	0.75	0.84	9.8	1	196.8
Cereal, Nutri-Grain, wheat, rte, dry	1 oz	28	101	2.4	0	0.1	0	24	1.8	8	0.8	190	0	0.36	0.42	4.9	15	98.84
Cereal, oatmeal, unsalted, ckd w/water	½ cup	120	74	3.1	1	0.2	0	13	2	10	0.8	1	19	0.13	0.02	0.2	0	4.8

Food	Amount	Weight (g)	Calories	Protein (g)	Fat (g)	Sat. Fat (g)	Choles- terol (g)	Carbo- hydrate (g)	Fiber (g)	Cal- cium (mg)	Iron (mg)	Sodium (mg)	Vit A (IU)	Thia- min (Vit B₁) (mg)	Ribo- flavin (Vit B₂) (mg)	Niacin (mg)	Vit C (mg)	Folate (mcg)
Cereal, raisin bran, rte, dry	1 cup	49	155	3.9	1	0.1	0	38	6.4	22	9	299	623	0.31	0.35	4.2	0	82.81
Cereal, Shredded Wheat, sml biscuits, rte, dry	1 cup	19	68	2.1	0	0.1	0	15	1.9	7	0.8	2	0	0.05	0.05	1	0	9.5
Cereal, Smacks, rte, dry	1 cup	37	141	2.4	1	0.4	0	32	1.3	4	2.5	70	1028	0.52	0.59	6.8	21	136.9
Cereal, Special K, rte, dry	1 cup	21	78	4.3	0	0	0	15	0.7	3	5.9	169	508	0.36	0.4	4.7	10	63
Cereal, Total, wheat, rte, dry	1 cup	33	116	3.3	1	0.2	0	26	2.9	284	19.8	218	1375	1.65	1.87	22.1	66	439.8
Cereal, Wheaties, rte, dry	1 cup	29	106	3.1	1	0.2	0	23	2	53	7.8	215	725	0.36	0.41	4.8	14	96.57
Cheese Puffs/Cheetos	1 oz	28	155	2.1	10	1.8	1	15	0.3	16	0.7	294	74	0.07	0.1	0.9	0	33.6
Cheese Spread, low fat, low sod	1 pce	34	61	8.4	2	1.5	12	1	0	233	0.1	2	92	0.01	0.13	0	0	3.06
Cheese, American, proc, shredded	1 oz	28	105	6.2	9	5.5	26	0	0	172	0.1	401	339	0.01	0.1	0	0	2.18
Cheese, blue	1 oz	28	99	6	8	5.2	21	1	0	148	0.1	391	202	0.01	0.11	0.3	0	10.19
Cheese, cheddar, diced	1 oz	28	113	7	9	5.9	29	0	0	202	0.2	174	297	0.01	0.11	0	0	5.1
Cheese, feta	1 oz	28	74	4	6	4.2	25	1	0	138	0.2	313	125	0.04	0.24	0.3	0	8.96
Cheese, monterey jack, shredded	1 oz	28	105	6.9	8	5.3	25	0	0	209	0.22	150	266	0	0.11	0	0	5.1
Cheese, mozzarella, part skm milk, low moist, shredded	1 oz	28	78	7.7	5	3	15	1	0	205	0.1	148	197	0.01	0.1	0	0	2.77
Cheese, parmesan, grated	1 Tbs	5	23	2.1	2	1	4	0	0	69	0	93	35	0	0.02	0	0	0.4
Cheese, ricotta, part skm	1 oz	28	39	3.2	2	1.4	9	1	0	76	0.1	35	121	0.01	0.05	0	0	3.67
Cheese, Swiss, shredded	1 oz	28	105	8	8	5	26	1	0	269	0	73	237	0.01	0.1	0	0	1.79
Cheesecake	1 pce	85	273	4.7	19	8.4	47	22	0.4	43	0.5	176	465	0.02	0.16	0.2	0	15.3
Cherries, sweet, fresh	10 ea	75	54	0.9	1	0.2	0	12	1.7	11	0.3	70	160	0.04	0.04	0.3	5	3.15
Chicken, broiler/fryer, breast, rstd	1 ea	98	193	29.2	8	2.1	82	0	0	14	1	70	91	0.06	0.12	12.5	0	3.92
Chicken, broiler/fryer, dark meat, w/o skin, rstd	3 oz	85	174	23.3	8	2.3	79	0	0	13	1.1	79	61	0.06	0.19	5.6	0	6.8
Chicken, broiler/fryer, drumstick, rstd	1 ea	52	112	14.1	6	1.6	47	0	0	6	0.7	47	52	0.04	0.11	3.1	0	4.16
Chicken, broiler/fryer, meat only, w/o skin, rstd	3 oz	85	162	24.6	6	1.7	76	0	0	13	1	73	45	0.06	0.15	7.8	0	5.1
Chips, corn	1 oz	28	151	1.8	9	1.3	0	16	1.4	36	0.4	176	26	0.01	0.04	0.3	0	5.6
Chips, tortilla, chili & lime	18 pce	28	110	2	2	0	0	22	2	60	3.6	200	0				0	
Chips, tortilla, plain	1 oz	28	140	2	7	1.4	0	18	1.8	43	0.4	148	55	0.02	0.05	0.4	0	2.8
Cod, batter fried	3½ oz	100	173	17.4	8	1.6	50	7	0.2	29	0.7	91	30	0.07	0.1	2.3	2	8.71
Cod, stmd/poached	3½ oz	100	102	22.4	1	0.1	46	0	0	4	0.3	80	28	0.02	0.05	2.2	3	6.6
Coffee, brewed	¾ cup	180	4	0.2	0	0	0	1	0	4	0.1	4	0	0	0	0.4	0	0.18
Collards, ckd w/o add salt	½ cup	95	25	2	0	0	0	5	2.7	113	0.4	9	2973	0.04	0.1	0.5	17	88.35
Cone, ice cream, wafer/cake type	1 ea	115	480	9.3	8	1.4	0	91	3.4	29	4.1	164	0	0.29	0.41	5.1	0	117.3
Cookie, chocolate chip, prep w/marg f/rec	2 ea	20	98	1.1	6	1.6	6	12	0.6	8	0.5	72	127	0.04	0.04	0.3	0	6.6
Cookie, chocolate sandwich, creme filled	4 ea	40	189	1.9	8	1.5	0	28	1.3	10	1.6	242	1	0.03	0.07	0.8	0	17.2
Cookie, fig bar	4 ea	56	195	2.1	4	0.6	0	40	2.6	36	1.6	196	18	0.09	0.12	1	0	15.12
Cookie, oatmeal raisin, prep f/rec	2 ea	26	113	1.7	4	0.8	9	18	0.8	26	0.7	140	167	0.06	0.04	0.3	0	7.8
Cookie, peanut butter, prep f/rec	2 ea	24	114	2.2	6	1.1	7	14	0.5	9	0.5	124	144	0.05	0.05	0.8	0	13.2
Cookie, shortbread, cmrcl, plain	4 ea	32	161	2	8	2	6	21	0.6	11	0.9	146	28	0.11	0.11	1.1	0	18.88
Cookie, vanilla, wafer type, 12–17% fat	10 ea	40	176	2	6	1.5	20	29	0.8	19	1	125	11	0.11	0.13	1.2	0	20
Coriander, raw	¼ cup	4	1	0.1	0	0	0	0	0.1	4	0.1	1	111	0	0	0	1	0.41
Corn, yellow, vac pack, cnd	½ cup	83	66	2	0	0.1	0	16	1.7	4	0.3	226	200	0.03	0.06	1	7	40.92
Cornbread, prep f/dry mix	1 ea	60	188	4.3	6	1.6	37	29	1.4	44	1.1	467	123	0.15	0.16	1.2	0	33
Cornmeal, yellow, degermed, enrich, dry	½ cup	120	439	10.2	2	0.3	0	93	8.9	6	5	4	496	0.86	0.49	6	0	224.4
Cottage Cheese, 2% fat	½ cup	113	101	15.5	2	1.4	9	3	0	77	0.2	459	79	0.03	0.21	0.2	0	14.8
Cottage Cheese, creamed, sml curd	½ cup	105	109	13.1	5	3	16	3	0	63	0.1	425	171	0.02	0.17	0.1	0	12.81
Crab, blue, cnd, drained	1 cup	135	134	27.7	2	0.3	120	0	0	136	1.1	450	7	0.11	0.11	1.8	4	57.38
Crackers, cheese	1 ea	10	50	1	3	0.9	1	6	0.2	15	0.5	100	16	0.06	0.04	0.5	0	8
Crackers, graham, plain/honey, 2½ square	2 ea	14	59	1	1	0.2	0	11	0.4	3	0.5	85	0	0.03	0.04	0.6	0	8.4
Crackers, matzoh, plain, svg	1 ea	28	111	2.8	0	0.1	0	23	0.8	4	0.9	1	0	0.11	0.08	1.1	0	32.76

Food	Amount	Weight (g)	Calories	Protein (g)	Fat (g)	Sat. Fat (g)	Cholesterol (mg)	Carbohydrate (g)	Fiber (g)	Calcium (mg)	Iron (mg)	Sodium (mg)	Vit A (IU)	Thiamin (Vit B1) (mg)	Riboflavin (Vit B2) (mg)	Niacin (mg)	Vit C (mg)	Folate (mcg)
Crackers, rye, wafers	2 ea	14	47	1.3	0	0	0	11	3.2	6	0.8	111	1	0.06	0.04	0.2	0	6.3
Crackers, saltine	1 ea	11	48	1	1	0.3	0	8	0.3	13	0.6	143	0	0.06	0.05	0.6	0	13.64
Crackers, standard, reg snack type, round	1 ea	3	15	0.2	1	0.1	0	2	0.5	4	0.1	25	0	0.01	0.01	0.1	0	2.31
Crackers, triscuit	1 ea	5	24	0.5	1	0.2	0	3	0.5	1	0.2	26	0	0.01	0.01	0.1	0	0.36
Crackers, wheat	1 ea	2	9	0.2	0	0.1	0	1	0.1	1	0.1	16	0	0	0.06	0	0	3.7
Cream Cheese	1 oz	28	98	2.1	10	6.2	31	1	0	22	0.3	83	400	0	0.06	0	0	0.34
Cream, light	1 Tbs	15	29	0.4	3	1.8	10	1	0	14	0	6	95	0	0.02	0	0	0.56
Cream, whipping, heavy	1 Tbs	15	52	0.3	6	3.5	21	0	0	10	0	6	221	0	0.02	0	0	
Croissant, butter	1 ea	57	231	4.7	12	6.6	38	26	1.5	21	1.2	424	424	0.22	0.14	1.2	0	35.34
Cucumber, w/o skin, raw, sliced	½ cup	60	7	0.3	0	0	0	2	0.4	8	0.1	1	44	0.01	0.01	0.1	2	8.4
Dates, fresh, whole	10 ea	83	228	1.6	0	0.2	0	61	6.2	27	1	2	42	0.07	0.08	1.8	0	10.46
Dinner, chicken, cacciatore, w/noodles, low cal, fzn	1 ea	308	311	22.5	10	2.4	59	33	3.4	29	3.2	934	732	0.28	0.4	8	26	32.22
Doughnut, cake	1 ea	47	198	2.3	11	1.7	17	23	0.7	21	0.9	257	27	0.1	0.11	0.9	0	22.09
Doughnut, raised, glazed	1 ea	60	242	3.8	14	3.5	4	27	0.7	26	1.2	205	8	0.22	0.13	1.7	0	25.8
Egg Substitute, Egg Beaters, new	¼ cup	61	30	6	0	0	0	1	0	20	1.1	125	300	0	0.85	0	0	32.0
Egg Whites, raw	1 ea	33	16	3.5	0	0	0	0	0	2	0.6	54	0	0.03	0.15	0	0	0.99
Egg Yolks, raw, lrg	1 ea	17	61	2.8	5	1.6	212	0	0	23	0.6	7	331	0.03	0.11	0	0	24.82
Eggs, hard ckd/bld, lrg	1 ea	50	78	6.3	5	1.6	212	1	0	25	0.6	62	280	0.03	0.26	0	0	22
Eggs, scrambled, plain, lrg	1 ea	64	106	7.1	8	2.4	225	1	0	45	0.8	179	436	0.03	0.28	0.1	0	19.2
Eggs, whole, fried	1 ea	46	92	6.2	7	1.9	211	1	0	25	0.7	162	394	0.03	0.24	0	0	17.48
Entree, lasagna, w/meat, prep f/rec	1 pce	220	352	20.7	14	7.2	52	36	2.5	243	2.8	351	902	0.21	0.3	3.8	13	17.82
Entree, macaroni & cheese, prep f/rec w/margarine	½ cup	100	215	8.4	11	4.4	21	20	0.6	181	0.9	543	430	0.1	0.2	0.9	0	5.15
Entree, meatloaf, beef	1 pce	111	232	20.2	14	5.6	107	5	0.2	37	2.1	185	148	0.06	0.28	3.3	1	14.28
Entree, quiche, lorraine	1 pce	242	724	20.5	56	25.9	304	34	1	318	2.6	303	1323	0.36	0.67	2.8	1	26.48
Entree, spaghetti, w/meatballs, prep f/rec	1 cup	248	332	18.6	12	3.3	74	39	7.7	124	3.7	1009	1587	0.25	0.3	4	22	9.99
Entree, spaghetti, w/tomato sauce & cheese, prep f/rec	1 cup	250	260	8.8	9	2	8	37	2.5	80	2.2	955	1075	0.25	0.17	2.2	12	8
Figs, dried, unckd	1 ea	21	54	0.6	0	0	0	14	2.5	30	0.5	2	28	0.01	0.02	0.1	0	1.57
Fish Sticks/Portions, heated f/fzn, 4x1x.5	2 ea	56	152	8.8	7	1.8	63	13	0	11	0.4	326	59	0.07	0.1	1.2	0	10.19
Flour, all purpose, white, bleached, enrich	1 cup	125	455	12.9	1	0.2	0	95	3.4	19	5.8	6	0	0.98	0.62	7.4	0	192.5
Flour, whole wheat	1 cup	120	407	16.4	2	0.4	0	87	14.6	41	4.7	6	0	0.54	0.26	7.6	0	52.8
Frankfurter/Hot Dog, beef & pork, 10 pack	1 ea	57	182	6.4	17	6.1	28	1	0	6	0.7	638	0	0.11	0.07	1.5	0	2.28
Frankfurter/Hot Dog, beef, 8 pack	1 ea	57	180	6.8	16	6.9	35	1	0	11	0.8	585	0	0.03	0.06	1.4	0	2.28
Frankfurter/Hot Dog, turkey	1 ea	45	102	6.4	8	2.7	48	1	0	48	0.8	642	0	0.02	0.08	1.9	0	3.6
Frozen Yogurt, vanilla/strawberry, nonfat, sml scoop	4 oz	113	112	5.6	0	0.1	2	22	0	196	0.1	75	7	0.05	0.23	0.1	1	11.99
Fruit Cocktail, in heavy syrup, cnd	1 cup	245	179	1	0	0	0	46	2.5	15	0.7	15	502	0.04	0.05	0.9	5	6.37
Fruit Cocktail, in juice	1 cup	248	114	1.1	0	0	0	29	2.5	20	0.5	10	756	0.03	0.04	1	7	6.2
Fruit Punch, prep f/pwd	1 cup	240	89	0	0	0	0	23	0.2	38	0.1	34	0	0	0	0	28	0.24
Fudge, chocolate, prep f/rec	1 oz	28	107	0.5	2	1.4	4	22	0	12	0.1	17	53	0	0.02	0	0	0.56
Grapefruit, pink, fresh, 3¾" diameter	½ ea	123	37	0.7	0	0	0	9	1.7	14	0.1	0	319	0.04	0.02	0.2	47	15.01
Grapes, tokay/empress/red flame, fresh	10 ea	50	36	0.3	0	0.1	0	9	0.5	6	0.1	1	36	0.05	0.03	0.2	5	1.95
Haddock, fillet, brd, fried	3 oz	85	184	17.1	9	1.9	65	7	0.2	53	1.5	145	69	0.08	0.09	3.7	0	11.6
Halibut, Greenland, fillet, bkd/brld	3 oz	85	203	15.7	15	2.6	50	0	0	3	0.7	88	51	0.06	0.09	1.6	0	0.85
Honey, strained, extracted	1 Tbs	21	64	0.1	0	0	0	17	0	1	0.1	1	0	0	0.01	0	0	0.42
Hot Cocoa/Choc, prep f/rec w/whole milk	1 cup	250	192	9.8	6	3.6	20	29	2	315	1.1	128	515	0.1	0.44	0.4	2	15
Hummus/Hummos, raw	1 cup	246	421	12.1	21	3.1	0	50	12.5	123	3.9	600	62	0.23	0.13	1	19	146.1
Instant Breakfast, prep f/dry mix w/nonfat milk	1 cup	282	216	15.7	1	0.7	9	36	0.2	407	4.8	268	2343	0.4	0.42	5.5	31	118.2

Food	Amount	Weight (g)	Calories	Protein (g)	Fat (g)	Sat. Fat (g)	Cholesterol (g)	Carbohydrate (g)	Fiber (g)	Calcium (mg)	Iron (mg)	Sodium (mg)	Vit A (IU)	Thiamin (Vit B_1) (mg)	Riboflavin (Vit B_2) (mg)	Niacin (mg)	Vit C (mg)	Folate (mcg)
Instant Breakfast, prep f/dry mix w/whole milk	1 cup	281	280	15.4	9	5.4	38	36	0.2	396	4.9	262	2151	0.41	0.47	5.5	31	117.7
Jam/Preserves, pkt	1 ea	14	39	0.1	0	0	0	10	0.2	3	0.1	4	2	0	0	0	1	4.62
Jelly	1 Tbs	18	51	0	0	0	0	13	0.2	1	0.5	5	3	0	0	0.1	0	0.18
Juice, apple, unswtnd, cnd/btld	½ cup	124	58	0.1	0	0	0	14	0.1	9	0.5	4	1	0.03	0.02	0.1	1	0.12
Juice, cranberry cocktail	1 cup	253	144	0	0	0	0	36	0.3	8	0.4	5	10	0.02	0.02	0.1	90	0.51
Juice, grape, unswtnd, btld/cnd	½ cup	127	77	0.7	0	0	0	19	0.1	11	0.3	4	10	0.03	0.05	0.3	0	3.3
Juice, grapefruit, unswtnd, cnd	½ cup	124	47	0.6	0	0	0	11	0.1	9	0.2	1	9	0.05	0.02	0.3	36	12.9
Juice, grapefruit, unswtnd, prep f/fzn conc	1 cup	247	101	1.4	0	0	0	24	0.2	20	0.3	2	22	0.1	0.05	0.5	83	8.89
Juice, lemon, fresh	1 Tbs	15	4	0.1	0	0	0	1	0.1	1	0	0	3	0	0	0	7	1.94
Juice, orange, prep f/fzn	½ cup	125	56	0.9	0	0	0	13	0.2	11	0.1	1	98	0.1	0.02	0.3	49	54.75
Juice, prune, w/o pulp	½ cup	88	60	0.7	0	0	0	14	0.5	2	0.9	4	54				3	
Juice, tomato, w/salt, cnd	1 cup	244	41	1.9	0	0	0	10	1	22	1.4	881	1357	0.11	0.08	1.6	45	48.56
Kale, ckd w/o add salt, drained	½ cup	55	15	1	0	0	0	3	1.1	40	0.5	13	4070	0.03	0.04	0.3	23	7.32
Kiwifruit/Chinese Gooseberries, fresh, med	1 ea	76	46	0.8	0	0	0	11	2.6	20	0.3	4	133	0.02	0.04	0.4	74	28.88
Lamb, leg, whole, lean, rstd, choice, ¼" trim	3 oz	85	162	24.1	7	2.3	76	0	0	7	1.8	58	0	0.09	0.25	5.4	0	19.55
Lamb, loin chop, lean, brld, choice, ¼" trim	3 oz	84	181	25.2	8	2.9	80	0	0	16	1.7	71	0	0.09	0.24	5.8	0	20.16
Lemonade, white, fzn conc	12 oz	340	615	1	1	0.1	0	160	1.4	24	2.4	14	0	0.09	0.33	0.3	60	34
Lentils, sprouts, stir fried	1 cup	124	125	10.9	1	0.1	0	26	4.8	17	3.8	12	51	0.27	0.11	1.5	16	83.08
Lentils, unsalted, ckd	1 cup	200	232	18	1	0.1	0	40	15.8	38	6.7	4	16	0.34	0.15	2.1	3	361.6
Lettuce, butterhead, Boston/bibb, leaf, raw	2 pce	15	2	0.2	0	0	0	0	0.2	5	0	1	146	0.01	0.01	0.1	1	11
Lettuce, romaine, raw, chpd	1 cup	55	8	0.9	0	0	0	1	0.9	20	0.6	4	1430	0.06	0.06	0.3	13	74.64
Lobster, northern, stmd	1 cup	145	142	29.7	1	0.2	104	2	0	88	0.6	551	126	0.01	0.1	1.6	0	16.1
Lunchmeat Spread, liverwurst, cnd	1 oz	28	87	3.6	7	2.5	33	2	0.5	3	2.3	193	3818	0.05	0.04	0.7	1	1.4
Lunchmeat, bologna, beef & pork	1 pce	28	88	3.3	8	3	15	2	0	3	0.4	285	0	0.05	0.09	2	0	3.99
Lunchmeat, bologna, turkey	2 pce	57	113	7.8	9	2.9	56	1	0	48	0.9	500	0	0.03	0.09		0	
Lunchmeat, roast beef, deli style, pouch	3 oz	85	96	17.2	3	1.1	41	1	0	5	1.6	860	0				0	
Lunchmeat, turkey breast, rstd, fat free	1 pce	28	24	4.2	0	0.1	9	1	0	3	0.3	334	0				0	
Mayonnaise, imit, low cal	1 Tbs	15	35	0.1	3	0.5	4	2	0	1	0	75	14	0	0	0	0	
Mayonnaise, soybean oil, w/salt	1 tsp	5	36	0.1	4	0.6	3	0	0	1	0	28	0	0	0	0	0	0.38
Melon, cantaloupe/musk, med 5" diameter	¼ ea	239	84	2.1	1	0.2	0	20	1.9	26	0.5	22	7705	0.09	0.05	1.4	101	40.63
Melon, honeydew, fresh, wedge, 1/8 melon	1 pce	129	45	0.6	0	0	0	12	0.8	8	0.1	13	52	0.1	0.02	0.8	32	7.74
Milk Shake, chocolate, fast food	10 fl-oz	340	432	11.6	13	7.9	44	70	2.7	384	1.1	330	316	0.2	0.83	0.5	1	11.9
Milk, evaporated, whole, w/add vit A, cnd	½ cup	126	169	8.6	10	5.8	37	13	0	329	0.2	133	500	0.06	0.4	0.2	2	9.95
Milk, low fat, 1%, w/add vit A	1 cup	244	102	8	2	1.6	10	12	0	300	0.1	123	500	0.1	0.41	0.2	2	12.44
Milk, low fat, 2%, chocolate	1 cup	250	179	8	5	3.1	17	26	1.2	284	0.6	150	500	0.09	0.41	0.3	2	12
Milk, low fat, 2%, w/add vit A	1 cup	244	121	8.1	5	2.9	18	12	0	297	0.1	122	500	0.1	0.4	0.2	2	12.44
Milk, nonfat/skim, w/add vit A	1 cup	245	86	8.4	0	0.3	4	12	0	302	0.1	126	500	0.09	0.34	0.2	2	12.74
Milk, whole, 3.3%	1 cup	244	150	8	8	5.1	33	11	0	291	0.1	120	307	0.09	0.4	0.2	2	12.2
Milkshake, strawberry, fast food	10 fl-oz	340	384	11.6	10	5.9	37	64	1.4	384	0.4	282	408	0.15	0.66	0.6	3	10.2
Mixed Vegetables, cnd, drained	1 cup	182	86	4.7	1	0.1	0	17	5.5	49	1.9	271	21198	0.08	0.09	1.1	9	42.95
Muffin, English, plain	1 ea	57	134	4.4	1	0.1	0	26	1.5	99	1.4	264	0	0.25	0.16	2.2	0	46.17
Muffin, English, plain, tstd	1 ea	52	133	4.4	1	0.1	0	26	1.5	98	1.4	262	0	0.2	0.14	2	0	38.48
Muffin, wheat bran, prep f/rec w/whole milk	1 ea	45	130	3.2	6	1.2	16	19	3.2	84	1.9	265	363	0.15	0.2	1.8	4	23.4
Mushrooms, raw, pces/slices	1 cup	35	9	1	0	0	0	1	0.4	2	0.4	1	0	0.03	0.15	1.4	1	4.2
Mustard Greens, ckd w/o add salt, drained	½ cup	70	10	1.6	0	0	0	1	1.4	52	0.5	11	2122	0.03	0.04	0.3	18	51.38
Nuts, almonds, dried, unblanched, whole	¼ cup	36	208	7.7	18	1.4	0	7	4.2	89	1.5	0	4	0.09	0.29	1.4	0	10.44
Nuts, Brazil, dried, shelled, 32 kernels	1 oz	28	184	4	19	4.5	0	4	1.5	49	1	1	0	0.28	0.03	0.5	0	1.12
Nuts, cashews, dry rstd, salted	1 cup	137	786	21	63	12.5	0	45	4.1	62	8.2	877	0	0.27	0.27	1.9	0	94.8
Nuts, coconut, unswtnd, dried	½ cup	65	429	4.5	42	37.2	0	16	10.6	17	2.2	24	0	0.04	0.06	0.4	1	5.85

Food	Amount	Weight (g)	Calories	Protein (g)	Fat (g)	Sat. Fat (g)	Cholesterol (g)	Carbohydrate (g)	Fiber (g)	Calcium (mg)	Iron (mg)	Sodium (mg)	Vit A (IU)	Thiamin (Vit B$_1$) (mg)	Riboflavin (Vit B$_2$) (mg)	Niacin (mg)	Vit C (mg)	Folate (mcg)
Nuts, peanuts, oil rstd, unsalted, chpd	1 oz	28	163	7.4	14	1.9	0	5	1.9	25	0.5	2	0	0.07	0.03	4	0	35.2
Nuts, pecans, dried, halves	1 oz	28	193	2.6	20	1.7	0	4	2.7	20	0.7	0	22	0.18	0.04	0.3	0	6.16
Nuts, walnuts, black, dried, chpd	1 oz	28	170	6.8	16	1	0	3	1.4	16	0.9	0	83	0.06	0.03	0.2	1	18.34
Oil, canola	1 cup	218	1927	0	218	15.5	0	0	0	0	0	0	0	0	0	0	0	0
Oil, corn	1 Tbs	15	133	0	15	1.9	0	0	0	0	0.1	0	0	0	0	0	0	0
Oil, olive	1 Tbs	15	133	0	15	2	0	0	0	0	0.1	0	0	0	0	0	0	0
Oil, peanut	1 cup	216	1909	0	216	36.5	0	0	0	0	0	0	0	0	0	0	0	0
Oil, safflower, greater than 70% linoleic	1 Tbs	15	133	0	15	0.9	0	0	0	0	0	0	0	0	0	0	0	0
Oil, soybean	1 tsp	5	44	0	5	0.7	0	0	0	0	0	0	0	0	0	0	0	0
Okra, bindi, ckd w/o add salt f/raw, drained, pods	8 ea	85	27	1.6	0	0	0	6	2.1	54	0.4	4	489	0.11	0.05	0.7	14	38.85
Olives, w/o pits, ripe, lrg, cnd	10 ea	44	51	0.4	5	0.6	0	3	1.4	39	1.5	384	177	0	0	0	0	0
Olives, w/o pits, ripe, sml, cnd	10 ea	32	37	0.3	3	0.5	0	2	1	28	1.1	279	129	0	0	0	1	0
Onions, yellow, ckd w/o add salt, drained, chpd	½ cup	105	46	1.4	0	0	0	11	1.5	23	0.3	3	0	0.04	0.02	0.2	5	15.75
Oranges, fresh, med	1 ea	180	85	1.7	0	0	0	21	4.3	72	0.2	0	369	0.16	0.07	0.5	96	54.54
Oysters, eastern, brd, fried, med	1 ea	45	89	3.9	6	1.4	36	5	0.1	28	3.1	188	136	0.07	0.09	0.7	2	13.95
Oysters, eastern, raw, wild	½ cup	120	82	8.5	3	0.9	64	5	0	54	8	253	120	0.12	0.11	1.7	4	12
Pancake, buckwheat, prep f/incomplete dry mix, 4"	1 ea	27	56	2.1	2	0.5	18	8	0.6	69	0.5	144	63	0.05	0.07	0.4	0	4.59
Pancake, plain, homemade, 4"	1 ea	73	166	4.7	7	1.5	43	21	1.1	160	1.3	320	143	0.15	0.21	1.1	0	27.74
Papaya, fresh, med	½ ea	227	89	1.4	0	0.1	0	22	4.1	54	0.2	7	645	0.06	0.07	0.8	140	86.26
Pasta, egg noodles, enrich, ckd	½ cup	80	106	3.8	1	0.2	26	20	0.9	10	1.3	6	16	0.15	0.07	1.2	0	51.2
Pasta, macaroni noodles, enrich, ckd	½ cup	70	99	3.3	0	0.1	0	20	0.9	5	1	1	0	0.14	0.07	1.2	0	49
Pasta, spaghetti noodles, enrich, salted, ckd	1 cup	140	197	6.7	1	0.1	0	40	2.4	10	2	140	0	0.29	0.14	2.3	0	98
Pasta, spaghetti noodles, whole wheat, ckd	1 cup	125	155	6.7	1	0.1	0	33	5.6	19	1.3	4	0	0.14	0.06	0.9	0	6.25
Pastry, cinnamon danish	1 ea	110	443	7.7	25	6.2	23	49	1.4	78	2.2	408	13	0.33	0.29	3.2	0	68.2
Peaches, fresh, sliced	½ cup	85	37	0.6	0	0	0	9	1.7	4	0.1	0	455	0.01	0.03	0.8	6	2.89
Peaches, in heavy syrup, cnd	½ tsp	96	71	0.4	0	0	0	19	1.2	3	0.3	6	319	0.01	0.02	0.6	3	3.07
Peaches, in juice, cnd, whole	½ tsp	77	34	0.5	0	0	0	9	1	5	0.2	3	293	0.01	0.01	0.4	3	2.62
Peanut Butter, smooth, salted	1 Tbs	32	190	8.1	16	3.3	0	6	1.9	12	0.6	149	0	0.03	0.03	4.3	0	23.68
Pears, bartlett, fresh, med	1 ea	180	106	0.7	1	0	0	27	4.3	20	0.4	0	36	0.04	0.07	0.2	7	13.14
Pears, in heavy syrup, cnd, halves	½ ea	103	76	0.2	0	0	0	20	1.6	5	0.2	5	0	0.01	0.02	0.2	1	1.24
Pears, in juice, cnd, halves	½ ea	77	38	0.3	0	0	0	10	1.2	7	0.2	3	5	0.01	0.01	0.2	1	0.92
Peas, cnd, drained	½ cup	85	59	3.8	0	0.1	0	11	3.5	17	0.8	214	653	0.1	0.07	0.6	8	37.65
Peas, green, ckd f/fzn w/o add salt, drained	½ cup	80	62	4.1	0	0	0	11	4.4	19	1.3	70	534	0.23	0.08	1.2	8	46.88
Peppers, bell, green, sweet, raw, med	1 ea	200	54	1.8	0	0.1	0	13	3.6	18	0.9	4	1264	0.13	0.06	1	179	44
Peppers, bell, red, sweet, raw, sml	1 ea	74	20	0.7	0	0	0	5	1.5	7	0.3	1	4218	0.05	0.02	0.4	141	16.28
Peppers, bell, yellow, sweet, raw, lrg	1 ea	186	50	1.9	0	0.1	0	12	1.7	20	0.9	4	443	0.05	0.05	1.7	341	48.36
Pickles, dill	1 ea	135	24	0.8	0	0.1	0	6	1.6	12	0.7	1731	444	0.02	0.04	0.1	3	1.35
Pickles, sweet, med	1 ea	35	41	0.1	0	0	0	11	0.4	1	0.2	329	44	0.01	0.01	0.1	0	0.35
Pie, apple, bkd f/fzn, 1/6th of 8"	1 pce	118	280	2.2	13	4.5	0	40	1.9	13	0.5	314	146	0.03	0.03	0.3	4	25.96
Pie, bluberry, prep f/rec, 1/8th of 9"	1 pce	158	387	4.3	19	4.6	0	53	2.2	11	1.9	292	66	0.24	0.21	1.9	1	36.34
Pie, cherry, prep f/rec, 1/8th of 9"	1 pce	118	319	3.3	14	3.5	0	45	1.8	12	2.2	225	483	0.17	0.15	1.5	1	31.86
Pie, chocolate cream, rts, 1/6th of 8"	1 pce	175	532	4.5	34	8.7	9	59	3.5	63	1.9	238	0	0.06	0.19	1.2	0	22.75
Pie, lemon meringue, rts, 1/6th of 8"	1 pce	140	375	2.1	12	2.5	63	66	1.7	78	0.9	204	245	0.09	0.29	0.9	4	18.2
Pie, pecan, rts, 1/6th of 8"	1 pce	138	552	5.5	26	4.9	44	79	4.8	23	1.4	585	242	0.13	0.17	0.3	2	37.26
Pie, pumpkin, rts, 1/6th of 8"	1 pce	114	239	4.4	11	2	23	31	3.1	68	0.9	321	3915	0.06	0.17	0.2	1	22.8
Pineapple, chunks, fresh	½ cup	78	38	0.3	0	0	0	10	0.9	5	0.3	1	18	0.07	0.03	0.3	12	8.27
Pineapple, in heavy syrup, cnd, tidbits	½ cup	128	100	0.4	0	0	0	26	1	18	0.5	1	18	0.12	0.03	0.4	9	5.89
Pineapple, in juice, cnd	½ cup	125	75	0.5	0	0	0	20	1	18	0.3	1	48	0.12	0.02	0.4	12	6
Popcorn, air popped, plain	1 cup	6	23	0.7	0	0	0	5	0.9	1	0.2	0	12	0.01	0.02	0.1	0	1.38

Food	Amount	Weight (g)	Calories	Protein (g)	Fat (g)	Sat. Fat (g)	Cholesterol (mg)	Carbohydrate (g)	Fiber (g)	Calcium (mg)	Iron (mg)	Sodium (mg)	Vit A (IU)	Thiamin (Vit B₁) (mg)	Riboflavin (Vit B₂) (mg)	Niacin (mg)	Vit C (mg)	Folate (mcg)
Popcorn, ckd in oil, salted	1 cup	11	55	1	3	0.5	0	6	1.1	1	0.3	97	17	0.01	0.01	0.2	0	1.87
Pork, bacon/cracklings, brld/pan fried/rstd	2 pce	15	86	4.6	7	2.6	13	0	0	2	0.2	239	0	0.1	0.04	1.1	0	0.75
Pork, cured, ham, reg, 11% fat, rstd	3 oz	85	151	19.2	8	2.7	50	0	0	7	1.1	1275	0	0.62	0.28	5.2	0	2.55
Pork, ham, whole, rstd	3 oz	85	232	22.8	15	5.5	80	0	0	12	0.9	51	8	0.54	0.27	3.9	0	8.5
Pork, ribs, spareribs, brsd	3 oz	85	337	24.7	26	9.5	103	0	0	40	1.6	79	8	0.35	0.32	4.7	0	3.4
Potato Chips, plain, salted	10 pce	20	107	1.4	7	2.2	0	11	0.9	5	0.3	119	0	0.03	0.04	0.8	6	9
Potatoes, au gratin, prep w/milk & butter f/dry mix	1 cup	245	228	5.6	10	6.3	37	31	2.2	203	0.8	1076	522	0.05	0.2	2.3	8	16.17
Potatoes, baked, w/flesh & skin, long	1 ea	202	220	4.6	0	0.1	0	51	4.8	20	2.7	16	0	0.22	0.07	3.3	26	22.22
Potatoes, hash browns, prep f/fzn	½ cup	78	170	2.5	9	3.5	0	22	1.6	12	1.2	27	0	0.09	0.02	1.9	5	5.07
Potatoes, mashed, w/whole milk	½ cup	105	81	2	1	0.3	2	18	2.1	27	0.3	318	20	0.09	0.04	1.2	7	8.61
Potatoes, sweet, flesh, bkd in skin, med, peeled	1 ea	146	150	2.5	0	0	0	35	4.4	41	0.7	15	31860	0.11	0.19	0.9	36	33
Pretzels, hard, salted, twisted	1 oz	28	107	2.5	1	0.2	0	22	0.9	10	1.2	480	0	0.13	0.17	1.5	0	47.88
Prunes, dried	5 ea	61	146	1.6	0	0	0	38	4.3	31	1.5	2	1212	0.05	0.1	1.2	2	2.26
Pudding, choc, rte, 5oz can	5 oz	142	189	3.8	6	1	4	32	1.4	128	0.7	183	51	0.04	0.22	0.5	3	4.26
Pudding, tapioca, 5oz can	5 oz	142	169	2.8	5	0.9	1	28	0.1	119	0.3	226	0	0.03	0.14	0.4	1	4.26
Pudding, vanilla, 5oz can	5 oz	142	185	3.3	5	0.8	10	31	0.1	125	0.2	192	30	0.03	0.2	0.4	1	0
Raisins, seedless, unpacked	1 oz	28	84	0.9	1	0	0	22	1.1	14	0.6	3	2	0.04	0.02	0.2	1	0.92
Raspberries, fresh	1 cup	123	60	1.1	1	0	0	14	8.3	27	0.7	0	160	0.04	0.11	1.1	31	31.98
Raspberries, swtnd, fzn	1 cup	250	400	10	15	9.1	12	62	5.5	368	3.1	245	400	0.09	0.53	0.8	1	27.5
Rice, brown, ckd	½ cup	96	107	2.5	1	0.2	0	22	1.7	10	0.4	5	0	0.09	0.02	1.5	0	3.84
Rice, white, reg, ckd	½ cup	103	134	2.8	0	0.1	0	29	0.4	10	1.2	1	0	0.17	0.01	1.5	0	59.74
Rice, wild, ckd	½ cup	100	101	4	0	0	0	21	1.8	3	0.6	3	0	0.05	0.09	1.3	0	26
Rolls, hard, white	1 ea	50	146	4.9	2	0.3	0	26	1.1	48	1.6	272	0	0.24	0.17	2.1	0	47.5
Salad Dressing, blue cheese/roquefort	1 Tbs	15	76	0.7	8	1.5	3	1	0	12	0.1	164	32	0	0.02	0	0	1.21
Salad Dressing, french	1 Tbs	16	69	0.1	7	1.5	0	3	0	2	0.1	219	208	0	0	0	0	0.67
Salad Dressing, French, low cal	1 Tbs	15	20	0	1	0.1	0	3	0	2	0.1	118	195	0	0	0	0	0
Salad Dressing, Italian	1 Tbs	15	70	0.1	7	1.1	0	2	0	2	0	118	12	0	0	0	0	0.73
Salad Dressing, Italian, diet, 2cal/tsp, cmrcl	1 Tbs	15	16	0	1	0.2	1	1	0	0	0	118	0	0	0	0	0	0
Salad Dressing, ranch	1 Tbs	15	80	0	8	1.2	5	0	0	0	0	105	0	0	0	0	0	0
Salad Dressing, thousand island	1 Tbs	15	57	0.1	5	0.9	4	2	0.2	2	0.1	105	48	0	0	0	0	0.94
Salad Dressing, thousand island, low cal	1 Tbs	15	24	0.1	2	0.2	2	2	0.2	2	0.1	150	48	0	0	0	0	0.84
Salad, chicken, w/celery	½ cup	78	268	10.6	25	3.1	48	1	0.2	16	0.6	201	155	0.03	0.07	3.3	1	8.46
Salad, pasta, garden primavera, prep f/dry	¾ cup	142	280	8	12	2.5	2	34	2	80	1.8	730	200	0.15	0.17	2	1	
Salad, potato	½ cup	125	179	3.4	10	1.8	85	14	1.6	24	0.8	661	261	0.1	0.07	1.1	12	8.38
Salad, tuna	1 cup	205	383	32.9	19	3.2	27	19	0	35	2	824	199	0.06	0.14	13.7	5	16.4
Salami, beef & pork, dry	1 oz	28	117	6.4	10	3.4	22	1	0	2	0.4	521	0	0.17	0.08	1.4	0	0.56
Salmon, pink, w/bone, cnd, not drained	3 oz	85	118	16.8	5	1.3	47	0	0	181	0.7	471	47	0.02	0.16	5.6	0	13.09
Salmon, sockeye, fillet, bkd/brld	3 oz	85	184	23.2	9	1.6	74	0	0	6	0.5	56	178	0.18	0.15	5.7	0	4.25
Salsa, homemade, Mexican sauce	1 Tbs	15	3	0.1	0	0	0	1	0.2	1	0	1	57	0.01	0	0.1	2	1.74
Sandwich, bacon, lettuce & tomato, on soft white	1 ea	130	323	10.8	18	4.7	22	30	1.7	54	2.1	619	271	0.36	0.2	3.4	12	35.5
Sandwich, egg salad, on soft white	1 ea	111	361	9.1	24	4.2	149	29	1.2	67	2.1	499	239	0.25	0.3	1.9	0	35.39
Sandwich, peanut butter & jam, on soft white, unsalted	1 ea	100	348	11.5	15	3.1	2	46	3	60	2.2	290	2	0.27	0.17	5.3	0	40.04
Sandwich, reuben, grilled	1 ea	237	458	27.6	29	9.8	80	25	2.2	286	4.2	1933	453	0.21	0.34	2.8	13	37.79
Sardines, Atlantic, w/bones, cnd in oil, drained	1 oz	28	58	6.9	3	0.4	40	0	0	107	0.8	141	63	0.02	0.06	1.5	0	3.3
Sauce, soy, made f/soy & wheat	1 Tbs	16	9	1.3	0	0	0	1	0.1	3	0.3	871	0	0.01	0.03	0.4	0	2.56
Sauce, teriyaki, rts	1 Tbs	18	15	1.1	0	0	0	3	0	4	0.3	690	0	0.01	0.01	0.2	0	3.6
Sauerkraut, w/liquid, cnd	½ cup	118	22	1.1	0	0	0	5	2.9	35	1.7	780	21	0.02	0.03	0.2	17	27.97

Food	Amount	Weight (g)	Calories	Protein (g)	Fat (g)	Sat. Fat (g)	Cholesterol (g)	Carbohydrate (g)	Fiber (g)	Calcium (mg)	Iron (mg)	Sodium (mg)	Vit A (IU)	Thiamin (Vit B_1) (mg)	Riboflavin (Vit B_2) (mg)	Niacin (mg)	Vit C (mg)	Folate (mcg)
Sausage, pork, smkd, link	1 ea	68	265	15.1	22	7.7	46	1	0	20	0.8	1020	0	0.48	0.17	3.1	1	3.4
Scallops, brd, fried, mixed species, lrg	2 ea	31	67	5.6	3	0.8	19	3	0	13	0.3	144	23	0.01	0.03	0.5	1	11.47
Seaweed, spirulina, dried	1 cup	119	345	68.4	9	3.2	0	28	4.3	143	33.9	1247	678	2.83	4.37	15.3	12	111.8
Shrimp/Prawns, brd, fried, lrg	7 ea	85	206	18.2	10	1.8	150	10	0.3	57	1.1	292	161	0.11	0.12	2.6	1	6.89
Shrimp/Prawns, ckd, lrg	3 oz	85	84	17.8	1	0.2	166	0	0	33	2.6	190	186	0.03	0.03	2.2	2	2.98
Soda, cola	12 fl-oz	369	151	0	0	0	0	38	0	11	0.1	15	0	0	0	0	0	0
Soda, cola/Coke, diet, w/sacc, low sod	12 fl-oz	340	0	0	0	0	0	0	0	14	0.1	54	0	0	0	0	0	0
Soda, ginger ale	12 fl-oz	366	124	0	0	0	0	32	0	11	0.7	26	0	0	0	0	0	0
Soda, lemon lime	12 fl-oz	340	136	0	0	0	0	35	0	7	0.2	37	0	0	0	0.1	0	0
Soda, root beer	12 fl-oz	340	139	0	0	0	0	36	0	17	0.2	44	0	0	0	0	0	0
Sole/Flounder, fillet, bkd/brld	3 oz	85	99	20.5	1	0.3	58	0	0	15	0.3	89	32	0.07	0.1	1.9	0	7.82
Soup, beef bouillon/broth, cnd, prep w/water	1 cup	240	17	2.7	1	0.3	0	0	0	14	0.4	782	0	0	0.05	1.9	0	4.8
Soup, chicken noodle, prep w/water	1 cup	241	75	4	2	0.7	7	9	0.7	17	0.8	1106	711	0.05	0.06	1.4	0	21.69
Soup, clam chowder, Manhattan, prep f/cnd	1 cup	244	112	12.3	2	0	10	11	3.1	41	1.8	725	2297				4	
Soup, clam chowder, New England, prep w/milk	1 cup	248	164	9.5	7	3	22	17	1.5	186	1.5	992	164	0.07	0.24	1	3	9.67
Soup, cream of chicken, prep w/milk	1 cup	248	191	7.5	11	4.6	27	15	0.2	181	0.7	1047	714	0.07	0.26	0.9	1	7.69
Soup, cream of mushroom, prep w/milk	1 cup	245	201	6	13	5.1	20	15	0.5	176	0.6	906	152	0.08	0.28	0.9	2	9.8
Soup, minestrone, prep w/water	1 cup	241	82	4.3	3	0.6	2	11	1	34	0.9	911	2338	0.05	0.04	0.9	1	36.15
Soup, pea, split, w/ham, prep w/water	1 cup	245	184	10	4	1.7	7	27	2.2	22	2.2	975	431	0.14	0.07	1.4	1	2.45
Soup, tomato, prep w/milk	1 cup	248	161	6.1	6	2.9	17	22	2.7	159	1.8	744	848	0.13	0.25	1.5	68	20.83
Soup, tomato, prep w/water	1 cup	245	86	2.1	2	0.4	0	17	0.5	12	1.8	698	691	0.09	0.05	1.4	67	14.7
Soup, vegetable beef, prep w/water	1 cup	245	78	5.6	2	0.9	5	10	0.5	17	1.1	794	1899	0.04	0.05	1	2	10.54
Soup, vegetable, vegetarian, prep w/water	1 cup	250	75	2.2	2	0.3	0	12	0.5	22	1.1	852	3118	0.05	0.05	0.9	2	11
Sour Cream, cultured	1 Tbs	14	30	0.4	3	1.8	6	1	0	16	0	7	111	0	0.02	0	0	1.51
Spinach, ckd w/o add salt, drained	½ cup	103	24	3.1	0	0	0	4	2.5	140	3.7	72	8436	0.1	0.24	0.5	10	150.1
Spinach, raw, chpd	1 cup	55	12	1.6	0	0	0	2	1.5	54	1.5	43	3693	0.04	0.1	0.4	15	106.9
Spinach, w/o add salt, cnd, drained	½ cup	103	24	2.9	1	0.1	0	4	2.5	131	2.4	28	9039	0.02	0.14	0.4	15	100.7
Squash, acorn, ckd	1 cup	245	83	1.6	0	0	0	22	6.4	64	1.4	7	632	0.25	0.02	1.3	16	27.69
Squash, summer, ckd w/o add salt, drained	½ cup	90	18	0.8	0	0.1	0	4	1.3	24	0.3	1	258	0.04	0.04	0.5	5	18.09
Squash, winter, avg, bkd, mashed	½ cup	103	40	0.9	1	0.1	0	9	2.9	14	0.3	1	3664	0.09	0.02	0.7	10	28.84
Strawberries, fresh, whole	1 cup	149	45	0.9	1	0	0	10	3.4	21	0.6	1	40	0.03	0.1	0.3	84	26.37
Strawberries, slices, swtnd, fzn	1 cup	250	240	1.3	0	0	0	65	4.8	28	1.5	8	60	0.04	0.13	1	104	37.25
Stuffing, bread, prep f/dry mix	½ cup	70	125	2.2	6	1.2	0	15	2	22	0.8	380	219	0.1	0.07	1	0	70.7
Sugar, beet/cane, brown, packed	1 tsp	5	19	0	0	0	0	5	0	4	0.1	2	0	0	0	0	0	0.05
Sugar, white, granulated	1 tsp	4	15	0	0	0	0	4	0	0	0	0	0	0	0	0	0	0
Syrup, maple	1 Tbs	20	52	0	0	0	0	13	0	13	0.2	2	0	0	0	0	0	0
Taco Shells	1 ea	10	47	0.7	2	0.3	0	7	0.7	20	0.2	67	33			0.2	0	
Tangerines/Mandarin oranges, fresh, med	1 ea	116	51	0.7	0	0	0	13	2.7	16	0.1	1	1067	0.12	0.03	0.2	36	23.66
Tea, brewed	¾ cup	180	2	0	0	0	0	1	0	0	0	5	0	0	0.03	0	0	9.36
Tempeh	1 cup	166	320	30.8	18	3.7	0	16	9	184	4.5	15	0	0.13	0.59	4.4	0	39.67
Tofu, firm, silken	½ cup	126	78	8.7	3	0.5	0	3	0.1	40	1.3	45	0	0.13	0.1	0.3	0	
Tomatoes, red, ripe, raw, med, whole	1 ea	100	21	0.9	0	0	0	5	1.1	5	0.4	9	623	0.06	0.05	0.6	19	15
Tomatoes, red, ripe, w/o add salt, cnd, in liquid	½ cup	121	23	1.1	0	0	0	5	1.2	36	0.7	179	720	0.05	0.04	0.9	17	9.44
Tortilla/Taco/Tostada Shell, corn	1 ea	148	693	10.7	33	5	0	92	11.1	237	3.7	543	518	0.34	0.08	2	0	8.88
Trout, rainbow, fillet, bkd/brld, wild	3 oz	85	128	19.5	5	1.4	59	0	0	73	0.3	48	42	0.13	0.08	4.9	2	16.15
Tuna, light, cnd in oil, drained	3 oz	85	168	24.8	7	1.3	15	0	0	11	1.2	301	66	0.03	0.1	10.5	0	4.51
Tuna, light, cnd in water, drained	3½ oz	99	115	25.3	1	0.2	30	0	0	11	1.5	335	55	0.03	0.07	13.1	0	3.96
Turkey, average, w/o skin, rstd	3 oz	85	144	24.9	4	1.4	65	0	0	21	1.5	60	0	0.05	0.15	4.6	0	5.95

Food	Amount	Weight (g)	Calories	Protein (g)	Fat (g)	Sat. Fat (g)	Cholesterol (g)	Carbohydrate (g)	Fiber (g)	Calcium (mg)	Iron (mg)	Sodium (mg)	Vit A (IU)	Thiamin (Vit B₁) (mg)	Riboflavin (Vit B₂) (mg)	Niacin (mg)	Vit C (mg)	Folate (mcg)
Turnip Greens, ckd f/fzn, drained	½ cup	73	22	2.4	0	0.1	0	4	2.5	111	1.4	11	5822	0.04	0.05	0.3	16	28.76
Turnips, ckd w/ add salt, raw, cubes	½ cup	78	16	0.6	0	0	0	4	1.6	17	0.2	39	0	0.02	0.02	0.2	9	7.18
Veal, loin, brsd	3 oz	85	241	25.7	15	5.7	100	0	0	24	0.9	68	0	0.03	0.26	7.7	0	11.9
Veal, loin, lean, brsd	3 oz	85	192	28.5	8	2.2	106	0	0	27	0.9	71	0	0.04	0.29	8.5	0	12.75
Vinegar, balsamic, 60 grain	1 Tbs	15	21	1	1	0.1	0	5	0	2	0.1	3	0	0.08	0.08	0.1	0	
Watermelon, fresh, diced	1 cup	160	51	1	0	0.1	0	11	0.8	13	0.3	3	586	0.13	0.03	0.3	15	3.52
Wheat, bulgur, ckd	1 cup	135	112	4.2	0	0.1	0	25	6.1	14	1.3	7	0	0.08	0.04	1.4	0	24.3
Wheat, flakes, rolled, dry	1 cup	30	97	3.5	0	0	0	21	4.4	18	1	0	0	0.13	0.03	1.4	0	
Wheat, germ, tstd	1 Tbs	6	23	1.7	1	0.1	0	3	0.8	3	0.5	0	0	0.1	0.05	0.3	0	21.12
Whiskey, 90 proof	2 fl-oz	42	110	0	0	0	0	0	0	0	0.3	0	0	0	0	0	0	0
Wine, cooler	4 oz	113	56	0.1	0	0	0	7	0	6	0.3	9	1	0.01	0.01	0.1	2	1.34
Wine, red	½ cup	30	22	0.1	0	0	0	1	0	2	0.1	2	0	0	0.01	0	0	0.6
Wine, Rose	2 fl-oz	59	42	0.1	0	0	0	1	0	5	0.2	3	0	0	0.01	0	0	0.65
Wine, white, med	2 fl-oz	59	40	0.1	0	0	0	0	0	5	0.2	3	0	0	0	0	0	0.12
Yogurt, fruit, low fat, 10g prot/8 oz	1 cup	227	231	9.9	2	1.6	10	43	0	345	0.2	133	104	0.08	0.4	0.2	1	21.11
Yogurt, plain, low fat, 12g prot/8 oz	8 oz	226	143	11.9	4	2.3	14	16	0	413	0.2	159	149	0.1	0.48	0.3	2	25.31
FAST FOOD RESTAURANTS																		
General																		
Burrito, bean	1 ea	166	342	10.8	10	5.3	3	55	6.3	86	3.5	754	254	0.48	0.46	3.1	1	66.4
Chili, con carne	1 cup	255	258	24.8	8	3.5	135	22	4	69	5.2	1015	1675	0.13	1.15	2.5	2	45.9
Cole Slaw, fast food	1 cup	120	178	1.8	13	1.9	6	15	2	41	0.9	324	409	0.05	0.04	0.1	10	46.8
English Muffin, w/butter	1 ea	63	189	4.9	6	2.4	13	30	1.9	103	1.6	386	136	0.25	0.31	2.6	1	56.7
Entree, enchilada, cheese	1 ea	230	451	13.6	27	14.9	62	40		458	1.9	1106	1638	0.12	0.6	2.7	1	92
Hot Dog, plain	1 ea	98	242	10.4	15	5.1	44	18		24	2.3	670	0	0.24	0.27	3.6	0	48.02
Pancake, w/butter & syrup	2 ea	232	520	8.3	14	5.9	58	91	1.2	128	2.6	1104	281	0.39	0.56	3.4	3	51.04
Sandwich, chicken, fillet, plain	1 ea	157	444	20.8	25	7.4	52	33	1.1	52	4	826	86	0.28	0.2	5.9	8	86.35
Sundae, hot fudge, fast food	1 ea	164	295	5.9	9	5.2	21	49	0	215	0.6	189	230	0.07	0.31	1.1	2	9.84
Arby's																		
Salad, chef	1 ea	273	136	12.3	6	2.6	84	9		113	3.3	529	3321	0.26	0.25	4.6	35	
Sandwich, beef, Arby Q	1 ea	190	389	17.6	15	5.4	29	48		70	9.2	1268		0.27	0.39	9.2		
Sandwich, beef, French dip & swiss cheese	1 ea	154	369	24.7	16	7.5	58	31	0.9	232	3.6	1237	0	0.18	0.47	7.4	0	16.35
Sandwich, beef 'n cheddar	1 ea	194	508	24.6	26	7.7	52	43		150	6.1	1166		0.42	0.63	9.8	1	
Sandwich, chicken, grilled, deluxe	1 ea	195	365	20	17	3	37	35		59	2.1	764	339	0.27	0.25	11.5	7	
Sandwich, roast beef, regular	1 ea	155	383	22	18	6.9	43	35	1.1	60	4.9	936	0	0.28	0.48	11	1	14
Sauce, Arby's	½ oz	14	15	0.1	0	0	0	3			0.4	113						
Sauce, horsey	½ oz	14	110	0.1	5	1.2	0	3		20		105						
Burger King Corporation																		
Cheeseburger, Whopper	1 ea	294	730	33	46	16	115	46	3	250	4.5	1350	750	0.34	0.48	7	9	
Croissant, w/egg, sausage & cheese	1 ea	110	375	13.8	29	10	162	16	0.6	94	2.2	712	250				0	
Hamburger, Whopper	1 ea	270	640	27	39	11	90	45	3	80	4.5	870	500	0.33	0.41	7	9	
Onion Rings, reg svg	3 ea	30	75	1	3	0.5	0	10	1.5	24	0.3	196	0				0	
Potatoes, french fries, salted, med svg	1 ea	116	370	5	20	5	0	43	3	0	1.1	240	0				4	
Sandwich, chicken, broiler	1 ea	168	373	20.3	20	4.1	54	28	1.4	41	3.7	325	203				4	
Sandwich, fish, big	1 ea	255	700	26	41	6	90	56	3	60	2.7	980	100				1	
Dunkin Donuts, Inc.																		
Croissant, plain	1 ea	18	81	1.2	5	1.2	2	8	0	6	0.5	78	0				0	
Hidden Valley																		
Salad Dressing, ranch, reduced fat & cal	2 Tbs	28	58	0.5	5	0.9	10	2	0	11	0.1	237	15				0	
International Dairy Queen Inc.																		
Frozen Yogurt Cone, med	4 oz	113	148	5.1	1	0.3	3	32	0	143	1	91	0	0.05	0.2	1	1	
Frozen Yogurt, nonfat	4 oz	113	133	4	0	0		28	0	133	1	93	0				0	

Food	Amount	Weight (g)	Calories	Protein (g)	Fat (g)	Sat. Fat (g)	Cholesterol (mg)	Carbohydrate (g)	Fiber (g)	Calcium (mg)	Iron (mg)	Sodium (mg)	Vit A (IU)	Thiamin (Vit B₁) (mg)	Riboflavin (Vit B₂) (mg)	Niacin (mg)	Vit C (mg)	Folate (mcg)
Hamburger, homestyle	1 ea	138	290	17	12	5	45	29	2	60	2.7	630	200	0.29	0.25	3.9	4	
Ice Cream Cone, vanilla, med	1 ea	142	237	5.7	6	4.3	22	38	0	179	1.3	115	538	0.06	0.26	0.1	2	
Milk Shake, vanilla, med	1 ea	397	520	12	14	8	45	88	0.3	400	1.4	230	400	0.12	0.6	0.8	0	
Onion Rings, svg	3 oz	85	241	3.8	12	3	0	29	2.3	15	1.1	135	0	0.09	0.05	0.4	0	
Sandwich, fish, fillet	1 ea	182	396	17.1	17	3.7	48	42	2.1	43	1.9	674	0	0.32	0.24	3.2	0	
Sundae, chocolate, med	1 ea	184	315	6.3	8	4.7	24	56	0	197	1.1	165	590	0.06	0.27	0.3	0	
Jack In the Box																		
Bowl, chicken, teriyaki	1 ea	502	670	26	4	1	15	128	3	100	4.5	1730	6500				24	
Cheeseburger, Jumbo Jack	1 ea	296	640	31	38	15	105	44	2	250	4.5	1340	750	0.44	0.54	2	9	
Hamburger	1 ea	104	250	12	9	3.5	30	30	2	100	3.6	610	0	0.16	0.28	2.1	0	
Hamburger, sourdough, jack	1 ea	233	690	34	45	15	105	37	2	200	4.5	1180	750	0.68	0.5	8.4	9	
Sandwich, chicken, supreme	1 ea	305	830	33	49	7	65	66	3	200	3.6	2140	500	0.49	0.4	13.7	9	
Kentucky Fried Chicken Corporation																		
Chicken, leg, original recipe	1 ea	54	124	11.5	8	1.8	66	4		18	0.6	374	89				1	1
Chicken, wing, hot & spicy	1 ea	55	210	10	15	4	55	9	1	20	0.7	350	100				1	1
Chicken, wing, original recipe	1 ea	45	134	8.6	10	2.4	53	5	0	19	0.3	396	96				1	1
Long John Silver's																		
Dinner, fish & fries, batter fried, 2pce	1 ea	261	610	27	37	7.9	60	52		40	1.8	1480		0.38	0.34	8	9	
McDonald's Nutrition Information Center																		
Biscuit, sausage & egg	1 ea	175	541	17.7	36	9.8	241	34	1	98	2.7	1140	295	0.53	0.57	4.1	0	27.73
Cheeseburger	1 ea	115	304	14.3	12	5.7	38	33	1.9	190	2.6	779	285	0.31	0.29	3.6	2	22.37
Cheeseburger, Quarter Pounder	1 ea	186	493	26	28	12.1	88	35	1.9	279	4.2	1200	465	0.37	0.4	6.3	2	31.06
Chicken, nuggets, McNuggets, 4 pce, svg	1 ea	71	190	12	11	2.5	40	10	1.1	9	0.7	340	0	0.08	0.11	5	0	
Danish, apple	1 ea	115	394	5.5	18	5.5	44	56		88	1.2	318	548	0.33	0.19	2.2	1	
Frozen Yogurt Cone, vanilla, low fat	3 oz	85	142	3.8	4	2.8	19	22	0	94	0.3	71	283			1	1	
Hamburger, Big Mac	1 ea	204	529	24.6	29	9.4	80	42	2.8	236	4.2	1011	283	0.46	0.42	5.7	3	46.53
Hamburger, Quarter Pounder	1 ea	160	391	21.4	20	7.4	65	34	1.9	140	4.2	763	93	0.37	0.3	6.3	2	25.63
McMuffin, egg	1 ea	138	294	17.2	12	4.6	238	27	1	203	2.7	802	507	0.5	0.45	3.3	1	33.47
McMuffin, sausage	1 ea	135	434	15.7	28	9.6	54	31	1.2	241	2.2	892	241	0.68	0.33	4.5	0	18.95
Milk Shake, vanilla, sml	1 ea	289	355	10.8	9	5.9	39	58	0	345	0.4	246	296	0.12	0.5	0.3	1	
Muffin, apple bran, fat free	1 ea	75	197	3.9	2	0.3	0	40	2	66	0.9	250	0	0.14	0.14	1.3	1	5.03
Pie, apple	3 oz	307	1037	12	52	14	0	136	4	80	4.3	797	548	0.71	0.43	5.6	96	33.16
Potatoes, french fries, sml svg	1 ea	68	210	3	10	1.5	0	26	2	9	0.4	135	0	0.05	0	1.9	9	25.57
Potatoes, hash browns	1 ea	55	135	1	8	1.6	0	15	1	7	0.4	342	0	0.08	0.02	0.9	2	8.64
Salad, garden, shaker	1 ea	149	100	7	6	3	75	4	2	150	1.1	120	1500				15	
Sandwich, Filet O Fish	1 ea	131	378	13.4	21	3.8	42	35	1.7	126	1.5	731	168	0.29	0.21	2.3	0	26.73
Sauce, sweet & sour, pkt 1	1½ oz	32	57	0	0	0	0	13	0	2	0.2	160	343	0	0.01	0.1	0	
Pizza Hut, Inc.																		
Pizza, cheese, pan, med, 12"	2 pce	205	495	22.8	21	9.5	47	53	3.8	273	2.8	951	1000	0.57	0.61	5.2	7	
Pizza, cheese, thin n' crispy, med, 12"	2 pce	148	350	18.8	14	6.8	43	36	3.4	247	1.8	911	922	0.39	0.39	4.8	5	
Pizza, pepperoni, pan, med, 12"	2 pce	211	539	22.4	24	8.1	49	57	4.1	209	3.3	1157	966	0.63	0.49	5.4	8	0
Pizza, pepperoni, personal pan	1 ea	255	637	27	28	10	55	69	5	250	4	1339	1164	0.56	0.66	8.2	10	
Pizza, supreme, pan, med, 12"	2 pce	255	581	28	28	11.2	56	52	5.6	219	4.3	1428	912	0.8	0.79	6	10	
Subway International																		
Sandwich, chicken breast, rstd, on white, 6"	1 ea	246	332	26	6	1	48	41	3	35	3	967	617				15	
Sandwich, Italian bmt, on white, 6"	1 ea	246	445	21	21	8	56	39	3	44	4	1652	753				15	
Sandwich, meatball, on white, 6"	1 ea	260	404	18	16	6	33	44	3	32	4	1035	712				16	
Sandwich, roast beef, deli style	1 ea	180	245	13	4	1	13	38	2	23	3	638	565				14	
Sandwich, tuna, w/lt mayonnaise, on wheat, 6"	1 ea	253	391	19	15	2	32	46	3	38	3	940	729				15	
Sandwich, turkey, on white, 6"	1 ea	232	273	17	4	1	19	40	3	30	4	1391	601				15	

Food	Amount	Weight (g)	Calories	Protein (g)	Fat (g)	Sat. Fat (g)	Cholesterol (g)	Carbohydrate (g)	Fiber (g)	Calcium (mg)	Iron (mg)	Sodium (mg)	Vit A (IU)	Thiamin (Vit B$_1$) (mg)	Riboflavin (Vit B$_2$) (mg)	Niacin (mg)	Vit C (mg)	Folate (mcg)
Taco Bell Inc.																		
Burrito, beef, big supreme	1 ea	298	520	24	23	10	55	54	11	150	2.7	1520	3000				5	
Burrito, seven layer	1 ea	234	438	13.2	19	5.8	21	55	10.7	165	3	1058	1240				5	
Burrito, supreme	1 ea	255	440	17	19	8	35	51	10	150	9	1230	2500	0.4	2.1	2.9	5	
Taco	1 ea	83	192	9.6	11	4.3	27	13	3.2	85	1.1	351	532	0.05	0.15	1.3	0	
Taco, soft	1 ea	92	225	9.2	10	4.1	26	12	3.1	82	1.1	337	511	0.39	0.22	2.7	0	
Wendy's Foods International																		
Cheeseburger, w/bacon, jr	1 ea	170	393	20.5	19	7.5	58	35	1.9	171	3.6	895	390	0.31	0.32	6.6	9	28.85
Chicken, nuggets	6 pce	94	292	13.9	20	3.6	37	14	0	24	0.5	589	0	0.15	0.14	9	1	
Frosty, dairy dessert, med	1 ea	298	440	11	11	7	50	73	0	410	1.4	260	1000	0.14	0.62	0.4	0	22.9
Hamburger, bacon classic, big	1 ea	251	517	30.1	26	10.7	88	41	2.4	206	4.5	1298	622	0.4	1.36	5.3	13	
Salad, caesar, w/o dressing, side	1 ea	130	151	12.4	8	3.4	25	9	2	190	1.6	538	2501				22	
Salad, chicken, grilled, w/o dressing	1 ea	338	195	22.1	8	1.7	46	10	4	188	2.1	676	5872				35	
Salad, garden, deluxe, w/o dressing	1 ea	271	110	6.7	6	1	1	10	3.9	189	1.5	319	5883				35	
Salad, taco, w/o chips	1 ea	510	411	28.7	20	10.5	69	31	8.7	403	4.5	1132	2582	0.29	0.5	3.2	28	88.27
Sandwich, chicken, brd	1 ea	208	433	27.4	16	3.1	54	47	1.8	93	2.7	754	217	0.43	0.32	13.3	13	
Sandwich, chicken, club	1 ea	220	483	30.6	20	4.4	64	48	1.9	95	2.9	957	222				14	
Sandwich, chicken, grilled	1 ea	177	283	22.6	7	1.5	61	34	1.8	84	2.7	698	201				9	
CONVENIENCE FOODS & MEALS																		
El Charrito																		
Entree, enchilada, beef, family size, 6 pack	1 ea	200	353	11.8	17	6.5	33	39	5.2	196	2.4	837	1961				3	
Healthy Choice																		
Dinner, fish, herb baked, fzn	1 ea	273	300	14.1	6	1.3	31	48	4.4	35	0.6	424	2650				0	
Dinner, meatloaf, traditional, fzn	1 ea	340	316	15.3	5	2.5	37	52	6.1	48	2.2	459	745				55	
Entree, burrito, chicken, con queso, fzn	1 ea	216	253	10.1	4	1.8	25	43	4.3	29	1.3	426	1084				4	
Entree, lasagna, roma, fzn	1 ea	284	311	19.3	7	2.2	26	44	4.4	111	2.7	430	371	0.22	0.19	1.5	4	
Entree, spaghetti, bolognese, fzn	1 ea	284	280	14	6	2	30	43	5	40	3.6	470	500				15	
Lean Cuisine																		
Entree, chow mein, chicken, w/rice	1 ea	241	198	12.3	5	0.9	33	26	1.9	19	0.3	482	95	0.14	0.16	4.7	6	
Entree, lasagna, w/meat sauce	1 ea	291	270	19	6	2.5	25	34	5	150	1.8	560	500	0.15	0.25	3	12	
Entree, ravioli, cheese	1 ea	241	250	12	8	3	55	32	4	200	1.1	500	750	0.06	0.25	1.2	6	
Entree, spaghetti, w/meatballs, fzn	1 ea	290	322	19.4	8	2.2	6	43	4.9	102	2.6	502	0					48
The Budget Gourmet																		
Dinner, chicken, teriyaki, 3 dish	1 ea	340	360	20	12		55	44		80	1.4	610	1500	0.15	0.34	6	12	
Dinner, veal, parmigiana, 3 dish	1 ea	340	440	26	20		165	39		30	4.5	1160	5000	0.45	0.6	6	6	
Entree, beef, sirloin tips, w/country gravy	1 ea	334	365	18.8	21		47	25		71	0.4	670	882	0.18	0.2	4.7	3	
Entree, linguini, w/shrimp	1 ea	284	330	15	15		75	33		10	3.6	1250	5000	0.3	0.17	3	2	
The Budget Gourmet-Slim Select																		
Entree, stroganoff, beef	1 ea	238	269	17.3	10		58	28		58	2.6	537	288	0.25	0.33	3.8	9	
Weight Watchers																		
Entree, chow mein, chicken	1 ea	255	200	12	2	0.5	25	34	3	40	0.7	430	1499				36	

This food composition table has been prepared for West-Wadsworth Publishing Company and is copyrighted by ESHA Research in Salem, Oregon—the developer and publisher of the Food Processor®, Genesis® R&D, and the Computer Chef® nutrition software systems. The major sources for the data are from the USDA, supplemented by more than 1200 additional sources of information. Because the list of references is so extensive, it is not provided here, but is available from the publisher.

Computer
Data
Form

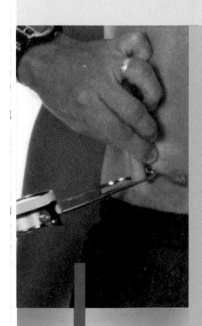

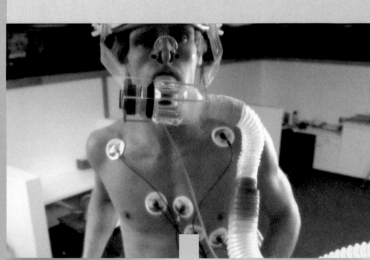

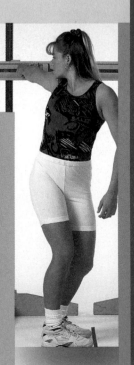

Preliminary Information

Data Disk Drive   A   B   C   (circle drive)

Pre-test _____   Post-test _____

Date (mm-dd-year)   _____-_____-_____

Course name _____

Section number _____

Instructor _____

General Information

Name _____

I.D. (9 digits or less) _____

Age _____

Male or female (circle one)   M   F

Body weight (pounds)   _____

Resting heart rate   _____

Systolic blood pressure   _____

Diastolic blood pressure   _____

Cardiorespiratory Endurance (circle one)

1. 1.5-mile run   Time _____:_____
2. 1.0-mile walk   Time _____:_____   HR _____
3. Step test   Recov. HR _____

4. Astrand test   WLoad _____
   5th min HR _____   6th min HR _____   Avg. HR _____
5. 12-min swim test   Distance _____

Muscular Strength (circle 1 or 2)

1. Muscular strength and endurance

Exercise	BW	×	%BW	= Resist.	Reps
			MEN WOMEN		
Lat pull down	_____:_____	×	.70 .45	= _____	_____
Leg extension	_____:_____	×	.65 .50	= _____	_____
Bench press	_____:_____	×	.75 .45	= _____	_____
Abd curl/crunch	_____:_____		NA		_____
Leg curl	_____:_____	×	.32 .25	= _____	_____
Arm curl	_____:_____	×	.35 .18	= _____	_____

2. Muscular endurance

MEN		WOMEN	
Bench jumps	_____	Bench jumps	_____
Chair dips	_____	Mod. push-ups	_____
Abd curl/crunch	_____	Abd curl/crunch	_____

Muscular Flexibility

Sit and reach   _____:_____

Right or left body rotation (circle one)   R   L

Right body rotation   _____:_____

Left body rotation   _____:_____

Shoulder width   _____:_____

Shoulder rotation   _____:_____

Body Composition (circle 1 2 or 3)

1. Skinfolds

MEN		WOMEN	
Chest	_____	Triceps	_____
Abdomen	_____	Suprailium	_____
Thigh	_____	Thigh	_____

2. Girth measurements

MEN (use inches)		WOMEN (use cm)	
Waist	_____	Upper arm	_____
Wrist	_____	Hip	_____
		Wrist	_____

3. Other technique
   Indicate percent body fat   _____

Skill Fitness

Agility	_____	Power	_____ ft. _____ in.
Balance	_____	Reaction time	_____
Coordination	_____	Speed	_____

Cardiovascular Disease (see pp. 329–332)

CHD risk score: _____

Cancer Risk (see pp. 344–353)

Rate each site from 1 to 3.

Low risk = 1   Moderate risk = 2   High risk = 3

	MEN	WOMEN
Lung	_____	_____
Colon-Rectum	_____	_____
Skin	_____	_____
Breast		_____
Cervical		_____
Endometrial		_____
Prostate	_____	
Testicular	_____	
Pancreatic	_____	_____
Kidney and bladder	_____	_____
Oral	_____	_____
Esophageal and stomach	_____	_____
Ovarian		_____
Thyroid	_____	_____
Liver	_____	_____
Leukemia	_____	_____
Lymphomas	_____	_____

Stress

Life Experiences Survey (p. 289)   _____

Type A personality assessment (p. 289) _____

Stress vulnerability (p. 295)   _____

Smoking (circle one)

Never smoked	= 1
Quit smoking	= 2
Cigarette smoker	= 3
Pipe smoker	= 4
Cigar smoker	= 5
Chew or dip tobacco	= 6

NUTRIENT ANALYSIS DATA

Use the computer form provided on page 87 and follow the instructions on page 60 of the book.

CARDIORESPIRATORY EXERCISE PRESCRIPTION DATA

Date (mm-dd-year)   _____-_____-_____

Name _____

Age _____

Resting heart rate _____

Male or female (circle one)   M   F

Current cardiorespiratory fitness (circle one)

Excellent = 1   Average = 3   Poor = 5
Good = 2   Fair = 4

EXERCISE LOG DATA

Use the activity list provided on page 126. Keep track of the exercise date, body weight, mode of exercise (activity), duration of exercise and exercise heart rate. Then simply follow the computer instructions.

Preliminary Information

Data Disk Drive   A   B   C   (circle drive)

Pre-test _____   Post-test _____

Date (mm-dd-year)   _____-_____-_____

Course name _____

Section number _____

Instructor _____

General Information

Name _____

I.D. (9 digits or less) _____

Age   _____

Male or female (circle one)   M   F

Body weight (pounds)   _____

Resting heart rate   _____

Systolic blood pressure   _____

Diastolic blood pressure   _____

Cardiorespiratory Endurance   (circle one)

1. 1.5-mile run   Time _____:_____
2. 1.0-mile walk   Time _____:_____   HR _____
3. Step test   Recov. HR _____
4. Astrand test   WLoad _____
   5th min HR _____   6th min HR _____   Avg. HR _____
5. 12-min swim test   Distance _____

Muscular Strength   (circle 1 or 2)

1. Muscular strength and endurance

Exercise	BW	×	%BW	= Resist.	Reps
	MEN WOMEN				
Lat pull down	_____:_____	×	.70 .45	= _____	_____
Leg extension	_____:_____	×	.65 .50	= _____	_____
Bench press	_____:_____	×	.75 .45	= _____	_____
Abd curl/crunch	_____:_____			NA	_____
Leg curl	_____:_____	×	.32 .25	= _____	_____
Arm curl	_____:_____	×	.35 .18	= _____	_____

2. Muscular endurance

MEN		WOMEN	
Bench jumps	_____	Bench jumps	_____
Chair dips	_____	Mod. push-ups	_____
Abd curl/crunch	_____	Abd curl/crunch	_____

Muscular Flexibility

Sit and reach   _____:_____

Right or left body rotation (circle one)   R   L

Right body rotation   _____:_____

Left body rotation   _____:_____

Shoulder width   _____:_____

Shoulder rotation   _____:_____

Body Composition   (circle 1 2 or 3)

1. Skinfolds

MEN		WOMEN	
Chest	_____	Triceps	_____
Abdomen	_____	Suprailium	_____
Thigh	_____	Thigh	_____

2. Girth measurements

MEN (use inches)		WOMEN (use cm)	
Waist	_____	Upper arm	_____
Wrist	_____	Hip	_____
		Wrist	_____

3. Other technique
   Indicate percent body fat   _____

Skill Fitness

Agility	_____	Power _____ ft. _____ in.	
Balance	_____	Reaction time	_____
Coordination	_____	Speed	_____

Cardiovascular Disease   (see pp. 329–332)

CHD risk score: _____

Cancer Risk   (see pp. 344–353)

Rate each site from 1 to 3.

     Low risk = 1   Moderate risk = 2   High risk = 3

	MEN	WOMEN
Lung	_____	_____
Colon-Rectum	_____	_____
Skin	_____	_____
Breast		_____
Cervical		_____
Endometrial		_____
Prostate	_____	
Testicular	_____	
Pancreatic	_____	_____
Kidney and bladder	_____	_____
Oral	_____	_____
Esophageal and stomach	_____	_____
Ovarian		_____
Thyroid	_____	_____
Liver	_____	_____
Leukemia	_____	_____
Lymphomas	_____	_____

Stress

Life Experiences Survey (p. 289)   _____

Type A personality assessment (p. 289)_____

Stress vulnerability (p. 295)   _____

Smoking   (circle one)

Never smoked	= 1
Quit smoking	= 2
Cigarette smoker	= 3
Pipe smoker	= 4
Cigar smoker	= 5
Chew or dip tobacco	= 6

NUTRIENT ANALYSIS DATA

Use the computer form provided on page 87 and follow the instructions on page 60 of the book.

CARDIORESPIRATORY EXERCISE PRESCRIPTION DATA

Date (mm-dd-year)   _____-_____-_____

Name _____

Age   _____

Resting heart rate   _____

Male or female (circle one)   M   F

Current cardiorespiratory fitness (circle one)

Excellent	= 1	Average	= 3	Poor	= 5
Good	= 2	Fair	= 4		

EXERCISE LOG DATA

Use the activity list provided on page 126. Keep track of the exercise date, body weight, mode of exercise (activity), duration of exercise and exercise heart rate. Then simply follow the computer instructions.

Glossary

A

Acquired immunodeficiency syndrome (AIDS) Any of a number of diseases that arise when the body's immune system is compromised by HIV.

Action stage Stage of change in which people are actively changing a negative behavior or adopting a new, healthy behavior.

Activities of daily living Everyday behaviors that people normally do to function in life (cross the street, carry groceries, lift objects, do laundry, sweep floors).

Acupuncture Chinese medical system that requires body piercing with fine needles during therapy to relieve pain and treat ailments and diseases.

Adenosine triphosphate (ATP) A high-energy chemical compound that the body uses for immediate energy.

Addiction Compulsive and uncontrollable behavior(s) or use of substance(s).

Adequate Intakes (AI) The recommended amount of a nutrient intake when sufficient evidence is not available to calculate the EAR and subsequent RDA.

Adipose tissue Fat cells in the body.

Aerobic Exercise that requires oxygen to produce the necessary energy (ATP) to carry out the activity.

Agility Ability to change body position and direction quickly and efficiently.

Air displacement Technique to assess body composition by calculating the body volume from the air displaced by an individual sitting inside a small chamber.

Alcohol (ethyl alcohol) A depressant drug that affects the brain and slows down central nervous system activity; has strong addictive properties.

Alcoholism Disease in which an individual loses control over drinking alcoholic beverages.

Allopathic medicine See conventional Western medicine.

Altruism True concern for the welfare of others.

Alveoli Air sacs in the lungs where gas exchange (oxygen and carbon dioxide) takes place.

Amenorrhea Cessation of regular menstrual flow.

Amino acids Chemical compounds that contain nitrogen, carbon, hydrogen, and oxygen; the basic building blocks the body uses to build different types of protein.

Amotivational syndrome A condition characterized by loss of motivation, dullness, apathy, and no interest in the future.

Amphetamine Powerful central nervous system stimulants.

Anabolic steroids Synthetic versions of the male sex hormone testosterone, which promotes muscle development and hypertrophy.

Anaerobic Exercise that does not require oxygen to produce the necessary energy (ATP) to carry out the activity.

Angina pectoris Chest pain associated with coronary heart disease.

Angiogenesis Formation of blood vessels, or capillaries.

Angioplasty A procedure in which a balloon-tipped catheter is inserted, then inflated, to widen the inner lumen of one or more arteries.

Anorexia nervosa An eating disorder characterized by self-imposed starvation to lose and maintain very low body weight.

Anthropometric techniques Measurement of body girths at different sites.

Anticoagulant Any substance that inhibits blood clotting.

Antioxidants Compounds such as vitamins C and E, beta-carotene, and selenium that prevent oxygen from combining with other substances in the body to which it may cause damage.

Aquaphobic Having a fear of water.

Arrhythmias Irregular heart rhythms.

Atherosclerosis Fatty/cholesterol deposits in the walls of the arteries leading to plaque formation.

Atrophy Decrease in the size of a cell.

Autogenic training Stress management technique using a form of self-suggestion, wherein an individual is able to place him/herself in an autohypnotic state by repeating and concentrating on feelings of heaviness and warmth in the extremities.

Ayurveda Unconventional Hindu system of medicine based on herbs, diet, massage, meditation, and yoga to help the body boost its own natural healing.

B

Balance Ability to maintain the body in proper equilibrium.

Ballistic stretching Exercises done with jerky, rapid, bouncy movements.

Basal metabolic rate (BMR) The lowest level of oxygen consumption necessary to sustain life.

Behavior modification The process to permanently change negative behaviors in favor of positive behaviors that will lead to better health and well-being.

Benign Noncancerous.

Bioelectrical impedance Technique to assess body composition by running a weak electrical current through the body.

Biofeedback A stress-management technique in which a person learns to reliably influence physiological responses of two kinds: either responses that are not ordinarily under voluntary control or responses that ordinarily are easily regulated but for which regulation has broken down because of trauma or disease.

Blood lipids (fat) Cholesterol and triglycerides.

Blood pressure A measure of the force exerted against the walls of the vessels by the blood flowing through them.

Bod Pod Commercial name of the equipment used for the assessment of body composition through the air displacement technique.

Body composition The fat and nonfat components of the human body; important in assessing recommended body weight.

Body mass index (BMI) Ratio of weight to height used to determine thinness and fatness.

Bradycardia Slower heart rate than normal.

Breathing exercise A stress management technique wherein the individual concentrates on "breathing away" the tension and inhaling fresh air to the entire body.

Bulimia nervosa An eating disorder characterized by a pattern of binge eating and purging in an attempt to lose weight and maintain low body weight.

C

Calorie The amount of heat necessary to raise the temperature of 1 gram of water 1 degree Centigrade; used to measure the energy value of food and cost (energy expenditure) of physical activity.

Cancer Group of diseases characterized by uncontrolled growth and spread of abnormal cells into malignant tumors.

Capillaries Smallest blood vessels carrying oxygenated blood to body tissues.

Carbohydrate loading Increasing intake of carbohydrates during heavy aerobic training or prior to aerobic endurance events that last longer than 90 minutes.

Carbohydrates A classification of dietary nutrient containing carbon, hydrogen, and oxygen; the major source of energy for the human body.

Carcinogens Substances that contribute to the formation of cancers.

Carcinoma in situ Encapsulated malignant tumor that has not spread.

Cardiac output Amount of blood pumped by the heart in one minute.

Cardiomyopathy A disease affecting the heart muscle.

Cardiorespiratory endurance The ability of the lungs, heart, and blood vessels to deliver adequate amounts of oxygen to the cells to meet the demands of prolonged physical activity.

Cardiovascular diseases The array of conditions that affect the heart and the blood vessels.

Carotenoids Pigment substances in plants that are often precursors to vitamin A. Over 600 carotenoids are found in nature and about 50 of them are precursors to vitamin A, the most potent one being beta-carotene.

Catecholamines "Fight-or-flight" hormones, including epinephrine and norepinephrine.

Cellulite Term frequently used in reference to fat deposits that "bulge out"; these deposits are nothing but enlarged fat cells from excessive accumulation of body fat.

Chiropractics Health care system that believes that many diseases and ailments are related to misalignments of the vertebrae and emphasizes the manipulation of the spinal column.

Chlamydia A sexually transmitted disease, caused by a bacterial infection, that can cause significant damage to the reproductive system.

Cholesterol A waxy substance, technically a steroid alcohol, found only in animal fats and oil; used in making cell membranes, as a building block for some hormones, in the fatty sheath around nerve fibers, and in other necessary substances.

Chronic diseases Illnesses that develop and last a long time.

Chronological age Calendar age.

Chylomicron Triglyceride-transporting molecules.

Circuit training Alternating exercises by performing them in a sequence of three to six or more.

Cirrhosis A disease characterized by scarring of the liver.

Cocaine 2-beta-carbomethoxy-3-betabenozoxytropane, the primary psychoactive ingredient derived from coca plant leaves.

Cold turkey Eliminating a negative behavior all at once.

Complementary and alternative medicine A branch of medicine concerned with treatments and health care practices not widely taught in medical schools, not generally used in hospitals, and not usually reimbursed by medical insurance companies.

Complex carbohydrates Carbohydrates formed by three or more simple sugar molecules linked together; also referred to as "polysaccharides."

Concentric Shortening of a muscle during muscle contraction.

Contemplation stage Stage of change in which people are considering changing behavior in the next 6 months.

Controlled ballistic stretching Exercises done with slow, short, and sustained movements.

Conventional Western medicine Traditional medical practice based on methods that are tested through rigorous scientific trials.

Cool-down Tapering off an exercise session slowly.

Coordination Integration of the nervous and the muscular systems to produce correct, graceful, and harmonious body movements.

Coronary heart disease (CHD) Condition in which the arteries that supply the heart muscle with oxygen and nutrients are narrowed by fatty deposits, such as cholesterol and triglycerides.

Creatine An organic compound derived from meat, fish, and amino acids that combines with inorganic phosphate to form creatine phosphate.

Creatine phosphate (CP) A high-energy compound that is used by the cells to resynthesize ATP during all-out activities of very short duration.

Cruciferous vegetables Plants that produce cross-shaped leaves (cauliflower, broccoli, cabbage, Brussels sprouts, and kohlrabi); seem to have a protective effect against cancer.

D

Daily Values (DV) Reference values for nutrients and food components used in food labels.

Dentist Practitioner who specializes in diseases of the teeth, gums, and oral cavity.

Deoxyribonucleic acid (DNA) Genetic substance of which genes are made; molecule that bears cell's genetic code.

Diabetes mellitus A disease in which the body doesn't produce or utilize insulin properly.

Diastolic blood pressure Pressure exerted by blood against walls of arteries during relaxation phase (diastole) of the heart; lower of the two numbers in blood pressure readings.

Dietary fiber A complex carbohydrate in plant foods that is not digested but is essential to the digestion process.

Dietary Reference Intakes (DRIs) A general term that describes four types of nutrient standards, which establish adequate amounts and maximum safe nutrient intakes in the diet. These standards are Estimated Average Requirements (EAR), Recommended Dietary Allowances (RDA), Adequate Intakes (AI), and Tolerable Upper Intake Levels (UL).

Disaccharides Simple carbohydrates formed by two monosaccharide units linked together, one of which is glucose. The major disaccharides are sucrose, lactose, and maltose.

Distress Negative stress: Unpleasant or harmful stress under which health and performance begin to deteriorate.

Dopamine A neurotransmitter that affects emotional, mental, and motor functions.

Dynamic training Strength-training method referring to a muscle contraction with movement.

Dysmenorrhea Painful menstruation.

E

Eccentric Lengthening of a muscle during muscle contraction.

Elastic elongation Temporary lengthening of soft tissue.

Electrocardiogram (ECG or EKG) A recording of the electrical activity of the heart.

Emotional wellness The ability to understand your own feelings, accept your limitations, and achieve emotional stability.

Endorphins Morphine-like substances released from the pituitary gland in the brain during prolonged aerobic exercise; thought to induce feelings of euphoria and natural well-being.

Energy-balancing equation A principle holding that as long as caloric input equals caloric output, the person will not gain or lose weight. If caloric intake exceeds output, the person gains weight; when output exceeds input, the person loses weight.

Environmental wellness The capability to live in a clean and safe environment that is not detrimental to health.

Enzymes Catalysts that facilitate chemical reactions in the body.

Essential fat Minimal amount of body fat needed for normal physiological functions; constitutes about 3 percent of total weight in men and 12 percent in women.

Estimated Average Requirements (EAR) The amount of a nutrient that meets the dietary needs in half the people.

Estrogen Female sex hormone; essential for bone formation and conservation of bone density.

Eustress Positive stress: Health and performance continue to improve, even as stress increases.

Exercise A type of physical activity that requires planned, structured, and repetitive bodily movement with the intent of improving or maintaining one or more components of physical fitness.

Exercise intolerance Inability to function during exercise because of excessive fatigue or extreme feelings of discomfort.

F

Fast-twitch fibers Muscle fibers with greater anaerobic potential and fast speed of contraction.

Fats Nutrients containing carbon, hydrogen, some oxygen, and sometimes other chemical elements.

Ferritin Iron stored in the body.

Fight or flight Physiological response of the body to stress that prepares the individual to take action by stimulating the vital defense systems.

Fixed resistance Type of exercise in which a constant resistance is moved through a joint's full range of motion.

Flexibility The ability of a joint to move freely through its full range of motion.

Folate One of the B vitamins.

Free weights Barbells and dumbbells.

Frequency How often a person engages in an exercise session.

Functional capacity The ability to perform ordinary and reasonably unusual demands of daily life without limitations and excessive fatigue or injury.

Functional independence Ability to carry out activities of daily living without assistance from other individuals.

G

Genital herpes A sexually transmitted disease caused by a viral infection of the herpes simplex virus Types I and II. The virus can attack different areas of the body, but commonly causes blisters on the genitals.

Genital warts A sexually transmitted disease caused by a viral infection.

Girth measurements Technique to assess body composition by measuring circumferences at specific body sites.

Glucose intolerance A condition characterized by slightly elevated blood glucose levels.

Glycemic index An index that is used to rate the plasma glucose response of carbohydrate-containing foods with the response produced by the same amount of carbohydrate from a standard source, usually glucose or white bread.

Glycogen Form in which glucose is stored in the body.

Goal The ultimate aim toward which effort is directed.

Gonorrhea Sexually transmitted disease caused by a bacterial infection.

H

Health A state of complete well-being, and not just the absence of disease or infirmity.

Health fitness standards The lowest fitness requirements for maintaining good health, decreasing the risk for chronic diseases, and lowering the incidence of muscular-skeletal injuries.

Health-related fitness Fitness programs that are prescribed to improve the overall health of the individual.

Healthy Life Expectancy (HLE) Number of years a person is expected to live in good health. This number is obtained by subtracting ill-health years from the overall life expectancy.

Heart rate reserve (HRR) The difference between the maximal heart rate and the resting heart rate.

Heat cramps Muscle spasms caused by heat-induced changes in electrolyte balance in muscle cells.

Heat exhaustion Heat-related fatigue.

Heat stroke Emergency situation resulting from the body being subjected to high atmospheric temperatures.

Hemoglobin Protein–iron compound in red blood cells that transports oxygen in the blood.

Herbal medicine Unconventional system that uses herbs to treat ailments and disease.

Heroin A potent drug that is a derivative of opium.

High density lipoproteins (HDLs) Cholesterol-transporting molecules in the blood ("good" cholesterol) that help clear cholesterol from the blood.

Homeopathy System of treatment based on the use of minute quantities of remedies that in large amounts produce effects similar to the disease being treated.

Homocysteine An amino acid that, when allowed to accumulate in the blood, may lead to plaque formation and blockage of arteries.

Human immunodeficiency virus (HIV) Virus that leads to acquired immunodeficiency syndrome (AIDS).

Hydrostatic weighing Underwater technique to assess body composition; considered the most accurate of the body composition assessment techniques.

Hypertension Chronically elevated blood pressure.

Hypertrophy An increase in the size of the cell (for example, muscle hypertrophy).

Hypokinetic Lacking physical activity.

Hypotension Low blood pressure.

Hypothermia A breakdown in the body's ability to generate heat; a drop in temperature below 95 degrees F.

I

Insulin Hormone secreted by the pancreas; essential for proper metabolism of blood glucose (sugar) and maintenance of blood glucose level.

Insulin resistance The inability of the cells to respond appropriately to insulin.

Intensity In cardiorespiratory exercise, how hard a person has to exercise to improve or maintain fitness.

Intensity (for flexibility exercises) Degree of stretch when doing flexibility exercises.

International unit (IU) Measure of nutrients in foods.

Isokinetic training Strength-training method in which the speed of the muscle contraction is kept constant because the equipment (machine) provides an accommodating resistance to match the user's force (maximal) through the range of motion.

Isometric training Strength-training method referring to a muscle contraction that produces little or no movement, such as pushing or pulling against an immovable object.

L

Lactic acid End product of anaerobic glycolysis (metabolism).

Lactovegetarians Vegetarians who eat foods from the milk group.

Lean body mass Body weight without body fat.

Life expectancy Number of years a person is expected to live based on the person's birth year.

Life Experiences Survey Questionnaire used to assess sources of stress in life.

Lipoproteins Lipids covered by proteins, they transport fats in the blood; types are LDL, HDL, and VLDL.

Locus of control A concept examining the extent to which a person believes he or she can influence the external environment.

Low-density lipoproteins (LDLs) Cholesterol-transporting molecules in the blood ("bad" cholesterol) that tend to increase blood cholesterol.

M

Maintenance stage Stage of change in which people maintain behavioral change for up to 5 years.

Magnetic therapy Unconventional treatment that relies on magnetic energy to promote healing.

Malignant Cancerous.

Mammogram Low-dose X rays of the breasts used as a screening technique for the early detection of breast cancer.

Marijuana A psychoactive drug prepared from a mixture of crushed leaves, flowers, small branches, stems, and seeds from the hemp plant *cannabis sativa.*

Massage therapy The rubbing or kneading of body parts to treat ailments.

Maximal heart rate (MHR) Highest heart rate for a person, related primarily to age.

Maximal oxygen uptake (VO_{2max}) Maximum amount of oxygen the body is able to utilize per minute of physical activity, commonly expressed in ml/kg/min. The best indicator of cardiorespiratory or aerobic fitness.

Meditation A stress management technique used to gain control over one's attention by clearing the mind and blocking out the stressor(s) responsible for the increased tension.

Mediterranean diet Typical diet of people around the Mediterranean region that focuses on olive oil, red wine, grains, legumes, vegetables, and fruits, with limited amounts of meat, fish, milk, and cheese.

Megadoses For most vitamins, 10 times the RDA or more; for vitamins A and D, 5 and 2 times the RDA, respectively.

Melanoma The most virulent, rapidly spreading form of skin cancer.

Mental wellness A state in which your mind is engaged in lively interaction with the world around you.

MET Represents the rate of resting energy expenditure at rest; MET is the equivalent of 3.5 ml/kg/min.

Metabolic fitness Denotes improvements in the metabolic profile through a moderate-intensity exercise program in spite of little or no improvement in physical fitness standards.

Metabolic profile A measurement to assess risk for diabetes and cardiovascular disease through plasma insulin, glucose, lipid, and lipoprotein levels.

Metabolic syndrome *See* Syndrome X.

Metabolism All energy and material transformations that occur within living cells; necessary to sustain life.

Metastasis The movement of cells from one part of the body to another.

Methamphetamine A more potent form of amphetamine.

Minerals Inorganic elements found in the body and in food; essential for normal body functions.

Mitochondria Structures within the cells where energy transformations take place.

Mode Form of exercise.

Moderate physical activity Activity that uses 150 calories of energy per day, or 1,000 calories per week.

Monogamous A sexual relationship in which two people have sexual relations only with each other.

Monosaccharides The simplest carbohydrates (sugars) formed by five- or six-carbon skeletons. The three most common monosaccharides are glucose, fructose, and galactose.

Morbidity A condition related to or caused by illness or disease.

Motivation The desire and will to do something.

Motor neurons Nerves connecting the central nervous system to the muscle.

Motor unit The combination of a motor neuron and the muscle fibers that neuron innervates.

Muscular endurance The ability of a muscle to exert submaximal force repeatedly over time.

Muscular strength The ability of a muscle to exert maximum force against resistance (for example, 1 repetition maximum [or 1 RM] of the bench press exercise).

Myocardial infarction Heart attack; damage to or death of an area of the heart muscle as a result of an obstructed artery to that area.

Myocardium Heart muscle.

N

Naturopathic medicine Unconventional system of medicine that relies exclusively on natural remedies to treat disease and ailments.

Negative resistance The lowering or eccentric phase of a repetition during the performance of a strength training exercise.

Nicotine Addictive compound found in tobacco leaves.

Nitrosamines Potentially cancer-causing compounds formed when nitrites and nitrates, which are used to prevent the growth of harmful bacteria in processed meats, combine with other chemicals in the stomach.

Nonallopathic medicine See complementary and alternative medicine.

Nonmelanoma skin cancer Cancer that spreads or grows directly from the original site but does not metastasize to other regions of the body.

Nurse Health care practitioner who assists in the diagnosis and treatment of health problems and provides many services to patients in a variety of settings.

Nutrient density A measure of the amount of nutrients and calories in various foods.

Nutrients Substances found in food that provide energy, regulate metabolism, and help with growth and repair of body tissues.

Nutrition Science that studies the relationship of foods to optimal health and performance.

O

Obesity An excessive accumulation of body fat, usually at least 30 percent above recommended body weight.

Objectives Steps required to reach a goal.

Occupational wellness The ability to perform one's job skillfully and effectively under conditions that provide personal and team satisfaction and adequately reward each individual.

Olestra Fat substitute made from sugar and fatty acids; provides no calories to the body because it passes through the digestive system without being absorbed.

Oligomenorrhea Irregular menstrual cycles.

Omega-3 fatty acids Polyunsaturated fatty acids found primarily in cold-water seafood, flaxseed, and flaxseed oil; thought to lower blood cholesterol and triglycerides.

Oncogenes Genes that initiate cell division.

One repetition maximum (1 RM) The maximum amount of resistance an individual is able to lift in a single effort.

Ophthalmologist Medical specialist concerned with diseases of the eye and prescription of corrective lenses.

Opportunistic diseases Diseases that arise in the absence of a healthy immune system, which would fight them off in healthy people.

Optometrist Health care practitioner who specializes in the prescription and adaptation of lenses.

Oral surgeon A dentist who specializes in surgical procedures of the oral-facial complex.

Orthodontist A dentist who specializes in the correction and prevention of teeth irregularities.

Osteopath A medical practitioner with specialized training in musculoskeletal problems who uses diagnostic and therapeutic methods of conventional medicine in addition to manipulative measures.

Osteoporosis Softening, deterioration, or loss of bone mass.

Overload principle Training concept that the demands placed on a system (cardiorespiratory or muscular) must be increased systematically and progressively over time to cause physiological adaptation (development or improvement).

Overweight Excess weight according to a given standard, such as height or recommended percent body fat; less than obese.

Ovolactovegetarians Vegetarians who include eggs and milk products in their diet.

Ovovegetarians Vegetarians who allow eggs in their diet.

Oxygen free radicals Substances formed during metabolism that attack and damage proteins and lipids, in particular the cell membrane and DNA, leading to diseases such as heart disease, cancer, and emphysema.

P

Pelvic inflammatory disease (PID) An overall designation referring to the effects of other STDs, primarily chlamydia and gonorrhea.

Percent body fat Proportional amount of fat in the body based on the person's total weight; includes both essential and storage fat.

Peripheral vascular disease Narrowing of the peripheral blood vessels (excludes the cerebral and coronary arteries).

Peristalsis Involuntary muscle contractions of intestinal walls that facilitate excretion of wastes.

Physical activity Bodily movement produced by skeletal muscles; requires expenditure of energy and produces progressive health benefits.

Physical fitness The ability to meet the ordinary as well as the unusual demands of daily life safely and effectively without being overly fatigued and still have energy left for leisure and recreational activities.

Physical fitness standards A fitness level that allows a person to sustain moderate to vigorous physical activity without undue fatigue and the ability to closely maintain this level throughout life.

Physical wellness Good physical fitness and confidence in one's personal ability to take care of health problems.

Physician assistant A health care practitioner trained to treat most standard cases of care.

Physiological age The biological and functional capacity (age-related) of the body.

Phytochemicals Chemical compounds thought to prevent and fight cancer; found in large quantities in fruits and vegetables.

Plastic elongation Permanent lengthening of soft tissue.

Plyometric exercise Explosive jump training, incorporating speed and strength training to enhance explosiveness.

Positive resistance The lifting, pushing, or concentric phase of a repetition during the performance of a strength-training exercise.

Power The ability to produce maximum force in the shortest time.

Precontemplation stage Stage of change in which people are unwilling to change behavior.

Preparation stage Stage of change in which people are getting ready to make a change within the next month.

Primary care physician A medical practitioner who provides routine treatment of ailments; typically, the patient's first contact for health care.

Process of change Actions that help you achieve change in behavior.

Progressive muscle relaxation A stress management technique that involves progressive contraction and relaxation of muscle groups throughout the body.

Progressive resistance training A gradual increase of resistance over a period of time.

Proprioceptive neuromuscular facilitation (PNF) Stretching technique in which muscles are stretched out sequentially with intermittent isometric contractions.

Proteins Complex organic compounds containing nitrogen and formed by combinations of amino acids; the main substances used in the body to build and repair tissues.

Pro-vitamin A compound that can be converted into a vitamin.

Q

Quackery/Fraud The conscious promotion of unproven claims for profit.

R

Range of motion Entire arc of movement of a given joint.

Rate of perceived exertion (RPE) A perception scale to monitor or interpret the intensity of exercise.

Reaction time The time required to initiate a response to a given stimulus.

Recommended body weight Body weight at which there seems to be no harm to human health; healthy weight.

Recommended Dietary Allowances (RDA) The daily amount of a nutrient (statistically determined from the EARs) considered adequate to meet the known nutrient needs of almost 98 percent of all healthy people in the United States.

Recovery time Amount of time the body takes to return to resting levels after exercise.

Registered dietician (RD) A person with a college degree in dietetics who meets all certification and continuing education requirements by the American Dietetic Association or Dietitians of Canada.

Relapse To slip or fall back into unhealthy behavior(s) or failure to maintain healthy behaviors.

Repetitions Number of times a given stretch is performed.

Resistance Amount of weight that is lifted.

Resting heart rate (RHR) Heart rate after a person has been sitting quietly for 15–20 minutes.

Resting metabolism Amount of energy (expressed in milliliters of oxygen per minute or total calories per day) an individual requires during resting conditions to sustain proper body function.

Reverse cholesterol transport A process in which HDL molecules attract cholesterol and carry it to the liver, where it is changed to bile and eventually excreted in the stool.

Ribonucleic acid (RNA) Genetic material that guides the formation of cell proteins.

Risk factors Lifestyle and genetic variables that may lead to disease.

S

Sedentary A person who is relatively inactive and whose lifestyle is characterized by a lot of sitting.

Semivegetarians Vegetarians who include milk products, eggs, and fish and poultry in the diet.

Set A fixed number of repetitions. One set of bench presses might be 10 repetitions.

Setpoint Weight control theory that the body has an established weight and strongly attempts to maintain that weight.

Sexually transmitted diseases (STDs) Communicable diseases spread through sexual contact.

Shin splints Injury to the lower leg characterized by pain and irritation in the shin region or front of the leg.

Side stitch A sharp pain in the side of the abdomen.

Simple carbohydrates Formed by simple or double sugar units with little nutritive value; divided into monosaccharides and disaccharides.

Skill-related fitness Fitness components important for success in skillful activities and athletic events; encompasses agility, balance, coordination, power, reaction time, and speed.

Skinfold thickness Technique to assess body composition by measuring a double thickness of skin at specific body sites.

Slow-sustained stretching Exercises in which the muscles are lengthened gradually through a joint's complete range of motion.

Slow-twitch fibers Muscle fibers with greater aerobic potential and slow speed of contraction.

Social wellness The ability to relate well to others, both within and outside the family unit.

Specificity of training Principle that training must be done with the specific muscle the person is attempting to improve.

Speed The ability to propel the body or a part of the body rapidly from one point to another.

Sphygmomanometer Inflatable bladder contained within a cuff and a mercury gravity manometer (or aneroid manometer) from which the pressure is read.

Spiritual wellness The sense that life is meaningful, that life has purpose, and that some power brings all humanity together; the ethics, values, and morals that guide us and give meaning and direction to life.

Spot reducing Fallacious theory that exercising a specific body part will result in significant fat reduction in that area.

Sterols Derived fats, of which cholesterol is the best known example.

Storage fat Body fat in excess of essential fat; stored in adipose tissue.

Stress The mental, emotional, and physiological response of the body to any situation that is new, threatening, frightening, or exciting.

Stress electrocardiogram An exercise test during which the workload is gradually increased (until the subject reaches maximal fatigue) with blood pressure and 12-lead electro-cardiographic monitoring throughout the test.

Stressor Stress-causing event.

Stretching Moving the joints beyond the accustomed range of motion.

Stroke volume Amount of blood pumped by the heart in one beat.

Structured interview Assessment tool used to determine behavioral patterns that define Type A and B personalities.

Subluxation Partial dislocation of a joint.

Substrate Substance acted upon by an enzyme (examples: carbohydrates and fats).

Sun protection factor (SPF) Degree of protection offered by ingredients in sunscreen lotion; at least SPF 15 is recommended.

Supplements Tablets, pills, capsules, liquids, or powders that contain vitamins, minerals, amino acids, herbs, or fiber that are taken to increase the intake of these nutrients.

Syndrome X An array of metabolic abnormalities that contribute to the development of atherosclerosis triggered by insulin resistance. These conditions include low HDL-cholesterol, high triglycerides, high blood pressure, and an increased blood clotting mechanism.

Synergistic action The effect of mixing two or more drugs, which can be much greater than the sum of two or more drugs acting by themselves.

Synergy A reaction in which the result is greater than the sum of its two parts.

Syphilis A sexually transmitted disease caused by a bacterial infection.

Systolic blood pressure Pressure exerted by blood against walls of arteries during forceful contraction (systole) of the heart; higher of the two numbers in blood pressure readings.

T

Tachycardia Faster-than-normal heart rate.

Tar Chemical compound that forms during the burning of tobacco leaves.

Techniques of change Methods or procedures used to aid with each process of change.

Telomerase An enzyme that allows cells to reproduce indefinitely.

Telomeres A strand of molecules at both ends of a chromosome.

Termination/adoption stage Stage of change in which people have eliminated an undesirable behavior or main-tained a positive behavior for over 5 years.

Thermogenic response Amount of energy required to digest food.

Transfatty acid Solidified fat formed by adding hydrogen to monounsaturated and polyunsaturated fats to increase shelf life.

Triglycerides Fats formed by glycerol and three fatty acids.

Tumor suppressor genes Genes that deactivate the process of cell division.

Type A Behavior pattern characteristic of a hard-driving, overambitious, aggressive, at times hostile, and overly competitive person.

Type B Behavior pattern characteristic of a calm, casual, relaxed, and easy-going individual.

Type C Behavior pattern of individuals who are just as highly stressed as the Type A but do not seem to be at higher risk for disease than the Type B.

Type I diabetes Insulin-dependent diabetes mellitus (IDDM), a condition in which the pancreas produces little or no insulin. Also known as juvenile diabetes.

Type II diabetes Non-insulin-dependent diabetes mellitus (NIDDM), a condition in which insulin is not processed properly. Also known as adult-onset diabetes.

U

Ultraviolet B rays (UVB) Portion of sunlight that causes sunburn and encourages skin cancers.

Unconventional medicine See complementary and alternative medicine.

Underweight Extremely low body weight.

V

Variable resistance Training using special machines equipped with mechanical devices that provide differing amounts of resistance through the range of motion.

Vegans Vegetarians who eat no animal products at all.

Vegetarians Individuals whose diet is of vegetable or plant origin.

Very low-density lipoproteins (VLDLs) Triglyceride, cholesterol, and phospholipid-transporting molecules in the blood that tend to increase blood cholesterol.

Vigorous activity Any activity that requires a MET level equal to or greater than 6 METs (21 ml/kg/min); 1 MET = energy expenditure at rest, 3.5 ml/kg/min.

Vigorous exercise Cardiorespiratory exercise that requires an intensity level above 60 percent of maximal capacity.

Vitamins Organic nutrients essential for normal metabolism, growth, and development of the body.

W

Waist-to-hip ratio A measurement to assess potential risk for disease based on distribution of body fat.

Warm-up Starting a workout slowly.

Weight-regulating mechanism (WRM) A feature of the hypothalamus of the brain that controls how much the body should weigh.

Wellness The constant and deliberate effort to stay healthy and achieve the highest potential for well-being. It encom-passes seven dimensions—physical, emotional, mental, social, environmental, occupational, and spiritual—and integrates them all into a quality life.

Workload Load placed on the body during physical activity, which determines the intensity of exercise.

Y

Yo-yo dieting Constantly losing and gaining weight.

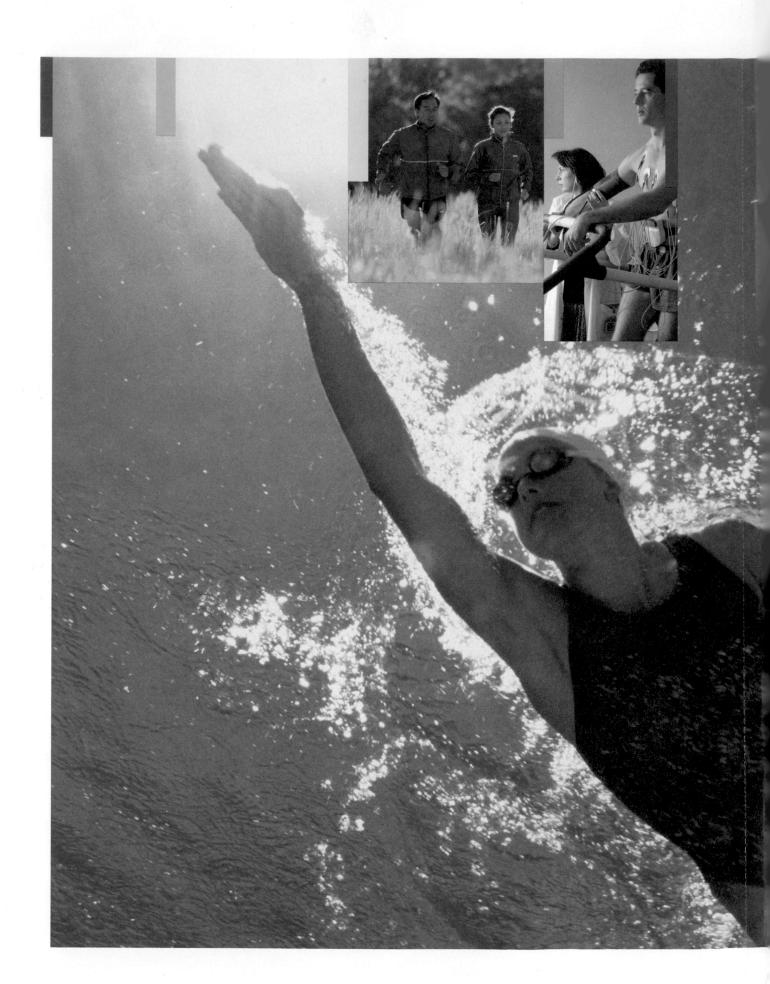

Principles and Labs
For Fitness and Wellness

SIXTH EDITION